COMPARATIVE CLINICAL HAEMATOLOGY

COMPARATIVE CLINICAL HAEMATOLOGY

EDITED BY

R. K. ARCHER

MA, PhD, ScD, FRCVS

Director, Equine Research Station,
Balaton Lodge, Newmarket CB8 7DW

AND

L. B. JEFFCOTT

BVetMed, PhD, MRCVS

Clinician, Equine Research Station,
Balaton Lodge, Newmarket CB8 7DW

WITH A FOREWORD BY

H. LEHMANN

MD, PhD, ScD, FRCP, FRS, FRIC, FRCPath

Professor of Clinical Biochemistry,
University of Cambridge,
Addenbrooke's Hospital, Cambridge CB2 2QR

BLACKWELL SCIENTIFIC PUBLICATIONS

OXFORD LONDON EDINBURGH MELBOUBNE

© 1977 Blackwell Scientific Publications
Osney Mead, Oxford OX2 0EL
8 John Street, London WC1N 2ES
9 Forest Road, Edinburgh, EH1 2QH
P.O. Box 9, North Balwyn, Victoria, Australia.

First published 1977

British Library Cataloguing in Publication Data
Comparative clinical haematology.
    1. Veterinary haematology
    I. Archer, Richard Kendray   II. Jeffcott, L. B.
    599′.02′113   SF769.5

ISBN 0–632–00289–1

Printed in Great Britain
at the Alden Press, Oxford
and bound by
Kemp Hall Bindery

CONTENTS

CONTRIBUTORS

R. K. ARCHER, MA, PhD, ScD, FRCVS *Director, Equine Research Station, Balaton Lodge, Newmarket, CB8 7DW*

D. I. CHAPMAN, PhD, MIBiol, FRIC, CChem *'Larkmead', Barton Mills, Bury St Edmunds, Suffolk*

C. le Q. DARCEL, MA, PhD, MRCVS *Head of Virology, Animal Diseases Research Institute (W), PO Box 640, Lethbridge, Alberta, T1J 3Z4 Canada*

D. L. DOXEY, BVM&S, PhD, MRCVS *Lecturer, Department of Veterinary Medicine, Royal (Dick) School of Veterinary Studies, Veterinary Field Station, Easter Bush, nr Roslin, Midlothian*

ENID ECCLESTON *Safety of Medicines Department, Imperial Chemical Industries Ltd, Mereside, Alderley Park, Macclesfield, Cheshire SK10 4TG*

B. GREENWOOD, MB, BS, BSc, PhD, MRCS, LRCP *Member of the scientific staff, ARC Institute of Animal Physiology, Babraham, Cambridge*

CHRISTINE HAWKEY, PhD *Senior Research Fellow, Head of Haematology Section, Nuffield Institute of Comparative Medicine, The Zoological Society of London, Regent's Park, London NW1*

R. D. HODGES, BSc, PhD *Lecturer in Physiology, Wye College (University of London)*

P. IMLAH, PhD, MSc, MRCVS *Senior Lecturer, Department of Animal Health, Royal (Dick) School of Veterinary Studies, Veterinary Field Station, Easter Bush, nr Roslin, Midlothian*

L. B. JEFFCOTT, BVetMed, PhD, MRCVS *Clinician, Equine Research Station, Balaton Lodge, Newmarket, CB8 7DW*

S. M. LEWIS, BSc, MD, FRCPath, DCP *Reader in Haematology, Royal Postgraduate Medical School and Consultant Haematologist, Hammersmith Hospital, London W12*

LINDSAY J. MACKEY, BVMS, PhD, MRCVS, MRCPath *Senior Lecturer, Department of Veterinary Pathology, University of Glasgow, currently Guest Professor, Division of Haematology, Department of Medicine, University of Geneva*

H.S. McTAGGART, BA, BSc, MRCVS *Senior Lecturer, Department of Veterinary Medicine, Royal (Dick) School of Veterinary Studies, Veterinary Field Station, Easter Bush, nr Roslin, Midlothian*

N. W. SPURLING, MIBiol *Senior Scientist, Department of Toxicology and Pathology, Medical Division, Allen and Hanburys Research Limited, Ware, Hertfordshire, SG12 0DJ*

FOREWORD

PROFESSOR H. LEHMANN

No living tissue of man and animals has been investigated so intensively as their blood. This not only because one can obtain samples without harming the donor but also because subtle changes can be observed easily and at short intervals in the investigation of diseases and their cures. This ease of access applies not only to the morphological parameters but also to the chemistry of cells and plasma. Indeed, one may wonder how much of the nineteenth-century work on mammalian metabolism, and particularly on nutrition, could have been speeded up if it had been possible to study blood rather than urine. This book is orientated towards the help comparative haematology can give to diagnosis of diseases of animals. This requires a review of what is known of the normal state, and the reader is regaled by a vista of the blood of man and of many animals as well as some birds. It is a fascinating story because, be it that the knowledge of blood is so detailed, be it that blood is so highly specialized an organ, there are described very many intriguing differences all designed to serve 'the creatures where nature (or selection!) ordered their estate'. It would be difficult to imagine such a widely varied fare in a book on comparative osteology or even on the liver or the heart. Thus, quite apart from the usefulness of this volume to practitioners of veterinary medicine, the differences between bloods can be considered an invitation to the zoologist, and one could think of no better help for him to prepare searching questions.

A glance at the contents table will tell the reader that he can expect a thorough preparation of the background of haematology with descriptions of investigations and technical methods all to support chapters on individual animals as well as one chapter on birds in general and one on avian leucosis in particular. This is a book which is dealing with the treatment of animals, and for that reason perhaps rabbit, rat and mouse are, at least at this stage, less considered. The various surveys are masterly and each one is complete in itself. Seeing them side by side one is impressed by the wealth of knowledge available, but one also notes that there are still many gaps. These must be starting points for comparative haematologists for further progress and no doubt an important role of this book will be to present this challenge. With the additional generous support of some 2,000 references, this volume is bound to become a standard work to be widely consulted. Drs Archer and Jeffcott and their colleagues will have earned themselves the gratitude of a readership well beyond the veterinary world for which the book is primarily intended.

H. LEHMANN

PREFACE

Our objective in editing this book has been to try and assemble as much practical information on comparative clinical haematology and its related techniques as possible. Since the whole field of clinical haematology has been studied much more extensively in human medicine, we felt that a broadly-based chapter on the clinical haematology of man would form a useful basis for comparison with other species and would highlight some of the areas where information is lacking. We hope that the book will be of interest to all those concerned with the maintenance of the health of animals, particularly when it is necessary to handle a species with which the worker may not, by custom, be familiar. We believe the task has not been tackled in this way before, and we are most grateful to our contributors who have made it possible.

ACKNOWLEDGEMENTS

We are indebted to Mrs Molly Wood for the time and care she has spent checking the bibliography. The task of writing and editing a textbook such as this would be impossible without excellent secretarial assistance, and we have been very fortunate in the considerable help we have received from our secretaries, Mrs Daphne Krombacher and Mrs Jane Waddell. Our thanks are also due to Mrs Anna Taylor for help with the proof reading and cross-checking the references.

The help and assistance given by the publishers, Blackwell Scientific Publications Ltd, is gratefully acknowledged, in particular Mrs Lis Bartlett for sub-editing the text and preparing the work for the press. Our printers have produced the cleanest proofs we have yet had the good fortune to see. Finally, may we thank Professor Hermann Lehmann for writing the foreword and for his encouraging remarks.

THE NATURE OF BLOOD AND
ITS DISORDERS

R. K. ARCHER

The study of haematology is undertaken for one of two general purposes; the first is the pursuit of knowledge about blood itself, as a part of a physiological appreciation of life; the second depends on the fact that small samples of blood are easily obtainable during the life of the subject and can be examined to help in assessment of health status of that subject. This book is concerned almost exclusively with the second purpose: that of a practical aid to diagnosis.

The nature of blood appears to differ according to one's particular point of view. Surgeons have been known to remark that it is a scarlet fluid with a remarkable propensity for obscuring the field; priests have regarded it from time immemorial as a life-containing fluid; some nomadic tribes still bleed their animals to obtain a nourishing food and drink. However, only very rarely is blood considered as an organ.

Blood is an organ, just as the liver, kidneys or brain. The obvious difference is that blood has a fluid matrix rather than a solid or semi-solid one. Indeed this fluid organ reaches almost every part of the body save the hair, teeth and cornea of the eyes. Because of this it is modified in its passage through the various organs of the body in ways which sometimes differ: certainly they may differ quite profoundly in disease as opposed to health. Here it is that one of the greatest aids to diagnosis arises, since blood is altered during circulation. Differences which can be revealed by appropriate laboratory tests are applicable to clinical medicine. Only fairly rarely are such tests diagnostic of a particular disease or state of wellbeing, but as more tests become available with increasing sensitivity, more and more information can be extracted and applied in the art of diagnosis.

There are limitations to the use of information which can be obtained from haematological examinations. These are most easily defined with an appreciation in general terms of the nature of blood.

1.1   THE STRUCTURE OF BLOOD AS AN ORGAN

In common with other organs, blood consists of several distinct cell types suspended or supported by a matrix. The fluid matrix is in fact an extremely complex mixture of proteins and other compounds in water with a closely controlled pH and osmotic pressure. A study of the structure of blood plasma is considered much more fully in textbooks of clinical chemistry, but for haematological studies it is usual to include the protein polymorphisms associated with blood types, enzymes which are dependent upon organs other than blood (e.g. the liver or the skeletal muscles), blood coagulation factors and paraproteinaemias associated with malignancy of cell lines such as lymphocytes or plasma cells. Of the cells there are more erythrocytes or red cells than all others together, five different kinds of leucocytes and platelets.

1.1.1   ERYTHROCYTES

The red blood cells are concerned with oxygen transport from lungs to other tissues. They are remarkably specialized cells, of relatively simple structure by light microscopy, but decidedly complex by electron microscopy, especially scanning electron microscopy after etching (Lewis *et al* 1968). Unusually, the erythrocytes are not nucleated in the circulating blood of mammals, but they are in fish, amphibia, reptiles and birds. As a generality there are some 500 erythrocytes in the blood for each leucocyte and about 20 for each platelet.

1.1.2 LEUCOCYTES

The several different kinds of leucocytes differ in their structure and functions, although in some cases these functions are very poorly understood. The *neutrophils* are associated with phagocytic activity, especially for bacterial invaders. When the collection of these cells is very great, frank pus is formed. The *basophils* correspond to the tissue mast cells and contain much histamine and heparin. When basophils are degranulated, this histamine and heparin is released. *Eosinophils* are increased in the blood whenever there is an increase in released histamine, which attracts the cells chemotactically either itself or through an additional chemical mediator, whether the histamine be increased in a tissue or much more rarely in circulating blood itself. Their functions are associated with the limitation and modification of the effects attributable to the release of chemical mediators of inflammation (histamine, 5-hydroxytryptamine, bradykinin, etc.). *Lymphocytes* are complicated by the existence of two distinct function types of similar morphology. The first are the T cells or thymus-dependent lymphocytes associated with antibody production and the ability to transform to blast forms or primitive undifferentiated cells in the bone marrow or the reticuloendothelial system. The second are the B cells or blood lymphocytes classically increased in certain virus-induced diseases and in chronic conditions associated with acid-fast bacterial infections. And finally, the *monocytes* are again phagocytic cells concerned with the removal of tissue debris, like the tissue macrophages, especially where the tissue damage is associated with chronic disorders associated with certain viral diseases.

1.1.3 PLATELETS

There is a controversy as to whether blood platelets are cells or just fractions of cells. They are formed by budding off cytoplasmic fragments from megakaryocytes in the bone marrow and, save in birds, are not nucleated. Avian thrombocytes appear likely to consist rather of nuclear fragments from megakaryocytes with only vestigial cytoplasm (Archer 1971). As to function, platelets are associated with the ability to become adhesive when the blood circulation suffers injury, so sticking to damaged or incomplete vascular endothelium and to each other. In this way a rapidly formed, flexible mat develops which, together with blood coagulation, usually successfully maintains the integrity of the circulatory system.

1.1.4 PLASMA

The suspending fluid of blood cells is the plasma. It is a complex mixture of proteins and other compounds in aqueous solution, with albumin and globulins predominating, fibrinogen also being present. Plasma is subject to changes attributable to passage through the organs since compounds may both be added to it or removed from it. Whilst many such changes can and do occur, the tendency for homeostasis of the plasma is remarkable, frequently involving large shifts of fluid to maintain it.

1.1.5 ORIGIN OF BLOOD CELLS

All the cells of circulating blood, including the platelets, arise in the adult by haematopoiesis in the bone marrow. It is unusual for haematopoiesis to occur elsewhere than the marrow in health: in certain disorders, haemolytic anaemias for example, it may occur in spleen or liver. In the fetus, distinct haematopoiesis may be seen in several organs, but at or near term it is generally confined to the red bone marrow. As the subject gets older, areas of active haematopoiesis are reduced and replaced within the bones by yellow, fatty marrow.

1.2 THE STRUCTURE OF CAPILLARY WALLS

The larger blood vessels, be they arteries or veins, are generally impermeable to the blood circulating within them. At the capillary level, however, the circumstances are quite different since the walls of capillaries are pervious not only to plasma but also, in certain circumstances, to blood cells. The studies of Leblond (1973) have clearly shown something of the structure of the sinusoids of the spleen and the bone marrow of normal rats. Using scanning electron microscopy, Leblond has demonstrated that the sinusoidal walls in the spleen are thin and lattice-like, the pores being some 0·5 to 2·5 μ diameter (Figs 1.1–1.4). These pores are smaller than the red cell diameter (about 5 μ) but the membrane is so thin that they can easily be distended to permit the passage of an erythrocyte. Clearly the much more easily deformed leucocytes could pass through such pores and it has to be assumed that they are normally 'closed' to cells by electrostatic means.

Leblond showed additionally that in the rat bone marrow the sinusoidal walls did not have visible perforations. It is suggested that these walls may have breakages permitting the passage of blood cells. Information on the possible pores occurring in other capillaries would be of considerable interest and is an area in which additional research would be likely to prove most interesting. The message at this time, however, is clear: it must be assumed that blood cells can and do cross capillary or sinusoidal walls without damage to those walls.

As to blood plasma, it is clear that fairly free passage across capillary walls can take place and it is for this reason that the measurement of circulating

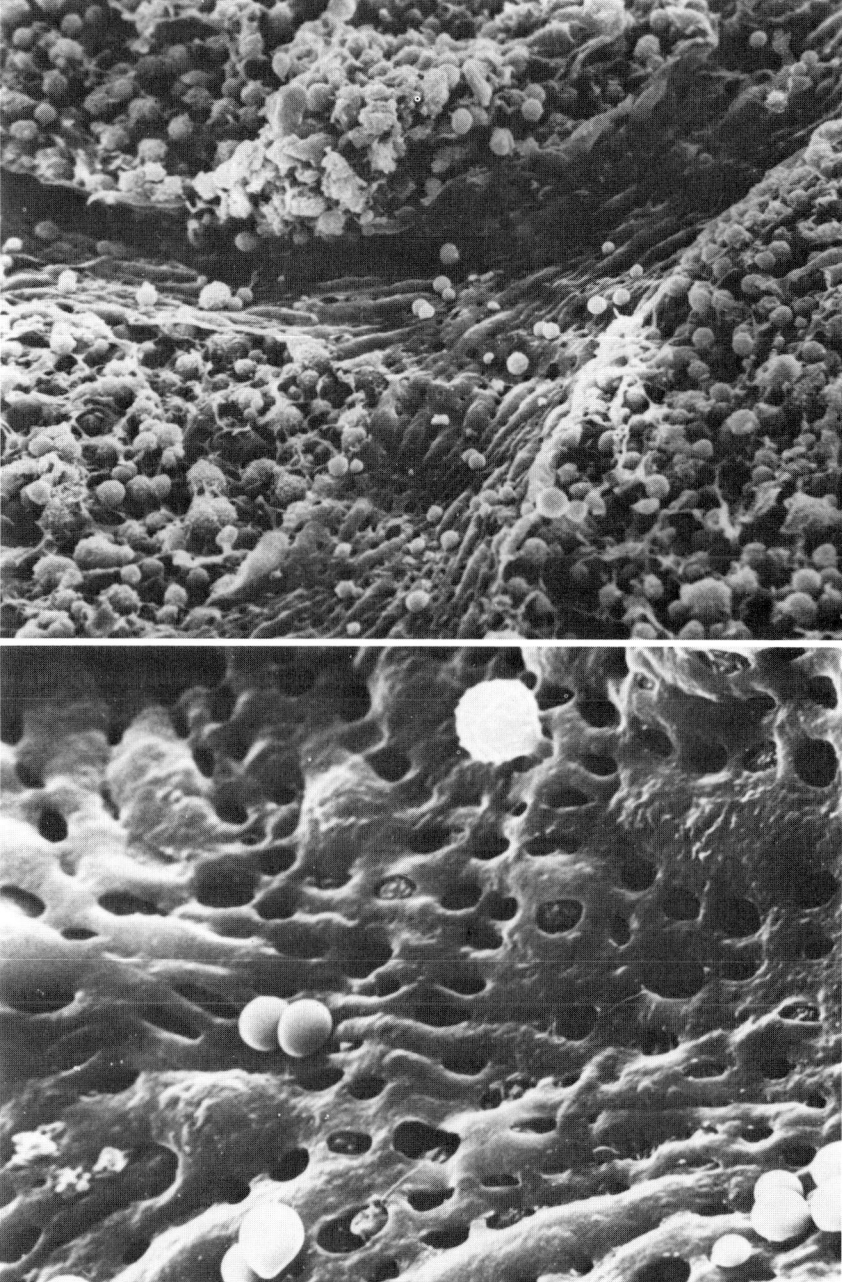

Fig. 1.1 Normal spleen. General view of a sinusoid dividing into two branches
(×700). (Figs 1.1–1.4 are reproduced from P. F. Leblond (1973) *Nouvelle Revue
Francaise d'Haematologie*, **13,** 771–6.)

   Fig. 1.2 Normal spleen. Showing the pores of the sinusoid (×3000).

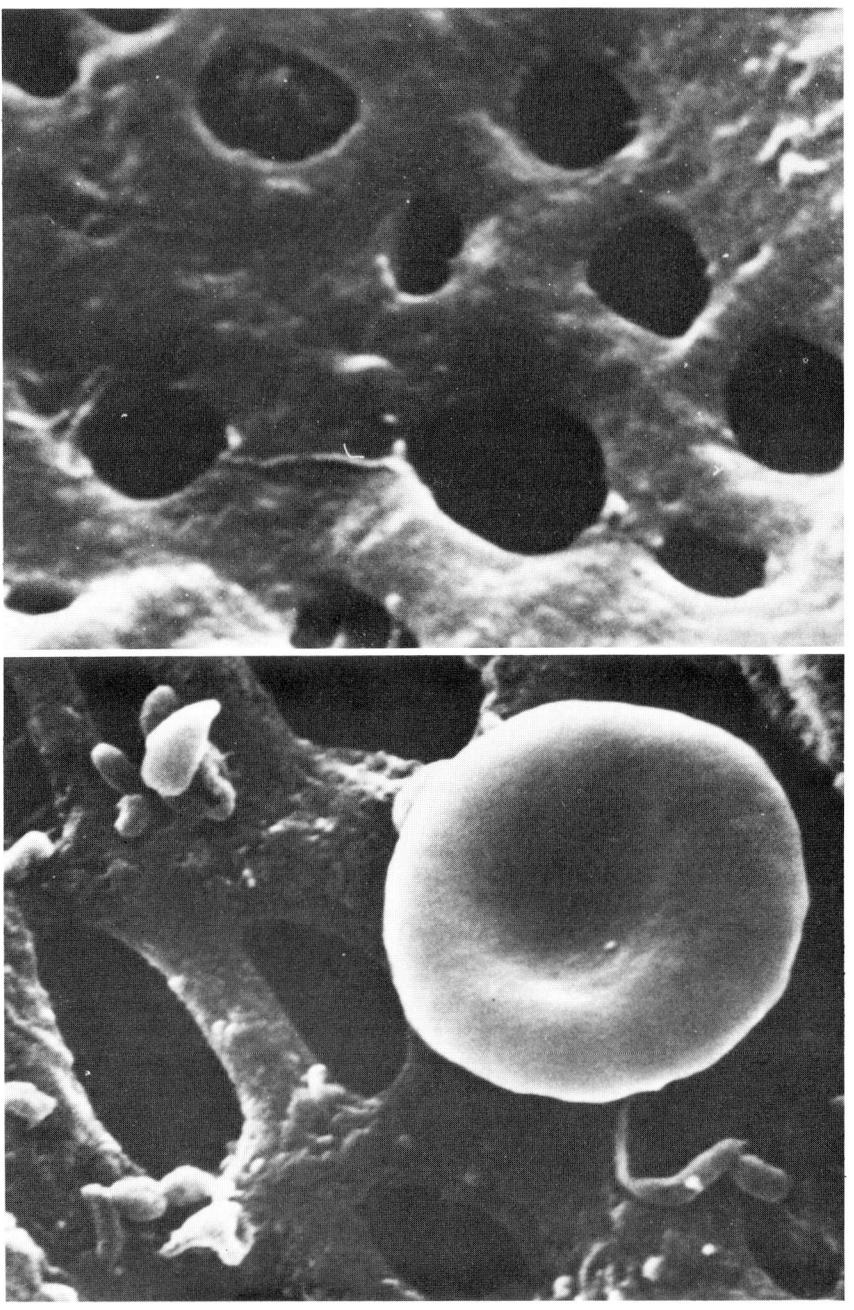

Fig. 1.3   Normal spleen. Higher magnification (× 9800).

Fig. 1.4   Normal spleen. To compare the diameter of an erythrocyte with an adjacent orifice (× 11,200).

plasma volume is fraught with difficulty. The molecules of albumin, one of the chief constituents of blood plasma, have a shape not unlike a corkscrew, which appears ready to traverse the capillary wall. Thus, most measurements of plasma volume in fact record the 'albumin space'.

1.3 THE INTERPRETATION OF HAEMATOLOGICAL LABORATORY TESTS

Whenever laboratory tests are to be interpreted in their application to clinical medicine it is absolutely necessary to be aware of their limitations. These limitations are of two kinds: firstly the limits to which laboratory tests are accurate and reproducible, and secondly those attributable to the status of the individual being tested.

In general, the accuracy and repeatability of established tests used in haematological laboratories far exceeds the needs of clinical medicine so long as quality control methods are applied. Such controls are essential to detect drift or failed calibration in laboratory equipment (see Chapter 14, p. 537). None the less, variations occur between laboratories making counts and other tests on aliquots of the same samples of blood, especially where quality control is not regularly and properly undertaken. Inter-laboratory comparisons without such controls may be impossible to interpret.

The status of an individual may greatly influence the figures that are obtained from laboratory examination of blood. Generally the objective will be to distinguish between health and disease, and in many diseases the distinction from health is marked. Apart from this, the blood of an individual may be changed from the known normal of that individual: here quite a small change can be closely observed and interpreted.

The effect of exertion must be kept closely in mind. Any exercise changes circulating blood and produces both an increase in circulating cells, particularly erythrocytes, and a decrease in plasma volume. Some individuals respond even to the sight of another being exerted; some individuals cannot be bled freely at rest without excitation or exertion to a degree; others may be so unconcerned that they almost sleep during the sampling process. Some quantitation of the effect of exercise can be achieved, but in some species, deer for example (see Chapter 9) only specimens from excited animals can be obtained. None the less the closer it is possible to approach standardization of the exertion state of individuals within a given species, the more often will it be possible to detect abnormalities. Generally the easiest standardization in this sense is 'alert rest'—that is to say, an animal neither exerted, excited for fighting, but rather alert and taking interest. The time from the last meal is frequently most relevant as hungry animals are hardly ever relaxed.

Bearing in mind the variations between individuals of a species, groups in that species and between different species, it is at once apparent that knowledge and skill are required to obtain useful meaning from haematological laboratory tests. Besides these, account must be taken of the fact that the blood circulation is not a closed piped system, but rather has extensive perforations and variations in distribution which can quickly change. Again, almost all blood samples collected for examinations are venous and from one of the greater veins: they are therefore mixed organ effluent blood. From this it follows that small changes in peripheral blood revealed by laboratory tests will either be meaningless or uninterpretable unless care has been taken to minimize the effects of the controllable variables: laboratory results by quality control, exertion state of the individual, knowledge of that individual (or a group as closely like as possible) in good health and a good clean puncture of the vessel used to take the sample to avoid contamination with other tissue. With these cautions, however, a great deal of information about an individual can be obtained by examining blood samples from it in the laboratory.

1.4 SOME CHARACTERISTIC CHANGES OF BLOOD

At this point it may be useful to consider some of the disorders of blood in general terms. Relatively few of these are primary disorders of blood: most are secondary to some more general condition such as malnutrition. Other conditions, which are certainly not disorders of the blood itself, are fairly easily identified by characteristic changes of circulating blood, and serial observations of blood samples from the same individual can give most valuable information about the progress of an illness.

1.4.1 ANAEMIA

More correctly, this should be termed 'hypoaemia' since there is no oxygen transport in the complete absence of erythrocytes. Anaemias can take several forms and can be classified in detail. Speaking generally, all arise either from failure to form enough erythrocytes or excessive destruction or loss of these cells. For example, in every half litre of blood there is about 250 mg of iron and, in man, about 5 mg is the maximum amount absorbable daily from a normal diet. If, therefore, the relatively trivial loss of some 10 ml blood occurs each day, iron deficiency will develop. Iron, however, is very well conserved within the body and supplementation of the diet is only rarely necessary, but the balance is a fine one.

Some forms of anaemia appear to be restricted to a single species. Pernicious anaemia, for example, has been described convincingly only in man. Certain anaemias which respond to therapy with vitamin B_{12} other than in man are rare: indeed several such anaemias appear to depend upon cobalt deficiency rather than vitamin B_{12} deficiency. Again, there is an infectious anaemia of horses attributable to virus infection: other species appear to be quite unaffected.

Biopsy examination of bone marrow is frequently diagnostic when an anaemia is of uncertain aetiology. Such an examination can distinguish between normal erythropoiesis and the megaloblastic erythropoiesis which is typical of pernicious anaemia. It can also indicate a maturation arrest of developing cells or erythroid hypoplasia as occurs in anaemias attributable to blood loss.

1.4.2 LEUCOPENIA

A reduction in the number of circulating leucocytes can occur if there is failure to develop the cells or if there is abnormally high tissue demand for them outside the blood itself. Failures of leucopoiesis are rare but can be determined by examination of the bone marrow. This type of examination is of great value to detect toxic effects of therapeutic agents. Reduced numbers of all kinds of leucocytes are uncommon, but are a feature of overwhelming infections, particularly in the newborn and young. Single kinds of leucocytes may be reduced when the demand for that particular kind is large and sudden. This may occur with neutrophils in very early, peracute bacterial infections; with eosinophils in shock; or with monocytes in a few acute viral infections. In such cases the cells leaving circulating blood are usually accumulating in the injured or invaded tissues.

1.4.3 PANCYTOPENIA

This is to be distinguished carefully from leucopenia, since in such cases both erythrocytes and leucocytes are decreased in the circulating blood. Generally this is a reflection of fluid shift, retention of water in the plasma, and not an impairment in cell development or reduction in life span.

1.4.4 HAEMOCONCENTRATION

As in the case of pancytopenia, haemoconcentration is a consequence of fluid shift, in this case a loss of water, or plasma from the circulation. Probably the commonest cause is the normal, healthy response to exertion or excitement, sometimes leading to substantial increases in cell concentrations within one or two circulation times of peripheral blood. In some species, certainly man, polycythaemia vera occurs in which there is continued overproduction of cells, or prolongation of the life span of cells. Sometimes this may be associated with malfunction of the spleen. Polycythaemia can be distinguished from haemoconcentration since, in the latter, erythrocytes, leucocytes and platelets are all increased in direct proportion, but in polycythaemia one cell type predominates, usually erythrocytes. The bone marrow exhibits marked hyperplasia in true polycythaemia, but not in haemoconcentration.

1.4.5 LEUCOCYTOSIS

An increase in one or more types of leucocyte is seen in bacterial infections (neutrophils), some virus infections (lymphocytes or monocytes) and parasitic infestations (eosinophils). The circulating blood can be regarded as a roadway for leucocytes from the producer (bone marrow) to the consumers (body tissues). Observations of various blood samples are thus comparable to a traffic census and can indicate quite clearly the attempts being made to meet tissue demands.

A distinction should be drawn between leukaemia and a leukaemoid reaction. The latter is a massive leucocytic response in the blood, predominantly of mature cells, to a particular infection or disorder. A leukaemia on the other hand is a malignant disorder of the bone marrow leading to a great increase of leucocytes in circulating blood, including their precursors. Leukaemias occur in man, dog, cat, cattle and domestic fowl relatively frequently; they are very uncommon in horses and very rarely looked for in deer or exotic species. One of the most intriguing things to be found in this book is the differences in type and course of leukaemias in different animals and the fact that lymphosarcoma is quite frequently accompanied by leucocytosis of the blood.

1.4.6 ABNORMAL BLOOD COAGULATION

There are a number of protein fractions of blood plasma concerned with blood coagulation. Deficiency of any of these impairs the usually remarkable ability of blood to change from liquid to solid if there is damage to the vascular endothelium. There may be inherited deficiencies, partial but seldom absolute, of one or more factors, directly causing disease. Factor VIII deficiency for example, is the underlying cause of haemophilia; a disease confirmed in several species. Deficiencies may be acquired: a reduction in factor VII follows poisoning (or therapy) with the coumarin-like drugs including warfarin. Warfarin poisoning, provided the resultant haemorrhage is not so severe in itself to endanger life, can be completely treated by therapy with vitamin K_1, a precursor of factor VII which is readily metabolized by the liver.

Thrombocytopenia, or a deficiency of platelets in circulating blood, can arise where minor haemorrhages are repeated, leading to an abnormally high withdrawal of platelets from circulation. It can also arise from autoimmune disorders, which usually respond to therapy with cortico-steroids:

sometimes, and for reasons not yet clear, therapy in the young with ACTH is more effective.

Where blood coagulation is abnormally active, extremely serious disorders follow consequent upon intravascular clotting. Indeed, disseminated intravascular coagulation (DIC) may so consume clotting factors that defibrination is a consequence, leading to renewed abnormal bleeding. If a therapeutic agent is eventually found which genuinely does render normal blood hypercoagulable, or spontaneously coagulable without discontinuity of vascular endothelium, it would seem probable that DIC and even defibrination would follow: surely a therapeutic disaster.

Haematological therapy of deficient coagulation is limited at present to the replacement of missing factors or profactors on the one hand, and the reduction of poisons which may reduce coagulation factors on the other hand.

1.4.7 BLOOD GROUPS

The first-discovered and apparently simple blood group system of man referred to as Landsteiner ABO does not have equivalents in the lower animals that have yet been studied. There are, however, definite blood types consequent upon protein polymorphisms which are genetically inherited amongst the plasma proteins, and red cell systems, in some ways like the ABO, dependent upon inherited differences of erythrocyte membranes. Generally the antigenic power of systems other than the ABO is not great and transfusions of blood within a species are rarely followed by reaction on the first occasion. Subsequent transfusions of the same donor blood may provoke very violent reactions, however, if delayed sufficiently for antibodies to develop in the recipient's blood. A detailed consideration of animal blood groups is outside the intentions of this volume.

1.4.8 PARAPROTEINAEMIAS

On occasion the usual pattern of proteins in blood plasma is deranged by the presence of large amounts of a single, abnormal protein. This occurs classically in myeloma of man, associated with an abnormal protein synthesized by the population of malignant plasma cells which is a feature of the condition. Abnormal proteins are seen in animals with myeloma and also in some cases of lymphosarcoma: in either case there may or may not be abnormal cells in the blood or bone marrow.

1.4.9 SERUM ENZYMES

In this context those enzymes which are dependent upon tissue other than blood are for consideration where they may aid diagnosis. For example aspartate amino transferase (AAT) as found in blood serum is elevated where there is damage to liver or tissue trauma. Creatine kinase (CPK) is elevated when skeletal muscle is damaged but sorbitol dehydrogenase (SDH) shows an increase in liver disorders. These and other clinical chemical tests are frequently invaluable in assessment of the site or organ damage, but a detailed consideration of them is beyond the scope of this book.

2

HAEMATOLOGICAL INVESTIGATION AS AN AID TO DIAGNOSIS

L. B. JEFFCOTT

2.1 INTRODUCTION

A good, working knowledge of clinical pathology is essential in order to make the most of haematology as an aid to diagnosis. Further, it is unwise to interpret haematological results without the support of a good clinical appreciation of the case. Scores of misdiagnoses have undoubtedly been made because of insufficient cognisance of these points. This chapter is intended to give a cursory, but none the less overall, view of the role of haematology as an aid to clinical diagnosis. I shall try to outline the present-day scope of haematological investigation and point out some of the limitations.

The art of medical or clinical diagnosis necessitates the use of all the senses of the physician; the path to achieve this objective is often complicated and may involve a number of steps (Fig. 2.1). If the optimum results of laboratory haematological tests are to be obtained, it is essential to bear three things in mind. Firstly, a good appreciation of the specific techniques and what they can be expected to detect. Secondly, a series of queries posed by examiner to which laboratory tests can provide an answer (e.g. can the clinical evidence of anaemia in a subject be confirmed by a low red blood count, RBC)?

L. B. Jeffcott

or does a case of suspected infection exhibit a raised white cell count (WBC) and can further diagnostic or prognostic information be determined from its

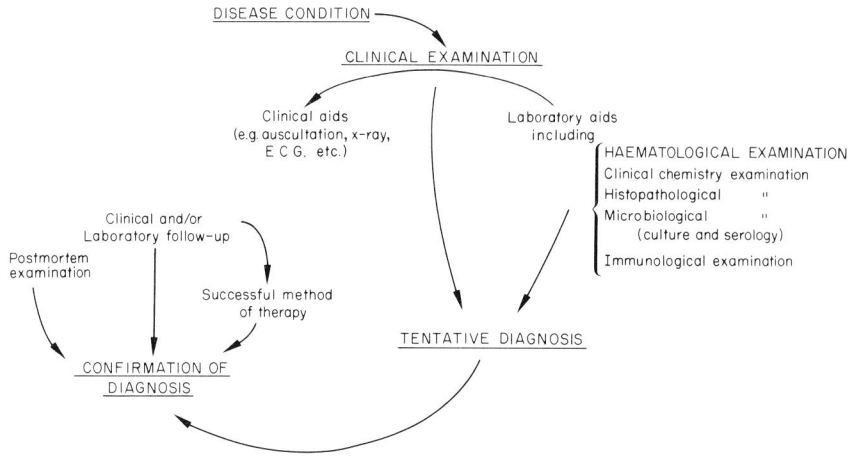

Fig. 2.1 Systematic approach to clinical diagnosis.

degree and differential?). Thirdly, a good knowledge of the nature of blood and its own disorders is required.

2.2   RANGE OF TESTS AVAILABLE

The range of tests applicable to haematological investigation is extensive (Table 2.1), although methods for all of them are not yet available for all the species covered in this book. Most of the techniques were first evaluated on and used for man and there is a temptation to use man as the reference species. This is perhaps especially true concerning some of the tests for blood clotting, and is further complicated if reagents from different species are mixed, so making correct interpretation almost impossible. This book is intended to draw attention both to the differences and to the similarities between man and other species. For instance, man is one of the few animals that is known to exhibit anaemia due to true nutritional deficiency of folate or vitamin B_{12}. Then there is the phenomenon of red cell sickling which is associated in man with a severe normochromic anaemia and an abnormal haemoglobin (Hb-S). However, it is not seen in other species except deer, and occasionally in sheep, where the haemoglobin is not abnormal and the phenomenon is unaccompanied by any known clinical or haematological effects. The presence of a distinct fetal haemoglobin (Hb-F) occurs in man and some animals (e.g. ruminants) but is not present in other species (e.g. horses). The erythrocyte metabolism of man and other animals shows great variation particularly

Table 2.1 Haematological tests available as aids to diagnosis

CELLS	PLASMA (or SERUM)
Red cell concentration (RBC)	Plasma viscosity (PV)
Haemoglobin concentration (Hb)	Plasma osmotic pressure (POP)
Packed cell volume (PCV)	Protein constituents:
Red cell morphology:	*Fibrinogen*
Anisocytosis	*Haptoglobin*
Poikilocytosis	*Serum proteins*
Sickling	Enzymes:
Parasites	*Non-specific enzymes*
Red cell indices:	*Organ-specific isoenzymes*
Mean corpuscular haemoglobin (MCH)	Ions and other serum constituents:
Mean cell volume (MCV)	*Iron*
Mean corpuscular haemoglobin	*Folate*
concentration (MCHC)	*Vitamin B_{12}*
Mean cell diameter (MCD)	*Total iron bind capacity* (TIBC)
Leucocyte concentration (WBC)	Clotting factors
Differential white cell count	Blood groups (serum polymorphisms)
Platelet concentration	
Erythrocyte sedimentation rate (ESR)	
Bone marrow biopsy	
Total blood volume	
Red cell metabolites (2,3-DPG, ATP etc.)	
Red blood antigens (blood types)	

in respect to oxygen affinity and the interaction of haemoglobin and 2,3-diphosphoglycerate (2,3-DPG). Many of the human complex congenital and hereditary forms of haematological abnormalities have not yet been recognized in lower animals (e.g. thalassaemia, hereditary elliptocytosis, G-6-PD deficiency etc.). There are even considerable differences in the bone marrow response to blood loss, anaemia and other diseases between man and some of the other species. All these examples and many more besides emphasize the importance of a comparative approach to haematological interpretation.

A valuable role of the clinical haematologist can be to advise on the most appropriate sample to take (e.g. blood, bone marrow or lymph node biopsy etc.) the bottles and anticoagulant to use and which tests seem most applicable. Before a proper decision can be made on the particular haematological test to be carried out in a case, it is imperative that the laboratory be given some details of the subject and its history. A few words of explanation are all that is necessary in cases where a fairly straightforward clinical diagnosis is required to be confirmed. In more obscure cases a discussion with the laboratory, before taking blood samples, often proves very useful and may save a good deal of time. There is little point in sending samples in an anticoagulant like EDTA (sequestrene) if an analysis of clotting is required. Samples sent by post may reach the laboratory in poor condition making it impossible to perform differential counts due to autolysis of the white cells. These samples may also show increased tendency to haemolysis which will obviously affect the red cell indices and seriously impair analysis of the anions (K^+, Na^+, etc.).

A knowledge of the accuracy and reproducibility of the various tests is especially relevant. For example, the erythrocyte sedimentation rate (ESR) is a technique which lacks sensitivity and rarely has diagnostic value in those species which show rouleaux formation of the red cells. On the other hand some of the serum enzymes are so sensitive that quite substantial increases may be detected in the absence of clinical signs.

The importance of adequate laboratory quality control is something frequently disregarded in veterinary haematology. Since the introduction of electronic particle counters and sophisticated biochemical equipment, it is feasible to maintain standardized results and to expect results from different laboratories to be in fairly close agreement. On the medical side the DHSS run a quality control scheme for over 400 haematological laboratories in the UK and aim to keep the results within about half a standard deviation of the national mean for normal blood.

The accuracy of manual counting of erythrocytes is inevitably difficult to standardize and may give rise to problems with interpretation. The commonest of these is a tendency to give lower readings for RBC than those determined by particle counting. This will also affect the red cell indices, principally the mean cell volume (MCV) and a diagnosis of apparent macrocytic anaemia may therefore be made erroneously. On the other hand the use of particle counters, calibrated for human erythrocytes, can give most obscure results for other species with widely different erythrocyte MCV.

2.3 COLLECTION OF SAMPLES FOR LABORATORY ANALYSIS

The technique of collection of blood samples from the various species is given in detail in Chapter 14, but there are a few general points that can be made at this time. It should be remembered that not only the method by which the sample was taken (e.g. arterial or venepuncture), but also the anticoagulant employed, and even the container used may affect the results. The effect of stress or exercise will cause appreciable haemoconcentration in most species and this could mask an anaemic condition. Some exotic animals are only sampled under the influence of sedative or anaesthetic agents and allowances for this must, of course, be made. The phenothiazine tranquillisers (e.g. acepromazine and promazine hydrochloride) are hypotensive drugs and their influence may result in depression of red cell figures simulating a normo-chromic anaemia.

The anticoagulant used may also affect the haematological results. The most widely used is EDTA (ethylenediamine tetra-acetic acid, usually as the di-K salt); however, this is not suitable for examination of plasma osmotic pressure (POP), some methods of platelet counting and for assessment of clotting function. For some biochemical estimations (e.g. serum Fe, Mg and Co) it may be necessary to use chemically clean glass sampling bottles. There is a danger with the widely used vacuum evacuated tubes (e.g. Vacu-tainer, Becton-Dickinson & Co, USA) as blood samples from some species collected into those tubes show increased cellular fragility and any resultant haemolysis then affects the final blood count.

To sum up it will be seen that the quality of the haematological results expected is limited by the state of the subject when bled and of the quality of the blood samples taken as well as the reliability or reproducibility of the tests employed.

2.4 INTERPRETATION OF HAEMATOLOGICAL DATA

This section, which deals with some of the basic principles of haematological interpretation, is best considered under the following sub-headings:

2.4.1 UNITS

The various units for haematological and biochemical analysis have always caused concern and even frustration to many veterinary clinicians. For this reason I thought it worthwhile to give a short explanation of the units employed in this book and to mention the merit of the International System of Units (SI) which has been adopted in hospital laboratories over the last few years.

The Système International d'Unités was devised to limit the confusion that arose from the diversity of units being introduced for expressing results of medical and scientific measurements. It was approved in 1960 by the Conférence Générale des Poids et Mesures and is generally accepted throughout the fields of haematology and clinical chemistry. It is based on the metric system and was designed to provide a coherent system of units that ensured uniformity of presentation of quantities, whilst minimizing the number of multiples and sub-multiples in common use (Baron *et al* 1974). SI units are based on seven base units of physical quantity and derived SI units are obtained by appropriate combination of these base units. Some of the derived

Table 2.2   Some of the more commonly used units and abbreviations in this book

PARAMETER	ABBREVIATION	UNITS
Red cell concentration	RBC	$10^{12}/l$
Haemoglobin	Hb	g/dl
Packed cell volume (haematocrit)	PCV	l/l
Total leucocyte concentration	WBC	$10^9/l$
Platelet count	—	$10^9/l$
Reticulocyte count	—	%RBC or $10^9/l$
Mean corpuscular haemoglobin	MCH	pg
Mean corpuscular volume	MCV	fl
Mean corpuscular haemoglobin concentration	MCHC	g/dl
Mean cell diameter	MCD	μm
Erythrocyte sedimentation rate	ESR	mm/h
Plasma viscosity	PV	centipoises
Serum proteins (including fibrinogen)	—	g/l
Serum haptoglobin	—	g/dl
Bilirubin	—	mg/100 ml
Serum folate	—	μg/l
Serum iron	—	μmol/l
Total iron binding capacity	TIBC	μmol/l
Serum ions (e.g. Ca, PO_4, Mg, K, Cl)	—	m mol/l
Serum enzymes (e.g. AAT, SDH, AP)	—	iu/l (μmol/min/l)
Other serum constituents (blood urea, glucose etc.)	—	g/l

SI units are used now in most medical and scientific journals. Further information may be obtained from a useful booklet published by the Royal Society of Medicine (1972) entitled 'Units, Symbols and Abbreviations. A Guide for Biological and Medical Editors and Authors'. A list of the more commonly used parameters in this book with their abbreviations and units is given in Table 2.2.

The measurements of enzyme activity do not fall within the scope of the SI system and the current trend is to quote them in International Units per litre (iu/l). The International Unit of activity is defined as that amount

Table 2.3 Nomenclature of the commonly used serum enzymes in this book

Enzyme	Abbreviation	International Enzyme Classification (1972)	Previous or alternative names
Alkaline phosphatase	AP	E.C. 3.1.3.1.	SAP
Amino aspartate transferase	AAT	E.C. 2.6.1.1.	Glutamic-oxaloacetic transaminase GOT or SGOT
Alamine aspartate transferase	Al-AT	E.C. 2.6.1.2.	Glutamic-pyruvic transaminase GPT or SPGT
Creatine kinase	CPK	E.C. 2.7.3.2.	Creatine phosphokinase
Glutamate dehydrogenase	GD	E.C. 1.4.1.2.	—
Lactate dehydrogenase	LDH	E.C. 1.1.1.27.	—
Ornithine carbamoyltransferase	OCT	E.C. 2.1.3.3.	SOCT
Sorbitol dehydrogenase	SDH	E.C. 1.1.1.14.	—

of enzyme which under given assay conditions will catalyse the conversion of 1 mol of substrate per minute. Unless identical methods are used by different laboratories they cannot be objectively compared. The common serum enzymes quoted in this book are listed in Table 2.3, together with their enzyme classification and alternative nomenclature (see Enzyme Nomenclature, 1972).

2.4.2   NORMAL OR REFERENCE VALUES

Normal ranges for all haematological and biochemical parameters are essential for detecting abnormalities associated with damage or disease. These values are usually calculated from the results obtained from a healthy population and individual figures are judged to be abnormal if they fall more than two standard deviations from the mean.

There are a number of snags and errors that can arise in the establishment of normal ranges. If the samples are not subjected to strict quality control during testing the results may be inaccurate and give an abnormally wide range. The same will be true if the number of samples collected is too small or they were obtained from a narrow or artificial cross section of the population (e.g. exotic animals in captivity, breeding colonies of laboratory or small animals kept under specialized conditions etc.). Another problem may be the naturally wide variation between individual animals and in these instances perhaps one should only refer to reference values for that one animal.

2.4.3   PROFILE TESTING

The introduction of profile testing has found particular importance in dairy cattle and the horse in recent years. The metabolic profile as a means of monitoring productivity and detecting early or subclinical disease has proved of considerable value. Basically it involves periodic testing of a series of biochemical and haematological parameters on a herd basis and will be discussed in more detail in Chapter 6.

In the thoroughbred racehorse the introduction of regular haematological profiles as fitness tests is proving quite popular. It is often anticipated that these tests can give some useful assessment of expected performance and potential. However, in our present state of knowledge they should probably be better termed as 'unfitness checks', as the best they can achieve is to inform the clinician which horses are unlikely to perform well!

2.4.4   IMPORTANCE OF CLINICAL HISTORY

As I have already said it is unfair to expect a consultant haematologist to make a diagnosis without knowledge of the subject's history. There may, of course, be quite marked haematological differences associated with the age, sex of the animal, the time of sampling in relation to exercise, feeding and time of day. Various transient haematological changes can be easily misinterpreted without a history. An example of this is demonstration of haemoconcentration which is without clinical significance if the sample is taken during stress or excitement. Again, alterations of the total and differential leucocyte counts may occur after travelling, exertion or following certain medication. For example an eosinopenia is frequently noted if the animal has recently been treated with corticosteroids.

2.4.5 DIAGNOSIS AND DIFFERENTIAL DIAGNOSIS

A thorough and careful assessment of all these facts is essential before reaching a tentative diagnosis. Two examples of the sort of step-by-step approach to haematological confirmation are given in Fig. 2.2a and b. There will, of course, be wide species variations between the usefulness and validity of some tests, and the ability to interpret the results, but the principle is the same. It is also very important to try to establish whether the haematological changes found are primary or secondary to the presenting clinical signs. A few examples will serve to illustrate this point as well as emphasizing the role of haematological data in differential diagnosis. As a clinical haematologist whose experience is chiefly limited to the horse I shall take specific examples of cases from this species.

Firstly the differentiation of bacterial or viral respiratory infection may be accomplished through haematological examination. In bacterial infections there will usually be a pronounced *neutrophilia*, sometimes with a *shift to the left*. On the other hand the initial response to virus infection is a *neutropenia* followed by leucocytosis due particularly to a lymphocytosis. In some of the equine respiratory virus infections (e.g. equid herpesvirus, EHV 1) there may be an associated increase of the liver sensitive *enzymes* (e.g. SDH and AAT). These biochemical changes are not usually seen with bacterial infections.

A second rather more complex example involves the animal which presents with a fairly normal appetite but progressive loss of bodily condition and pallor of the visible mucous membranes. The blood count may show a low RBC with associated raised WBC. Further information about the type of anaemia should be obtained to assist in deciding whether it is likely to be primary or secondary. Many of the anaemias with insidious onset are normocytic or normochromic, show hypoplasia of the bone marrow and develop secondarily to some systemic inflammatory or neoplastic condition.

Differentiation of the WBC may reveal the presence of neutrophilia possibly associated with increased *plasma viscosity* (PV), indicative of some abnormality of the plasma protein profile. These findings are rather non-specific but may signify a chronic inflammatory process. A markedly depressed

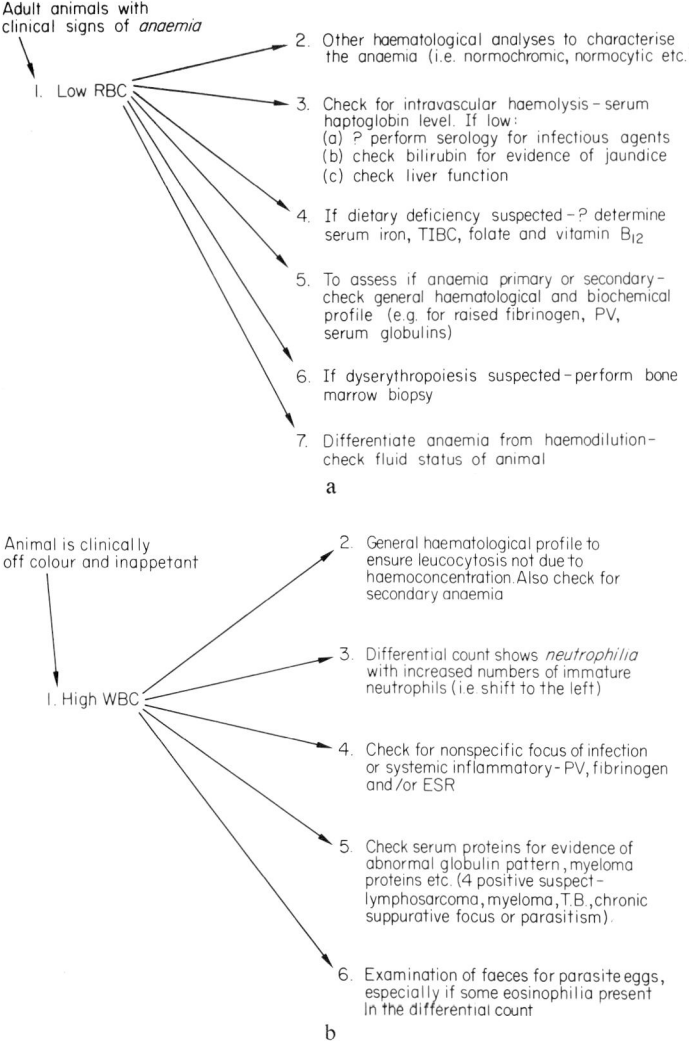

Fig. 2.2a, b An example of haematological analysis as an aid to diagnosis.

serum albumin with a compensatory rise in the globulin fractions may be seen in chronic liver damage. However, in the absence of raised liver specific serum enzymes (e.g. SDH, AAT, AP etc.) this finding is almost pathognomic of intestinal malfunction and a protein-losing enteropathy with leakage of serum proteins through the damaged intestinal epithelium into the lumen of the gut. The exact aetiology is often obscure but the condition has some similarity to Crohn's disease in man. The outcome of these cases in spite of treatment is always poor and unless progressive fall of serum albumin can be halted the prognosis is hopeless. Electropherograms with elevation of the serum globulins are more commonly found in horses with persistent neutrophilia. For instance, an elevation of α_2 *globulin* is frequently encountered if there is some chronic suppurative focus or extensive degenerative lesions of bone. A raised β_1 *globulin*, often accompanied by a circulatory eosinophilia, is seen in horses suffering from extensive larval migration due to *Strongylus vulgaris*. Increase of γ *globulin* are seen in some chronic bacterial infections (e.g. tuberculosis) or in some cases of cirrhosis and the presence of certain *paraproteinaemias* is occasionally seen in horses with multiple myeloma or lymphosarcoma.

Finally an example to illustrate the value of certain biochemical changes (i.e. serum enzymes) of such conditions as azoturia (also referred to as setfast, paralytic myoglobinuria and tying-up). In this syndrome there is acute and painful cramping of the muscles of the back and quarters. There are usually no changes in the blood count but marked increases of the enzymes, CPK and AAT. In knowing the serum half life of these enzymes and the time of onset of clinical signs a diagnosis can be made together with some appreciation of the extent of muscular damage. In addition by repeat blood sampling of the subject it should be possible to make a prognosis and to forecast when the animal may be returned to work.

2.4.6 FOLLOW-UP SAMPLES

The collection and analysis of follow-up blood tests in monitoring the progress of a case can obviously be important to the referring clinician. It is perhaps often forgotten how valuable they are to the haematologist who is frequently asked to give a prognosis for a variety of haematological conditions. Having already made a plea to give the laboratory sufficient history to help establish a diagnosis, it is just as helpful to receive follow-up reports from cases so that future cases can be coped with that much more effectively.

THE HAEMATOLOGY OF MAN

S. M. LEWIS

3.1 INTRODUCTION

It is a matter for debate whether man has entirely benefited from the way in which his blood has become adapted with his progress up the evolutionary scale. There is no doubt, however, that man is unique amongst the animals in the range of blood diseases and the diversity of environmental and nutritional factors which may affect his blood. In this chapter will be described the physiology of human blood, the pathogenesis and pathology of haematological abnormalities and some of the clinical manifestations of blood diseases. Human haematology has been studied extensively, and numerous monographs and textbooks are devoted to it. It is not intended to provide here a comprehensive treatise on the subject, nor an exhaustive bibliography, but this chapter has been included because an appreciation of human haematology might serve as a basis for understanding animal haematology. For detailed information on various aspects of human haematology, the reader should refer to the key references, mainly review articles, which are given in each section, or to one of the standard textbooks, (e.g. Hoffbrand & Lewis 1972, Williams *et al* 1972, Hardisty & Weatherall 1975, Dacie & Lewis 1975, Wintrobe 1974). In like manner, blood cell appearances in various diseases are illustrated in the figures but it has been impossible to include a comprehensive atlas of blood cell morphology, and the reader is referred to one of the several excellent atlases that are now available (e.g. McDonald *et al* 1970, Undritz 1973, and, especially for ultrastructural studies, Bessis 1973).

3.2 HAEMATOPOIESIS

Blood cells are formed in the bone marrow, spleen, liver and lymph nodes. Initially they are derived from a mesenchymal stem cell which first appears in the yolk sac in the embryo at 2 weeks (Fig. 3.1). At 6 weeks the liver becomes the chief haematopoietic organ and the mesenchymal cell differentiates into a reticulum cell and thence into a haemocytoblast. The liver becomes the main site of haematopoiesis by the 12–16th week and remains active until a few weeks before birth. At first this is confined to erythropoiesis but soon granulopoiesis also commences and by the 16th week the liver is an active site of granulocyte production.

The spleen is a relatively minor organ both for erythropoiesis and granulopoiesis; its activity starts at about the same time as the liver, continuing to the 20th week and then, to a small extent, until birth. The bone marrow becomes a site of haematopoiesis from about 20 weeks. At first it is involved chiefly in granulopoiesis but soon the multipotential mesenchymal cells which inhabit the marrow give rise also to erythroblasts, myeloblasts and megakaryocytes.

Lymphocytes are also mesenchymal in origin. There are two types of lymphocytes—thymus derived lymphocytes (T cells) and thymus independent lymphocytes (B cells)—which have different functional properties: the former play a central role in mediation of cellular immunity; the latter are equated with cells which occur in birds in the bursa of Fabricius and are responsible for antibody production. There is, however, strong evidence that all circulating lymphocytes are ultimately derived from the bone marrow stem cells. It has been shown that the spleen, lymph nodes and gut-associated lymphoid tissue (tonsils, appendix and Peyer's patches) are populated by cells which have originally migrated there from the blood, and that the lymphoid cells in the thymus, too, have migrated via the blood from the bone marrow.

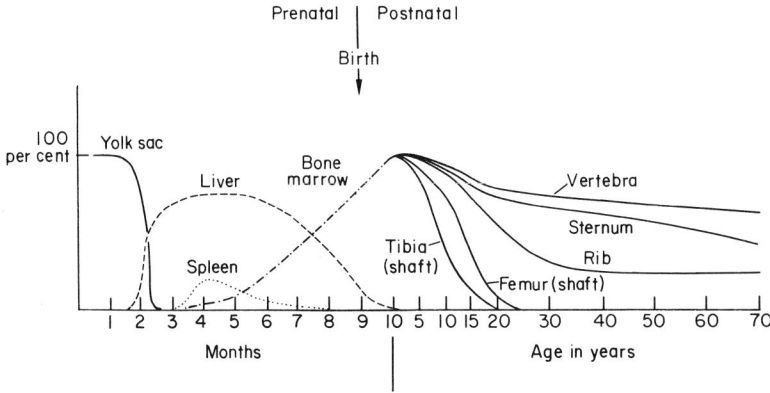

Fig. 3.1   Sites of erythropoietic tissue in fetus, childhood and adult life.

Monocytes are thought to stem from the same sites as lymphocytes. The majority are formed in the bone marrow and are derived from the same precursor cell as are myeloid cells.

3.2.1   POSTNATAL HAEMATOPOIESIS (Fig. 3.1)

At birth actively haematopoietic marrow occupies the entire capacity of the bone, and this remains so for 2–3 years. During this time, the spleen, liver and other extramedullary sites are inert, but because the marrow capacity is fully extended, any excessive demands for blood production caused by haemorrhage or haemolysis will result in reactivation of extramedullary haematopoiesis, initially, as a rule, by the spleen. From childhood, there is a gradual replacement of active (red) marrow by fatty (yellow) marrow. The long bones begin to develop fatty marrow at their diaphyseal ends, and then progressively from the distal to the proximal ends of bones so that by the age of 20–22 years red marrow is confined to the upper ends of femur and humerus and to the flat bones of the sternum, ribs, vertebrae, cranium and pelvis. In old age, these sites, too, become increasingly replaced by fatty marrow.

3.3 ERYTHROID CELL PROLIFERATION AND MATURATION

Cells of the erythroid series have the same fundamental capacity for growth and division as do all cells, and this is under the control of DNA and RNA. The erythroid cells, however, are unique on 2 counts: (a) they have the

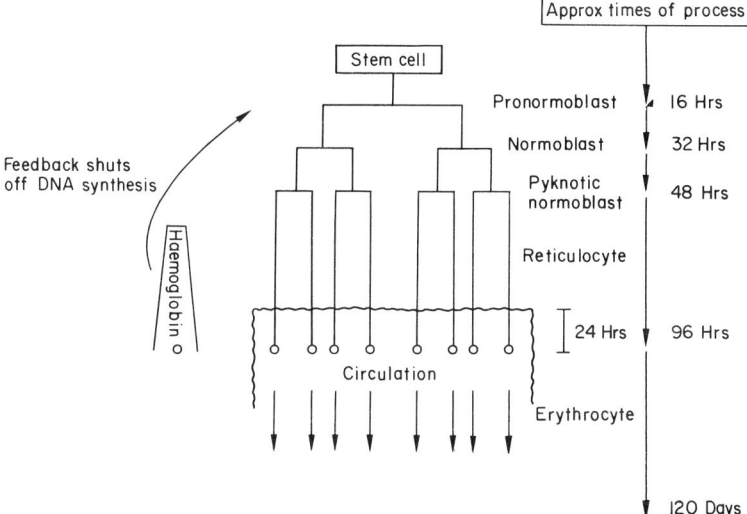

Fig. 3.2   Scheme illustrating erythroid cell proliferation and maturation.

capacity for haemoglobin synthesis and (b) as they mature they lose their nuclei, but remain functionally active in circulation for a length of time. The period of maturation and division is associated with the synthesis of lipo-proteins, nucleoproteins, carbohydrates, enzymes and haemoglobin. The sequence of events which leads to mitosis and maturation commences when a resting cell is triggered into a proliferative cycle. There are 3 mitotic divisions during the evolution of the pronormoblast to late (pyknotic) normoblast (Fig. 3.2). The interphase (intermitotic interval) is 16 hours so that matura-tion to the late normoblast takes 2 days. Haemoglobinization takes 2 to 4 days. When a critical haemoglobin concentration is reached, a feedback mechanism is triggered which shuts off further nucleic acid synthesis and cell division. Thus the number of divisions in a fixed interphase time is determined by the rate of haemoglobin synthesis: when haemoglobin synthesis is accelerated, critical haemoglobin concentration is reached more rapidly; in haemoglobin deficiency, the shut-off fails and this results in an increased number of divisions with the production of microcytes. As the cell matures the nucleus becomes pyknotic and it is then extruded by a process of cytoplasm cleavage for which active cell movement is required. The immature enucleated cell is known as the reticulocyte. The reticulocyte matures in 2–3 days, 24 hours of which are spent in the circulation. However, if the reticulocyte is released into circulation prematurely, its maturation time in circulation will be prolonged for up to 3 days. After the erythrocytes have matured they can survive in circulation for 100–120 days. At the end of this time they are destroyed by phagocytosis in the reticulo-endothelial system. This occurs partly in the spleen, but RE cells throughout the body are also involved; it is now thought that in normal subjects the marrow plays a major part in the process (Lajtha 1965, LoBue & Gordon 1967, Gordon 1970a, b, Stohlman 1970, Lozzio 1973, Wolstenholme & O'Connor 1973, Wickramasinghe 1975).

3.4   REGULATION OF ERYTHROPOIESIS

The very complex process of erythropoietic cell proliferation and maturation is dependent upon a number of important interrelated factors. Perhaps the most important factor for the control of erythropoiesis is erythropoietin and several hormones, notably androgens, play a part either directly or by stimulating the action of erythropoietin. Erythropoiesis also requires iron in a form which is usable for the production of haemoglobin, and a number of other nutrient agents, notably vitamin B_{12} and folate. Furthermore, correct integration of DNA, RNA and protein is necessary for the production of structurally normal haemoglobin chains, whilst for the mature erythrocyte to retain its shape and to remain alive and functional requires an integral cell membrane and an ability to derive energy and reducing power from glucose. Failure of one or more of these processes will cause anaemia. In the next section the various types of anaemia and their pathogenesis will be briefly described.

3.5   IRON METABOLISM AND IRON-DEFECTIVE ANAEMIA

A normal adult male has about 4 g of iron in his body, 65–70 per cent of which is present in the circulating haemoglobin. Most of the remainder is present as storage iron, either in the form of haemosiderin or ferritin.

Myoglobin contains 4–5 per cent of body iron and a small amount of iron is present in haem-containing enzymes such as cytochromes, catalase and peroxidase. Storage iron, including iron which is released following haemoglobin breakdown, is found mainly in the reticulo-endothelial cells of the

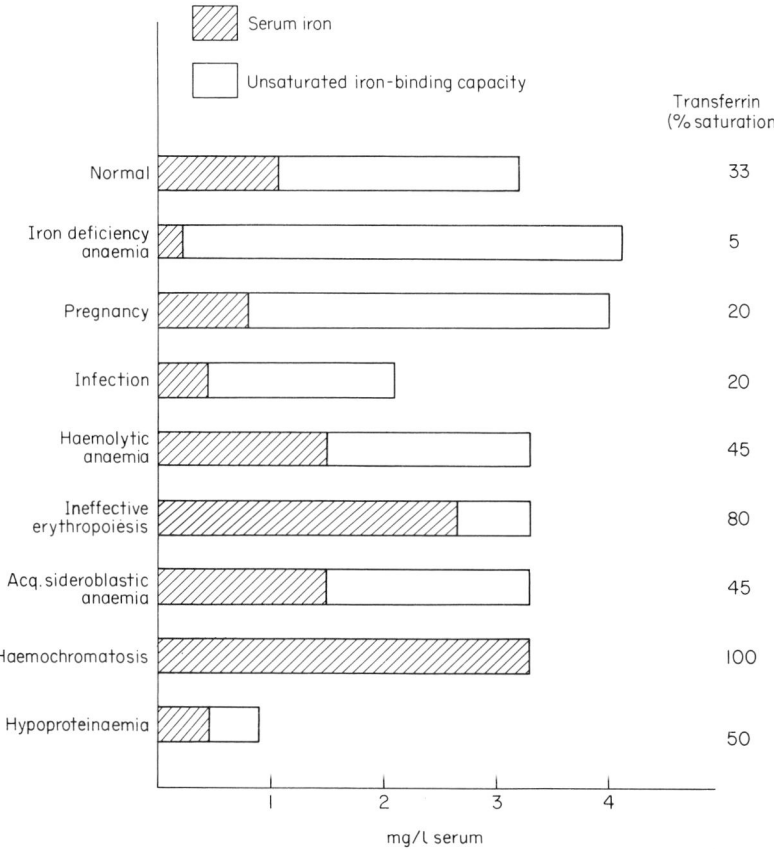

Fig. 3.3 Values found for serum iron, unsaturated iron binding capacity and percentage saturation in various conditions.

liver, spleen and bone marrow but it is also found in parenchymal cells, notably those of the liver, but also in the kidney, pancreas, thyroid, adrenals and other organs. Storage iron consists, as a rule, of approximately 65 per cent ferritin and 35 per cent haemosiderin. These 2 forms of iron differ from each other as follows: haemosiderin is a water-insoluble protein–iron complex containing about 37 per cent of iron by weight and existing as large particles which are visible by light microscopy and stain by prussian blue reaction; ferritin is a water-soluble protein–iron complex containing about 20 per cent of iron and consisting of a well-defined protein shell, apoferritin, together with colloidal ferric hydroxide and phosphate.

Iron is transported in plasma attached to a β-globulin protein, transferrin. The plasma concentration of transferrin is 1·2–2·0 g/l and it binds about 1·4 μg Fe per mg. Normally, a total of 4 mg of iron circulates bound in this form. It passes to the bone marrow where, at the surface of the erythroblast, the iron is released from its attachment and enters the cell. There most of the iron is rapidly converted to haem in the mitochondria. The non-haem residue is in the form of ferritin, and some is degraded into haemosiderin. The release of iron requires that transferrin should be attached to a specific site on the surface of developing red cells and to a less extent of other tissues of the body. Such sites are present in reticulocytes as well as in the nucleated erythroid cells, but are not present in mature red cells. Iron bound to proteins other than transferrin goes to the liver and other organs but not specifically to the marrow: large colloidal particles of iron are removed by the reticulo-endo-thelial system. The range of iron concentration in plasma is normally quite wide (0·7–1·8 mg/l); the iron-binding capacity is 2·5–4·0 mg/l, so that trans-ferrin is about one third saturated with iron. Alteration in the amount of transferrin in the plasma and in its percent saturation with iron occurs in various disorders (Fig. 3.3).

3.5.1 NORMAL IRON BALANCE

The mechanism by which the body maintains normal iron balance depends on the interrelationship of absorption, utilization and excretion. Iron is maxi-mally absorbed from the duodenum, less well from the jejunum and only tiny amounts are absorbed from the stomach and ileum. Inorganic iron is better absorbed than food iron and its absorption is favoured by any factor which helps to keep it soluble. The ferrous form is more soluble than the ferric form both in inorganic and organic complexes and low pH hydrochloric and ascorbic acids help to maintain iron in the ferrous form. Low molecular weight substances such as sugars, amino acids and succinates chelate iron; these iron chelates are highly soluble and facilitate attachment of iron to the intestinal mucosa. Some iron passes from the mucosal cell to bind to trans-ferrin in plasma while the remainder is thought to combine with apoferritin in the cell to form ferritin. The mechanism within the mucosal cell which determines the amount of iron transported to plasma is extremely sensitive to the iron requirements of the body. The iron which is absorbed is trans-ported round the body by the plasma and extravascular fluid, and joins the iron stores which have come from the breakdown of red cells at the end of their life span. About 90 per cent of the iron used by the marrow each day derives from the latter source and only 10 per cent is derived from the slow turnover of the storage pool and from absorption from the gut. Indeed, daily requirements of iron in the adult male are low in comparison to body stores, being about 1 mg. About half the normal loss of iron occurs in stools from shedding intestinal cells, bile and iron laden macrophages; a small amount is lost in the urine and by nails, hair and desquamated epithelial cells. In the growing child and in the menstruating female requirements are higher, whilst the highest requirements of all occur in pregnancy where the total daily requirement is 1·5–3·0 mg.

3.5.2 HAEM SYNTHESIS

The synthesis of haem is illustrated in Fig. 3.4. The enzyme ALA-synthetase probably is the major site of control since the amount of this enzyme seems to determine the amount of haem formed. The activity of ALA-synthetase increases in the basophilic normoblast to reach a peak in the polychromatic normoblast, and it then diminishes so that no activity is present in the mature

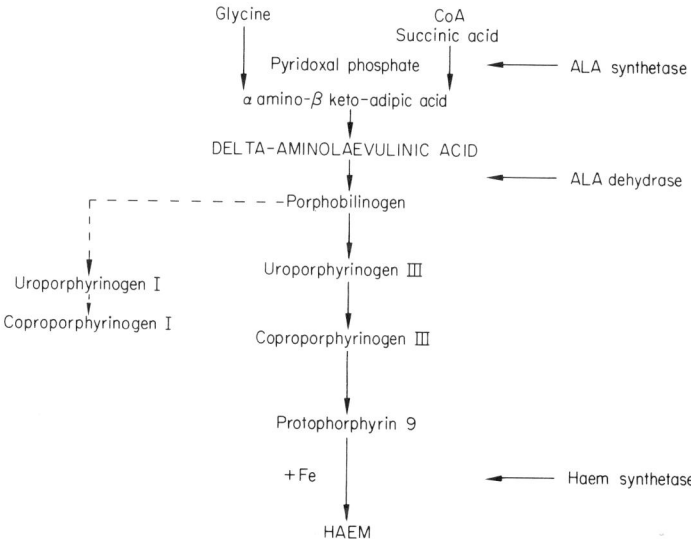

Fig. 3.4 Pathway of haem synthesis.

erythrocyte. ALA-synthetase is activated by low concentration of free organic iron, whereas high concentrations of iron inhibit the enzyme. Haem formation enhances globin formation and lack of haem reduces globin formation.

During haem synthesis several porphyrins are formed as intermediates. The normal red cells contain 40–520 μg/l protoporphyrin and 0–40 μg/l coproporphyrin. Increased amounts of both these products are found in iron deficiency anaemia, lead poisoning, sideroblastic anaemia and the anaemias of chronic infection and malignancy. Normally a small amount of copro-porphyrin is excreted in the urine (100–250 μg/day). It is increased when erythropoiesis is hyperactive as in haemolytic anaemias or when there is dyserythropoiesis as in pernicious anaemia and aplastic anaemia. This qualitative normal but excessive metabolism must be distinguished from a group of disorders associated with abnormal porphyrin metabolism. These are known as the porphyrias, 2 of which are of haematological importance, namely congenital erythropoetic porphyria and erythropoietic protopor-phyria. In the former, uroporphyrin and coproporphyrin are present in red cells and urine in increased amounts; in the latter, increased protoporphyrin is found in the red cells but the urine is normal.

3.5.3 IRON DEFICIENCY ANAEMIA

A state of latent iron deficiency may be present when the stores are depleted and no stainable iron is present in the bone marrow but nevertheless the serum iron may still be normal. With increasing iron deficiency, anaemia develops; the red cells become microcytic and hypochromic (Fig. 3.5) and there is a reduction in MCHC and MCH. In the bone marrow (Fig. 3.6) the

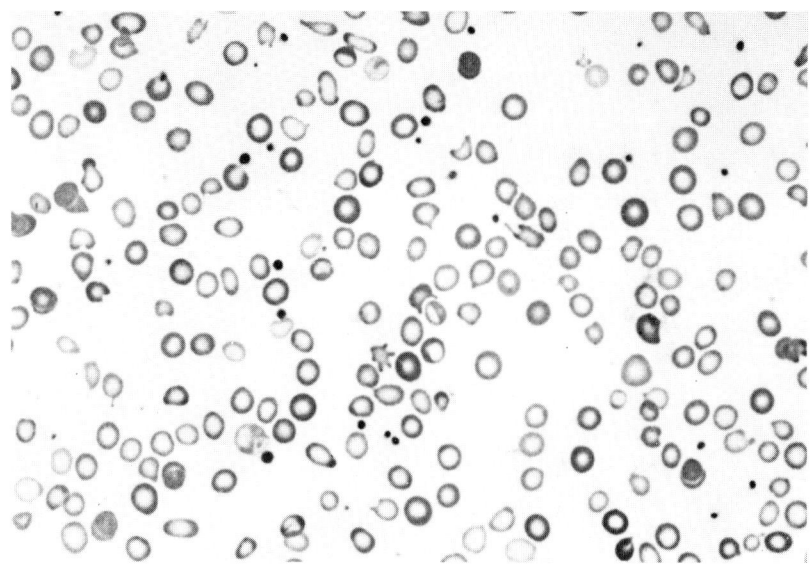

Fig. 3.5 Blood film in iron deficiency anaemia ($\times$ 500).

erythroblasts have a ragged vacuolated cytoplasm, pyknotic nuclei and various signs of dyserythropoiesis (see below). The serum iron concentration is usually low, and values below 0·3 mg/l are not uncommon. The total iron-binding capacity is usually increased and transferrin saturation is 35 per cent (Fig. 3.3). Iron deficiency affects not only the haemopoietic system, but widespread tissue changes also occur, giving rise to some of the clinical manifestations of severe iron deficiency anaemia, namely koilonychia ('spoon nail'), angular stomatitis and gastritis leading to gastric atrophy.

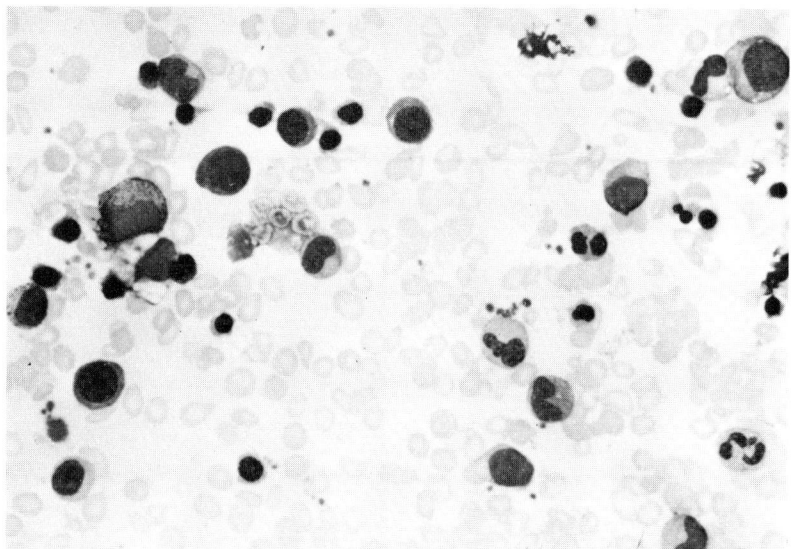

Fig. 3.6 Bone marrow film from patient with severe iron deficiency anaemia (×600).

3.5.4 IRON DEFECTIVE ANAEMIAS

Apart from iron deficiency, certain other conditions may give rise to a block in haem synthesis with the development of a hypochromic anaemia. This is the situation in the sideroblastic anaemias, a group of refractory anaemias in which there are hypochromic cells in the peripheral blood, an excess of iron in the bone marrow, with many of the developing erythroblasts containing iron granules arranged in a ring around the nucleus (ring sideroblast). The latter is the particular diagnostic feature.

Three forms of sideroblastic anaemia are recognized: (1) congenital, (2) primary acquired and (3) secondary.

3.5.4.1   Congenital sideroblastic anaemia

This is a rare disorder occurring mainly in males usually in childhood or adolescence. Inheritance is sex-linked, partly recessive. Patients present with a hypochromic anaemia, reduced MCV and MCHC. The serum iron is usually raised, the total iron binding capacity saturated, Hb-A$_2$ is low and Hb-F is normal.

3.5.4.2   Primary acquired sideroblastic anaemia

This is a disease predominantly of middle-aged and elderly subjects who usually present with symptoms of anaemia. The sexes are affected equally and

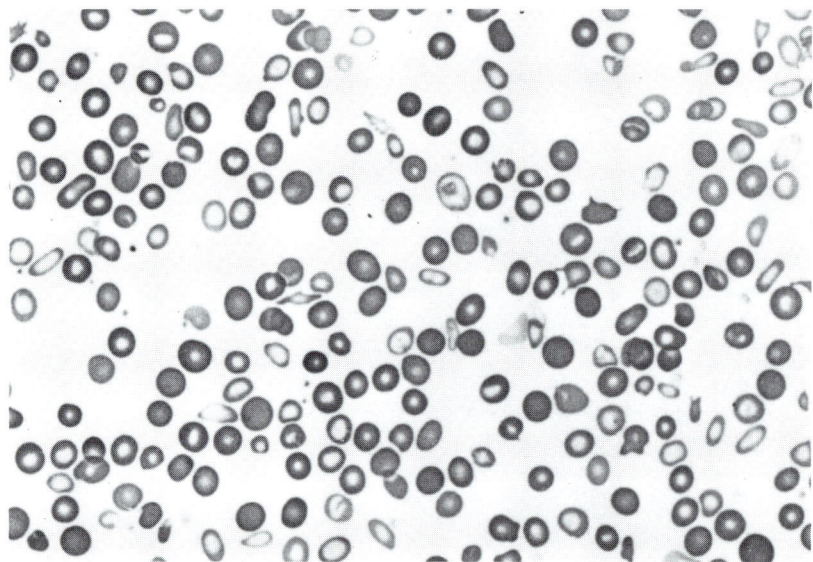

Fig. 3.7   Blood film in sideroblastic anaemia. There is a population of hypo-chromic cells alongside one of normochromic cells ($\times$ 500).

there is no family history. The disease may be present for many years before the diagnosis is made. The peripheral blood film is characteristically dimorphic (Fig. 3.7), and the proportion of hypochromic cells is usually lower than in the inherited disease. The serum iron is usually raised but may be normal. The bone marrow in both the inherited and acquired forms is usually hypercellular; the erythroblasts tend to be microcytic with ragged vacuolated cytoplasm resembling that seen in iron deficiency anaemia, but there are also present the characteristic ring sideroblasts, which are well demonstrated when film is stained for iron (Fig. 3.8).

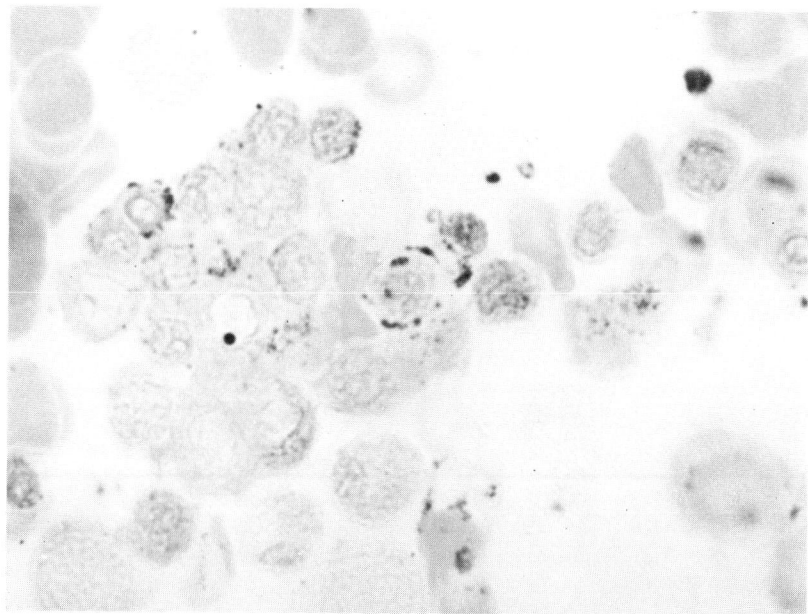

Fig. 3.8 Bone marrow in sideroblastic anaemia, stained by Perls's reaction for iron. Ring sideroblasts are present ($\times$ 1300).

3.5.4.3 Secondary sideroblastic anaemia

Sideroblastic anaemia may be present in patients with myeloid leukaemia, erythroleukaemia and myelomatosis and in myelosclerosis. It has been reported in patients with defective pyridoxine metabolism due to vitamin B_6 deficiency or following the administration of a vitamin B_6 antagonist (e.g. isoniazid, cycloserine, pyrazinamide); other causes include defects of enzymes in the haem pathway leading to a defect in the conversion of pyridoxine to pyridoxal, such as occurs in alcoholism, and in chloramphenicol toxicity. Lead is another common agent known to inhibit enzymes in the haem pathway, acting specifically on the mitochondria.

The haematological changes in lead poisoning are extremely variable. In severe cases, there is usually a moderate degree of anaemia with a slightly elevated reticulocyte count, polychromasia and, characteristically, punctate basophilia. The bone marrow shows erythroid hypoplasia and variable numbers of ring sideroblasts. Children with lead poisoning frequently have an associated iron deficiency but in adults the plasma iron level is often elevated. Red cell protoporphyrins and coproporphyrins are raised as is the urinary excretion of ALA-coproporphyrin 3 and uroporphyrin 1 (Bothwell & Charlton 1970, Hines & Grasso 1970, Dagg *et al* 1971, Goldberg 1971, Jacobs & Worwood 1974, Cartwright & Deiss 1975).

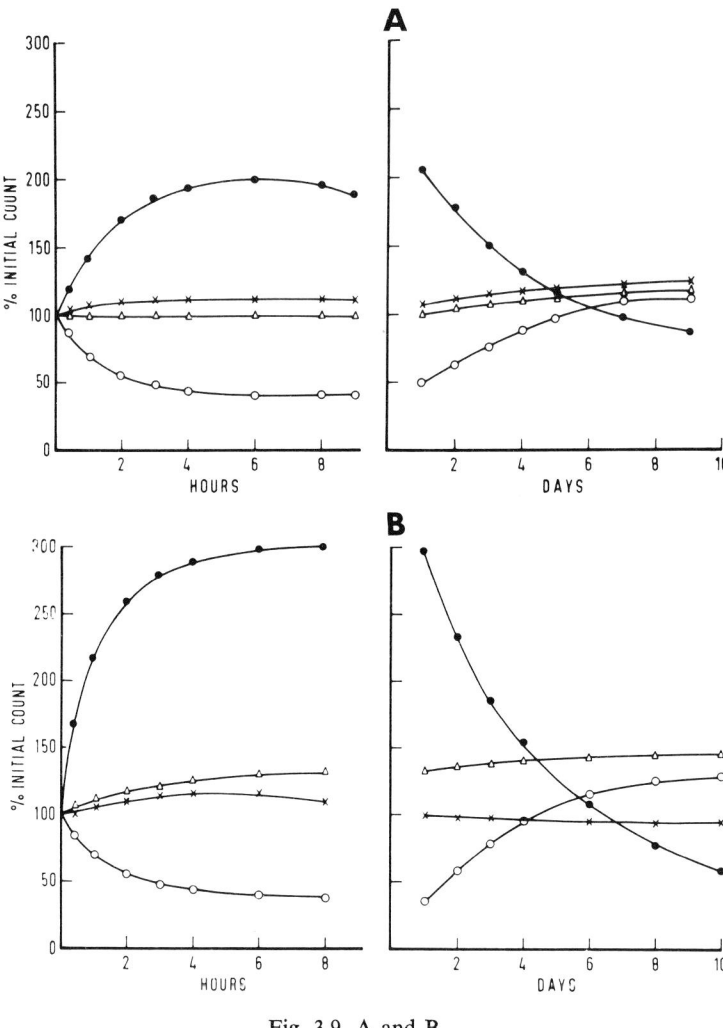

Fig. 3.9, A and B

Fig. 3.9 ^{59}Fe surface counting patterns. Following an intravenous injection of ^{59}Fe, radioactivity is measured over sacrum (●), spleen (△), liver (×) and heart (○). The patterns shown are characteristic of: (A) normal; (B) iron deficiency; (C) myelosclerosis with extramedullary erythropoiesis; (D) aplastic anaemia.

3.5.5 FERROKINETIC MEASUREMENTS

Ferrokinetic studies, usually with ^{59}Fe, enable one to determine the rate and efficiency of haemoglobin synthesis, to identify the site or sites of storage

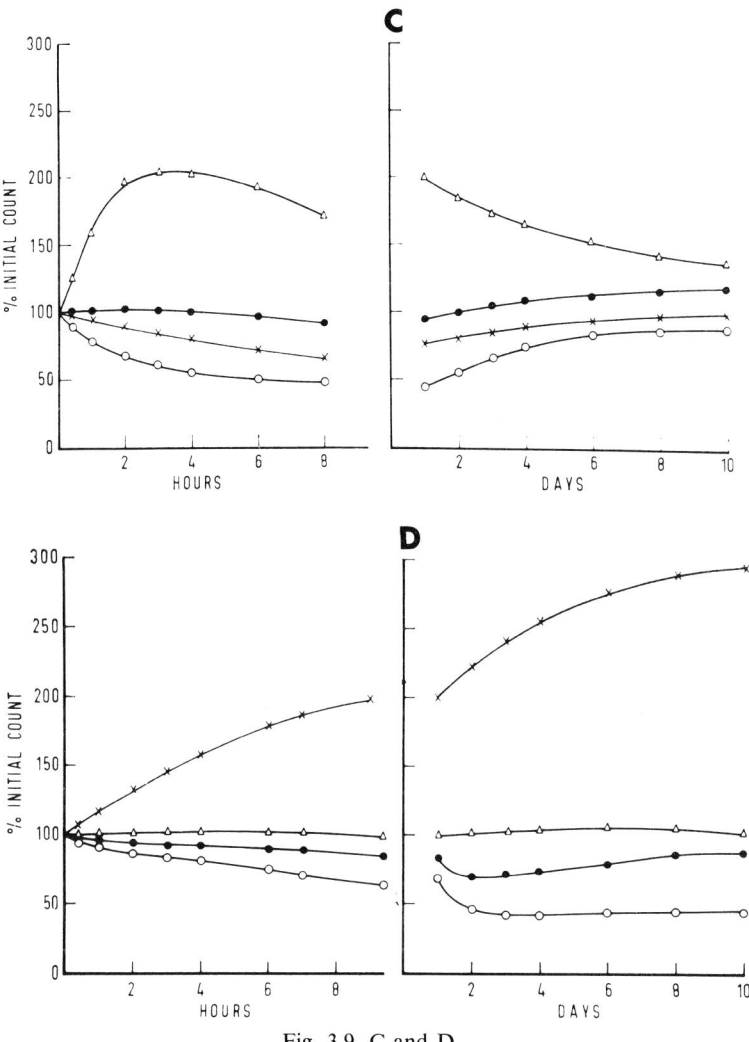

Fig. 3.9, C and D

and/or utilization of the iron, and to demonstrate whether erythropoiesis is taking place within the bone marrow or at extramedullary sites. The studies consist of (a) plasma iron clearance, (b) circulating iron incorporation (sometimes called iron utilization) and (c) surface counting. Plasma iron turnover (PIT) may be derived from iron incorporation and plasma iron concentration; erythrocyte iron turnover (RBCIT) may be derived from PIT and iron incorporation. The normal range of $T_{\frac{1}{2}}$ plasma clearance is 60–140 minutes. The turnover rate is 0·38–0·77 mg/dl of blood per day. The clearance rate is influenced by the intensity of erythropoiesis and also by the activity of the macrophages of the reticulo-endothelial system, especially in the liver, spleen and bone marrow. Rapid clearance occurs in iron deficiency anaemias, haemolytic anaemias, haemorrhagic anaemias and polycythaemia vera. The clearance rate is decreased in aplastic anaemia. Plasma iron turnover is increased in iron deficiency anaemia, haemolytic anaemias and myelosclerosis. It is increased also in ineffective erythropoiesis, particularly so in thalassaemia (Mediterranean anaemia). The appearance of the isotope in circulating erythrocytes is an indication of effective erythropoiesis: normally about 70–80 per cent of the administered iron is thus utilized. A rapid plasma clearance is usually associated with early and relatively complete utilization; this is the state which occurs in iron deficiency anaemia. Conversely, in aplastic anaemia a slow plasma clearance is associated with low utilization. Inconsistent results occur in megaloblastic anaemias and in haemoglobinopathies in which there is a variable degree of ineffective erythropoiesis, and also when there is extramedullary erythropoiesis (as in myelosclerosis) and when there is rapid haemolysis. Erythroid iron turnover provides a measure of effective erythropoiesis but it tends to give an underestimate if there is increased haemolysis.

Surface counting is a technique whereby the administration of ^{59}Fe-labelled transferrin is followed by measurement of the amount of radioactivity over the liver, spleen, heart and bone marrow (usually sacrum) by means of a collimated scintillation counter. This technique is particularly useful in determining the site of iron sequestration and whether there is extramedullary erythropoiesis. Characteristic patterns can be seen in a number of conditions (Fig. 3.9). The extent of erythropoietic activity is perhaps better demonstrable by radioactive screening after administration of ^{52}Fe or ^{99m}Tc, using a scanning couch or a positron scintillation camera (Anger & Van Dyke 1964, Van Dyke *et al* 1967, Finch *et al* 1970, Kniseley 1972, Jacobs & Worwood 1974).

3.6 MEGALOBLASTIC ANAEMIAS

Megaloblastic anaemias are caused by a deficiency of either Vitamin B_{12} or folate, resulting from inadequate intake or malabsorption. The only source of B_{12} available to humans is food of animal origin. A normal Western diet contains 5–13 μg daily; daily loss (mainly in urine and faeces) is 1–3 μg and as the body does not have the ability to degrade Vitamin B_{12}, daily requirements are also about 1–3 μg. Stores are of the order of 2–3 mg, and this is sufficient for three to four years if supplies are completely cut off. There are 2 mechanisms for absorption of vitamin B_{12} in man; the usual process is an active absorption through the ileum, mediated by gastric intrinsic factor. The second mechanism is a passive one through the jejunum and ileum but this is extremely inefficient, and less than 1 per cent of an oral dose of vitamin B_{12} is absorbed in this way. The intrinsic factor (IF) associated with active absorption is a glycoprotein produced in gastric parietal cells in the fundus and body of the stomach. The IF-B_{12} complex passes to the ileum where the vitamin B_{12} is then absorbed. The B_{12} becomes bound to a carrier protein known as a transcobalamin: one type of transcobalamin (TC1) is an α globulin which carries nearly all the vitamin B_{12} normally present and acts as a storage protein. Another form (TC2) serves mainly to carry vitamin B_{12} from one organ to another and it readily gives up its B_{12} to bone marrow and other tissues.

Folic acid (pteroylglutamic acid) is the parent substance of a large family of compounds called 'folates'. These occur in most foods, notably in liver, yeast, nuts and various greens. The total folate content of an average Western diet is about 650 μg daily but folate is easily destroyed by heating, particularly in large volumes of water as in boiling vegetables, and over 90 per cent may be lost by this process. Total body folate in the adult is 5–10 mg, stored predominantly in the liver, and daily requirement is about 100 μg. Up to 13 μg is lost in the urine each day and some is lost by sweat and desquamation. In addition, breakdown products of degraded folate are also lost in the urine. Stores are only sufficient for 4 months in the normal adult and thus severe folate deficiency may develop quite rapidly.

The principal site of folate absorption is the upper small intestine (i.e. duodenum and jejunum) with a falling off in absorption from jejunum to ileum. Absorption occurs by a process of diffusion with saturation; folic acid is more readily absorbed than folates, especially polyglutamate forms which must be hydrolysed to monoglutamates, either in the lumen of the gut or within the mucosa, before entering the portal blood on its way to storage in the liver.

Causes of vitamin B_{12} and folate deficiency are shown in Table 3.1. In man the most important cause of vitamin B_{12} deficiency, at least in Britain, is pernicious anaemia (PA). It is, as a rule, a disease of adults and can be defined as severe lack of intrinsic factor on the basis of atrophic gastritis possibly due to a local genetically determined cell-mediated autoimmune reaction. However, childhood PA does exist, in one of two forms: one type occurs in older children and resembles adult PA being associated with gastric atrophy, achlorhydria and serum intrinsic factor antibody. The second more common type has no demonstrable intrinsic factor but the child has a normal gastric mucosa and a normal secretion of acid.

Deficiency of intrinsic factor and vitamin B_{12} will inevitably follow total gastrectomy. After partial gastrectomy, a proportion of patients also develop deficiency: this usually manifests four years or more following the operation and occurs in about 10–15 per cent of patients. The explanation in these cases

Table 3.1 Causes of megaloblastic anaemia

	Vitamin B_{12} deficiency	Folate deficiency	Other
Nutritional	Vegans	Poor diet Kwashiorkor	Vitamin E deficiency
Malabsorption Gastric	Pernicious anaemia Congenital Acquired Total gastrectomy Partial gastrectomy	Partial gastrectomy	
Intestinal	Crohn's disease Tropical sprue Ileal resection Stagnant-loop syndrome Jejunal diverticulosis Ileo-colic fistula Intestinal stricture Selective malabsorption with proteinuria	Crohn's disease Tropical sprue Coeliac disease Jejunal resection Dermatitis herpetiformis Specific malabsorption	

Excess utilization	Fish tapeworm infestation	Pregnancy Lactation Haemolytic anaemias Erythroleukaemia Malignant disease
Drugs (interfering with absorption)	Colchicine Para-aminosalicylic acid Neomycin Alcohol	Diphenylhydantoin Primidone Cycloserine Barbiturates Alcohol
Drugs (interfering with nucleoprotein synthesis)	Methotrexate	Cytosine arabinoside 5-fluorouracil Hydroxyurea *Also:* Erythroleukaemia Other leukaemias Sideroblastic anaemias

is that the operation results in atrophy of the remaining stomach and possible inhibition of secretion of intrinsic factor by bile. Malabsorption of vitamin B_{12} independent of intrinsic factor may occur following ileal resection especially if more than 4 feet of the terminal ileum is removed. Another cause is colonization of the upper small intestine by faecal organisms. This may occur in patients with jejunal diverticulosis, when there is an anatomical blind loop due to Crohn's disease, or following an operation. The cause of malabsorption is thought to be due to the utilization of dietary vitamin B_{12} by the organisms which probably compete with intrinsic factor for the vitamin.

Nearly all patients with acute and subacute tropical sprue show malabsorption of vitamin B_{12}; this may persist as the principal abnormality in the chronic form of the disease and the patient may present with megaloblastic anaemia or neuropathy due to vitamin B_{12} deficiency.

Diphyllobothrium infestation is another well-known cause of vitamin B_{12} deficiency. This fish tapeworm lives in the small intestine of man, mainly in the ileum, and it accumulates vitamin B_{12} from food, rendering it unavailable for absorption. Expulsion of the worm by therapeutic means causes a spontaneous improvement in both serum vitamin B_{12} level and vitamin B_{12} absorption.

As daily requirement of folate is high relative to stores and to dietary intake, nutritional folate deficiency is common. This is especially the case with people who are liable to take inadequate amounts of folate in their diet for socio-economic reasons, namely the old, edentulous, poor, alcoholics, and also with patients who suffer from anorexia or have dietary fads. Malabsorption occurs in tropical sprue, coeliac disease (sometimes associated with dermatitis herpetiformis) and in a rare congenital condition of selective malabsorption. Minor degrees of malabsorption occur following jejunal resection, partial gastrectomy and in Crohn's disease.

Deficiency of folate consequent on excess utilization occurs, notably, in pregnancy when the daily requirement increases by 100–300 μg because of transfer of the vitamin to the fetus, and also during lactation. Folate deficiency also occurs in chronic haemolytic anaemias, in myelosclerosis where there is considerably increased turnover of nucleic acids, and in various chronic inflammatory conditions, such as tuberculosis, rheumatoid arthritis, psoriasis and chronic bacterial infections, where deficiency is caused both by increased demands and loss of appetite.

3.6.1 CLINICAL FEATURES OF MEGALOBLASTIC ANAEMIAS

The clinical features are those of anaemia together with anorexia and there may be weight loss, diarrhoea or constipation. Other more specific features include glossitis, jaundice of the unconjugated type, and skin pigmentation.

If the platelet count is low, this may lead to bleeding manifestations. Patients with vitamin B_{12} deficiency may also present with neurological disease as well as, or instead of, anaemia. The usual symptoms are parasthesia in the hands or feet, difficulty in walking and, more rarely, in the use of the hands. These symptoms arise because of a peripheral neuropathy associated in some cases with degeneration of the posterior and lateral tracts of the spinal cord, primarily as a result of demyelinization. Visual disturbances occur with retrobulbar neuritis or optic neuropathy. Mental symptoms also occur, although they are usually mild, consisting of forgetfulness, irritability and inertia, but on rare occasions an organic dementia with delirium may occur.

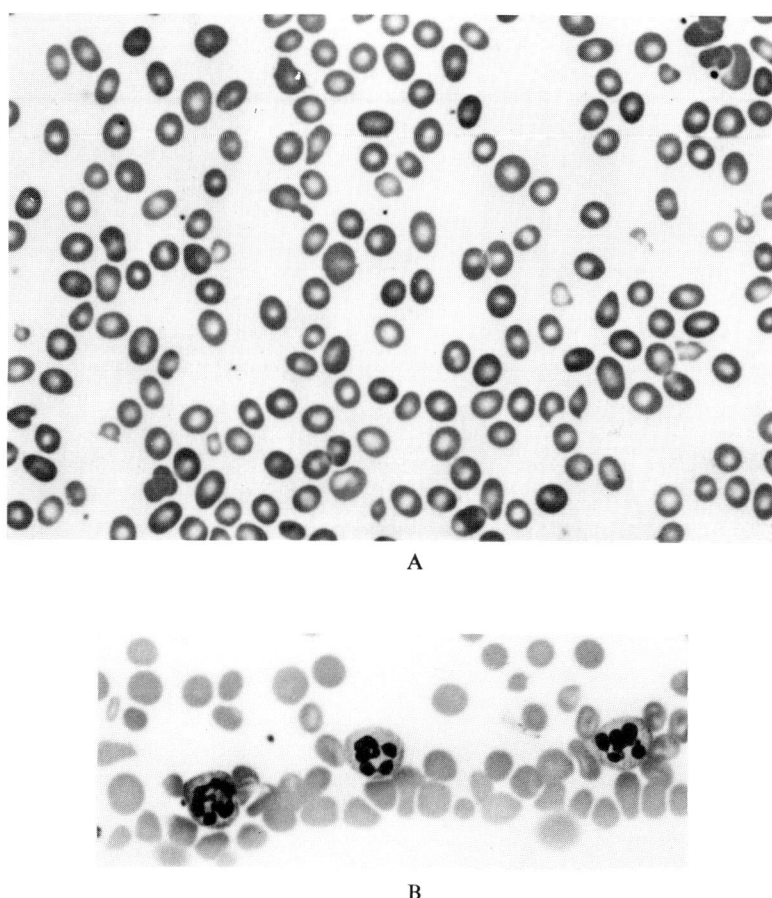

A

B

Fig. 3.10 Blood films from patients with megaloblastic anaemia: (A) characteristic red cell morphology; (B) hypersegmented neutrophil ($\times$ 500).

3.6.2 HAEMATOLOGICAL FEATURES OF MEGALOBLASTIC ANAEMIAS

The diagnostic feature in a peripheral blood film is the presence of oval macrocytes with a considerable degree of anisocytosis and poikilocytosis (Fig. 3.10). MCV is raised: the reticulocytes are usually less than 5 per cent. In severe anaemia nucleated red cells may appear in the blood; they are morphologically abnormal (see below). Neutrophils show hypersegmentation

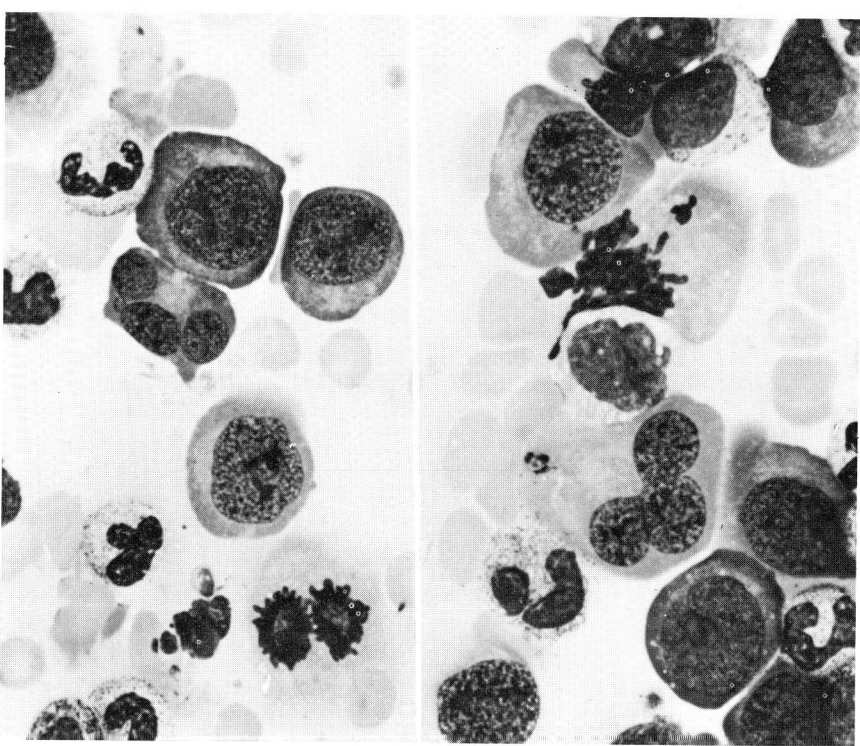

Fig. 3.11   Megaloblasts in bone marrow (× 960).

of the nucleus. The total white cell count tends to fall as a result of reduction of granulocytes and lymphocytes. The platelet count may be moderately reduced although in severe cases it may be as low as $40 \times 10^9/l$ or less. The bone marrow is hypercellular, the myeloid:erythroid ratio is normal or reduced and there is an accumulation of primitive cells as there is selective intra-medullary death of the more mature forms. There is a dissociation between nucleus and cytoplasm in the erythroblasts, and this gives the characteristic morphological features of megaloblasts (Fig. 3.11). The myeloid cells also show dyshaemopoietic changes—giant metamyelocytes and hypersegmented polymorphs.

3.6.3 DIAGNOSIS OF VITAMIN B_{12} OR FOLATE DEFICIENCY

There are 4 main methods used clinically to diagnose vitamin B_{12} deficiency: (1) therapeutic trial, (2) measurement of serum vitamin B_{12} level, (3) methylmalonic acid secretion, (4) absorption studies. Other methods of value which have recently begun to be used include direct measurement of intrinsic factor and intrinsic factor antibodies.

3.6.3.1 Therapeutic trial

This is undertaken by studying the haematological response to a physiological dose of vitamin B_{12} (e.g. 1 μg i.m. daily), an optimal response is shown by reticulocytosis which begins on the 3rd day and reaches a peak on the 6th or 7th day of therapy, while erythropoiesis begins to become normoblastic after 48 hours and leucopoiesis becomes normal by the 12th to 14th day. The haemoglobin should rise by about 1 g/dl per week and the leucocyte and platelet counts should become normal after about 7 days.

3.6.3.2 Serum vitamin B_{12} level

This is measured by means of microbiological assay using *Lactobacillus leichmannii*, *Euglena gracilis* or other suitable test organism. The results vary depending on the method used and other factors which have to be taken into account (see Dacie & Lewis 1975). With the *Euglena gracilis* method, the normal range in humans is 160–925 ng/l. There is also a radio-isotope assay based on competitive protein binding when radioactive B_{12} is added to serum.

3.6.3.3 Methylmalonic acid excretion

This is estimated in urine by a chromatographic method. Urinary excretion is raised in vitamin B_{12} deficiency and normal in folate deficiency.

3.6.3.4 Investigation of vitamin B_{12} absorption

An important step in the study of a patient suffering from B_{12} deficiency is to establish whether or not he has the capacity to absorb the vitamin normally. This is best accomplished with the aid of vitamin B_{12} labelled with an isotope of cobalt, either ^{58}Co or ^{57}Co. The original method was that described by Schilling who measured urinary excretion of an oral dose of radioactive B_{12} followed by a dose given together with intrinsic factor. The normal urinary excretion is greater than 10 per cent of the test dose in the first 24 hours; in patients with pernicious anaemia or with vitamin B_{12} deficiency associated with intestinal malabsorption, excretion is less than 5 per cent. In the latter case excretion will be unaffected by adding intrinsic factor concentrate to the second dose, whereas in pernicious anaemia this manoeuvre will result in normal absorption and excretion. Alternatively, it is possible to calculate the extent of absorption by measuring faecal excretion or plasma radioactivity, by whole body counting or by surface counting in order to identify hepatic uptake.

Folate deficiency may usually be surmised in a patient with megaloblastic haematopoiesis and a normal serum vitamin B_{12} level. It is possible to confirm the diagnosis of folate deficiency by a number of procedures similar to those for vitamin B_{12}.

THERAPEUTIC TRIAL

If the patient has uncomplicated megaloblastic anaemia due to folate deficiency, there will be a satisfactory haematological response to physiological dosage of folic acid (100–200 μg daily). Response to a larger dose is not diagnostic since patients with vitamin B_{12} deficiency may respond haematologically to 400 μg or more of folic acid daily. If malabsorption of folate is suspected, physiological doses of folic acid should be given parenterally for the therapeutic trial. A poor response may be due to an associated deficiency of vitamin B_{12} or iron or to infection. It may also occur in diseases where there is increased folate utilization (e.g. haemolytic anaemia or myelosclerosis) where demands for folate may be as much as 10 times normal.

3.6.3.5 Serum folate assay

Folate activity of serum is due mainly to the presence of a folic acid coenzyme 5-methyltetrafolic acid. Because this compound is microbiologically active for *Lactobacillus casei* but not for *Streptococcus faecalis*, the former organism is used for the assay of naturally occurring folates in serum and red cells. The normal range of serum folate is 6–21 μg/l, and the normal range of red cell folate is 160–640 μg/l.

3.6.3.6 Folic acid absorption

Folic acid absorption may be measured in a way similar to that for vitamin B_{12}. The test can be carried out with non-radioactive folic acid and subsequent measurement of folic acid in serum by microbiological assay (using *Streptococcus faecalis*). Alternatively tritium-labelled folic acid can be administered and absorption determined by the measurement of urinary excretion.

3.6.4 MEGALOBLASTIC ANAEMIA DUE TO FACTORS OTHER THAN B$_{12}$ OR FOLATE DEFICIENCY

Vitamin B$_{12}$ and folate deficiencies are thought to cause megaloblastic anaemia by depriving the marrow of one of the major bases of DNA, namely thymine. Folate deficiency deprives cells of purine and pyriminine precursors whilst B$_{12}$ deficiency acts by disturbing foliate metabolism. Megaloblastic anaemia can also occur if there is a shortage of thymine or one of the other bases of DNA (adenine, guanine or cytosine) irrespective of cause. A block in DNA synthesis resulting in a megaloblastic anaemia may thus occur as a result of drugs such as cytosine arabosine, 5-fluorouracil and hydroxy-urea which inhibit DNA synthesis at various points (Chanarin 1969, Herbert 1970, Hoffbrand 1971, Mollin & Waters 1971, Dacie & Lewis 1975, Hoffbrand 1975).

3.7 MISCELLANEOUS NUTRITIONAL ANAEMIAS

Anaemia occurs as a result of severe protein malnutrition in kwashiorkor, and in the protein–calorie malnutrition state of marasmus. In these conditions, the anaemia is usually normochromic and normocytic; reticulocyte count is normal or low and the marrow is of normal or reduced cellularity. Marrow may, however, be frankly megaloblastic or may show megaloblastic changes in the leucocytes such as giant metamyelocytes and hypersegmented neutrophils. The way in which protein deficiency causes anaemia is uncertain. Lack of protein does not seem to reduce haemoglobin synthesis directly but it is possible that it acts by diminution of erythropoietin secretion.

Other nutrients which are necessary for the integrity of erythropoiesis include ascorbic acid and vitamin E. A number of minerals (in addition to iron) are present in the erythrocyte. These include copper, zinc, manganese and cobalt. However, the possible requirements of the marrow for these elements has been the subject of discussion over a number of years and there is no clear evidence that deficiency of any of these induces anaemia in man.

3.7.1 HORMONES

These have a significant influence in the regulation of erythropoiesis. The most important is erythropoietin; this is a glycoprotein hormone which is produced by the action of a renal erythropoietic factor derived from the mitochondria of the kidney. Increased amounts of erythropoietin are found in hypochromic, megaloblastic, haemolytic and aplastic anaemias; it may also be increased in hypoxia and in renal tumours, and in these situations this leads to the development of polycythaemia. Erythropoietin output is said to be decreased by hypertransfusion, hyperoxia and by a reduction in tissue oxygen requirements. Primarily, erythropoietin is thought to control the rate at which the marrow stem cells give rise to pronormoblasts and to influence the rate of maturation, haemoglobin synthesis and the release of cells from the marrow into circulation. There is some evidence that the microenvironment plays a part; an increased circulation in a part of the skeleton results in increased haematopoiesis in that same part: this is possibly due to the fact that developing erythroblasts require adequate oxygenation for a maximal response and/or that erythropoietin and other factors essential for haematopoiesis might become available only when there is adequate vascularity for their local transport.

An association of sex hormones with regulation of erythropoiesis is suggested by the relationship of haemoglobin to age and sex. Testosterone is known to cause a rise in haemoglobin and androgens have been shown to be beneficial in at least some patients with aplastic anaemia. There appears to be a direct relationship between administration of androgens and increased levels of erythropoietin; this may be due to an action of the androgen on the kidney causing increased erythropoietin production on any given stimulus, or androgen may not only stimulate the production of erythropoietin but also potentiate the action of erythropoietin on stem cells.

Adrenocorticotrophic hormone and corticosteroids, thyrotrophic hormone and thyroxine are also associated with erythropoietic stimulus. This may be by direct effect of increasing erythropoietin production by acting as an intermediary for erythropoietin action or indirectly by reason of the fact that these hormones increase the general metabolism resulting in increased oxygen need. Evidence for the association of hormones with erythropoiesis comes from the fact that anaemia may occur in hypothyroidism, pituitary disease and Addison's disease.

A complex situation occurs in pregnancy. There is an increase in erythropoietic activity, possibly stimulated by lactogenic hormones. However, this is countered by an increase in plasma volume which leads to a haemodilution anaemia (pseudo-anaemia), and also by the frequent occurrence of true anaemia caused by iron and/or folate deficiency (Jepson & Lowenstein 1967, Fisher 1968, Naets & Wittek 1968, Gordon 1970a, Gordon 1971, McClugage *et al* 1971, Sanchez-Medal 1971).

3.8 THE STRUCTURE AND FUNCTION OF HAEMOGLOBIN

The main function of the red cell is to transport oxygen to the tissues and carbon dioxide to the lungs. In order to do so the cell consists largely of haemoglobin and its metabolic pathway has been adapted in order to maintain the function of the haemoglobin molecule. In man the normal adult erythrocyte contains about 30 pg of haemoglobin. The haemoglobin has a molecular weight of 64,000 and the molecule consists of 4 haem groups with two α-polypeptide chains, each of 141 amino acid molecules, and 2 β-polypeptide chains, each with 146 amino acid molecules. Although the synthesis of each globin chain and of haem are ordered by different genes, they occur in a close interaction so that normally there is no excess production of haem or of globin and the chains come to lie symmetrically with α chains on top

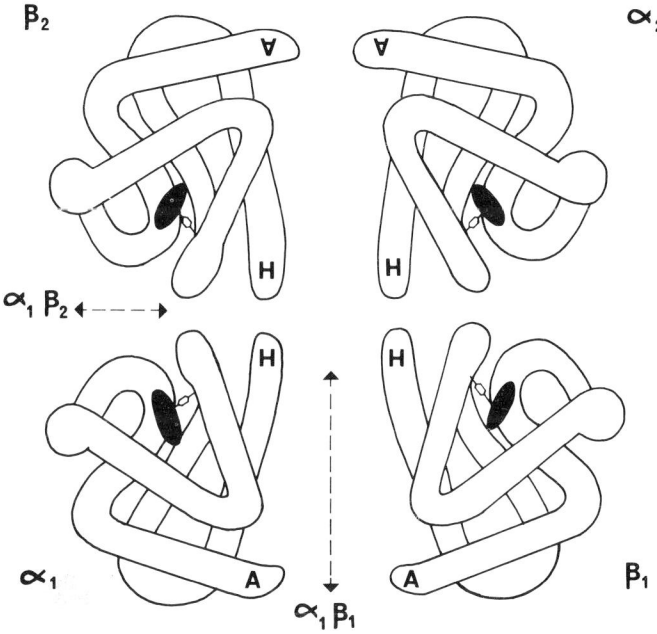

Fig. 3.12 Diagrammatic representation of the relationship between the α and β chains in the haemoglobin tetramer. The α, β, (α₂ β₂) contact is the stabilizing one; the α₁ β₂ (α₂ β₁) is the contact across which the β chains slide during oxygenation and deoxygenation. Reproduced by courtesy of Professor J. M. White.

of a pair of symmetrically placed β chains (Fig. 3.12). When oxygen is bound to the haemoglobin, polypeptide chains pivot on each other in such a way that the space between the β chains is reduced. Conversely, the space is expanded when the oxygenation has taken place, resulting in the respiratory-like movement of the haemoglobin molecule.

It is by its iron (ferrous) component that haemoglobin is an oxygen carrier. In its functional state, a haemoglobin molecule with its four haem molecules can combine with four molecules of oxygen. It is essential that when haemoglobin takes up oxygen it does not itself undergo oxidation in the process. Nearly all the amino acids which form the part of the globin chain to which the iron is attached have non-polar side chains which exclude water molecules from the haem pocket and thus maintain haem iron in the reduced state. Despite this protective pocket some haemoglobin is slowly oxidized to methaemoglobin. In health only about 0·4 per cent of the haemoglobin is so converted to methaemoglobin although in a number of diseases larger amounts of methaemoglobin may be produced by one or other mechanism under which haemoglobin undergoes oxidation or by failure of the metabolic enzyme system which converts methaemoglobin back to functional haemoglobin.

3.8.1   OXYGEN AFFINITY

The relationship between the concentration of the environmental oxygen (the partial pressure of oxygen) and the degree of oxygenation of haemoglobin (its saturation with oxygen) is expressed by the oxygen dissociation curve (Fig. 3.13). The affinity of adult haemoglobin for oxygen is such that, under normal conditions, haemoglobin becomes almost fully saturated with oxygen in the lungs and is able to give up this oxygen readily in the tissues. A decrease in this oxygen affinity prevents the complete oxygenation in the lungs, whereas an increased affinity would make it more difficult for the tissues to obtain their oxygen requirement. Oxygen affinity is influenced by pH changes: carbon dioxide decreases oxygen affinity and thus ensures that in the lungs, where CO_2 is eliminated, oxygen affinity is greater than in the tissues where more ready dissociation is required. Another influence is the presence within the cell of a relatively large amount of 2,3-diphosphoglycerate (2,3-DPG). Reduced haemoglobin readily binds 2,3-DPG and in doing so its molecular configuration is fixed in such a way that there is a lowered affinity for oxygen. Accordingly, an increased amount of haemoglobin within the erythrocyte lowers the level of 2,3-DPG; this stimulates the production of more 2,3-DPG. Thus the presence of an increased amount of reduced haemoglobin leads to increased formation of 2,3-DPG, a lowered oxygen affinity and consequently a more efficient passage of oxygen to the tissues. The level of 2,3-DPG in the cells is of particular importance in adaptation to high altitude and to hypoxia.

Certain amino acid substitutions also have a profound effect on the position of the oxygen dissociation curve. Thus, for instance, in Hb-S the curve is markedly shifted to the right, whereas in Hb Köln the curve is shifted to the left. The oxygen affinity of the molecule must always be taken into account when considering the effect of anaemia in the patient. Thus, for example, a patient with low affinity haemoglobin can exist normally with a haemoglobin value of 8 g/dl because this type can give up far more oxygen than will

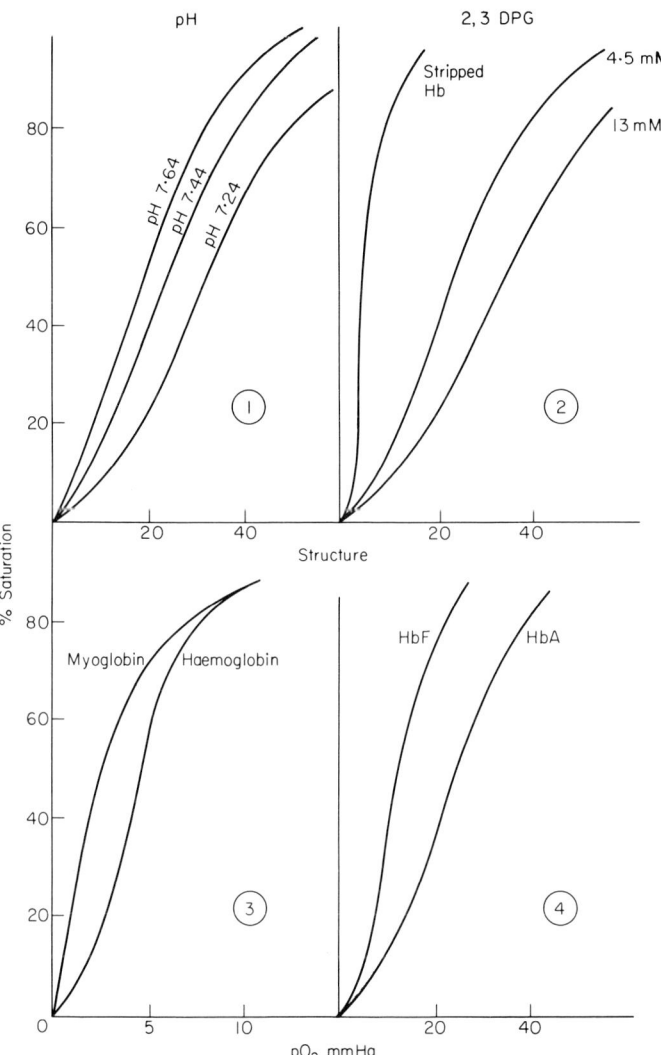

Fig. 3.13 Factors affecting the oxygen affinity and slope of the oxygen dissociation curve:

1. Bohr effect, in which decreasing pH shifts the curve to the right (lower affinity).
2. Effect of 2,3-DPG deficiency ('Slipped Hb') which results in a high oxygen affinity. The curve shifts back towards normal with addition of increasing amounts of 2,3-DPG, and the affinity is normal when the concentration of 2,3-DPG is 13 mM.
3. Comparison between myoglobin (hyperbolic curve) and haemoglobin (sigmoid curve).
4. Comparison between Hb-F and Hb-A. The high affinity of Hb-F is due to its inability to bind 2,3-DPG. Reproduced by courtesy of Professor J. M. White.

Hb-A for the same pO_2. It is of interest also to note that stored blood has a low 2,3-DPG content which is not restored until several hours after transfusion. Thus, transfused blood may be relatively ineffective in its function if it has a high oxygen affinity and does not give up oxygen readily to tissues.

3.8.2 FETAL AND EMBRYONIC HAEMOGLOBINS

There are two polypeptide chains, ε and ζ, that are specific to the embryonic period. They occur in 3 embryonic forms of haemoglobin, Hb Gower 1, Hb Gower 2 and Hb Portland 1, which are found in the human embryo during the first few weeks. By the 10th week of pregnancy they are replaced by Hb-F. This fetal haemoglobin consists of 4 polypeptide chains, 2 α and 2 γ. The α chains are identical to those from Hb-A but the γ chains have a different amino acid sequence than β chains of the adult. Fetal red cells transport oxygen from placenta to fetal tissues and they have a high oxygen affinity which helps in the transport. This higher oxygen affinity is due to a difference in interaction of 2,3-DPG with Hb-F as compared to that with Hb-A which it binds to a greater degree. The proportion of Hb-F in fetal blood reaches a maximum of about 95 per cent of total haemoglobin during the second 3 months of pregnancy and it begins to fall from about the 34th week of pregnancy. In cord blood of full term infants it forms 70–90 per cent of total haemoglobin. Chain synthesis is genetically determined and there are regulator genes responsible for the switch from γ to β chain production at birth. After birth Hb-F continues to fall and has virtually disappeared within 12 months of birth. In hereditary persistence of fetal haemoglobin (HPFH) and in thalassaemia, Hb-F synthesis continues beyond this time and it may reappear to some extent in certain acquired haematological disorders, notably aplastic anaemia, megaloblastic anaemias, erythroleukaemia and other forms of leukaemia. The occurrence of Hb-F in disease can be due either to delayed disappearance of Hb-F or reactivation of γ chain synthesis.

3.8.3 PATHOLOGICAL VARIANTS OF HAEMOGLOBIN

Well over a hundred pathological variants of haemoglobin have been recognized up to the present time. Only a proportion of these result in disease and there are two types of haematological abnormality which are produced by the haemoglobin variants: (a) a haemolytic anaemia due to haemoglobin becoming insoluble and (b) alteration in the function of the molecule as an oxygen transporter. The first of these defects can arise either because of a decrease

Fig. 3.14   Blood film in sickle cell anaemia.
(a) Light microscope ($\times 500$).
(b) Scanning electron microscope ($\times 5000$).

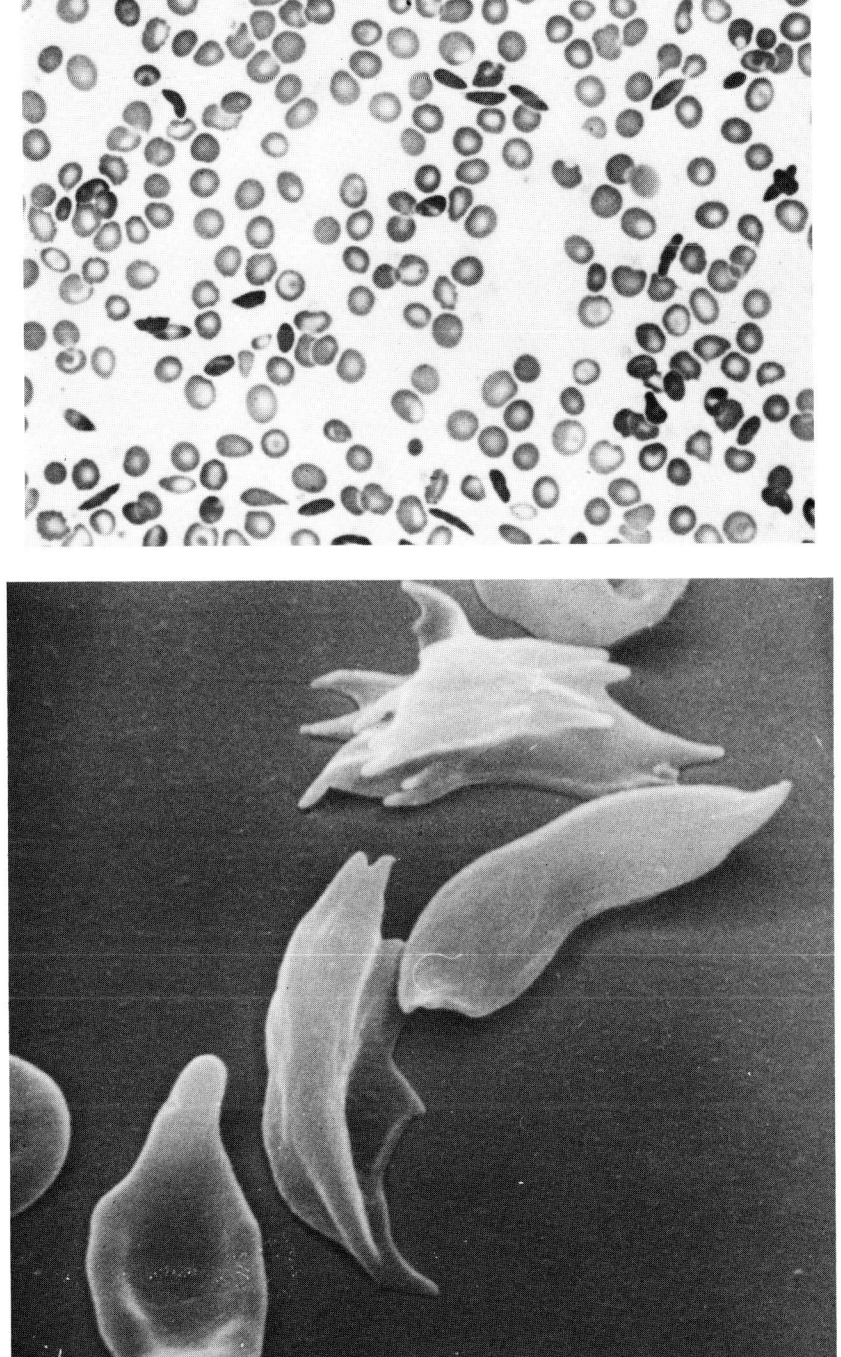

S. M. Lewis

in the solubility of the protein at low oxygen tension (e.g. Hb-S) or because of denaturation of the haemoglobin (unstable haemoglobins). The second defect is due either to the presence of methaemoglobin (Hb-M) or to an alteration in the oxygen affinity as described above.

Structural variants are due to substitution of the externally sited (polar) and of the internally sited (non-polar) amino acids.

3.8.3.1 Hb-S

This is the best known haemoglobin variant which results from substitution of external amino acids. In homozygous sickle cell disease nearly all the red cell haemoglobin is in the form of Hb-S and the balance is largely Hb-F. There is a severe normochromic anaemia with target cells, microcytes and up to 20 per cent are irreversibly sickled in peripheral blood films (Fig. 3.14).

Sickling takes place especially in the small capillaries of the tissues where pO_2 is low and the blood is relatively stagnant. Sickling increases the stagnation, and this leads to a further fall in pO_2 in the tissue and thus further sickling. If the cell is sickled for a short time only, the process is probably reversible, but after prolonged sickling haemoglobin will interact with the cell membrane resulting in the development of a rigid cell—this cell is irreversibly sickled and will be removed from circulation.

Hb-S trait is the heterozygous condition in which the Hb is a mixture of normal Hb-A together with Hb-S. This is a benign disease associated with little anaemia and only a slight reduction in red cell survival. Sickling does not usually occur in vivo, but can be demonstrated *in vitro* by exposing a blood sample to a reducing agent. The trait is potentially harmful during deep anaesthesia, following thrombosis and during air travel.

3.8.3.2 Hb-C

This is another substitution variant which is common in Africa. In the homozygous condition, there is usually moderate anaemia and the blood film shows many target cells (Fig. 3.15). Hb-AC disease is a benign condition in which the blood film shows many target cells but without anaemia. A common combination is that of Hb-SC which results in many if not all the features of Hb-SS disease.

Other external amino acid substitutions result in Hb-D which is found sporadically in several parts of the world and Hb-E which is found in southeast Asia.

3.8.3.3 Variants resulting from substitution of internal amino acids

These variants can be divided into 3 broad groups: Hb-M, altered affinity

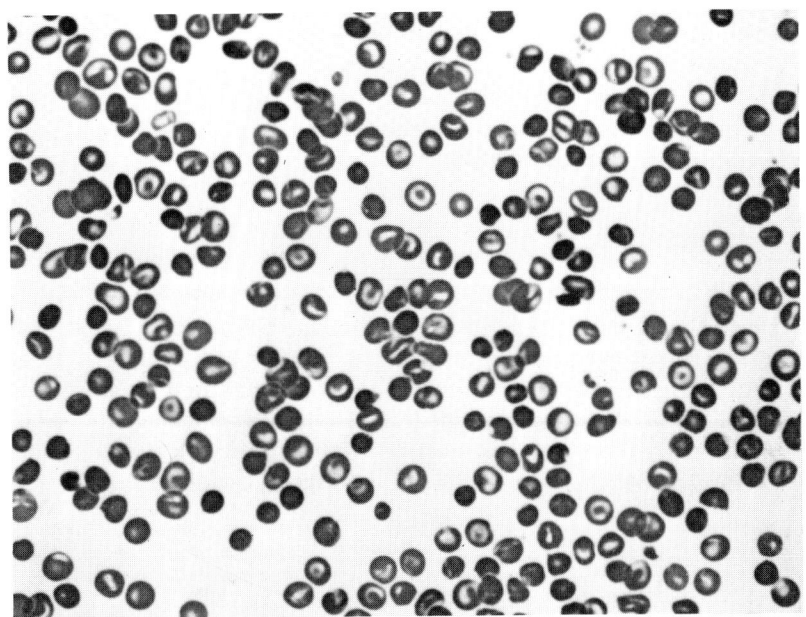

Fig. 3.15   Blood film in Hb-C disease (× 500).

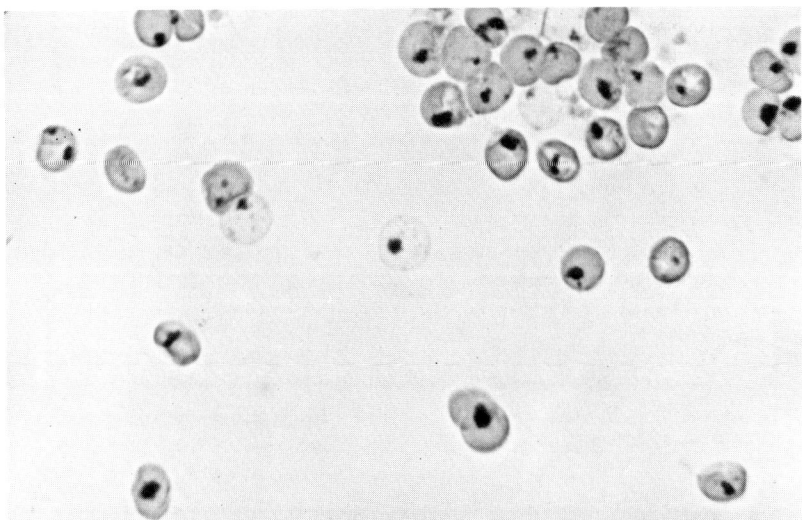

Fig. 3.16   Blood film from unstable haemoglobin (Hb-Köln) after splenectomy.
Stained supravitally with methyl violet to demonstrate Heinz bodies (× 500).

haemoglobins, and unstable haemoglobins. Hb-M variants have been dis-covered in many parts of the world and they have been named appropriately (e.g. Hb Boston, Hb Saskatoon, Hb Hyde Park). They cause methaemo-globinaemia and the patient may become cyanosed. The only other clinical abnormality, as a rule, is development of polycythaemia due to high oxygen affinity of the haemoglobin. It is necessary to distinguish Hb-M anomaly from congenital methaemoglobinaemia and from chronic methaemoglobin-aemia due to intake of oxidant drugs such as phenacetin (see p. 63 and Fig. 3.20). Altered affinity of the haemoglobin molecule occurs as a result of certain substitutions. Some cause high oxygen affinity (e.g. Hb Chesapeake), with tissue hypoxia, and this gives rise to polycythaemia. At least one variant (Hb Kansas) is a low oxygen affinity haemoglobin and this results in cyanosis and anaemia.

The unstable haemoglobins form the largest group of abnormal variants resulting in clinical disease and there are about 30 different types known (including Hb Köln and Hb Hammersmith). All affected patients suffer from a haemolytic anaemia, one form of the so-called congenital non-spherocytic haemolytic anaemias. The peripheral blood will show numerous Heinz bodies after splenectomy (Fig. 3.16) and they can also be generated by in-cubating the blood for 24 hours, or for a shorter time in the presence of a redox dye such as New methylene blue. The specific test for the abnormal haemoglobin is the demonstration that it is heat-precipitable, usually at 50°C.

3.8.3.4   Thalassaemia

Thalassaemia is a disorder which arises because of defective synthesis of one of the pair of globin chains. Two main forms of thalassaemia occur; in β-thalassaemia there is reduced production of β chains and in α-thalassaemia there is reduced synthesis of α chains with consequent production of Hb Barts (γ chains alone) or Hb H (β_4). β-thalassaemia occurs in a homozygous or heterozygous state with varying degrees of anaemia. There is defective haemo-globinization of the red cells and intracellular precipitation of the α chains which are synthesized in excess. This gives rise to the characteristic appear-ances of the blood film (Fig. 3.17) and to haemolysis. At its mildest, there may be only minimal anaemia and no outward physical findings. Indeed, this condition of thalassaemia minor may be missed for many years and will only be identified if, for some reason, a blood film is examined, as this will reveal the characteristic features of a mild hypochromic anaemia with target cells and basophilic stippling.

Thalassaemia major results from the homozygous state of the β-thalas-saemia gene. The disease is usually extremely serious and death frequently occurs in childhood. Anaemia is usually severe; the blood film shows a marked hypochromic anaemia with many target cells and some normoblasts; the bone marrow shows the morphological features of ineffective haemoglobin-ization and dyserythropoiesis. One characteristic feature is the presence in haemoglobin defective erythroblasts of pale blue inclusion bodies which are free α chains. As mentioned above, Hb-F persists in thalassaemia. In the homozygote it may well be present to as much as 60–100 per cent, and it will be accompanied by Hb-A$_2$ without any normal Hb-A. In the heterozygote, however, Hb-F may be normal or only slightly increased although Hb-A$_2$ will usually be increased.

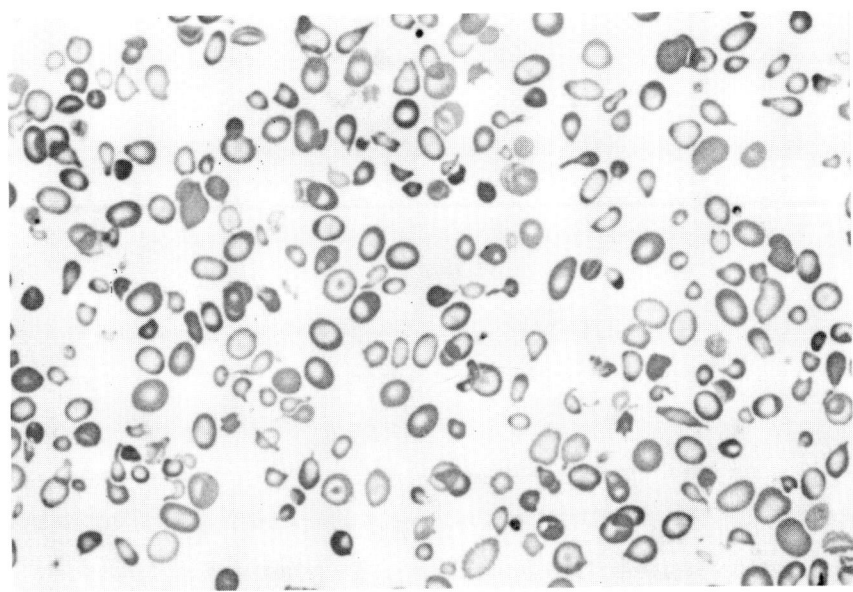

Fig. 3.17   Blood film in severe thalassaemia ($\times$ 500).

Thalassaemia is predominantly a disease of the Mediterranean area with high frequency in Italy and Greece but extending also to the Middle East and to India and the Far East.

α-Thalassaemia is a much less common disorder, without a specific geographic distribution. There are 2 types of α-thalassaemia genes, and the interaction between them results in the clinical syndromes which vary in severity and expression. The severe form of the homozygous state results in hydrops foetalis with fetal death usually by the 32nd week. The hetero-zygous state is either asymptomatic and harmless or clinically mild (Weatherall 1969, Huehns 1970, White & Dacie 1971, Weatherall & Clegg 1972, Forget 1974, Lehmann & Huntsman 1974, Ranney 1974).

S. M. Lewis

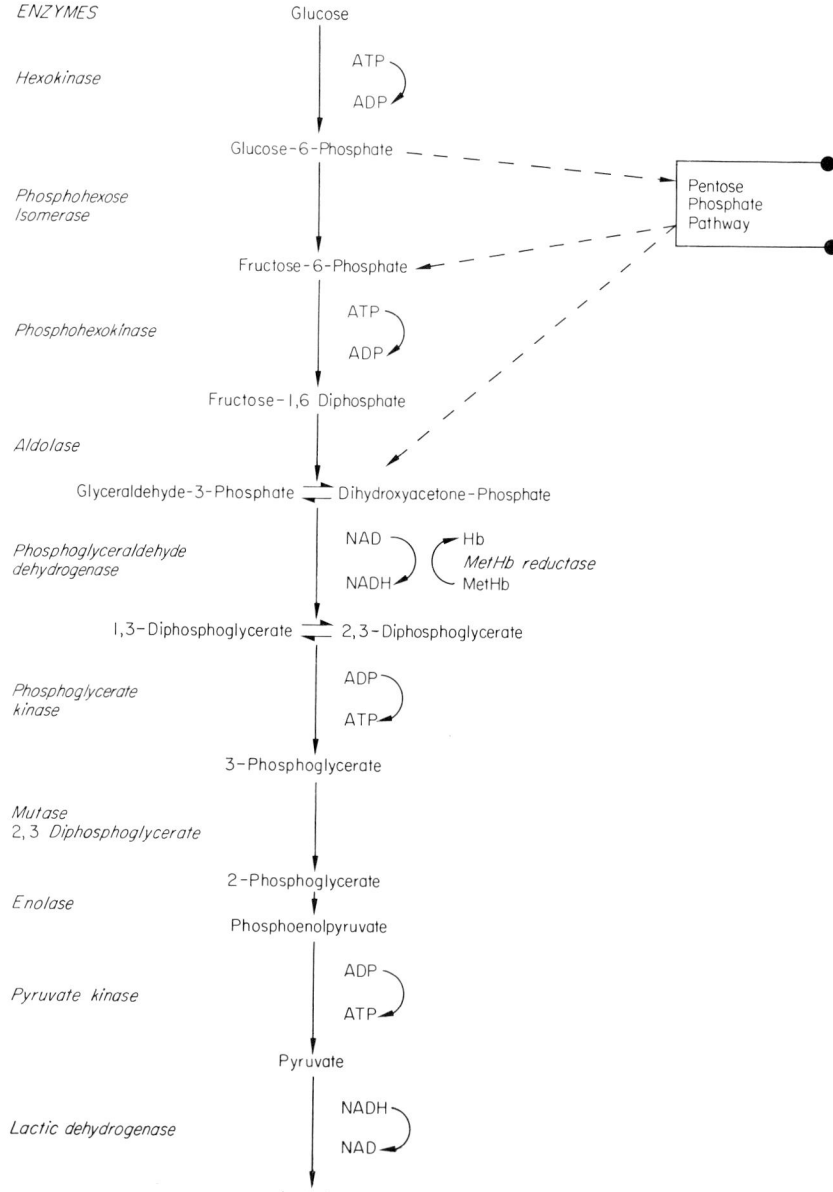

Fig. 3.18 The Embden-Meyerhof anaerobic pathway of glycolysis: ATP = adenosine triphosphate; ADP = adenosine diphosphate; NAD = oxidized nicotinamide-adenine-dinucleotide; NADH = reduced nicotinamide-adenine-dinucleotide.

3.9 RED CELL METABOLISM

Because the erythrocyte has no nucleus, it exists at a lower level of metabolism than any other body cell. It cannot synthesize proteins or lipids and as it has no mitochondrial apparatus for oxidative metabolism it relies on the surrounding medium of its environment for maintaining its metabolic integrity. The erythrocyte does not use the oxygen which it carries in its haemoglobin for production of the energy that is required for its maintenance. Instead, its energy is derived from the anaerobic breakdown of glucose to pyruvate and

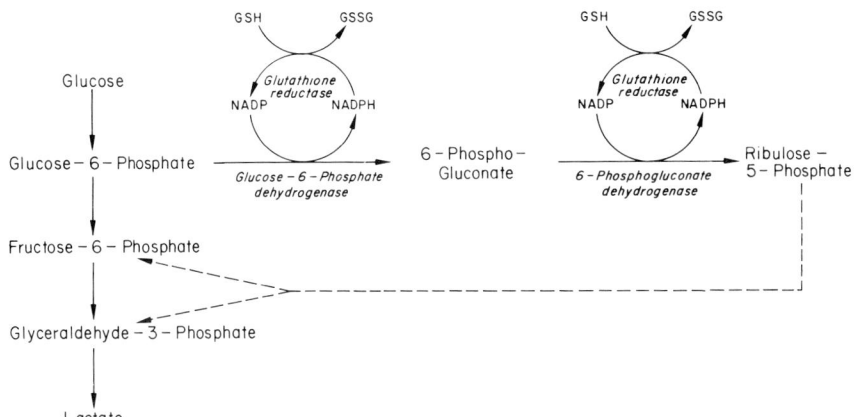

Fig. 3.19 The pentose phosphate aerobic pathway of glycolysis: GSH = reduced glutathione; GSSG = oxidized glutathione; NADP = oxidized nicotinamide-adenine-dinucleotide phosphate; NADPH = reduced nicotinamide-adenine-dinucleotide phosphate

lactate by the Emden-Meyerhof pathway of glycolysis (Fig. 3.18). In this cycle each mole of glucose yields 2 moles of adenosine triphosphate (ATP). This is the source of energy responsible for preserving the cell's biconcave shape, for maintaining the membrane lipids and for running the metabolic pump which controls sodium and potassium flux and thus the osmotic integrity of the cell. ATP production is lowered in certain congenital lesions of glycolysis; when this occurs there is a markedly reduced survival of the erythrocytes.

Whilst the Emden-Meyerhof pathway with its ATP production is the factor responsible for the preservation of the integrity of the cell itself, there is also need for a process to ensure the integrity of function of its haemoglobin. This is achieved by another glycolytic pathway, the pentose phosphate or phosphogluconic shunt (Fig. 3.19); this is an oxidative process in which haemoglobin is protected against oxidation by the oxidative process being

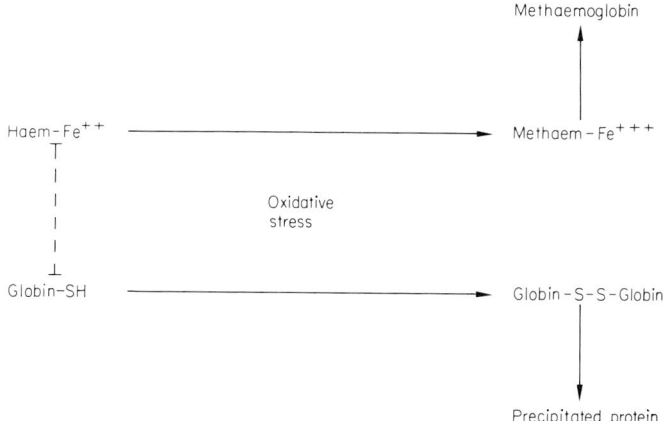

Fig. 3.20 The effects of oxidation of haemoglobin resulting from defect in reduction mechanism.

Table 3.2 Hereditary defects in red cell metabolism

A. *Disorders of membrane function*
    Hereditary spherocytosis
    Hereditary elliptocytosis
    Acanthocytosis
    Congenital pyknocytosis

B. *Disorders of energy production and utilization*
    Deficiency of glycolytic enzymes
        Pyruvate kinase
        Hexokinase
        Triosephosphate isomerase
        Diphosphoglycerate mutase
        Phosphoglycerate kinase
        Phosphoglucose isomerase
    Deficiency of ATPase

C. *Disorders of oxido-reduction system*
    Glutathione reduction
        Deficiency of glucose-6-phosphate dehydrogenase
        glutathione reductase
        glutathione synthetase
        glutathione peroxidase
        6-phosphogluconate dehydrogenase
    Methaemoglobin reduction
        Deficiency of methaemoglobin reductase
    Extrinsic
        Deficiency of vitamin E

used for the production of reduced glutathione (GSH) from oxidized glutathione (GSSG) in a reaction that is catalysed by the enzyme glutathione
reductase. This pathway plays a relatively small part in glycolysis but it
becomes increasingly active when there is an increased need for reducing
potential within the cells, as for example, when the cell is challenged by an
oxidant drug. When an enzyme of the oxidative pathway is deficient or defective the reduction mechanism may be inadequate to cope with the excess
stress of such a drug challenge and haemoglobin will then become oxidized
(Fig. 3.20). This results in the production of methaemoglobin and in precipitation of globin into Heinz bodies which then attach themselves as large aggregates to the inner part of the cell membrane and lead to lysis of the cell.

Disorders of red cell metabolism occur as a result of disorders of membrane function, disorders of energy production and utilization and disorders
of the oxido-reduction system. The main clinically important red cell defects
which result from these disorders are illustrated in Table 3.2. Some of these
are described below.

3.9.1 HEREDITARY SPHEROCYTOSIS

This familial disorder is characterized by the presence of microspherocytes
in the peripheral blood (Fig. 3.21), a shortened red cell life span and splenomegaly. The spleen plays an essential role in the pathogenesis of haemolysis

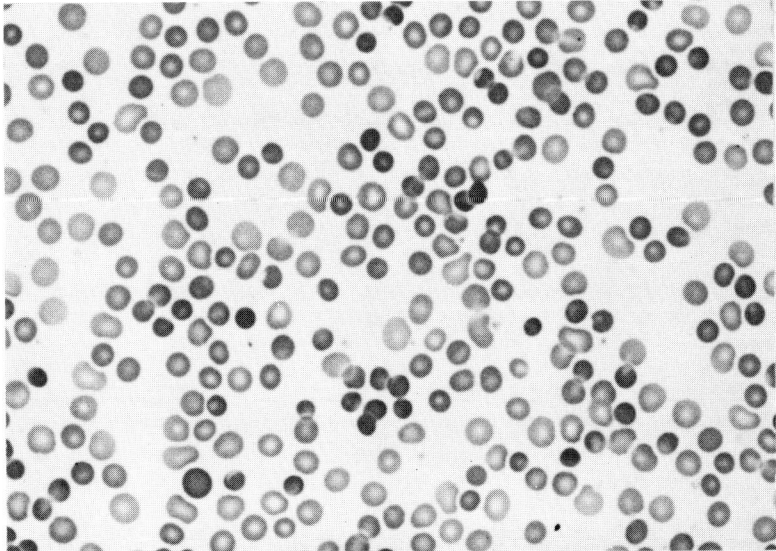

Fig. 3.21 Blood films from patient with hereditary spherocytosis showing microspherocytes (× 500).

S. M. Lewis

in this disease and splenectomy cures the haemolysis. This is because HS cells are trapped in the splenic cords, probably because they are unable to deform easily for passage from the cord to the splenic sinus. While thus trapped the cells are subjected to unfavourable metabolic conditions of glucose lack and acidosis, both of which decrease the production of energy in the form of ATP. Possibly as a result of both these effects of splenic trapping, the HS cell loses part of its membrane by phagocytosis during the passage through the spleen and so develops a smaller surface area to volume ratio, and becomes micro-spherocytic. The more spherocytic the cell becomes, the less is it able to de-form and the longer is it trapped in the spleen, until eventually the whole cell is engulfed by splenic macrophages and destroyed.

3.9.2 HEREDITARY ELLIPTOCYTOSIS

The trait for this condition is not uncommon, but the majority of patients have no abnormal symptoms or signs, or at most only a mild anaemia. By

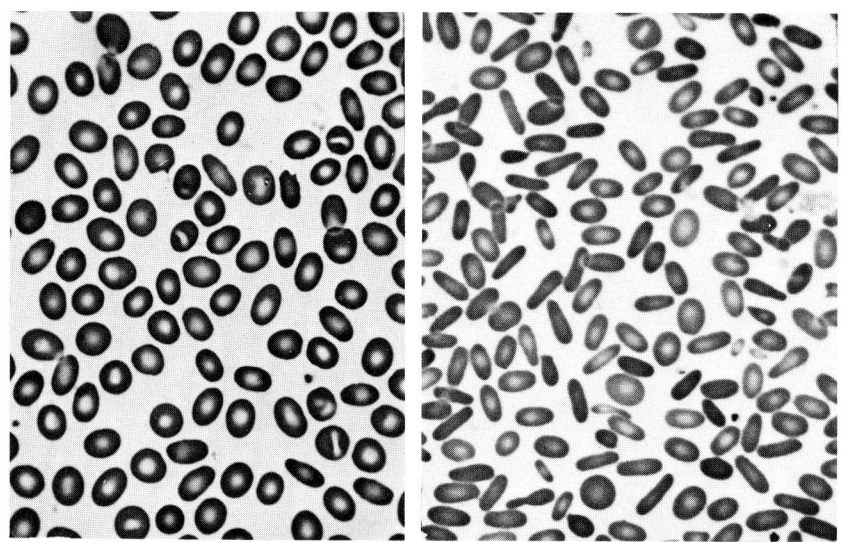

Fig. 3.22   Blood films showing various grades of elliptocytosis (× 600).

contrast, in the less common homozygous state patients have marked haemo-lysis and sometimes severe anaemia. The shape of the red cell varies from long rod-shaped cells to slightly oval ones (Fig. 3.22). As with hereditary sphero-cytosis, splenectomy will cure the haemolysis in hereditary elliptocytosis.

3.9.3 PYRUVATE KINASE DEFICIENCY

This is one of the commonest inborn errors of red cell metabolism. It is an important member of the group of conditions previously referred to as congenital non-spherocytic haemolytic anaemias. Pyruvate kinase catalyses the conversion of phosphoenopyruvate to pyruvate in the penultimate step of the glycolytic pathway. Deficiency or functional defect of PK has a marked effect on the overall glycolytic rate, on ATP production and on the level of metabolic intermediates. PK deficient cells are destroyed throughout the reticulo-endothelial system and not preferentially in the spleen. Clinically there is considerable variation in presentation, severity and response to treatment. There are no characteristic features in the blood film and there are no spherocytes, but there is a tendency for macrocytosis, and a high reticulocyte count. Osmotic fragility and incubation autohaemolysis are abnormal but results vary and specific diagnosis is, of course, made by PK assay.

3.9.4 GLUCOSE-6-PHOSPHATE DEHYDROGENASE (G-6-PD) DEFICIENCY

This is one of the most common genetically determined metabolic defects of the red cell. It came first to attention as the cause of pamaquine and primaquine-induced haemolysis in sensitive subjects and it was established that the sensitivity was familial and affected about 10 per cent of Negroes. There are four ways in which G-6-PD deficiency may present: (a) acute drug-induced haemolysis, (b) favism, (c) chronic haemolytic anaemia and (d) neonatal jaundice. Active drug-induced haemolysis occurs typically 3 days after taking the drug. Severity of haemolysis depends on the type of G-6-PD deficiency present, the dosage of the drug and the duration of its administration. The drugs which may cause haemolysis include antimalarials, sulphonamides and sulphones, analgesics, antihelminthics and a wide range of antibacterial substances. Acute infections, both bacterial and viral, may also cause haemolysis in susceptible patients.

Sensitivity of the blood to the broad bean, *Viscia fava,* has been recognized as a cause of drug-induced haemolytic anaemia for a long time. Attacks do not, however, occur on every contact with the fava bean and it is not clear what triggers off the reaction on any one occasion. Patients with favism are also sensitive to infections and to the oxidizing drugs which may induce an acute episode of haemolysis. A number of cases of chronic haemolytic anaemia have been described which result from G-6-PD deficiency and which do not require a specific drug action to induce haemolysis. They have in the past been included in the congenital non-spherocytic haemolytic anaemias (Dacie 1960, Beutler 1968, Yunis 1969, Brain 1971, Valentine 1971, Valentine 1972, Gordon-Smith & White 1974, Surgenor 1974, Prankerd & Bellingham 1975).

3.10 ACQUIRED HAEMOLYTIC ANAEMIAS

The acquired haemolytic anaemias fall into two main groups: (1) immune haemolysis in which antibodies and/or complement play a major role in the pathogenesis of red cell destruction or where there is an immune drug-induced haemolysis and (2) physical haemolysis which occurs as a result of fragmentation or chemical damage to the red cells.

The diagnosis of an autoimmune haemolytic anaemia depends primarily upon the demonstration of autoantibodies adsorbed to the patient's red cells. The autoantibodies are of two kinds: *warm antibodies* are associated with the appropriate antigen more quickly at 37°C than at lower temperatures whereas *cold antibodies* do not associate with the appropriate antibody at 37°C although they do so readily at temperatures below 30°C. The commonest type of warm auto-antibody which gives rise to an autoimmune haemolytic (AIHA) is an IgG globulin. Warm antibodies behave in vitro very similarly to Rh antibodies and, indeed, often seem to have Rh specificity. The commonest type of cold auto-antibody is an IgM antibody which agglutinates normal red cells to high titre at 4°C, and leads to the clinical syndrome of cold haemagglutinin disease (CHAD). Characteristically, the titre falls off markedly as the temperature rises.

Auto-immune haemolytic anaemias (AIHA) of the warm type can run an acute or a chronic course. The commonest physical findings are a slight to moderate splenomegaly often accompanied by some degree of hepatomegaly. Jaundice is always present if red cell destruction is rapid and it is accentuated if liver function is impaired. Although all patients with AIHA have haemolysis, sometimes the haemolysis is well compensated and there is little or no anaemia. When anaemia is severe there is often a very high reticulocyte count and a variable degree of spherocytosis which correlates to some extent with the severity of haemolysis. Warm type AIHA may be idiopathic or may occur in association with various other disorders, especially lymphoma, systemic lupus erythematosus and other auto-immune diseases.

The cold haemagglutinin disease (CHAD) may also be idiopathic or associated with well-defined disorders, especially lymphoma, reticulum cell sarcoma, and various infections, particularly atypical pneumonia due to Mycoplasma pneumoniae and, very occasionally, infectious mononucleosis. Chronic CHAD is a disorder of elderly people who present with a gradually developing anaemia which is much worse in cold weather. In addition to the anaemia and jaundice, these patients present, characteristically with Raynaud's phenomenon (pallor of the extremities) and haemoglobinuria. The appearance of the peripheral blood is characteristic. If the specimen is put in a refrigerator or if the room temperature is cold, agglutination occurs and the red cells may become a single mass. The films are difficult to spread and microscopically are seen to be grossly agglutinated (Fig. 3.23). However, if the

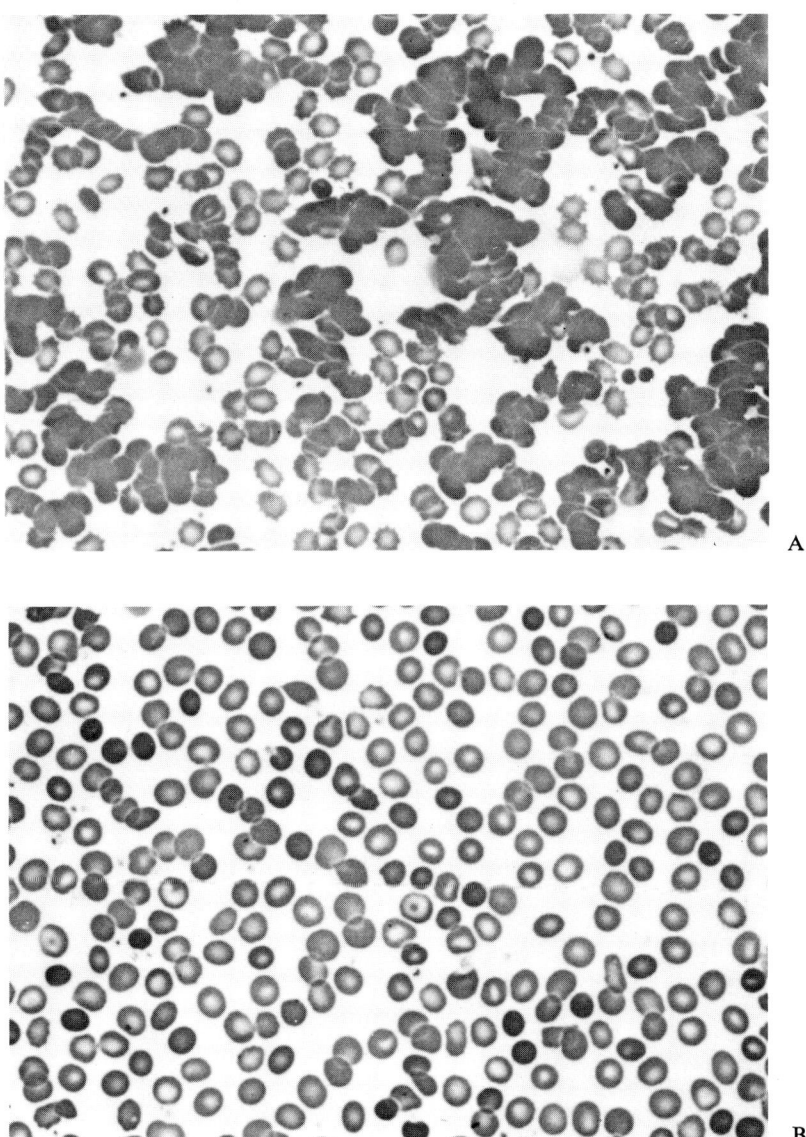

Fig. 3.23 Blood films from case of cold haemagglutinin disease: (A) Prepared at room temperature; (B) prepared at 37°C (× 500).

specimen is warmed to 37°C and blood films made on slides heated to this temperature, the auto-agglutination will generally disappear.

3.10.1 DRUG-INDUCED HAEMOLYTIC ANAEMIAS

These may be due to metabolic injury (see p. 63 and 65) or an immune reaction. The latter occur in 2 forms: (1) drug-induced immune haemolytic anaemias in which the patient's serum does not react with normal red cells unless the offending drug is also present and (2) drug-induced auto-immune haemolytic anaemias in which the drug provokes the development of auto-antibodies very similar to those seen in warm AIHA, and thereafter the reaction proceeds even without the presence of the drug. A wide range of drugs have been reported to lead to auto-immune haemolytic anaemia. These include, notably, phenacetin, sulphonamides, penicillin and some cephalosporins, PAS, quinine and quinidine.

3.10.2 PHYSICAL HAEMOLYTIC ANAEMIA

Under a number of conditions red cells may become chemically damaged in circulation and this leads to fragmentation, with helmet cells, burr cells, schistocytes, and microspherocytes (Fig. 3.24). The most common causes of this phenomenon are shown in Table 3.3. It should be emphasized that the

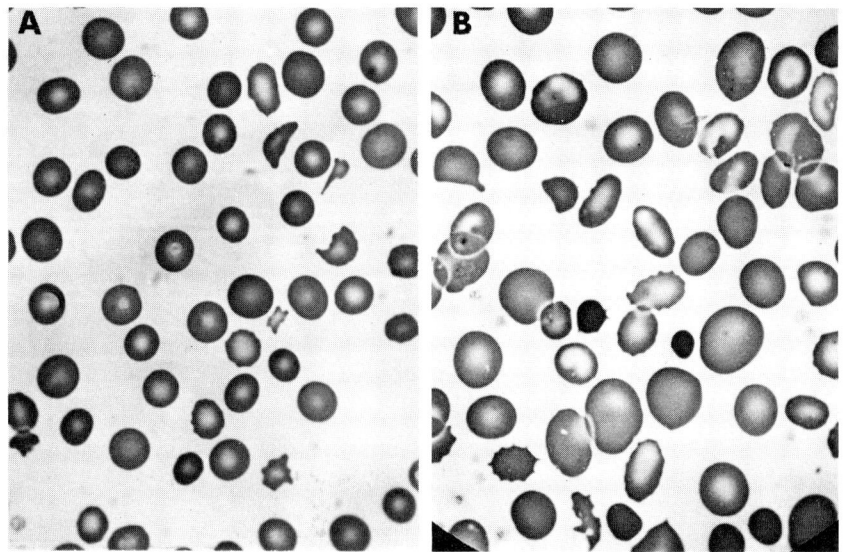

Fig. 3.24 Blood films from: (A) Cardiac haemolytic anaemia and (B) microangiopathic haemolytic anaemia (× 700).

pathogenesis is different in the different conditions. Thus, in cardiac haemolytic anaemia red cell fragmentation is due to direct damage as a result of shearing stress when a jet of blood impinges on the plastic surface of a valve replacement. By contrast, microangiopathic haemolytic anaemia is characteristically associated with widespread or localized damage to small vessels, with fibrin deposition, and it has been postulated that red cell damage occurs as a result of the blood flow through the fibrin mesh, with the red cells striking individual fibrin strands and undergoing mechanical fragmentation. Another condition, exertional haemoglobinuria, is confined almost entirely to young men who typically give a history of running or marching of some duration on hard surfaces, often without previous training. Immediately afterwards they void red urine which contains large amounts of haemoglobin, the soles

Table 3.3   Causes of physical (mechanical) haemolytic anaemia

Cardiac haemolytic anaemias
Exertional ('March') haemoglobinuria
Microangiopathic haemolytic anaemias
   Haemolytic uraemic syndrome
   Thrombotic thrombocytopenic purpura
   Malignant hypertension
   Polyarteritis nodosa
   Glomerular nephritis
   Antepartum haemorrhage
   Pre-eclampsia
   Septicaemias
   Carcinomas (especially mucin-secreting adenocarcinoma)
   Homograft rejection

of their feet feel hot and painful, and they experience nausea, abdominal pain and aching back and legs. The haemoglobinuria rapidly diminishes on subsequent passage of urine. The defect has been explained in simple mechanical terms to be due to stamping of the feet and it does not appear to be due to an intrinsic defect in the patient's red cells or capillary bed. Running on soft surfaces or wearing shock-absorbent footwear greatly reduces the in vitro haemolysis.

Whereas cardiac haemolytic anaemia and exertional haemoglobinuria have clear-cut aetiological factors and are easily recognizable, microangiopathic haemolytic anaemia may arise from a wide range of clinical associations. These include obstetric defibrination after abruptio placentae or amniotic fluid embolism, disseminated intravascular coagulation associated with septicaemias, malignant hypertension, the haemolytic uraemic syndrome in children, and thrombotic thrombocytopenic purpura. Microangiopathic haemolytic anaemia also occurs in association with mucin-forming adenocarcinomas (Dacie 1962, Dacie & Worlledge 1969, Marsh & Lewis 1969, Brain 1970, Worlledge 1973 Prankerd & Bellingham 1975, Swisher 1976).

3.10.3 ESTIMATION OF LIFE SPAN OF RED CELLS

This is a relatively laborious investigation; it is not as a rule included in the first order of investigations on a patient suspected of suffering from a haemolytic anaemia, but it provides the definitive information as to whether or not a patient has a haemolytic process (with or without anaemia) as well as being used to demonstrate whether the spleen is a predominant site of red cell destruction. Measurement of the mean red cell life is particularly useful in order to distinguish between anaemia due to failure of the marrow to respond normally and anaemia which occurs because of an excessive demand.

Several methods have been described for red cell survival studies. The most commonly used method today is by random labelling of circulating red cells with ^{51}Cr. The disadvantages of this method are that there may be an early loss of label over the first 1 to 3 days, and chromium elutes from circulating red cells. It is, however, possible largely to avoid the former error and correct for the latter error provided that a standardized method is used and meticulous attention is paid to technical detail. Mean red cell life span in health has generally been reported to be 100–120 days. Recent work has, however, suggested that the range is wider with a mean of 110 days and SD of 20 days.

When survival data are plotted on arithmetic or logarithmic graph paper, it is possible to obtain useful information from the actual pattern of the curve. Theoretically, normal red cell distribution is selectively determined by the age of the cells; and the cells are lost to circulation only at the end of their life span. This results in a survival curve, the slope of which is arithmetically linear. A similar pattern, more or less, occurs in hereditary haemolytic anaemias. On the other hand, in the auto-immune haemolytic anaemias red cell destruction is typically random, so that the curve of elimination is exponential and it will produce a straight line slope on semilogarithmic graph paper. In some cases of haemolytic anaemia the survival curve appears to consist of 2 components, an initial steep slope followed by a much less steeply falling slope. This double population is seen in sickle cell anaemia, paroxysmal nocturnal haemoglobinuria and in some cases of hereditary enzyme-deficiency haemolytic anaemias (International Committee for Standardization in Hematology, 1971, Dacie & Lewis 1975).

3.11 APLASTIC ANAEMIA

Aplastic anaemia is the term usually used to refer specifically to a condition in which there is pancytopenia in the peripheral blood, a bone marrow which shows reduced cellularity, and evidence of diminished erythropoietic activity by ferrokinetic studies (prolonged plasma iron clearance and reduced red cell utilization of ^{59}Fe). Patients present with signs and symptoms which relate to the severity of the anaemia, thrombocytopenia or neutropenia. If thrombocytopenia is sufficiently severe, there will be a bleeding tendency either as ecchymosis and purpura or retinal haemorrhages and bleeding into organs, especially cerebral haemorrhage. Infection may become serious during the course of the illness. The blood film shows anisocytosis, macrocytosis and the neutrophils often show morphological abnormalities in the form of coarse red cytoplasmic granules in Romanowsky-stained films and extremely high content of alkaline phosphatase when the film is stained by an appropriate cytochemical reaction. There is an absolute reticulocytopenia although this is not inevitable at all times and during the course of the illness the reticulocyte count (relatively at least) may be normal or even increased. This suggests that the marrow may not be uniformly affected and this is confirmed on biopsy, as in aplastic anaemia normal and even hypercellular marrow may be obtained at one site, whereas in an adjacent area the true picture of hypoplasia is found (Fig. 3.25). Where there is a cellular area, an outstanding feature is the presence of dyserythropoiesis: the erythroid cells show megaloblastosis and asynchrony of maturation between nucleus and cytoplasm, binucleated cells and various features of nuclear degeneration. These appearances illustrate the extent to which a qualitative defect of erythropoiesis occurs as part of the haematological pattern in aplastic anaemia.

The common type of aplastic anaemia is a chronic acquired form. In about a third of cases, there is a clear association with a drug or chemical, but the aetiological role of toxic agents, drugs or chemicals is not yet clearly understood. Some chemotherapeutic agents will invariably cause marrow depression with a direct dose effect relationship and when the drug is stopped the marrow usually recovers soon thereafter. There are other drugs that appear to be harmless to the bulk of the population in the usual therapeutic dose and which may only occasionally cause aplastic anaemia, as a direct dose related reaction may require a dose many times greater than that normally given. Thus, for example, one in sixty thousand patients risk developing aplastic anaemia as a result of chloramphenicol therapy, but there is no method available to detect susceptible subjects and the cause of individual susceptibility is not known.

There are a number of ways in which haematopoietic depression may occur: a number of drugs and toxins are known to affect nucleic acid and protein synthesis although the site of action varies. Chloramphenicol, for example, inhibits protein synthesis at a stage subsequent to the attachment of amino acids to transfer RNA (i.e. by blocking the transfer of amino acids to ribosomes). Benzene and a number of other chemicals inhibit DNA synthesis in erythroid cells at the stage of the basophilic normoblasts and in the

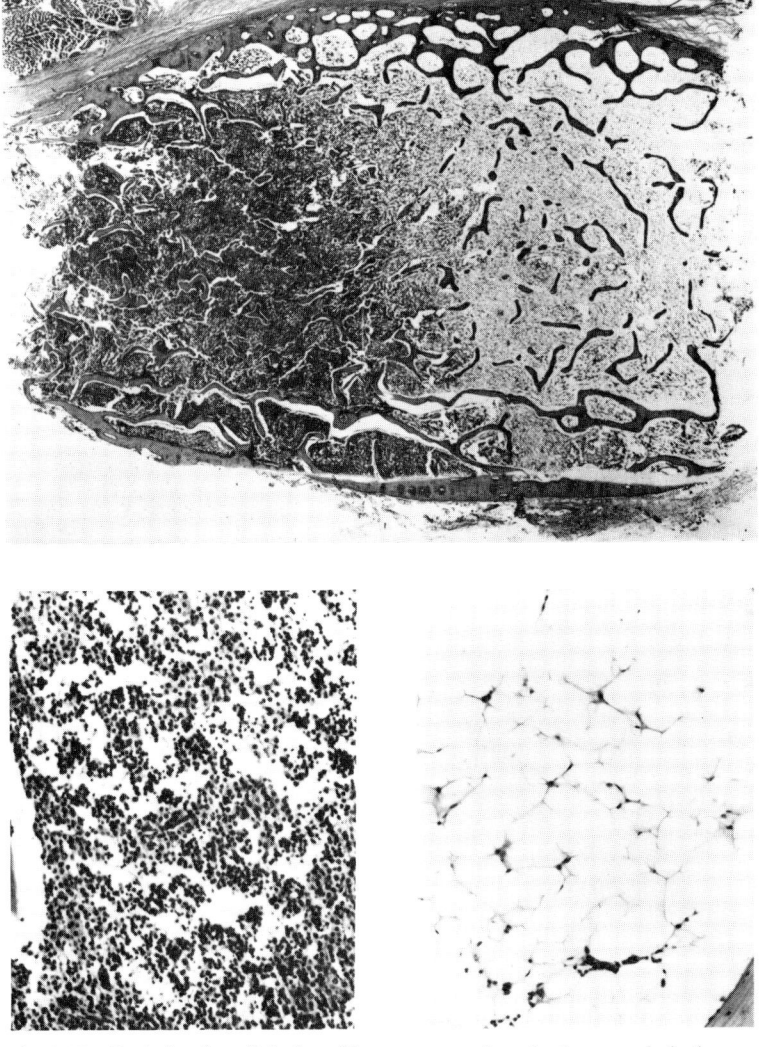

Fig. 3.25 Variation in cellularity of bone marrow in aplastic anaemia is demonstrated in this section of sternum obtained post mortem (× 5). Lower figures are high power views of two areas in upper figure (× 100).

myeloid line, at the stage of the myelocyte. Other toxins affect synthesis at the stage of the stem cell. Where no drug or toxin can be identified, the condition is referred to as 'idiopathic', but in reality it may not be possible to be sure whether a drug taken by a patient prior to the onset of the disease might be incriminated, especially in these days of therapeutic over-abundance, when few people are not subjected to a drug at some time or do not come into contact with potentially toxic environmental pollution. Another factor to be considered in the development of aplastic anaemia is the blood supply to the marrow itself. Haematopoiesis requires an adequate medullary microcirculation to support growth of haematopoietic tissue. Thus any toxic substance which destroys the sinusoidal structure of the marrow may result in aplastic anaemia with atrophy of haematopoietic tissue.

A less common form of aplastic anaemia is the congenital type known as Fanconi's anaemia. As acquired aplastic anaemia can occur at a very early age, the age of onset alone cannot be used to distinguish the 2 conditions. The clinical manifestations of Fanconi's anaemia include hyperpigmentation, skeletal malformations and other malformations such as microcephaly and mental retardation, deafness and strabismus and hypogonadism. In the majority of cases of Fanconi's anaemia, cytogenetic abnormalities are demonstrable. These are mainly chromatid type of abnormalities in the form of endoreduplication, chromatic exchange or gaps and breaks.

Aplastic anaemia (acquired or congenital) is liable to terminate in paroxysmal nocturnal haemoglobinuria or in leukaemia. 10–15 per cent of patients presenting with chronic aplastic anaemia develop PNH or PNH-like defects during the course of their disease. Leukaemia is a less common complication; it seems to be especially likely to occur following benzene toxicity and phenylbutazone, although any agent which causes aplastic anaemia is probably potentially leukaemogenic as the leukaemia probably develops as a result of chromosomal injury in the damaged bone marrow.

3.11.1 RED CELL APLASIA

As a rule, haematopoietic depression involves all cell lines. Pure red cell aplasia is less common, but occurs either as an acquired or a congenital condition. The acquired type appears to be due to an antibody directed specifically against erythroblasts and/or erythropoietic factors. It is often associated with a thymoma, occasionally with myasthenia gravis and in a proportion of cases it may be possible to demonstrate serum antinuclear factor, LE cells and a positive antiglobulin test.

The congenital or familial type is known as Diamond–Blackfan anaemia. In contrast to Fanconi's anaemia, in this condition there are no constitutional anomalies and the sole defect is that of red cell production. It becomes manifest soon after birth. The anaemia is normocytic and normochromic and may be severe while reticulocytes are usually less than 1 per cent. In the bone marrow, there is a remarkable absence of erythroid precursors but all other elements are normal. The cause of Diamond–Blackfan anaemia is not known but the familial incidence and early age of onset suggest that the abnormality is genetically determined. In some cases an abnormality of tryptophan metabolism has been described (Krantz 1973, Lewis 1971, Williams *et al* 1973).

3.12　DYSERYTHROPOIETIC ANAEMIAS

The term dyserythropoiesis is imprecise and does not refer to any one specific disorder or pathogenetic pathway. It embraces a number of conditions which primarily affect either the nucleus or the cytoplasm of the developing erythroid

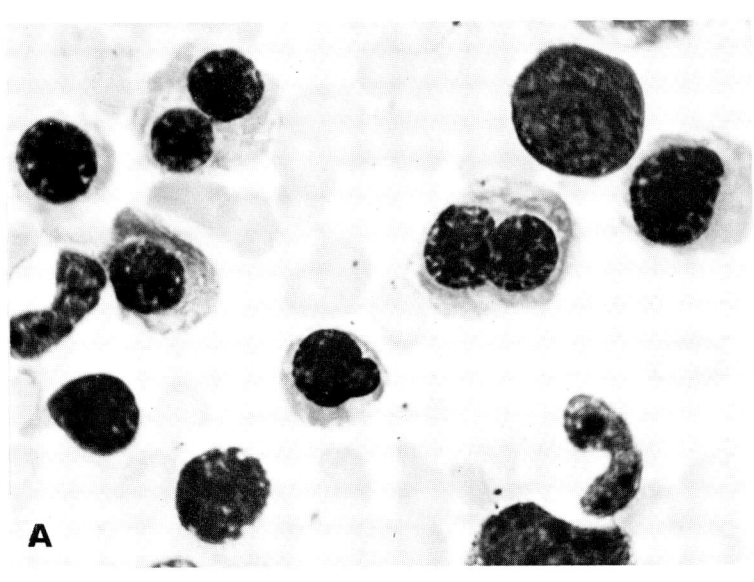

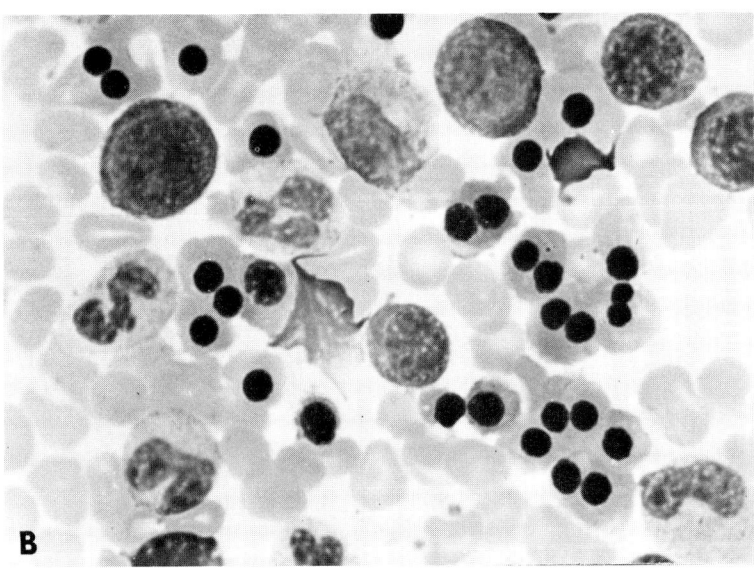

cell, or the environment in which erythropoiesis takes place. In some cases the cause of the defect is easily identified (e.g. deficiencies of vitamin B_{12} or folate, iron deficiency and defective haemoglobin synthesis). In other cases the cause of the dyserythropoiesis is more obscure and its role in the pathogenesis of the anaemia and the disease itself is often unclear. This situation occurs in aplastic anaemia, myelosclerosis and in infections. There is also a group of congenital disorders (see below). By using the term dyserythropoiesis, one underlines the fact that defect in erythropoiesis can lead to the production of abnormal erythroid cells, some of which are destroyed within the marrow during maturation (ineffective erythropoiesis) while those which reach maturity and

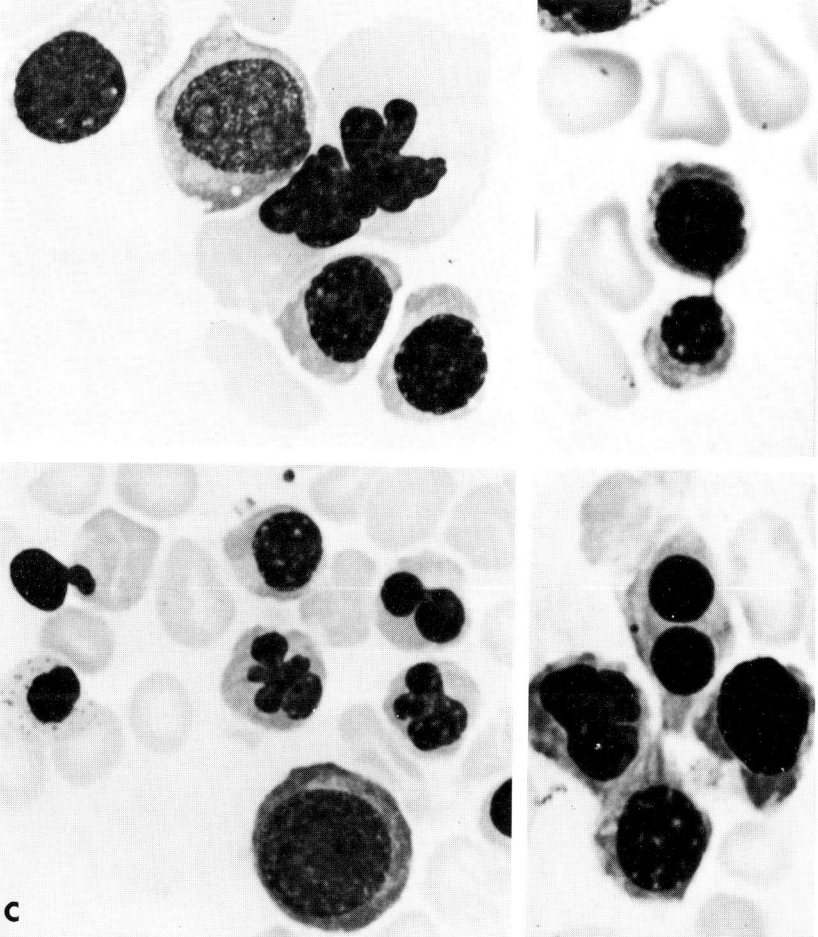

Fig. 3.26 Morphological features of dyserythropoiesis: (A) CDA Type 1 (B) CDA Type 2 (C) acquired forms (All at × 900).

enter circulation may show morphological abnormalities and have a shortened life span. Recent electron microscope studies have indicated that in dyserythropoiesis, nuclear membrane disruption seems to be one of the fundamental defects leading to other anomalies and probably to failure of DNA and RNA synthesis and RNA transport and thus to the production of cells which are morphologically and functionally abnormal. At the light microscope level the characteristics of dyserythropoiesis are binuclearity and multinuclearity sometimes with internuclear bridging, nuclear lobulation, budding and fragmentation associated with karyorrhexis and pyknosis, megaloblastic changes, cytoplasmic abnormalities including vacuolation, persistent cytoplasmic bridges, basophilic stippling and excess accumulation of iron in lyzosomes or mitochondria (Fig. 3.26).

3.12.1 CONGENITAL DYSERYTHROPOIETIC ANAEMIAS (CDA)

There are several related conditions which have been classified partly on the basis of their morphological features, into different types. In Type I the erythroblasts show megaloblastic changes and internuclear chromatin; in Type II there is binuclearity and multinuclearity with pluripolar mitosis and karyorrhexis, whilst Type III is characterized by gigantoblasts and multinuclearity with up to twelve nuclei. There is increasing evidence that although the types can still be broadly separated by electron microscopic studies they have many features in common and, as with other forms of dyserythropoiesis, a fundamental abnormality seems to be nuclear membrane disruption. CDA Type II has one unique feature in that cells lyse in acidified serum of a proportion of normal donors, hence the eponym by which it is usually known: HEMPAS—hereditary erythroblast multinuclearity with positive acidified serum. However, lysis by acidified serum does not occur with the patient's own serum and by contrast to PNH it is due to a markedly increased uptake of a naturally occurring iso-antibody which is deficient in HEMPAS serum and not primarily to increased sensitivity to complement action (Lewis & Verwilghen 1973, 1977).

3.12.2 PAROXYSMAL NOCTURNAL HAEMOGLOBINURIA (PNH)

Primarily PNH is a haemolytic anaemia but with overtones of marrow hypoplasia and dyserythropoiesis. The erythrocytes are destroyed intravascularly and if this is severe there will be haemoglobinuria. PNH occurs with more or less equal frequency in men and women. It is rare in children and is not familial. The presenting symptoms may be those of anaemia but may equally well be due to one of the complications of PNH such as thrombocytopenia, pancytopenia or venous thrombosis. Venous thrombosis occurs frequently in PNH and may even be the dominant clinical feature and give the greatest difficulties in management of the patient. When haemoglobinuria occurs, it will be recognized by the colour of the urine which may vary from pale red to black and, in classical cases, the early morning specimen will be especially affected. There is nothing characteristic in the blood picture: anaemia may be moderate or severe; red cells are usually normocytic and normochromic although they may also be hypochromic and the MCHC is normal or slightly low. The reticulocyte count is usually raised, at times markedly so, but in general the reticulocytosis is lower than might be expected when related to the degree of anaemia by comparison with other types of haemolytic anaemia.

There is an interrelationship of PNH and marrow hypoplasia. In the patients in whom haemolysis is the dominant feature, the anaemia may be associated with a relatively low reticulocyte count, leucopenia and mild thrombocytopenia. Other patients may have moderate or severe haemolysis and at the same time more definite evidence of chronic marrow hypoplasia and pancytopenia. In other patients again, aplastic anaemia has been the first diagnosis and they appear to be suffering from aplastic anaemia throughout their illness with PNH being present only as an incidental laboratory finding. In diagnosing PNH, haemoglobinuria must be distinguished from haematuria as a cause of red urine. In all cases, whether there is haemoglobinuria or not, haemosiderin will be excreted in the urine. Haemosiderinuria is, however, not specific and both haemoglobinuria and haemosiderinuria may occur in severe intravascular haemolysis, irrespective of the cause.

PNH red cells are unusually susceptible to lysis by complement and this can be demonstrated in vitro by a variety of tests (e.g. acidified serum (Ham), sucrose lysis, thrombin lysis and cold antibody lysis). The acidified serum test is considered to be the diagnostic test for PNH although sucrose lysis and other tests are useful as screening procedures (Dacie & Lewis 1972; Sirchia & Lewis 1975).

3.13 ABNORMALITIES OF LEUCOCYTES AND LEUCOPOIESIS

3.13.1 LEUCOPENIA

Leucopenia is defined as a reduction of leucocytes below $4 \times 10^9/l$ in the peripheral blood. In practice, this usually implies especially a reduction of the neutrophils. Leucopenia or neutropenia may follow on the administration of cytotoxic drugs in a dose-related effect or it may occur as a sensitivity reaction when a drug or toxic agent is administered to a susceptible person. By contrast to aplastic anaemia the neutropenia is usually reversible on withdrawal of the drug.

Cyclical neutropenia is a rare disorder characterized by episodes of neutropenia occurring at more or less regular intervals. The most commonly reported oscillation is 20–21 days. There is a cyclical reduction in the granulocyte proliferative pool in the bone marrow followed by the onset of neutropenia which may be so severe that granulocytes disappear completely from the peripheral blood. Family studies suggest that the disease may be transmitted as an autosomal dominant.

Agranulocytosis is a term used to describe a particularly severe condition when there is an almost total disappearance of the neutrophils from the peripheral blood. This condition is characterized by severe infection. It follows administration of a drug, often one of the antibiotics and it is believed that the mechanism of the neutropenia is immunological: circulating neutrophils become coated with a drug-antibody complex and they are preferentially removed by the reticuloendothelial system. The marrow is active and shows an abundant number of granulocyte precursors but the more mature forms (from myelocyte onwards) are missing. This is not, however, a 'maturation arrest' as it is due to depletion as the maturing cells emerge prematurely from the bone marrow or are destroyed in situ.

3.13.1   LEUCOCYTOSIS

In normal man the upper limit of the leucocyte count is $11 \cdot 0 \times 10^9/l$. There are approximately 40–75 per cent neutrophils, 20–45 per cent lymphocytes, 1–6 per cent eosinophils, 2–10 per cent monocytes and less than 1 per cent basophils. The term 'leucocytosis' refers to an increase in the total number of circulating leucocytes, irrespective of which cell type is responsible. 'Neutrophilia', or 'neutrophil leucocytosis', 'lymphocytosis', 'eosinophilia' and 'monocytosis', specify which cells are increased. It is, however, necessary to establish that the increase is an absolute one and not a relative one, due only to a decrease in the other cells. A neutrophil count above $7 \cdot 5 \times 10^9/l$ is an absolute neutrophilia, while in an absolute lymphocytosis, the lymphocytes are above $4 \cdot 0 \times 10^9/l$.

A moderate increase in the total leucocyte count, due mainly to neutrophilia, occurs as a normal response to exercise, following meals, as a result of emotional stress and during pregnancy. Strenuous exercise may cause a leucocytosis of up to $30 \times 10^9/l$, with an increase in the numbers of both neutrophils and lymphocytes. Leucocytosis also occurs in a wide range of pathological conditions. Neutrophil leucocytosis occurs in acute infections, in burns and in malignant disease. Pyogenic bacteria are liable to cause a particularly marked increase in the neutrophils leading to the so-called 'leukaemoid reaction' which must be distinguished from leukaemia. An eosinophil leucocytosis is a characteristic feature of parasitic infections, allergic reactions, skin diseases and certain neoplastic diseases including Hodgkin's disease.

An absolute lymphocytosis is less common than the relative lymphocytosis which is associated with a low neutrophil count. A true lymphocytosis is characteristic of chronic lymphocytic leukaemia (see p. 87). It also occurs in acute infectious lymphocytosis, in chronic infections such as tuberculosis and brucellosis, and in viral infections, including infectious hepatitis and infectious mononucleosis.

3.13.3 INFECTIOUS MONONUCLEOSIS

This is an acute illness that attacks mainly young adults. It is characterized by fever, sore throat, lymphadenopathy and splenomegaly. In the peripheral blood there is a moderately increased leucocyte count between 12 and

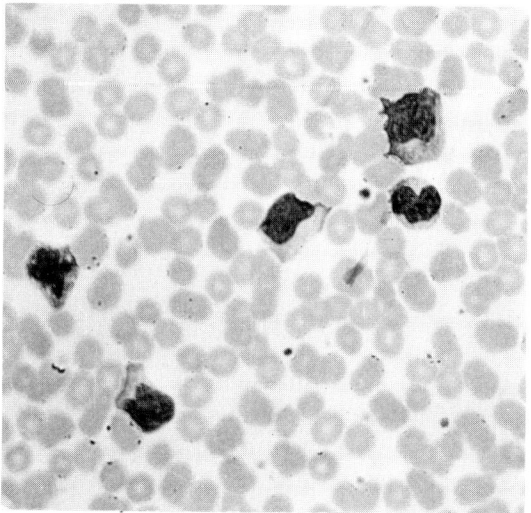

Fig. 3.27 Atypical mononuclear cells in blood film from case of infectious mononucleosis ($\times$ 500).

$18 \times 19^9/l$ and the increase is mainly due to the presence of mononuclear cells, many of which are atypical morphologically with abnormalities in the nuclear chromatin, whilst the cytoplasm is vacuolated or foamy in appearance, with an irregular outer border and deep blue staining periphery (Fig. 3.27). It should be noted that similar atypical lymphoid cells may also be seen though in lesser numbers in other virus diseases such as varicella and infectious hepatitis and some bacterial infections and sometimes in malignant disease. In infectious mononucleosis, a variety of antibodies appear in the serum. Characteristically, they include serum agglutinins, notably anti-sheep-cell haemagglutinins. These provide the basis for the diagnostic Paul–Bunnell test.

3.13.3 GRANULOCYTE VARIATIONS

There are a number of variations of neutrophil morphology which occur either in a congenital form or an acquired phenomenon. They are listed in Table 3.4 and some are illustrated in Fig. 3.28 (Davidson 1968, Mills & Cooperand 1971; Nathan & Baehner 1971, Stites & Leikola 1971, Pisciotta 1973, Cline 1974, 1975, MacKinney & Cline 1974, Bainton 1975, Lichtman 1975).

Table 3.4 Variations in neutrophil morphology

Eponym	Inheritance	Features	Occurrence of acquired form
Pelger-Huët	Dominant	Bilobed nuclei	Leukaemias Metastic carcinoma Infections
Hereditary hypersegmentation	Dominant	Neutrophil nuclei with 5 or more lobes	Megaloblastic anaemias Pyogenic infection
May-Hegglin	Dominant	Döhle bodies	Infection Burns Pregnancy
Alder-Reilly	Recessive	Prominent dark purple granules	Infection Burns ('Toxic granules')
Chediak-Higashi	Recessive	Giant granules	—
Chronic granulomatous disease	Recessive	Defective phagocytic function	—

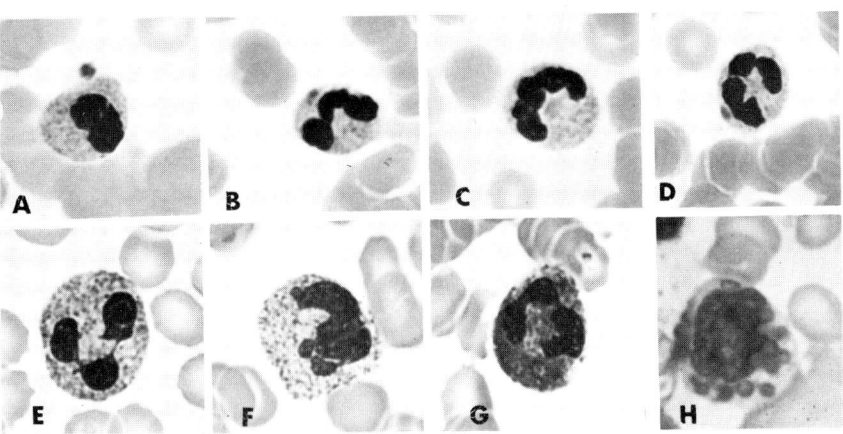

Fig. 3.28 Neutrophil anomalies (×900): (A) and (B) Pelger-Huët; (C) nuclear hypersegmentation; (D) Döhle bodies; (E), (F) and (G) excessive granulation; (H) Chediak-Higashi.

3.13.5 THE LEUKAEMIAS

3.13.5.1 Acute leukaemia

Leukaemia is a neoplastic disorder of bone marrow cells characterized by the preponderance of stem cells which bear a resemblance to normal myeloblasts, lymphoblasts etc. Deviations from normal morphology accompany the malignant changes and this may be marked, so that classification based on morphological description alone can at best be only approximate. It is possible, however, to classify the types of acute leukaemia on the basis of clinical features (especially age incidence), cytochemical tests, functional tests and ultrastructural features as seen by electron microscopy.

3.13.5.2 Lymphoblastic leukaemia

This is the most frequent malignancy of childhood and its incidence peaks at 3 to 5 years of age. The predominant cell is lymphoblast-like (Fig. 3.29),

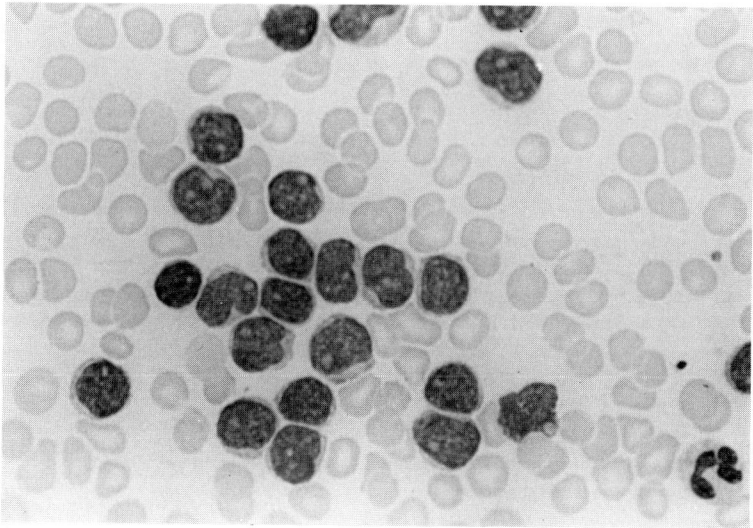

Fig. 3.29 Lymphoblastic leukaemia (× 600).

generally uniform in appearance but with some pleomorphism, and with tendency towards early lymphocytic differentiation. The majority of cases are identified with B cell lymphocytes. Peroxidase reaction is uniformly negative, PAS reaction is positive in a proportion of blasts, especially the usual type, although in the less common T cell type PAS reaction is negative or there are only some fine granules with a positive reaction. Similarly, acid-phosphatase is typically weakly positive, or negative in lymphoblastic leukaemia, but in the T cell type the reaction may be moderately to strongly positive.

3.13.5.3 Acute myeloid leukaemia

This condition is subdivided into a number of types. The least well differentiated type is called myeloblastic leukaemia; another type consisting mainly of promyelocytes is called promyelocytic. Then again, myeloid leukaemias

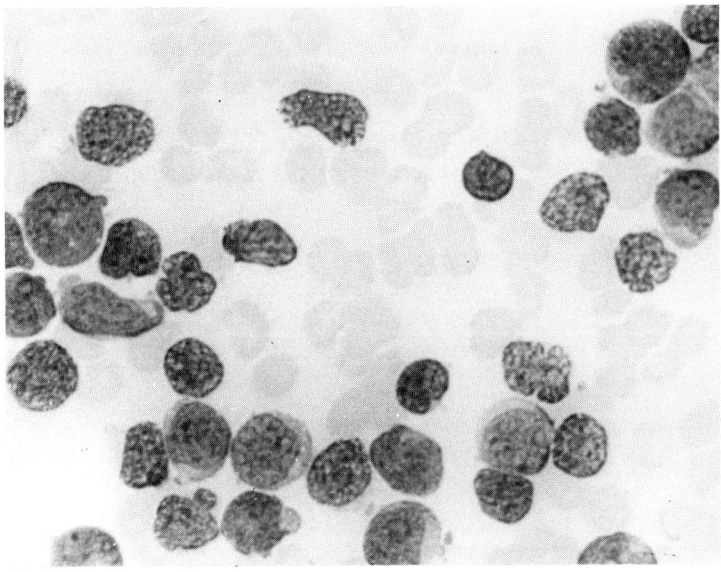

Fig. 3.30   Myeloblastic leukaemia (× 600).

often have a proportion of monocytoid cells in the bone marrow and peripheral blood. When almost all the cells resemble monocytes, the term monocytic leukaemia is used; when the monocytes are clearly aberrant granulocytic cells and co-exist with developing granulocytes, the term myelomonocytic leukaemia is used. In any sub-type of acute myeloid leukaemia, a variable admixture of erythroblasts is often present in the bone marrow or peripheral blood. The term erythroleukaemia (sometimes referred to as Di Guglielmo's syndrome) applies to those cases where leukaemic infiltration involves both erythroid and myeloid precursors, whilst when all the proliferating cells are erythroblasts, often of bizarre morphology, the disease is termed erythraemic myelosis. All these conditions, and especially myeloblastic leukaemia, may occur in children and infants but the incidence increases with age and they are usually considered to be the acute leukaemia of adults. The myeloblasts which fill the bone marrow and usually also the peripheral blood have disturbed morphological features: there are large bizarre nucleoli, and some cells contain Auer bodies which are azurophilic rod-like lysosomal structures characteristic of leukaemia (Fig. 3.30). In myelomonocytic leukaemia the bone marrow is infiltrated with typical myeloblasts and promyelocytes and also with atypical immature cells with indented or folded nuclei, poor chromatin clumping and nucleoli (Fig. 3.31). In the peripheral blood there are seen cells which have the features of both monocytes and bizarre metamyelocytes (Fig. 3.32). In acute myeloid leukaemias the reactions for

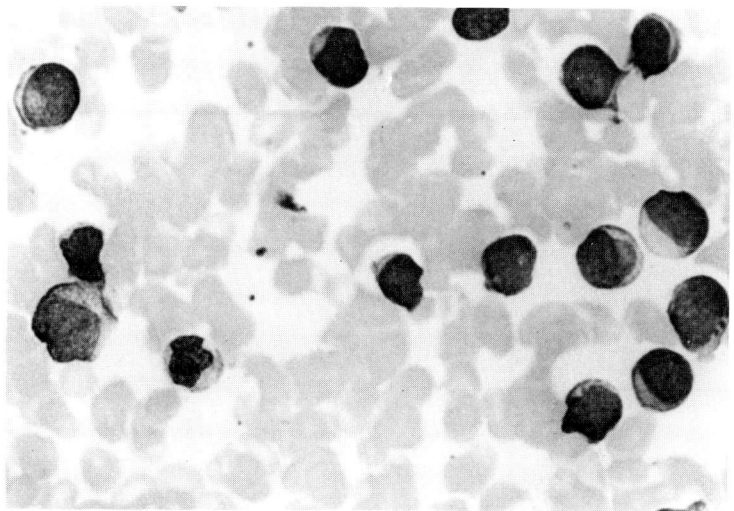

Fig. 3.31 Bone marrow in myelomonocytic leukaemia (×600).

peroxidase, Sudan Black B and chloracetate esterase are moderately to strongly positive in blasts which are differentiating to promyelocytes whilst the reactions for non-specific esterases with naphthol AS acetate and α naphthol acetate substrate are strongly positive where there is monoblastic–monocyte differentiation. The acid-phosphatase test is especially positive in the monocytic and to a lesser degree in the myelomonocytic leukaemias. The cytobacterial test for lysozyme is another simple method which helps to identify monocytic differentiation.

Erythroleukaemia is often characterized by a positive PAS reaction in the erythroblasts, whilst the erythroblasts themselves have atypical morphology: they are megaloblastic and have many features of dyserythropoiesis (Fig. 3.33).

Eosinophilic leukaemia is an extremely rare subtype of acute myeloid

S. M. Lewis

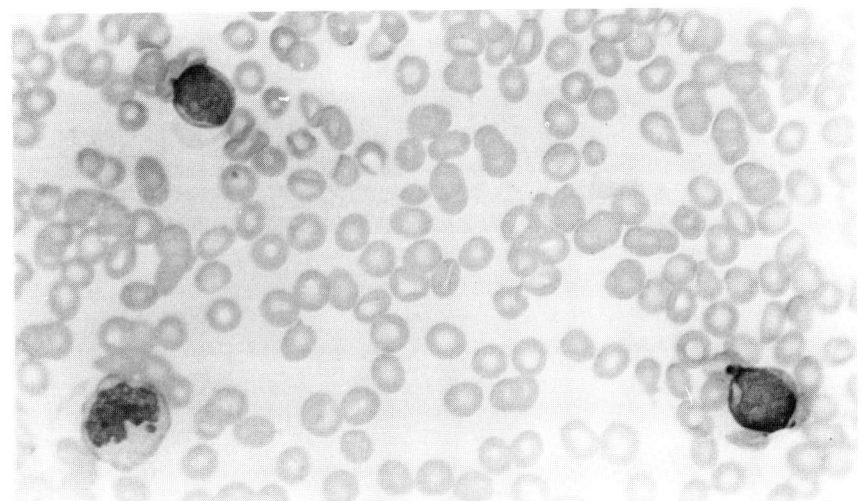

Fig. 3.32   Blood film in myelomonocytic leukaemia (× 550).

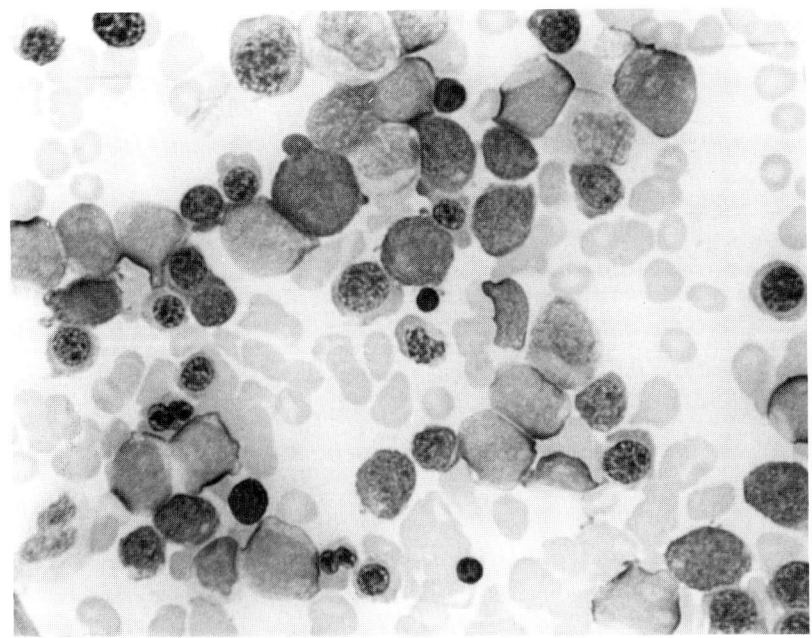

Fig. 3.33   Bone marrow in erythroleukaemia (× 600).

leukaemia; it is characterized by preponderance of eosinophils and eosinophil precursors many of which show morphological aberrations. In some leukaemias, especially chronic granulocytic leukaemia, a high basophil count may occur but these basophils should be distinguished from leukaemic cells as basophilic leukaemia is not recognized as an entity.

The major clinical manifestations of acute leukaemia stem from the bone marrow failure and from organ enlargement and infiltration by the tumour cells. Bone marrow failure results in anaemia, thrombocytopenia and granulocytopenia. The thrombocytopenia gives rise to ecchymosis and bleeding and the neutropenia leads to increased susceptibility to infection. The organs affected by enlargement are especially lymph nodes and the spleen. Central nervous system infiltration results in increased intracranial pressure, ocular disturbance and cranial and peripheral nerve palsies; these manifestations occur primarily in lymphoblastic leukaemia. Hypertrophy of the gums and oral ulcers are frequently noted in monocytic leukaemia. Another unusual manifestation, which occurs uniquely in promyelocytic leukaemia, is an unusually severe bleeding tendency, which occurs irrespective of the platelet count and unrelated to the thrombocytopenia. It is associated with plasma clotting factor deficiencies (hypofibrinogenaemia and low levels of Factor V and Factor VII) and is presumably due to a diffuse intravascular clotting triggered by thromboplastic material released from the leukaemic promyelocytes.

3.13.5.4 Chronic granulocytic leukaemia

Chronic granulocytic leukaemia (CGL) occurs with equal frequency in both sexes. It is most common in middle age, and is rare below the age of ten although in infants there occurs a disease similar to, although not identical with, chronic granulocytic leukaemia, originating from fetal myeloid stem cells and referred to as juvenile granulocytic leukaemia. The clinical features of CGL are usually due to anaemia; there may be excessive bruising or bleeding and this may occur even when the platelet count is normal or even elevated; enlargement of the spleen results in an increasingly obvious abdominal mass. In the peripheral blood the total leucocyte count is high, usually above $50 \times 10^9/l$ and often above $100 \times 10^9/l$ and in the typical case provides the characteristic appearances from which an immediate diagnosis may be made (Fig. 3.34). Mature granulocytes and metamyelocytes predominate in the blood smear, but myelocytes and promyelocytes are also readily found as is an occasional myeloblast. There is a varying degree of anaemia and relative marrow failure will be indicated by a low reticulocyte count. Thrombocytosis is not uncommon early in the disease but, as the disease progresses, thrombocytopenia occurs. The bone marrow reflects the peripheral blood leucocyte count: there is marked hypercellularity due to

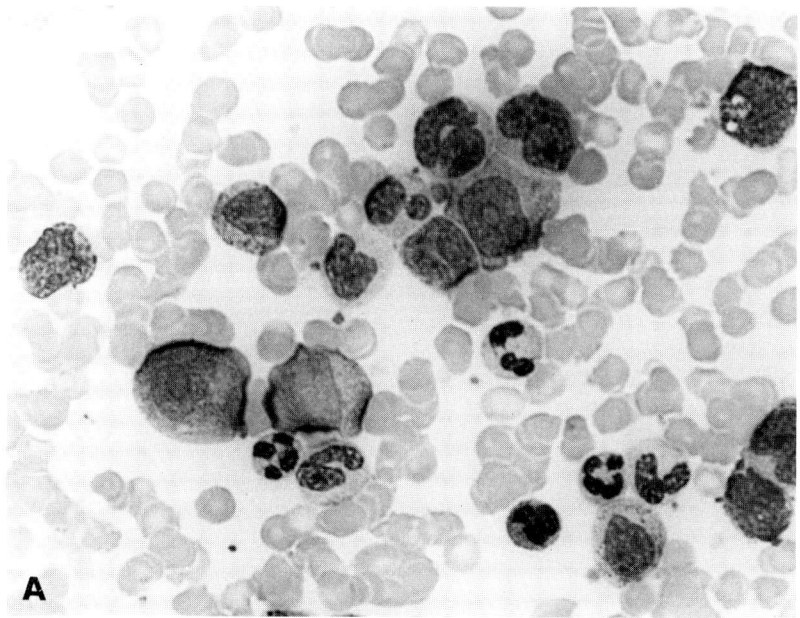

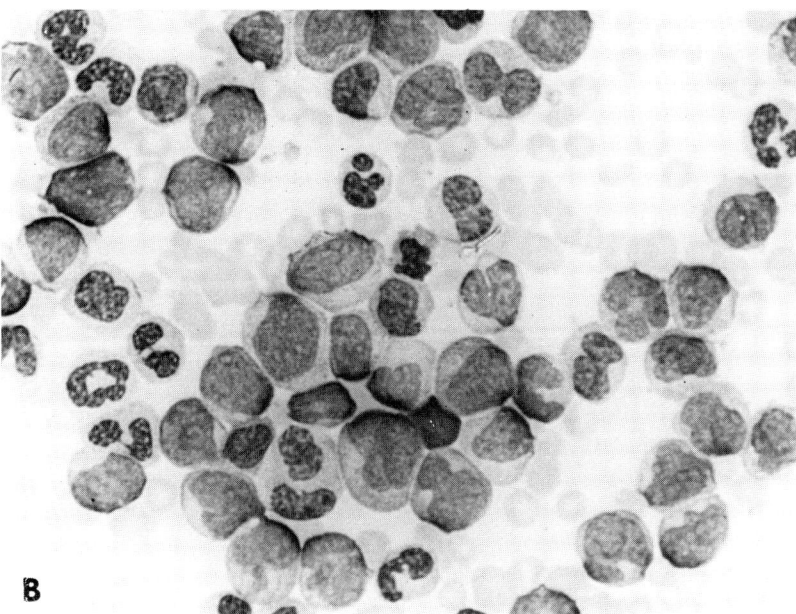

Fig. 3.34 Blood film (A) and bone marrow film (B) in chronic granulocvtic leukaemia (× 600).

intense granulocyte hyperplasia; myeloblast, promyelocytes and early myelocytes are prominent although abundant mature granulocytes are also seen;
eosinophils and basophils may be conspicuous; erythroid precursors are
fewer than normal. As a rule, cytochemical staining need not be called on for
diagnosing CGL although neutrophil alkaline phosphatase activity is of value
in distinguishing the high leucocyte count from a leukaemoid reaction which
occurs in certain infections. In the latter the alkaline phosphatase score is very
high whilst in CGL low scores are typical in the untreated cases, although the
initial score may change to normal or high during remission, after splenectomy
or when the patient undergoes blast cell transformation. One feature which
characterizes CGL is the presence of the Philadelphia (Ph[1]) chromosome.
This abnormal chromosome is present in 80–85 per cent of patients with
CGL and those cases in whom it is not found are thought to have an atypical
form of the disease which merges with chronic myelomonocytic leukaemia.
It may also occur, but only very rarely, in other diseases with myeloid metaplasia, such as myelofibrosis and polycythaemia vera.

Chronic myelomonocytic leukaemia is a sub-type which occurs in elderly
subjects. The course is often slowly progressive for a number of years. The
chief features are high absolute neutrophil and monocyte counts. The bone
marrow is highly cellular with gross granulocytic hyperplasia, and with
adequate numbers of megakaryocytes. There is a relatively high proportion
of metamyelocytes and neutrophils, together with promyelocytes and myelocytes, and often a far lower proportion of monocytes than would be expected
from the blood picture.

3.13.5.5   Chronic lymphocytic leukaemia (CLL)

This is characterized by a slow progressive accumulation of well differentiated
small lymphocytes of normal morphology. They infiltrate in all tissues in
which lymphocytes normally occur, and this leads to organ enlargement,
notably lymph nodes and spleen. The bone marrow is extensively infiltrated
and the circulating blood has an increased lymphocyte count to the order of
$200 \times 10^9/l$ to $500 \times 10^9/l$ or even higher (Fig. 3.35). Although the lymphocytes
appear normal they are not: they smudge easily when smeared and they are
functionally abnormal and non-reactive as demonstrable by their impaired
capacity to react to antigenic challenges by an appropriate immune response
and their failure to transform into blast cells when cultured with phytohaemagglutinin. Lymphocytes do not proliferate rapidly in chronic lymphocytic leukaemia. In some patients the disease progresses only very slowly over
years. Anaemia may be slight and peripheral adenopathy limited. In other
patients there is a gradually rising leucocyte count, increasing anaemia and
increasing lymphadenopathy.

Histologically CLL is indistinguishable from lymphocytic lymphoma and it is equally appropriate to consider CLL as a lymphoma or as a leukaemia.

Leukaemic reticuloendotheliosis is an uncommon condition characterized by an infiltration by mononuclear cells with unusual cytoplasmic villi which give it an eponym of 'hairy cell leukaemia'. From functional studies it seems likely that these cells are lymphocytic rather than histiocytic in origin and that the disease should be considered as lymphoproliferative, and related to CLL.

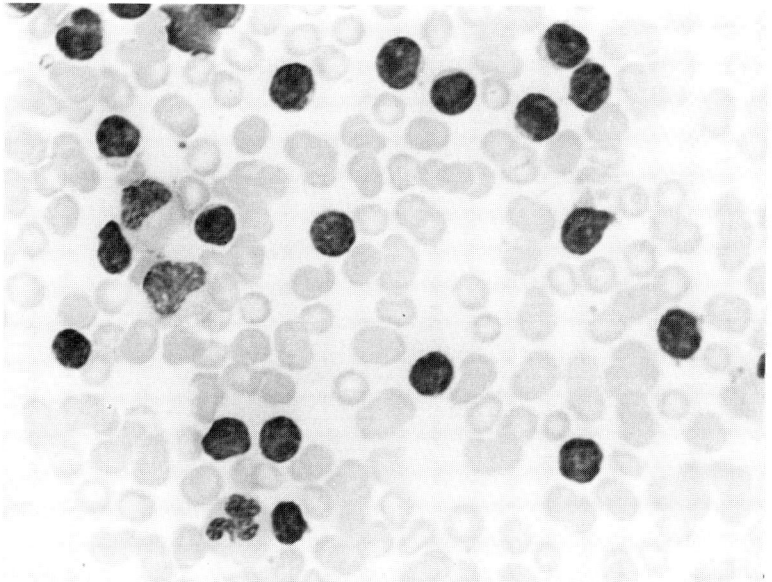

Fig. 3.35   Blood film in chronic lymphocytic leukaemia (× 600).

3.13.6   CHRONIC LYMPHOPROLIFERATIVE DISORDERS

The classification of the chronic lymphoproliferative disorders has been complicated by the use of different systems of classification, some based on histopathology and others on clinical features. A classification based entirely on histopathology is not entirely satisfactory, whereas a classification based on clinical features provides a framework on which can be built a methodical approach to investigation, diagnosis and the planning of treatment. This is illustrated in Table 3.5. Conditions include chronic lymphocytic leukaemia, malignant lymphomas and lymphosarcoma and in this classification it is extended to include Hodgkin's disease and myelomatosis. By contrast to CLL, the lymphomas are neoplasms of cells of the lymphoid tissue which arise focally, and metastasize by local infiltration and via lymphatics and blood stream. They most often begin in a lymph node but they can begin in lymphoid tissue in the alimentary canal and occasionally in other extranodal sites such as ovary, thyroid or salivary glands. Hodgkin's disease is included in the classification because the Reed-Sternberg cell which characterizes Hodgkin's disease is a malignant histiocyte, although the disease itself differs fundamentally from other lymphomas.

Immunoproliferative disorders or gammopathies are themselves a complex group of conditions which affect the plasma cells and lymphocytes and of which myelomatosis is the most common example.

Table 3.5 Classification of lymphomas and related disorders

A. *Lymphocytic*	
Systemic lymphoreticular neoplasms	Chronic lymphatic leukaemia
	Lymphocytic lymphoma
	Follicular lymphoma (benign phase)
Focally arising neoplasms	Lymphosarcoma
	Reticulum cell sarcoma
	Histiocytic medullary reticulosis
	Hodgkin's disease
Immunocytomas	Benign monoclonal macroglobulinaemia
	Idiopathic cold-antibody disease
	Waldenström's macroglobulinaemia
	Malignant lymphoma with macroglobulinaemia
B. *Plasmacytic*	
	Benign monoclonal hyperglobulinaemia
	Essential cryoglobulinaemia
	Myelomatosis
	Extramedullary plasmacytoma
	Plasma cell leukaemia

Myelomatosis is a malignant disease of plasma cells with early and wide dissemination, especially to the axial skeleton, leading to osteoporosis and lytic lesions in the vertebrae, pelvis, ribs and sternum. The tumour produces large amounts of Bence-Jones paraprotein, a monoclonal light protein, which causes renal tubular damage and leads to a reduction in normal immunoglobulins and impaired capacity to respond to primary antigenic stimulus.

Waldenström's macroglobulinaemia is another form of neoplastic disease with clinical and laboratory features intermediate between those of chronic lymphocytic leukaemia and myelomatosis. The specific feature is the presence of a homogeneous IgM macroglobulin which is synthesized by abnormal lymphoid cells. (Franklin 1973, Catovsky *et al* 1974, Gunz & Baikie 1974, Hamilton Fairley 1974, Rosenberg 1974, Galton 1977).

3.14 NON-LEUKAEMIC MYELOPROLIFERATIVE DISORDERS

The term 'myeloproliferative disorders' encompasses polycythaemia vera, myelosclerosis and essential thrombocythaemia; these disorders may co-exist or may merge into each other, and occasionally, some time may elapse before a bone marrow showing a myeloproliferative picture will alter sufficiently to indicate which cell line has been especially or specifically affected. Some of the disorders may run a relatively benign course which does not alter throughout the life of the patient. In other cases the disease may run an acute course from the beginning or may become malignant only after a considerable period of time. The interrelationship of the myeloproliferative disorders, arising from the common reticulum cell, is illustrated in Fig. 3.36.

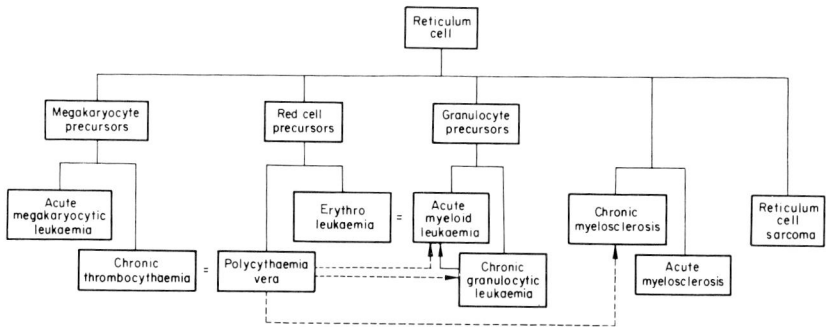

Fig. 3.36 Scheme illustrating relationship of various conditions that are included in the myeloproliferative disorders.

3.14.1 POLYCYTHAEMIA VERA

In polycythaemia vera (PV) there is an absolute increase in the red cell volume. As a rule, this results in a high RBC, Hb and PCV. In PV there is commonly a leucocytosis, thrombocytosis and enlargement of the spleen although these are not constant features. The bone marrow is, as one would expect, hypercellular. There is loss of fat spaces, and the marrow is crowded by erythroid cells, myeloid cells and also frequently by megakaryocytes.

An essential requirement for the diagnosis of PV is the demonstration of an absolute increase in the patient's circulating red cell mass. Measurement of haemoglobin, PCV and RBC provide information on the relative red cell concentration in the blood, but this does not take into account fluctuations in the plasma volume or total blood volume. It is thus necessary to distinguish between true polycythaemia and 'relative' or 'pseudo' polycythaemia; the latter may occur as a result of peripheral circulatory failure, dehydration, oedema or prolonged bed rest and also in the so-called 'stress polycythaemia' syndrome.

When the presence of a true erythrocytosis has been established it is further necessary to distinguish between PV and polycythaemia which is secondary to an underlying disease.

Secondary polycythaemia occurs either as a compensatory mechanism to meet the oxygen needs of the body or because of the presence of erythro-poietin-producing lesion. The former includes pulmonary cardiac disease when there is a reduced arterial PO_2, high altitude, congenital methaemo-globinaemia, abnormal haemoglobins with increased oxygen affinity (result-ing in tissue anoxia), Hb-M variants which result in excessive formation of methaemoglobin, and chemical or physical agents which cause sulphaemo-globinaemia and methaemoglobinaemia. Polycythaemia associated with excess erythropoietin production occurs with a variety of renal lesions, mainly carcinoma of the kidney and renal cystic conditions, and also several other tumours such as uterine fibromas and hepatomas.

3.14.2 ESSENTIAL THROMBOCYTHAEMIA

'Thrombocytosis' or an increased platelet count above the upper limit of normal (400×10^9/l) occurs as a result of acute blood loss, in acute infections,

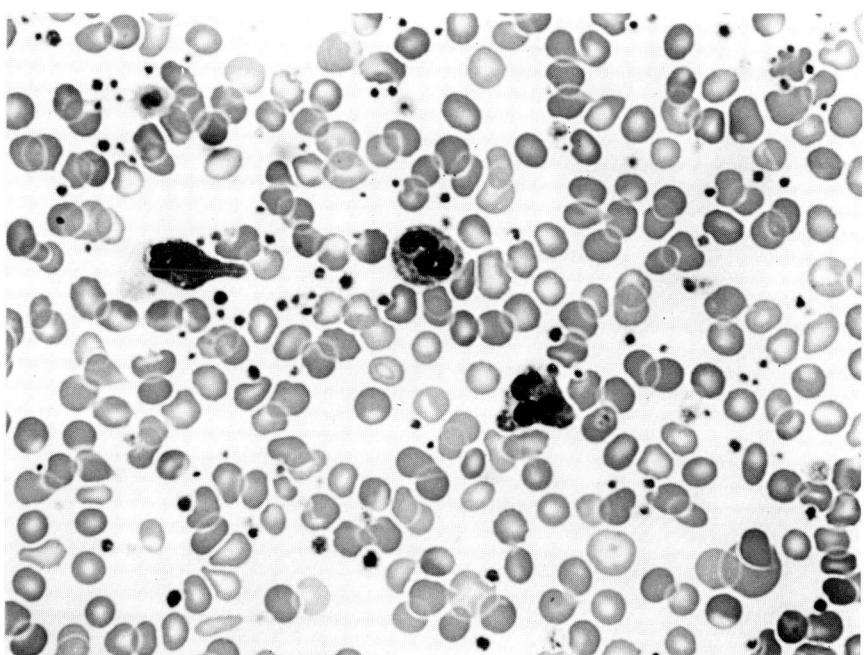

Fig. 3.37 Blood film in essential thrombocythaemia ($\times$ 700).

carcinoma, lymphoma and following operations. In none of these cases is the platelet count, as a rule, increased beyond $1000 \times 10^9/l$. A remarkably increased platelet count sustained at levels of over a million is more likely to be due to the myeloproliferative disorder known as thrombocythaemia. This condition is closely related to polycythaemia vera and, indeed, there is evidence that it might be merely a variant of the latter disease. None the less it is convenient and useful to consider it as a distinct clinical and haematological syndrome since the raised platelet count is the dominant feature; also, because haemorrhage is common, there is usually anaemia with a low MCH and MCHC. There is usually a leucocytosis which is more pronounced than in polycythaemia vera. The platelet count is not infrequently as high as 3000–$5000 \times 10^9/l$. The blood film is characterized by the abundance of platelets; many of the platelets are morphologically abnormal and giant forms or even megakaryocyte fragments may be seen (Fig. 3.37). Bone marrow is readily obtained by aspiration. There is, as a rule, hyperplasia of the marrow and especially striking is the increase in the numbers of megakaryocytes and platelets.

3.14.3   MYELOSCLEROSIS

In myelosclerosis the essential pathological feature of the marrow is the proliferation of fibroblasts with deposition of collagen and frequently an increase in osseous tissue. The blood count usually shows a normochromic or hypochromic anaemia of moderate severity. There is an anisocytosis and poikolocytosis, the latter with teardrop forms, a variable reticulocytosis and the features of a leuco-erythroblastic anaemia (normoblasts and myelocytes) (Fig. 3.38). Bone marrow aspiration is usually unsuccessful resulting in a so-called dry tap. Biopsy of the bone marrow (e.g. from the iliac crest) shows a gross increase in reticulum which takes the form of coarse wavy fibres which are thought to represent mature collagen (Fig. 3.39).

Not infrequently there is a history of preceding polycythaemia. In some cases the disease progresses very slowly, the blood picture remaining relatively stable and the spleen enlarging only very gradually. In such cases there are few if any symptoms and the patient can lead a normal or almost normal life without treatment. Eventually the patient will develop symptoms due to anaemia, splenic enlargement, bleeding or the constitutional effects of the disease. About 10–20 per cent of patients die with an acute termination which is similar to acute myeloblastic leukaemia.

In its classical form myelosclerosis presents with a characteristic and easily identifiable picture. However, a similar histopathological lesion may occur in tuberculosis and in malignant disease and it is, of course, important to exclude these when making the diagnosis of primary myelofibrosis (Lewis *et al* 1972, Videbaek 1975).

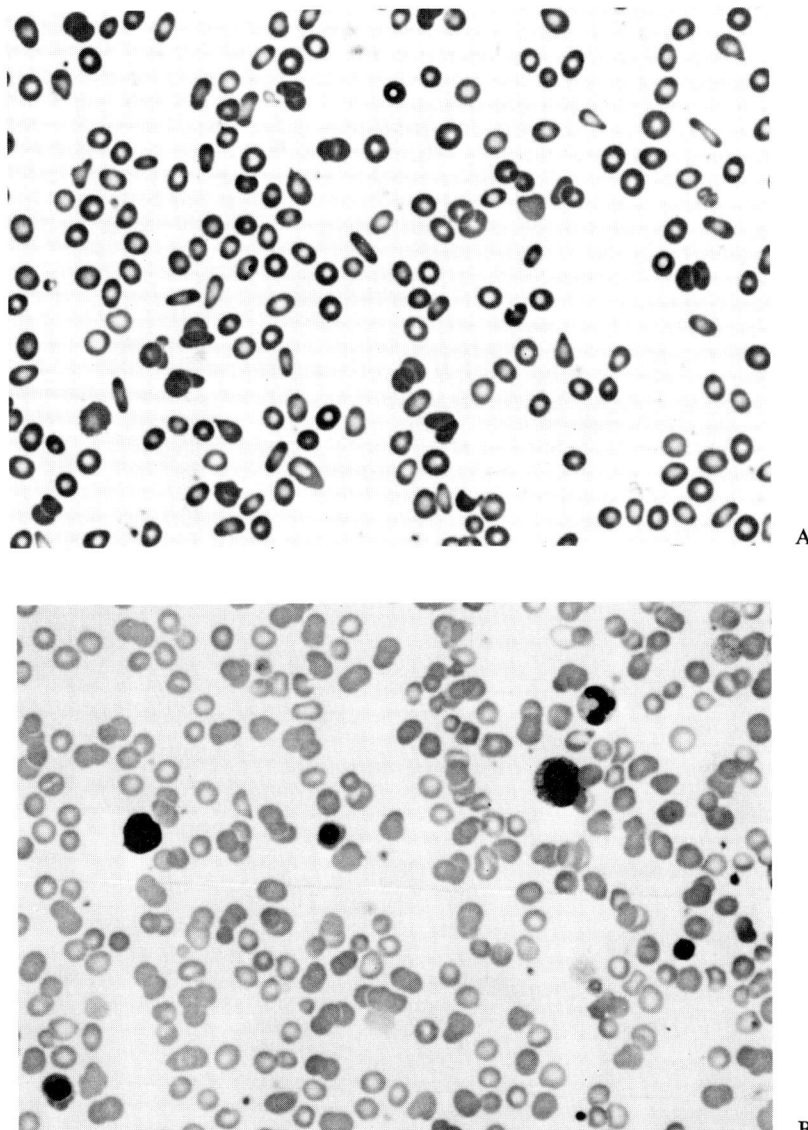

Fig. 3.38 Blood films in myelosclerosis: (A) Characteristic tear drop poikilocytes; (B) Leuco-erythroblastic anaemia (× 500).

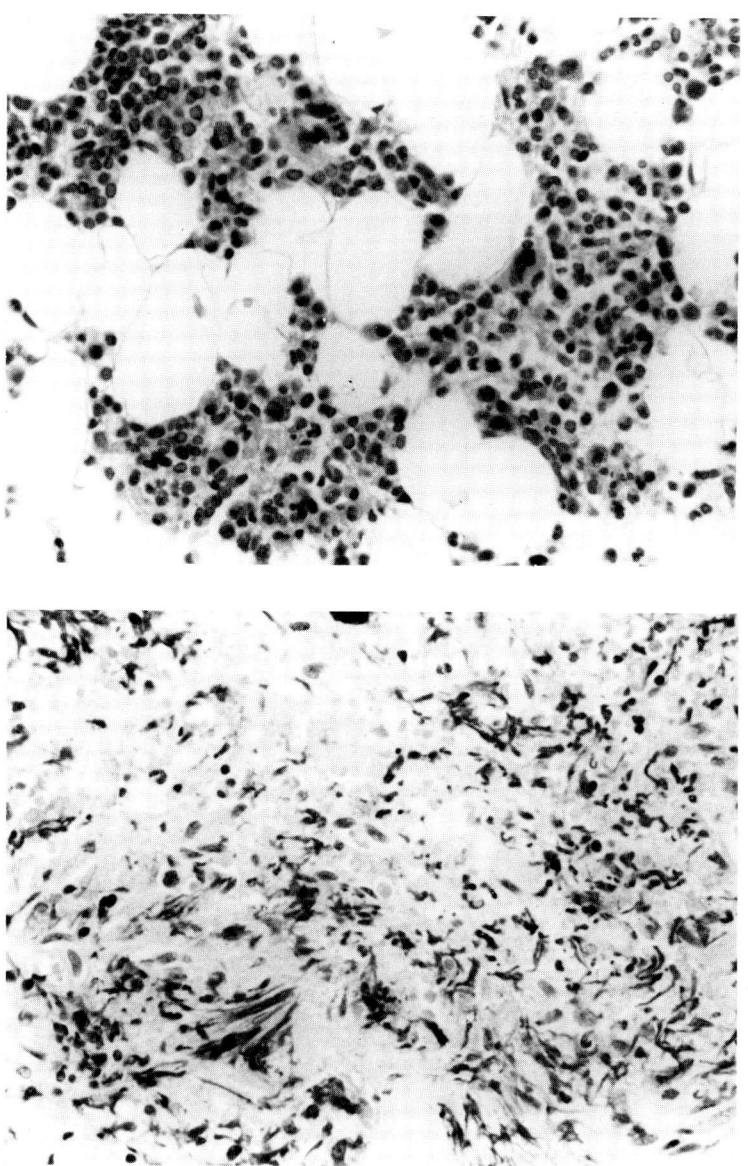

A

Fig. 3.39 Bone biopsy sections, stained: (A) by haematoxylin and eosin (× 200). (B) by silver impregnation to demonstrate reticulin (× 100). Top: normal. Lower: myelosclerosis.

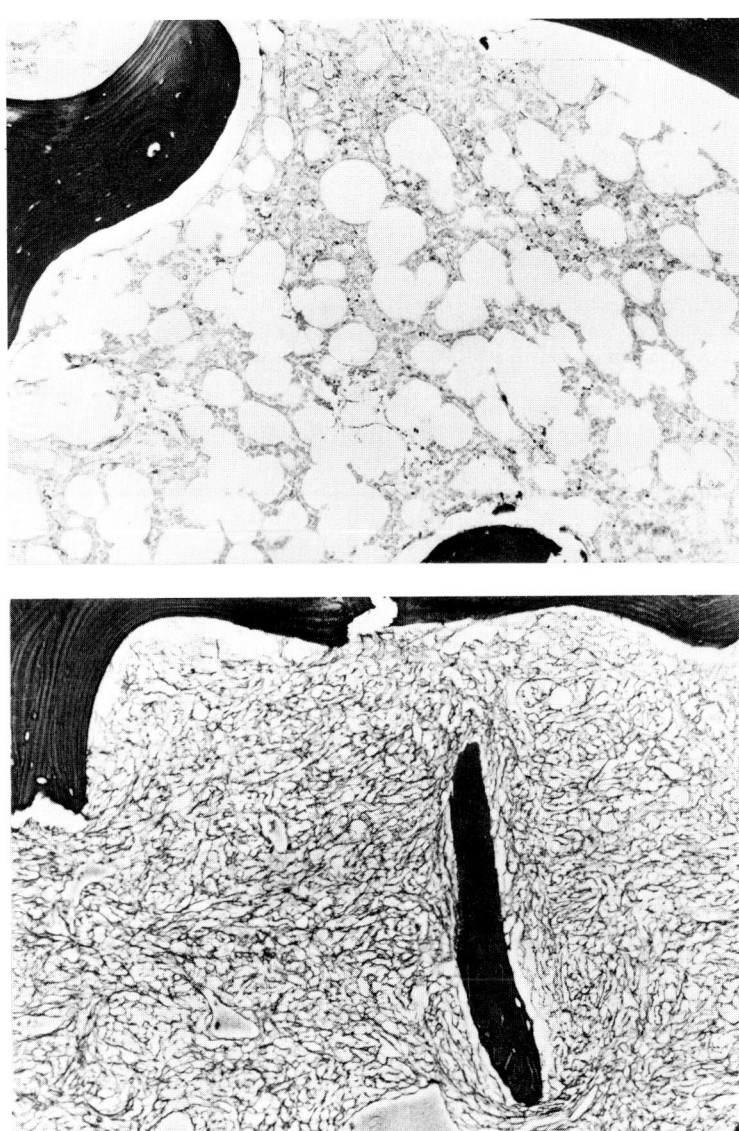

B

3.15   SPLENOMEGALY

With few exceptions disease involving the spleen will result in its enlargement, and splenomegaly is a frequent and important clinical sign in various haematological disorders. It is also enlarged as a result of infection, parasites, portal hypertension, amyloidosis, and lipid storage diseases. There are a number of disorders in which the effect of splenic enlargement comes to dominate the blood picture or at least is a significant factor in the anaemia, leucopenia and thrombocytopenia which occurs. The conditions in which splenomegaly, *per se*, is associated with a blood cytopenia are shown in Table 3.6.

The ways in which an enlarged spleen may contribute in the causation

Table 3.6   Important causes of splenomegaly

Inflammatory diseases
  Septicaemias
  Infective endocarditis
  Typhoid
  Infectious mononucleosis
  Tuberculosis
  Brucellosis
  Sarcoidosis
  Felty's syndrome
  Malaria
  Schistosomiasis
  Trypanosomiasis
  Tropical splenomegaly syndrome

Congestion
  Cirrhosis
  Portal hypertension
  Congestive cardiac failure

Reactive hyperplasia
  Chronic haemolytic anaemias
  Haemoglobinopathies
  Severe megaloblastic and iron deficiency
    anaemias
  Idiopathic thrombocytopenic purpura

Infiltrations
  Leukaemias
  Malignant lymphomas
  Histiocytic medullary reticulosis
  Malignant histiocytosis
  Myelofibrosis
  Polycythaemia vera
  (Non-tropical 'idiopathic'
    splenomegaly (?))
  Carcinoma
  Amyloidosis
  Lipid storage diseases

Cysts and Tumours
  Echinococcus
  Haemangioma
  Lymphangioma

of anaemia are now well established: three mechanisms come into play: (a) red cell pooling, (b) increased destruction of red cells and (c) expansion of plasma volume.

(a) RED CELL POOLING

By means of isotope studies it has been possible to measure the amount of blood concentrated in the spleen under different conditions. It has been shown that with normal spleens blood flow through the splenic circulation is 10–20 ml/min and when isotope-labelled blood is administered, equilibrium is reached within a few minutes. Splenic red cell volume is approximately 20–60 ml with a negligible amount in a slow mixing compartment. With enlargement of the spleen, splenic uptake kinetics indicate that in addition to the normal fast mixing compartment there is present a vascular slow mixing compartment which may have a half-mixing time as long as 30 minutes. When enlarged, the slowly exchanging pool may contain up to a third of the body red cell volume; this is particularly the case in myelosclerosis, hairy cell leukaemia and also, though to a lesser extent, in lymphoproliferative disorders.

(b) REDUCTION IN RED-CELL SURVIVAL

In most patients with enlarged spleens a mild or moderate reduction of red-cell survival can be demonstrated. This occurs even when there is no patent morphological abnormality of the red cell. Anatomically, red cell pooling occurs predominantly in the splenic cords, or when splenic enlargement is caused by malignant infiltration, in abnormal vascular channels created by the destruction of the normal splenic microcirculation. Because of plasma skimming, the stagnant concentrated masses of red cells in the pool are poorly perfused with circulating plasma and they have to compete unequally with metabolically superior nucleated cells of the red pulp for the available glucose. It has been suggested that as a result of glucose deprivation, the mature red cells are likely to suffer metabolic damage during the long periods spent in the splenic pool. With each return to the general circulation, the red cells have some capacity to recover but repetitious pooling will be deleterious and some of the cells will eventually develop irreversible metabolic damage.

(c) INCREASED PLASMA VOLUME

Splenomegaly, whatever the cause, is often associated with a rise in plasma volume which results in dilutional anaemia. The cause of this is unknown, but it is possible that the rise in plasma volume may be a readjustment which the body makes in an attempt to fill the increased vascular space. With increasing splenomegaly, a greater proportion of the total cardiac output is delivered to the splenic circulation, and the spleen may act as an arterio-venous fistula which in turn is responsible for the rise in blood volume.

3.15.1 IDIOPATHIC SPLENOMEGALY

Idiopathic splenomegaly occurs as a common condition in a number of tropical countries, notably in Uganda, Nigeria, New Guinea and the Congo. In some cases malaria has been incriminated but the disease is not the result of active malaria as parasitaemia is usually scanty and malaria pigment is not found in biopsy material from the liver and spleen. It seems more likely that it is an abnormal immunological reaction to malaria antigen. Clinically the tropical splenomegaly syndrome is an important cause of illness and death. Anaemia is often severe although leucopenia and thrombocytopenia tend to be only moderate.

There is also an idiopathic splenomegaly of a non-tropical nature, which is also known as 'primary hypersplenism'. Patients have moderate anaemia, leucopenia, neutropenia of a severe degree and moderate thrombocytopenia. The spleen is grossly enlarged and the liver may or may not be palpable. Histological findings have revealed splenic hyperplasia often with a disproportionate lymphoid proliferation, although not sufficient to justify a diagnosis of malignant lymphoma but suggestive thereof. It is thought that at least in some cases the patients may be suffering from a benign pre-lymphoma which has the potentiality of proceeding subsequently to overt malignancy (Pryor 1967, Blendis *et al* 1970, Weiss & Tavassoli 1970, Bowdler 1975).

3.16 THROMBOCYTOPENIA

Thrombocytopenia occurs when platelet destruction, utilization or sequestration exceeds the capacity of the marrow to produce platelets. There is a wide variation between patients in the level of platelet count associated with bleeding; in some patients spontaneous bleeding may occur when the platelet count is no less than $80 \times 10^9/l$ but in the majority of cases bleeding will occur only when the platelet count has fallen to $20–30 \times 10^9/l$. The functional capacity of the platelets may vary in different types of thrombocytopenia and as a result of dysthrombopoiesis. The disorders associated with thrombocytopenia are numerous and any attempt at a complete classification is not practical; in this chapter it is possible only to mention some of the more important causes of thrombocytopenia.

3.16.1 APLASTIC ANAEMIA AND MARROW INFILTRATION

Decreased marrow output of platelets will result when megakaryocytes are reduced in numbers as a result of haematopoietic failure in aplastic anaemia and when normal haemopoietic tissue is replaced by infiltration of the marrow by leukaemic or other malignant cells. The former condition may be idiopathic or associated with a drug or toxin known to cause marrow depression.

3.16.2 DRUG-INDUCED THROMBOCYTOPENIA

By contrast to aplastic anaemia another mechanism comes into play in the case of drug-dependent thrombocytopenia which occurs as a result of an immunological mechanism following the administration of a drug. A large number of drugs can cause this effect, notably quinidine, quinine and the sulphonamides. However, a much larger list of commonly used drugs including aspirin and codeine have been suspected of causing thrombocytopenia. The disorder is a self-limiting one and spontaneous recovery can be expected 2 weeks or less after cessation of the drug.

3.16.3 IDIOPATHIC THROMBOCYTOPENIC PURPURA (ITP)

This is a syndrome of unknown but presumably autoimmune aetiology characterized by bleeding manifestations, persistent thrombocytopenia and the presence of normal or increasing numbers of megakaryocytes in the bone marrow. Megakaryocytes are on average larger than normal so that the total megakaryocyte mass may be increased up to eight times normal. A number of megakaryocytes show absent or poor cytoplasmic granulation, and in the peripheral blood the few platelets which are seen may be abnormally large.

3.16.4 INTRAVASCULAR COAGULATION

Thrombocytopenia of severe degree is usual in acute defibrination syndromes. In subacute or chronic intravascular coagulation some degree of thrombocytopenia is usual and severe thrombocytopenic purpura and microangiopathic haemolytic anaemias. The cause of the thrombocytopenia is thought to be that platelets together with fibrin are deposited in the vascular system in the form of microthrombi, or the platelets may be absorbed to circulating or fixed immune complexes. Vascular damage particularly in the kidney may expose collagen and cause platelet adhesion and aggregation.

3.16.5 SPLENIC POOLING OF PLATELETS

As described above, splenomegaly with hypersplenism may result in thrombocytopenia. In health platelets released from the marrow appear both in a circulating platelet pool and in a splenic pool, the latter being about one-third the size of the circulating pool. In conditions associated with splenomegaly up to 90 per cent of the marrow output of platelets may be accommodated in the spleen, and this will lead to thrombocytopenia in the peripheral blood. The enlarged splenic pool exchanges constantly with circulating platelets and platelet life span may be nearly normal. However, as platelet production is controlled by the total blood platelet mass and not by the level of circulating platelets, there will be an underproduction of platelets.

3.16.6 ABNORMAL PLATELET FUNCTION

A number of conditions have been recognized in which a bleeding tendency occurs as a result of impaired platelet function rather than from reduced

S. M. Lewis

platelet numbers. The best known disorders in this group are thrombas-thenia (Glanzman's disease) and von Willebrand's disease. Mention should be made here also of thrombocythaemia: abnormal bruising and bleeding, especially from the gastrointestinal tract, occurs frequently in the myelo-proliferative disorders despite a high platelet count. The cause of the bleeding is not known but abnormalities of platelet behaviour have been demonstrated, notably impaired clot retraction, defective platelet factor III availability, reduced adhesiveness to glass and abnormal platelet aggregation (Hirsh & Doevy 1971, Turpie *et al* 1971, O'Brien 1972, Stuart 1975).

3.17 HAEMOSTASIS

The rapid arrest of haemorrhage following injury to the blood vessels requires a vascular response and a reaction which involves platelets and plasma constituents. The complex process whereby vasoconstriction occurs, platelets adhere to the exposed subendothelial tissue, a platelet fibrin plug forms and

Table 3.7 Properties of coagulation factors

Factor	Eponym	Storage stability	Present in serum	Adsorption by inorganic adsorbing agents	Effect of oral anticoagulant (coumarin; indanedione)
I	Fibrinogen	Stable	No	No	No effect
II	Prothrombin	Stable	No	Yes	Reduced
III	(Thromboplastin)				
IV	(Calcium)				
V	{ Proaccelerin { Labile factor	Labile	No	No	No effect
VI	Not used				
VII	{ Proconvertin { Stable factor	Stable	Yes	Yes	Reduced
VIII	{ Antihaemophilic factor { AHF	Labile	No	No	
IX	{ Christmas factor { Plasma thromboplastin component (PTC)	Stable	Yes	Yes	Reduced
X	Stuart Power factor	Stable	Yes	Yes	Reduced
XI	Plasma thromboplastin antecedent (PTA)	Stable	Yes	No	No effect
XII	{ Hageman factor { Contact factor	Stable	Yes	No	No effect
XIII	{ Fibrin stabilizing factor { Transamidase	Stable	Reduced	No	No effect

the blood coagulation mechanism becomes activated is well described in many standard textbooks. It would, indeed, be an impossible task to try to summarize the normal haemostatic mechanism and the detection of coagulation defects in this short chapter. The properties of some coagulation factors

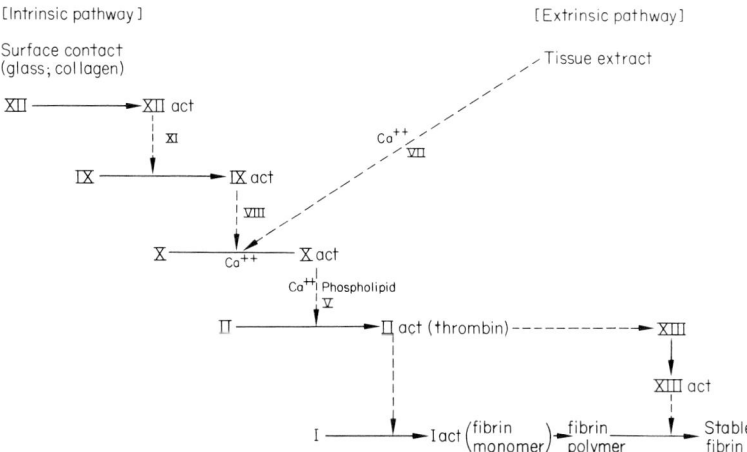

Fig. 3.40 Scheme to illustrate coagulation mechanism. The intrinsic pathway is activated by surface contact and involves specifically factors VIII, IX, XI and XII; the extrinsic pathway is activated by tissue extract and involves factor VII. The other factors are shared by both pathways.

Table 3.8 Causes of factor VIII deficiency

Congenital
    Haemophilia (sex-linked recessive)
    Female carriers of haemophilia
    Von Willebrand's disease (autosomal dominant)
    Combined factor V + VIII deficiency (autosomal recessive)
    Isolated factor VIII deficiency (autosomal dominant)

Acquired
    Factor VIII inhibitor
    Disseminated intravascular coagulation

---

are indicated in Table 3.7 and a scheme to illustrate the coagulation mechanism in Fig. 3.40.

    Disorders of haemostasis may be hereditary or acquired. Normally, all the hereditary disorders are due to a deficiency or an abnormality of a single clotting factor. By far the best known is haemophilia; this is due to factor

VIII deficiency caused by the synthesis of an abnormal protein with impaired biological activity. Other well-known disorders are Christmas disease which is due to a deficiency of factor IX and von Willebrand's disease where (by contrast to haemophilia) there is a true reduction in synthesis of factor VIII. Acquired coagulation defects are caused by disorders of synthesis, excessive utilization or inhibition of one or more of the coagulation factors. By contrast to the congenital disorders, acquired defects in synthesis of a single coagulation factor are almost unknown, and usually several coagulation factors are included together. Disorders occur as a result of abnormality of vitamin K metabolism, oral anticoagulant therapy, intestinal malabsorption or liver disease. Abnormal loss of coagulation factors occurs in intravascular coagulation and when there is a primary stimulation of fibrinolysis as during thrombolytic therapy with streptokinase. Inhibition of coagulation factors is the result of the action of antibodies directed against specific coagulation factors or by interference (e.g. by heparin) with some stage or stages of the coagulation mechanism. The complicated interrelationship of defects is illustrated in Table 3.8 which shows various forms of factor VIII deficiency which have been recognized, some congenital and others acquired. Combined deficiencies occur and this increases the complexity (Douglas 1973, Bennett 1974, Dacie & Lewis 1975, Biggs 1972, 1976).

4

THE HAEMATOLOGY OF EXOTIC MAMMALS

C. HAWKEY

4.1 INTRODUCTION

In this chapter the haematology of mammals other than the common domesticated and laboratory species is discussed. The animals included are mainly
those classified in the zoological orders Primates (monkeys and apes),
Carnivora (wolves, lions, bears, racoons, etc.), Perissodactyla (zebras,
rhinoceroses, tapirs), Artiodactyla (camels, giraffes, antelopes, wild cattle and
sheep), Cetacea (whales and dolphins), Pinnipedia (seals, sea lions), Rodentia
(porcupines, coypu, etc.) and Marsupialia (wallabies and kangaroos).
Domesticated and laboratory species are only mentioned for purposes of
comparison.

Comparative haematology at this level is a difficult subject, not only
because of the large number of species to be considered but also because
of the practical problem of obtaining blood samples from a large enough
number of healthy representatives of each species to establish normal ranges.
The information in the literature on the haematology of exotic mammals has
mostly been derived from study of captive animals and usually does not take
into account the effects of the captive environment and differences which
might be present in the natural habitat. Almost invariably, exotic mammals
studied in captivity or in the wild are subjected to a high degree of stress
which may influence the blood picture and the necessity of using anaesthetic
or tranquillizing drugs, often different for each species and usually with
unknown effects on the blood picture, imposes another variable on the findings. These problems must be constantly borne in mind when assessing the
results of comparative haematological studies. Other problems arise from
difficulties in determining the age, general health and sometimes even the sex
of exotic animals in the wild. Rarely have haematological studies on wild
mammals included large enough numbers to provide statistically valid normal
ranges subdivided for age and sex.

Comparative haematology is, however, an important subject since it provides a means of demonstrating basic haematological principles not evident
from the study of a single species. For example, it can be shown that, although
there is considerable variation in red cell count and size, the haemoglobin
level (Hb), packed cell volume (PVC) and MCHC are remarkably constant

throughout the Mammalia (Wintrobe 1934, Hawkey 1975) (Fig. 4.1). This illustrates the importance of the oxygen carrying capacity of the red cell in mammalian evolution and also suggests that the amount of haemoglobin per cell is functionally optimal. In addition, recognition of this principle contributes to the interpretation of results obtained on species for which normal values are not available since decrease or increase in Hb, PCV or MCHC beyond fairly narrow limits can be relied upon as evidence of anaemia or polycythaemia respectively. A second general principle which has become apparent from comparative studies is that, with regard to the red cell count, white count, neutrophil/lymphocyte ratio and measurable activity of blood clotting factors, closely related animals generally show similar values. For these parameters, findings from an animal for which the species normal is not known can therefore be interpreted with reference to the normal ranges of animals classified in the same family (see Fig. 4.2 and 4.3). Thus, by applica-tion of basic principles the difficulties arising from lack of established normal values for each individual mammalian species can to some extent be over-come. In addition, identification of basic principles must always be potentially useful as a contribution to the full understanding of theoretical haematology.

Most of the material to be discussed in this chapter has been derived from a survey of the haematology of healthy and sick mammals in the collection of the Zoological Society of London. The normal series has been described in detail elsewhere (Hawkey 1975). The discussion is approached from a general point of view and aims to describe the basic characteristics of mam-malian blood and the similarities and differences between the various groups of mammals. For reasons already stated, animals have mostly been grouped to their zoological order or family. Where possible, abnormal haematological findings associated with defined clinical signs are also discussed. Unfor-tunately, however, information on the clinical haematology of exotic mam-mals is even more difficult to obtain than normal values, partly because of the small numbers and selected populations available for study but also because of the practical difficulties associated with follow-up studies in species which must be subjected to the added trauma of handling and anaesthetization in order to obtain blood samples.

4.2 RED CELLS

4.2.1 GENERAL CONSIDERATIONS

The red cells of all mammals are anucleate and in all except members of the family Camelidae (camels, llamas, alpacas, etc.) they take the form of bicon-cave discs. In camels and their relatives the cells are oval and flattened. On stained smears and in wet preparations of blood, the red cells of normal mammals show little variation in size or shape. The presence of a significant

Table 4.1 Characteristics of normal red cells

	Polychromatic red cells	Reticulocytes % of red cells	Nucleated red cells	Howell-Jolly bodies	ESR mm/h (Wintrobe)
Primates					
Prosimii	+	1·1 (0·8–1·3)	+	+	<1
Cebidae	+	2·1 (0·4–7·9)	+	+	<1
Cercopithecidae	−	0·8 (0·1–1·6)	−	−	2·0 (0·1–1·2)
Pongidae	−	0·6 (0·2–0·8)	−	−	3·5 (0–9)
Carnivora					
Felidae	−	0·7 (0·2–2·0)	−	+	10·7 (4–19)
Canidae	−	0·7 (0·3–1·6)	−	−	2·0 (0·6–5)
Ursidae	−	0·3 (0·1–0·6)	−	−	2·5 (0–6)
Procyonidae	−	0·8 (0·4–1·0)	−	−	
Mustelidae	−	0·5	−	−	
Viverridae	−	0·5 (0·1·2)	+	+	1·0
Hyaenidae	−	0·5 (0·4–0·5)	−	−	
Artiodactyla					
Suidae	−	0·4 (0–1)	+	+	2·8 (2–4)
Camelidae	−	0·4 (0–1)	−	−	0
Cervidae	−	0·2 (0–0·5)	−	−	2·9 (0·5–8·0)
Bovinae	−	<0·1	−	(+)	1·0 (0–4)
Hippotraginae	−	<0·1 (0–0·3)	−	(+)	1·1 (0–4)
Caprinae	−	<0·1 (0–0·3)	−	−	1·1 (0–6)
Perissodactyla					
Equidae	−	<0·1 (0–0·1)	−	+	16·5 (2–30)
Ceratomorpha	−	<0·1 (0–0·1)	−	+	37·0 (7–59)
Proboscidea	−	<0·1 (0–0·1)	−	+	31·3 (21–40)
Rodentia					
Myomorpha	+	2·9 (1·7–4·2)	−	+	<1
Hystricomorpha	+	1·1 (0–1·8)	+	+	3·9 (2·8–6·0)
Cetacea	+	3·2	+	+	
Pinnipedia		1·9			
Marsupialia	+	1·0 (0–3·6)	−	+	6·0 (0–12)
Monotremata	−		−	+	7·3 (4–10)

degree of anisocytosis, poikilocytosis or hypochromia generally indicates an abnormality although at the present time there is not sufficient evidence to permit interpretation of these findings at the human level. Red cell rouleaux formation is marked in some species and virtually never seen in others and usually is not a useful clinical parameter. Polychromatic cells on a stained blood film, together with a high reticulocyte count are indicators of active erythropoiesis, but in some species are normally very common and in others are extremely rare; thus, the species or family normal must be known in order to assess their significance (Table 4.1). In some species a small number of nucleated red cells are generally present and in some, inclusion bodies similar in appearance to Howell-Jolly bodies are a normal finding. Again, the significance of their presence in individual animals must be assessed with regard to the species normal rather than to the human situation.

Red cell life span has not been measured in exotic species but judging by the reported variation in domestic and laboratory species (Schalm 1967), species differences would be expected. If it is assumed that a high reticulocyte count in normal animals reflects a rapid red cell turnover rate, then this is apparently increased compared with man in some New World monkeys, rodents and dolphins. However, such an assumption is not necessarily valid because, as has already been pointed out, in some groups of animals, for example the Perissodactyla, reticulocytes in the circulating blood are extremely rare, even in situations of acute blood replacement. In these animals it is likely that red cell maturation is completed in the bone marrow. At the other end of the scale, in those species with high reticulocyte counts, the reticulocytes may persist for an unusually long period in the circulation, thus contributing to the high count.

The main function of all red cells is oxygen transport and in all vertebrates, including mammals, the cells contain haemoglobin. As has already been mentioned, the amount of haemoglobin (MCHC) per unit mass of red cells is remarkably constant throughout the mammals (Fig. 4.1), the exception to this rule again being camels and their relatives. In these animals the MCHC is apparently increased; this may be partly due to the fact that their red cells are flat rather than biconcave and therefore presumably can hold extra haemoglobin molecules.

Throughout the mammals, electrophoretic analysis of the haemoglobin present shows much species variation and in many species, polymorphism is evident (Kitchen 1974). Knowledge of amino acid sequences of the globin moiety of the haemoglobin molecule has been used to establish evolutionary relationships amongst mammals and other animals (Goodman *et al* 1975). Although sickled red cells occur in deer and some carnivores, in these animals, unlike human patients with sickle cell disease, the condition is apparently non-pathological (Ball *et al* 1976) and in fact, haemoglobinopathies have not been described in any wild species.

In order to maintain a constant MCHC, haemoglobin levels and packed red cell volumes are also constant throughout the mammals (Fig. 4.1). As in man, decrease or increase of these values beyond a fairly narrow range

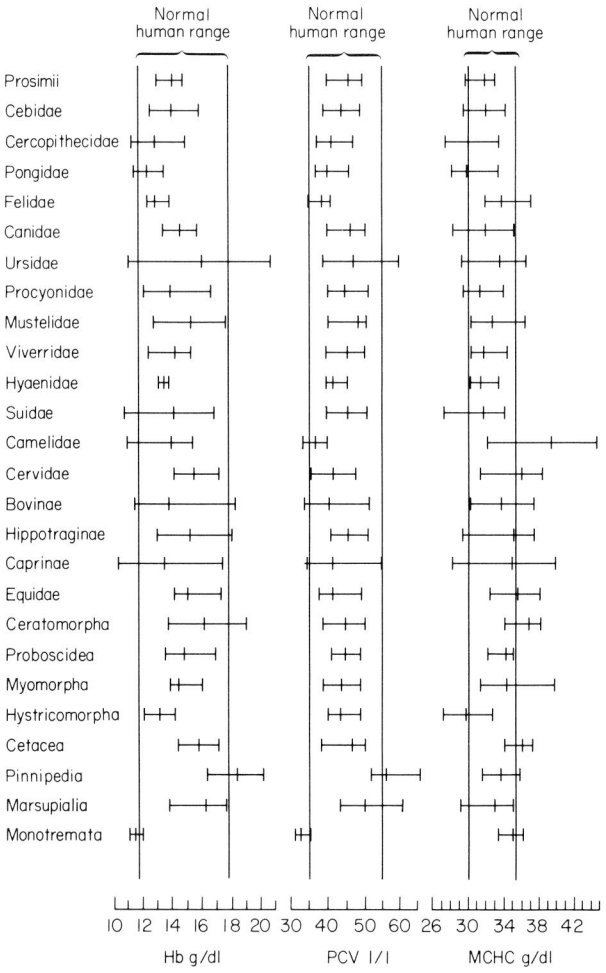

Fig. 4.1 Haemoglobin level, packed cell volume and mean cell haemoglobin concentration of normal mammals. Average values and ranges for normal animals in different zoological groups compared with the normal human ranges.

signifies anaemia or polycythaemia respectively. It should be noted, however, that the classification of the type of anaemia present in most mammals cannot be carried out with the degree of certainty usually possible in human patients. Because of the wide species variation in red cell size, to be discussed later, a morphological classification can only be used with reference to a firm knowledge of the species normal. Aetiologically, mammalian anaemias can be classified in broad terms into the 4 main categories, haemorrhagic, haemolytic, nutritional and aplastic or hypoplastic anaemia. However, within

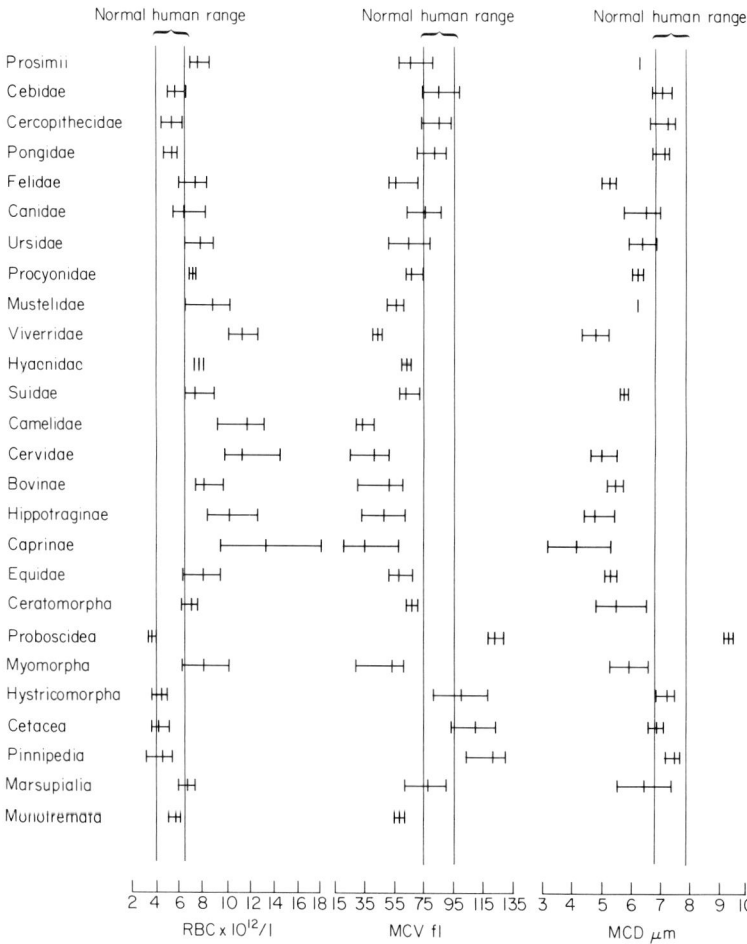

Fig. 4.2 Red cell counts and mean red cell volumes and diameters of normal mammals. Average values and ranges for normal animals in different zoological groups compared with the normal human ranges.

either of these classification schemes, methodological limitations and lack of information about species differences in factors controlling erythropoiesis impose great difficulties in the further stages of determining the exact cause or rational treatment of the condition. For example, an exact understanding of a haemolytic process occurring in an unusual species often demands a complete clinical history and species-specific diagnostic reagents, none of which are generally readily available. In the case of probable nutritional anaemias, it is known that, compared with man, some species require extra nutrient factors for normal erythropoiesis (Schalm 1967) and that some substances such as vitamin B_{12}, essential for human red cell production, are apparently without effect in other mammals (Siddons 1974b). Although mild or moderately severe anaemia is found with some frequency in captive wild mammals, much further information is required for a complete understanding of the aetiology and treatment of such cases.

At the other end of the scale, primary polycythaemia has not been reported in wild mammals but polycythaemia secondary to disrupted water balance or stress is relatively common and may mask underlying anaemia. It should always be borne in mind that sick animals are also stressed and, in addition, they often do not feel like drinking or may not be able to gain access to their source of water.

In contrast to the relatively constant values for haemoglobin and PCV, the red cell count in different groups of mammals is very variable (Fig. 4.2). There is an inverse relationship between red cell size and count, animals with low counts having large cells and vice versa, thus maintaining the constant PCV (Fig. 4.2). The smallest red cells yet described in mammals are found in the Malay chevrotain (*Tragulus javanicus*) and have a mean cell diameter (MCD) of $1\cdot5\,\mu$ (Duke 1963). The largest occur in elephants where the MCD is $8\cdot5$–$9\cdot7\,\mu$ (Hawkey 1975). It has been suggested that MCD is related to body weight (Wintrobe 1934) but this relationship does not hold good for mammals in general, although it may be applicable to species within an order. The presence of a large number of small cells increases the total surface area available for gaseous exchange and this would be advantageous in situations of low oxygen availability. It is interesting, therefore, that animals living at high altitudes often have small red cells. However, diving mammals such as dolphins and seals (Cetacea and Pinnipedia) which are periodically exposed to periods of low oxygen availability while submerged, have relatively large red cells which have a higher than usual average thickness. In these mammals the reduced rate of diffusion of oxygen out of the cells as a consequence of their greater thickness may be a means of ensuring a constant slow release of oxygen to essential organs during the dive.

At a practical level, species differences in red cell size must be appreciated when examining blood films from different animals. Whereas anaemia and polycythaemia can be diagnosed by applying basic haematological principles to the results of haemoglobin and PCV measurements, the red cell count, MCV and MCD can only be assessed in terms of the species normal. In this respect, species classified in the same zoological family usually have similar red counts, illustrating the general principle that for previously unstudied animals, some information can be gained about the expected normal values by studying figures for related species.

The last red cell parameter to be considered in general terms is the erythrocyte sedimentation rate (ESR). The rate at which red cells sediment under standard conditions is influenced by the size and number of cells and by their tendency to form rouleaux. Rouleaux formation is increased by high levels of fibrinogen and plasma globulins. In human blood, a raised ESR is considered to be a useful non-specific indication of a variety of chronic disorders and local inflammatory conditions. This test, however, cannot be used in the same way for other species. In some groups of animals, for example, members of the Perissodactyla, rouleaux formation is very marked in normal animals and the ESR is high by human standards. In others, such as some Artiodactyla, erythrocyte sedimentation is minimal even in grossly diseased animals. In addition to these predictable species variations, marked variation in ESR is often found in clinically normal animals of the same species. A comparative study of erythrocyte sedimentation should be useful in furthering the understanding of factors influencing this phenomenon.

4.2.2 RED CELLS OF NON-HUMAN PRIMATES

In recent years the use of non-human primates as laboratory animals has greatly increased and there has been a parallel increase of reports in the literature referring to their haematology. The reader is referred to the monograph on primate haematology by Huser (1970) for a comparative discussion of the subject.

In non-human primates the appearance of the red cells is very similar to those of man and, in general, human standards can be applied to monkey red cells. In the most primitive members of the group, the prosimians (lemurs, lorises, etc.) the MCD is slightly lower and the total red cell count correspondingly higher than in the more advanced groups. Some information on red cell survival time is given by Huser (1970). Although only a few species have been studied, judging by the frequency by which polychromatic cells and reticulocytes are found in the peripheral blood of normal animals it would appear that the rate of red cell production is higher in prosimians and New World monkeys (Cebidae) than in other primate groups.

Electrophoretic studies have shown that a single major component, indistinguishable from human haemoglobin A, occurs in chimpanzees, gorillas, gibbons and most Old World and New World species (see Huser, 1970 for review). In Pongidae and Cebidae a minor component similar to human HbA$_2$ is also present. Many species show haemoglobin polymorphism (Barnicot & Jolly 1966, Huser 1970); in some individuals (e.g. some orang utans, gibbons) a haemoglobin fraction moving closely together with human Hb-S is found, but these animals show no evidence of red cell sickling (Huser 1970).

This emphasizes the fact that similar electrophoretic mobility does not imply molecular identity. Haemoglobin polymorphism has not been associated with increased red cell destruction or any other haematological abnormality in non-human primates.

Physiological factors reported to influence the red count of non-human primates include seasonal and diurnal variation (Kuksova 1960), age, sex (Hodson *et al* 1967) and diet (Seymour Jones *et al* 1947). The latter effect may at least partly explain the findings that captive monkeys usually have higher Hb and PCV levels than animals studied in the wild (Allen & Carstens 1965, Foy *et al* 1965). Trypanosomes, microfilaria and malarial parasites are fairly commonly found in newly captured and imported monkeys (Capel-Edwards & Hall 1970, Wellde *et al* 1971). The blood picture is also influenced by stress (Ives & Dack 1956) and this fact, together with the possible effects of anaesthetic and tranquillizing drugs and frequency of bleeding (Wisecup *et al* 1968, Hawkey & Dean 1976) must be taken into account when assessing haematological findings in monkeys.

There is species variation in the degree of rouleaux formation present on stained films but marked rouleau is not seen in normal animals. The ESR is usually low but individuals with raised ESR in the absence of clinically abnormal signs are sometimes encountered. A raised ESR has been reported in pregnant rhesus monkeys (Allen & Seigfried 1966) and in the author's experience occurs sometimes, but not always, in animals with tuberculosis and other infections. The diagnostic usefulness of this test in infections has been discussed by Sauer and Fegley (1960). No correlation has been found between degree of parasitaemia and ESR in squirrel monkeys (Capel-Edwards & Hall 1970) and a normal ESR has been recorded in a gorilla with signs of rheumatoid arthritis (Clevenger *et al* 1971).

Individuals or groups of monkeys exhibiting a moderate degree of anaemia are fairly frequently found in captive populations. Haemorrhagic anaemia has been recorded in association with vitamin K deficiency of unknown aetiology in some new world species (Hawkey 1972), in prosimians with vitamin K deficiency in association with hypervitaminosis A (Rivers & d'Souza 1976) and in vitamin C deficient squirrel monkeys (Lehner *et al* 1968). Haemolytic anaemia has been encountered only in monkeys experimentally infected with malaria or with induced vitamin E deficiency (Hayes 1974). Folate deficiency in baboons is sometimes associated with macrocytic anaemia and megaloblastic marrow changes (Siddons 1974a) but vitamin B_{12} deficiency produces no haematological changes (Oxnard *et al* 1968, Siddons 1974b c). Macrocytic anaemia of pregnancy has been recorded in a few individuals and microcytic anaemia is a common finding in animals with secondary hyperparathyroidism.

Non-human primates are prone to haemoconcentration in association with gastro-intestinal upsets and occasionally with stress.

4.2.3 RED CELLS OF EXOTIC CARNIVORES

The red cells of carnivores are smaller than those of primates and the total red cell count is higher. Within the order the smallest red cells and highest count are found in members of the family Viverridae (genets, mongooses, civets, etc.) and the largest in canine animals. On stained films red cells of feline animals often appear crenated; this is thought to be an artefact produced by the anticoagulant used or during drying. In feline animals a small number of the red cells normally contain Howell-Jolly bodies. The haemoglobin level is often somewhat lower in the Felidae than in the Canidae and high levels are often found in ursine animals (bears). Haemoglobin polymorphism has been described in members of the Viverridae but not in other carnivores (Seal 1969). It is interesting that a non-pathological sickling tendency also occurs in three species of this family, the slender mongoose (*Herpestes sanguineus*) and spotted and blotched genets (*Genetta genetta* and *G. tigrina*) (Hawkey & Jordan 1967, Ball *et al* 1976).

It is reported in the literature that inclusion bodies resembling Heinz bodies occur in small numbers of the red cells of normal domestic cats and are increased in the presence of certain drugs and other chemical substances (Schalm 1965). This indicates a degree of instability of the haemoglobin molecule and this is apparently true of the haemoglobin molecule of other feline species since similar red cell inclusion bodies have been found in lions, tigers and pumas. The chemicals responsible for this finding have not been determined.

Physiological variables influencing the red cell count and PCV of domestic carnivores include age (Ederstrom & De Boer 1946, Anderson *et al* 1971), feeding (Reece & Wahlstrom 1970) and diet (Gower Smith 1944). Domestic carnivores are highly strung animals, particularly affected by stress and in stress situations a marked increase in red cell count and PCV occurs (Schalm 1967, Reece & Wahlstrom 1970). This phenomenon probably also operates in wild members of the order but is not evident in animals in which the blood sample is collected under anaesthetic. A significant degree of anaemia is apparently more common in captive wild Felidae than in Canidae. In both groups the cause is often difficult to define. Regenerative normocytic anaemia associated with haemorrhage has been found in lions, tigers and serval cats and is also reported in Aleutian disease of mink (Gorham *et al* 1965). In wild Felidae, normocytic anaemia without a reticulocyte response has been encountered in cases of hypothyroidism, renal failure and bacterial infection, and microcytic hypochromic anaemia in association with malignancy and hypoparathyroidism. Pregnant or lactating animals often show regenerative normocytic anaemia or slight macrocytosis. Seasonal variation in the red cell count of bears has been reported, possibly as a result of vitamin B_{12} or folate deficiency accruing during hibernation (Seal *et al* 1967). Microcytic hypo-

Christine Hawkey

chromic anaemia consistent with iron deficiency is apparently relatively common in American black bears (Youatt & Erickson 1958, Hock 1966, Seal *et al* 1967).

Normal ranges for the ESR have been worked out for domestic cats and dogs (Irfan 1961) but not for other carnivores. It appears that the red cells of Felidae normally sediment more rapidly than those of Canidae. In captive wild carnivores, erythrocyte sedimentation rates significantly more rapid than normal for the species and independent of co-existing anaemias, have been found in pregnancy (lion, New Guinea singing dog), malignant disease (lion, tiger, cheetah), traumatic injury (wolf, dingo, lynx, serval, leopard), hypothyroidism (coati, lion), bacterial infection (puma), arthritis (jaguar, cheetah), spondylosis (brown and striped hyaena) and renal failure (tiger). This list indicates that the test may give clinically significant results in wild Felidae and Canidae and warrants further study in this respect.

4.2.4   RED CELLS OF PERISSODACTYLA

The red cells of perissodactyls are smaller than those of man and the total red cell count is higher. Within the order, rhinoceroses (family Rhinocerotidae) have larger cells and lower counts than tapirs (family Tapiroidea) and equine animals (family Equidae). On stained blood films there is often some degree of anisocytosis and the cells may appear crenated. Rouleaux are always present to a high degree. Polychromatic cells are notably absent and in all animals in the order; reticulocytes are extremely rare, even in cases of severe regenerative anaemia. Howell-Jolly bodies are found in small numbers in zebras and rhinoceroses. In rhinoceroses, particularly in the white rhinoceros (Hawkey 1975) the red cells often contain single refractile bodies resembling Heinz bodies. These may be present in up to 50 per cent of the red cells without apparent clinical abnormality. Their presence has not been associated with any particular drug or chemical substance (Fig. 4.11).

In conjunction with the marked tendency for red cell rouleaux formation in perissodactyls, the ESR is normally high. This finding is well recognized in horses and for this species it is claimed that a 20-minute reading may be clinically significant, being decreased in some inflammatory conditions and increased in anaemia. These aspects of erythrocyte sedimentation have not been studied in wild perissodactyls.

The total red cell count is increased by stress and exercise in horses (see Chapter 5). Wild members of the group are, however, usually bled under anaesthetic which may obviate stress effects, but which introduces another variable factor. In horses the total red count is influenced by age and in wild equidae and rhinoceroses the red cell count is higher and the MCV lower in juveniles than in adults. Macrocytic anaemia of pregnancy has been noted in zebras. In equine animals and rhinoceroses newly imported from the wild red cell and Hb values are often lower than in animals maintained in captivity for some time, suggesting some degree of nutritional deficiency corrected by the captive diet. Clearly definable mild haemorrhagic anaemia associated with trauma is seen occasionally in these animals. Haemolytic anaemias have not been found in wild perissodactyls; the presence of Heinz bodies in rhinoceroses is not associated with reduced Hb levels although it must be admitted that red cell survival studies have not been carried out in these animals. The plasma of horses and other perissodactyls is often yellow in appearance (see p. 184). It is also important to remember that the reticulocyte count is not a useful parameter in the diagnosis of any form of anaemia in animals of this group.

An occasional finding in rhinoceroses is a moderate macrocytic anaemia associated with an increase in lobulation of the neutrophil nuclei. In one case the condition has apparently responded to vitamin B_{12}.

4.2.5   RED CELLS OF ARTIODACTYLA

This order includes several domesticated species for which the haematology is discussed elsewhere in this book (Pigs, Chapter 7; Cattle, Chapter 6; Sheep and Goats, Chapter 8; and Deer, Chapter 9). Within the order a clear distinction can be made between animals of the three sub-orders Suiformes (pigs and peccaries), Tylopoda (camels, llamas, etc.) and Ruminantia (chevrotains, deer, giraffes, antelopes and bovine animals). The red cells of the Suiformes are large compared with the average value for ruminants, while in camels and their relatives the cells are unique amongst mammals because of their oval shape. In all groups the inverse relationship between red cell size and number is well illustrated. The large number of small erythrocytes often found in ruminants has been related to the high altitude habitats often occupied by these animals. This group contains the animal with the smallest red cells yet described, the Malay chevrotain in which the MCD is 1·5 μm, but which is not, in fact, a mountain dweller.

On stained blood films the red cells of these animals usually show a slight degree of anisocytosis. The cells of the Suidae are often crenated and show some rouleaux formation. The oval cells of the Camelidae are unusual in several respects. They are flattened rather than biconcave and have a comparatively low mean cell average thickness (Bartels *et al* 1963). Their outline on stained films is less distinct than usual. They do not form rouleaux and their sedimentation rate is extremely slow. Cabot's rings occur with some frequency (Fig. 4.12) and Howell-Jolly bodies are sometimes present. A few reticulocytes are normally found in the circulating blood and the number is increased in anaemic animals where nucleated red cells are sometimes also present. Both reticulocytes and nucleated red cells tend to be disc-shaped rather than oval. Red cells of Camelidae have a high resistance to hypotonic salt solutions (Ponder *et al* 1928). This has been associated with a high water binding capacity of the red cell components (Perk 1963) and has been suggested as an adaptation to changes in the ionic strength of the plasma, resulting from infrequent but massive imbibition of water (Perk 1963).

The calculated MCHC for Camelidae red cells is invariably high compared with other mammals. This may be because the cells are flat rather than biconcave so that presumably there is more space for Hb molecules. Alternatively, the thin flat cells may pack more closely when centrifuged to obtain a haematocrit value, thus affecting the calculation. It has, however, been shown that the oxygen uptake per unit volume of these cells is 50% greater than in other mammals (Bartels *et al* 1963), suggesting that the high MCHC is a true finding.

In the Ruminantia the red cells are often small, but otherwise generally have no unusual features. An exception to this statement is provided by animals classified in the family Cervidae (deer) in which the red cells of most species exhibit a tendency to become sickle-shaped (Gulliver 1840, Hawkey 1975). Since the shape change occurs in oxygenated blood, sickled red cells are often present in small numbers on blood films dried in air or prepared from well-mixed EDTA blood samples. The subject of red cell sickling in deer is discussed further in Chapter 9.

Judging from basic haematological principles, captive wild ruminants belonging to the sub-families Bovinae and Caprinae often appear to be anaemic with relatively low Hb levels (Hawkey 1975). This finding may be a reflection of inadequacies of the captive environment but the groups include domestic cattle and sheep which also show comparatively low Hb levels (Ryan 1971a, Reda & Hathout 1957). Diurnal and cyclic variation in red cell count, possibly related to changes in water balance, have been recorded in cattle (Fiennes 1952), and may also occur in other bovine animals. Anaesthetic and tranquillizing drugs can also influence the red cell count; in wild impala and eland lower values for Hb, RBC and PVC have been found after anaesthetization with xylazine, alone or in combination with other drugs than in shot animals and this reduction has been explained by haemodilution with interstitial fluid correlated with drug-induced reduction in heart rate and blood pressure (Drevemo & Karstad 1974). These variables could explain some of the reported low values. If bovine and caprine animals do suffer from true low grade anaemia, the cause is not clear. Reduced MCHC appears to be relatively common, possibly associated with subclinical iron or copper deficiency or an excess of molybdenum. These animals are also prone to infection with intestinal parasites which may be responsible for chronic haemorrhagic anaemia. Macrocytic or normocytic anaemia has been recorded in pregnant Bovidae and in aged Bovinae, macrocytic anaemia is sometimes present.

Camels and llamas in captivity are also apparently prone to anaemia which is usually of a normochromic regenerative type. Unconfirmed haemolytic anaemia has been observed in captive llamas associated with Heinz body production and probably caused by chemical poisons. Interestingly, in this species, the Heinz bodies are not apparently associated with the red cell membrane but appear excentrically within the cells. Normocytic anaemia has been recorded in wild Suidae with bacterial infections and anaemia associated with grossly deformed red cells in newborn giraffes. Haemoconcentration is a relatively common finding in severely ill artiodactyls. This may mask underlying anaemia.

Although the ESR is not a clinically useful test in domestic cattle (Bunce 1954), results on captive wild ruminants suggest that in some species the test may function as a non-specific indicator of clinical abnormality as it does in man. Significant increases in ESR, independent of the red cell count, have been recorded in association with injury in deer and yaks, arthritis, acute enteritis and uterine cysts in deer and with general loss of condition in eland, nilgais, European bison, waterbuck, blackbuck, blesbok and wapiti. The test certainly warrants further study in these species. In Camelidae, as has already been mentioned, red cells show virtually no tendency to sediment even in grossly anaemic animals. In wild Suidae a small increase in ESR has been recorded in animals with acute bacterial infection.

4.2.6 RED CELLS OF ELEPHANTS

The red cells of elephants are amongst the largest yet described in mammals. The MCV is around 120 fl and the MCD often greater than 9·0 cu μ. In these animals the calculated mean cell average thickness is comparable with that of man and most other mammals. The total red cell count is around $3 \times 10^{12}/l$. Other than their large size, the red cells have no unusual features. Howell-Jolly bodies are occasionally seen. Adult African elephants have higher red cell count, Hb level and MCV than juveniles of the species and than Indian elephants. Reticulocytes are rare in both species. The red cells normally show a marked tendency for rouleaux formation and the ESR is rapid.

4.2.7 RED CELLS OF CETACEANS

There are several haematological adaptations to diving apparent in this group of mammals which involve the red cells. As well as an increased blood volume (Ridgway 1972) the Hb level is usually high, particularly in species such as Dall's porpoise which dive to the greatest depths (Ridgway *et al* 1970) and in these species the red cells are smaller than in, for example, the bottle-nosed dolphin (*Tursiops truncatus*) which is a relatively slow swimmer and shallow diver. Thus, in the deep divers, possession of comparatively smaller cells may be advantageous by providing an increased surface area for gaseous exchange although it should be noted that the cells are large compared with mountain dwelling species such as sheep and goats which are also exposed to conditions of low oxygen availability. Another adaptation to periods of anoxia experienced whilst diving may be the apparently greater than usual thickness of the red cells in cetaceans compared with most other mammals. It has been claimed that the red cells of man are of a thickness to permit maximum rate of oxygen diffusion out of the cell (Gibson *et al* 1955) and the fact that, irrespective of MCD, the red cells of most other mammals have a thickness comparable with those of man confirms the likelihood that a functional significance limits this value. Animals with thicker cells would be expected to have a reduced rate of O_2 diffusion; this may be advantageous in diving mammals where the cells could act as an important slow-releasing oxygen store during periods of submersion.

Thus, in cetaceans the high MCV is not paralleled by a high MCD. On stained films the red cells appear somewhat similar in size to those of man. Polychromasia is a regular finding and the reticulocyte count is normally greater than 3 per cent suggesting a fairly rapid red cell turnover rate. This fact is interesting because study of the red cell life span of laboratory and domesticated species (Schalm 1967) suggests a relationship between red cell survival time and body weight and therefore to basic metabolic rate, smaller animals having a faster turnover rate. The problems in using reticulocyte count as an indicator of rate of erythropoiesis have already been pointed out but it is remarkable that cetaceans are the only large mammals so far described which normally have a high reticulocyte count. These animals are also unusual in that their metabolic rate is higher than would be expected from their size (see Ridgway 1972). It would be interesting to study the red cell life span in these mammals.

Howell-Jolly bodies and, occasionally, nucleated red cells are seen in the peripheral blood of normal animals. Rouleaux formation is evident and the ESR is normally more rapid than in man. A trailing of reticulocytes is often seen when carrying out this test on cetaceans. There is no clear indication that the ESR is a clinically useful test in dolphins.

Stress does not appear to have a significant effect on red cell parameters in cetaceans (Andersen 1966, Geraci & Medway 1973). The MCV and Hb level often fall in newly captive dolphins but both return to normal with acclimatization. Little is known about iron metabolism in cetaceans but, compared with man, reported values for total iron binding capacity are high and the degree of saturation is relatively low (Ridgway *et al* 1970). Supplementation of the diet with iron, especially for newly captured animals, has been suggested (Andersen 1966, Ridgway *et al* 1970).

Haemorrhagic anaemia has been reported in the harbour porpoise secondary to haemoptysis and parasitic infestation (Andersen 1966) and the finding of 35 per cent nucleated red cells in the blood film of a wounded white whale after swimming for 6 days carrying a harpoon (Quay 1954) suggests

a massive marrow response to haemorrhage. Hypochromic and hyper-
chromic anaemia in animals suffering from parasitic infestation or dietary
inadequacies are relatively common (Andersen 1966). Haemoconcentration
associated with hepatic fibrosis of unknown origin has been reported (Medway *et al* 1966).

4.2.8 RED CELLS OF RODENTS

This order includes more than 1700 species, a small number of which are
commonly used as laboratory animals and are mentioned elsewhere in this
book (Chapter 15). The haematology of a few of the less accessible species has
been documented (Lord *et al* 1954, Strike 1970, Frankel *et al* 1972, Larkin
et al 1972, Hawkey 1975, Watson & Hawkey 1976). It is evident from the
information available that the variation in red cell count and size is wide, particularly in hystricomorph rodents (Hawkey 1975). This is perhaps not surprising since the blood picture of laboratory rodents is influenced by many
physiological and experimental factors and variation has been reported in different strains of mice (Russel *et al* 1951) and even in rats of the same strain
obtained from different dealers (Kozma *et al* 1969). Nevertheless, systematic
study of rodent haematology on a wide comparative basis may reveal interesting adaptations to the many and varied environmental conditions experienced
by these animals.

Generally speaking, the red cell turnover rate of rodents is rapid (Womack
1972, Schalm *et al* 1975) and reticulocytes, often occurring in clumps, are
common in the circulating blood. Nucleated red cells are sometimes seen
in normal myomorph rodents and in both myomorphs and hystricomorphs,
Howell-Jolly bodies in small numbers are present. Hystricomorphs usually
have larger red cells than myomorphs; the largest red cells yet described in
rodents are those of the capybara, the largest living rodent. In this species
sickled red cells have been noted (Hawkey 1975) but have not yet been studied
in detail. Rouleaux formation is not common in rodents and the ESR is
usually less than 3 mm in 1 hour.

Although congenital anaemias of various types have been well documented
in laboratory rodents (Bannerman *et al* 1973), these have not yet been identified in other rodent species.

4.3 WHITE CELLS

4.3.1 GENERAL CONSIDERATIONS

In all mammals the blood contains cells recognizable as neutrophilic, eosinophilic and basophilic granulocytes, lymphocytes and monocytes. There is,

however, much species variation in the total white cell count, the neutrophil/lymphocyte ratio, the morphology and staining characteristics of the cells in normal animals and in the response of the cells to physiological and pathogenic stimuli. In the following sections some of these differences will be discussed. It is evident that the white cell characteristics of closely related animals are generally similar and, as for red cells, animals of the same zoological order have been grouped together.

As far as is known, the white cells carry out the same functions in all

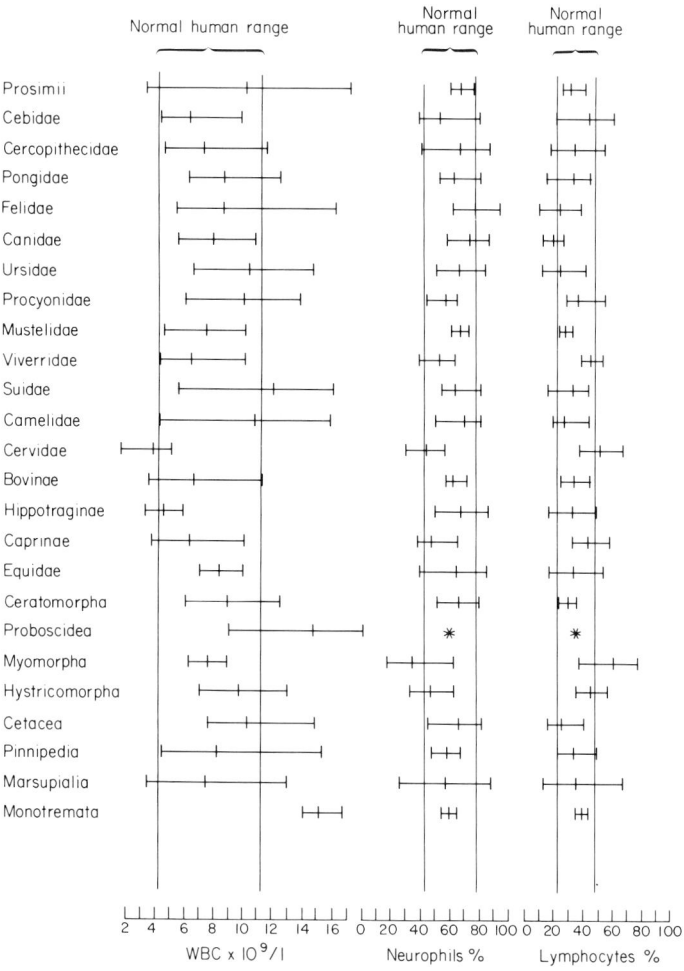

Fig. 4.3 White cell counts and percentages of neutrophils and lymphocytes of normal mammals. Average values and ranges for normal animals in different zoological groups compared with the normal human ranges.
* atypical mononuclear cells present

mammals. For domestic animals it has been shown that the degree of response to physiological and pathological stimuli is variable and this variation, as would be expected, extends to wild mammals. Generally speaking, species classified in the orders Primates, Carnivora and Cetacea show a marked leucocytosis and neutrophilia in response to bacterial infections while in Artiodactyla and Perissodactyla the response is less marked. In domestic animals there are also species differences in the effects of stress on the white count (Schalm 1967); this reaction has not been studied in wild species.

When interpreting the white cell picture in sick animals, results must be considered in relation to the species normal total count, which can vary from less than $2 \times 10^9/l$ in deer, for example, to $12 \times 10^9/l$ in elephants and some carnivores, and in relation to the expected response to pathogenic stimuli for the species. Unfortunately, data for most species with regard to the second of these criteria are not yet available. Of great importance is the examination of white cell morphology, particularly that of the neutrophils. In many instances this gives a better indication of the presence of toxic stimuli than the total white cell count and can also be used to distinguish stress effects. Toxic changes in neutrophils stained by Romanowsky techniques include the presence of early forms (a shift to the left), toxic granulation, blue-staining cytoplasm and cytoplasmic inclusions defined as Döhle bodies. Each of these variations requires comment and must itself be considered in relation to the species or group of animals under investigation. For example, a shift to the left may not be obvious in animals in which nuclear lobulation is not distinct, such as myomorph rodents and some artiodactyls or in species which normally have a low lobe count such as rhinoceroses (Fig. 4.9). Similarly, it must be borne in mind that in many groups (e.g. some primates, marsupials) the neutrophil nuclei are normally hyperlobulated compared with man. There is also much variation in neutrophil cytoplasmic granulation between the virtual absence of granules in some artiodactyls, through many degrees of moderate granulation which may be eosinophilic or basophilic or both, to the heavy eosinophilic granulation seen in rabbits and hystricomorph rodents and intense basophilic granulation described in the neutrophils of some primates and artiodactyls (Figs 4.6 and 4.8). Of these normal variations it appears that true toxic granulation is most frequently, but not always, found in moderately granular neutrophils; the apparently agranular types do not respond and in cells which normally show heavy basophilic granulation, a response is not distinguishable. Döhle bodies are useful indicators of bacterial infection in some species but have not been found in others.

For reasons already stated, little systematic information is available about the white cell response to disease in most wild species. In addition it must be appreciated that bacterial and parasitic infections encountered by wild animals in captivity probably bear little relationship to natural infections experienced in the wild. In the following sections, the normal white cell picture of animals in a number of mammalian orders is defined and the limited information about variation in response to bacterial infection and other pathogenic stimuli in captive wild mammals is discussed as a basis for further study.

4.3.2   WHITE CELLS OF NON-HUMAN PRIMATES

Figures quoted in the literature for the total white cell counts of normal monkeys are sometimes above the normal human range (Melville *et al* 1967, Huser 1970, Clevenger *et al* 1971). However, there is evidence that if strict care is taken to include only those individuals known to be clinically normal at the time of collecting the blood sample, normal ranges for most species are similar to those of man (Hawkey 1975). Physiological variables reported to influence the total white cell count include age and weight, sex and stress (Huser 1970). Some anaesthetic and tranquillizing drugs also produce an effect (Huser 1970). The count is usually above the adult count in newborn monkeys (Huser 1970) and, within the Primates as a whole, is often higher in prosimians than in New World and Old World monkeys and great apes. In great apes, like man, the neutrophil is the preponderant cell type in adults (Huser 1964, Hawkey 1975) whilst in other non-human primates there is considerable species variation in the neutrophil/lymphocyte ratio. Eosinophils, basophils and monocytes generally occur in numbers similar to those found in man.

When stained with Romanowsky stains, neutrophilic granulocytes show species differences in nuclear lobulation, types of granulation and in the staining properties of the cytoplasm. In most species the nucleus shows a larger number of lobes than is normally seen in man (Hall 1929, Huser 1970). Drumstick appendages are clearly apparent in females and other forms of nuclear appendages are relatively common in both sexes (Huser 1970).

The cytoplasm of the neutrophil granulocytes stains pale pink with Romanowsky stains. In most species the granules are small and pink. Heavy azurophilic granulation has, however, been described in neutrophils and other granulocytes of a few species, including the chimpanzee (Huser 1970). Döhle bodies are normally found in small numbers in some species.

The eosinophilic granulocytes, like the neutrophils, are characterized by the presence of hyperlobulated nuclei compared with those of man. There is species variation in the size, shape and staining characteristics of the eosinophilic granules and species variation in their ultrastructure has been demonstrated by electron microscopy (Huser 1970). In those species with heavy azurophilic granulation in the neutrophils, similar granules are also evident in the eosinophils. In some species the eosinophil count is often unaccountably higher than expected; an example of a species with a high eosinophil count is *Aotus trivirgatus*, the owl monkey, which is also interesting in that the granules of the circulating eosinophils are elongated although those in the marrow are spherical. In this species, reduction in eosinophil count can be a useful indication of stress.

Basophils compose about 1 per cent of the white cells in most species. Granulation is usually heavy, preventing the nuclear lobes from being counted. There is much species variation in size, shape and staining intensity of the granules. The cytoplasm when visible is pink in the great apes, as in man, but blue in Old and New World monkeys and prosimians. The relationship between species differences in the appearance of the basophilic granules and their classification as true basophils or circulating tissue mast cells has been discussed by Huser (1970) who concludes that the situation cannot be assessed without further study (Fig. 4.7).

On stained blood films the monocytes of non-human primates appear similar in size or smaller than the neutrophils. There is great morphological variability in the nucleus which may be round, indented, or may have 2–3 lobes. The nuclear chromation shows a coarsely linear pattern. The cytoplasm is abundant, greyish-blue in colour and may contain a number of small azurophilic granules. Transitional forms of monocytes have been described (Hall 1929, Huser 1970). In all primate species small and large lymphocytes are found, typically containing a well-defined, excentric nucleus, usually showing one or more indentations. The cytoplasm is clear blue and often contains fine azurophilic granules. Atypical lymphocytes occur in significant numbers; these include small forms in which the nucleus is deeply indented and may appear bilobed, large monocytoid forms with oval or indented nuclei and abundant cytoplasm reminiscent of the cells seen in human infectious mononucleosis and cells corresponding to human Türk cells in which the size is variable, the nucleus is round or oval, often with nucleoli and the cytoplasm is dark blue with a clear perinuclear area. These cell types are more frequently seen in normal non-human primates than in man.

Histochemical reactions of the white cells of non-human primates have been studied by Huser (1970). The results, summarized in Table 4.2, indicate interesting species differences in reaction.

The reaction of non-human primate white cells to infection and other types of pathogenic challenge can be difficult to evaluate because of the effects of physiological and experimental variables on the total white cell count. It has been claimed that counts as high as $30 \times 10^9/l$ can occur in healthy animals (Huser 1970), although this would appear to be exceptional. In the author's experience, neutrophilia in monkeys kept under standardized conditions and handled by experienced workers is usually associated with bacterial infection or trauma. In cases where the total white count is raised, the neutrophil morphology should be considered as an essential guide to the cause. A shift to the left has the same significance as in man but must be interpreted in the light of the fact that neutrophils of most monkeys have

Table 4.2 Histochemical reactions of primate white cells and platelets (summarized from Huser 1970)

	N	E	B	L	M	PL
Peroxidase						
Man	2–4	4	0	0	0–3	0
Great apes	2–4	4	0	1*	0–3	0
Old World monkeys	4	4	0	1*	0–3	0
New World monkeys	4	4	0	1*	0–3	0
Prosimians	4	4	0	1*	0–3	0
Alkaline phosphatase						
Man	1–2	0	0	0	0	0
Great apes	1–3**	0	0	1*	0	0
Old World monkeys	0–4**	0	0	1*	0	0
New World monkeys	0–4**	0	0	1*	0	0
Prosimians		0	0		0	0
Acid phosphatase						
Man	1	2	0	2	2	2
Great apes	1–3**	1	0	2	2	2
Old World monkeys	1–3**	3	3	2	2	2
New World monkeys	1	3	3	2	2	2
Prosimians	1	3	3	2	2	2
β glucuronidase						
Man	2–3	0–1	0	2	1–3	
Great apes	2–4	0–1	0	2	1–3	
Old World monkeys	0	0–1	0	1	0–1	
New World monkeys	0	0–1	0	1	0–1	
Prosimians	0–3		0	1	0–2	
Esterase						
Man	1	1	1	0	2–3	3–4
Non-human primates	2–4	2	4	1–2	1–2	3–4
Sudan black						
Man	1	1	0–1	0	1	
Non-human primates	1	1	0–1	1	1	
PAS						
All primates	4	1	4	1	1	

N = neutrophil, E = eosinophil, B = basophil, L = lymphocyte, M = monocyte, PL = platelets.

Key: 0 = negative
    1 = weakly positive
    2 = moderately positive
    3 = strongly positive
    4 = very strongly positive
* Some positive cells
** Species differences

higher lobe counts than human neutrophils. In these animals the presence of 3–5 per cent band forms is significant. Visible increase in basophilic granulation is associated with bacterial infection in those species in which granulation is normally obvious. Döhle bodies are found in healthy individuals of some species such as gorillas, but an increase in their numbers in neutrophils of species not showing obvious granulation is a reliable indication of infection. Neutrophil alkaline phosphatase levels are useful only in those species where the level is normally low or moderate; those with high normal levels cannot be expected to show a further increase.

Other clinical conditions reported to influence the white cells of non-human primates include folate deficiency which produces neutropenia associated with a shift to the right and the presence of giant metamyelocytes in baboons (Siddons 1974a). Vitamin B_{12} deficiency has no haematological manifestations in these monkeys (Siddons 1974b). In malarial infections, an increase in mononuclear cells is found with evidence of phagocytosis (Taliaferro & Klüver 1940). In aplastic anaemia of unknown aetiology, neutropenia with a marked shift to the left and toxic granulation has been recorded in Aotus monkeys.

Leukaemia in non-human primates is an important subject which cannot be discussed in detail in this chapter. Cases of spontaneous disease resembling chronic lymphocytic leukaemia in man have been reported and a case of myeloid leukaemia in a gibbon is discussed by Huser (1970). Radiation-induced acute myeloid leukaemia has been studied by Zalusky *et al* (1965) and Siegal *et al* (1968). Of major interest is the report by Lapin *et al* (1975) of induction of leukaemia in stump-tailed monkeys and baboons injected with material from human leukaemia patients. Lymphoproliferative diseases have been produced in some non-human primate species by Epstein-Barr virus (Epstein *et al* 1973a b) and herpesvirus (*Herpesvirus saimiri*) isolated from healthy squirrel monkeys has been shown to cause malignant lymphoproliferative disease in owl monkeys, marmosets and several other species (see McCarthy & Tosolini 1975). Recently the author has studied a case of spontaneous lymphoblastic leukaemia in a prosimian, the mouse lemur (*Microcebus murinus*).

4.3.3 THE WHITE CELLS OF EXOTIC CARNIVORES

The total white cell count of domestic carnivores (cats and dogs) is affected by stress and other physiological variables and reported normal ranges are usually wide. The influence of such variables on the white cells of wild carnivores has not been studied; these animals are usually tranquillized or anaesthetized before being bled and limited experiments on the effects of phencyclidine HCl, ketamine HCl or barbiturates have not demonstrated any significant differences. Normal averages and ranges for white cells of the families within the order Carnivora are given in Fig. 4.3. In most species neutrophils outnumber lymphocytes and age differences have not been noted. The neutrophil/lymphocyte ratio is higher in Canidae and Felidae than in Procyonidae and Viverridae.

Neutrophils stained with Romanowsky stains generally appear poorly granular although sometimes small pink granules are apparent. Nuclear lobulation is distinct and the number of lobes present is usually greater than seen in normal human neutrophils. Eosinophils contain closely packed, small round or oval granules and the cytoplasm, if visible, stains blue. Vacuolated eosinophils with dark blue cytoplasm are sometimes seen in wild Canidae and Ursidae; no clinical significance has yet been attributed to the presence of these cells. Generally speaking the granules are more intensely eosinophilic in feline than in canine animals. Basophils are rare in Canidae, Felidae and Ursidae but compose 1–2 per cent of the white cells in Procyonidae, Musteli-dae and Viverridae. Lymphocytes are represented by small and large forms and monocytes are relatively agranular.

In Canidae, Felidae and Viverridae the total white cell count is usually increased in response to bacterial infection, trauma and in malignant disease. In these animals counts of up to $45 \times 10^9/l$ are not uncommon, with marked neutrophilia and a shift to the left. Toxic granulation is not usually evident but the neutrophil cytoplasm may be blue-staining and, in Canidae, Döhle bodies are often present. The neutrophil response to bacterial infection appears to be less marked in Ursidae and Procyonidae but the number of animals studied in these groups is small and further experience may disprove this statement. A moderate neutrophilia without the presence of immature or toxic cells has been noted in bears with rheumatic disease and hyaenas with spondylosis. Eosinophilia is relatively common in most carnivores, sometimes in association with parasitic infestations or allergic dermatitis but often without detectable cause. Leukaemia has not been recorded in wild Carnivora.

4.3.4 THE WHITE CELLS OF PERISSODACTYLA

The normal average total white cell count is similar in members of the Equidae and Ceratomorpha and in both groups neutrophils are the predominant white cell in the circulating blood. A physiological neutrophilia occurs in horses in response to exercise and stress; this has not been studied in wild members of the group which are usually sedated before blood samples are collected.

When stained with Romanowsky stains the neutrophil cytoplasm is poorly granular. The nucleus is generally multilobed in Equidae but in Cerato-morphs rarely has more than two lobes. This is particularly evident in neutrophils of the white rhinoceros. Eosinophils of equine animals are striking for their relatively large, strongly eosinophilic spherical or oval granules whereas in ceratomorphs the granules are small, regular and spherical. In both groups, basophils are rare and only sparsely granular. Large lymphocytes are relatively common in all members of the order and in rhinoceroses the nucleus is pale staining and often bilobed. Monocytes are without unusual features.

In response to bacterial infections, a relative neutrophilia is usually evident; the total white cell count is generally less than $20 \times 10^9/l$, but occasionally counts of up to $40 \times 10^9/l$ are found. In Equidae the cells show a shift to the left but toxic granulation is not an obvious feature. In Indian rhinoceroses an increase in the number of nuclear lobes has been noted in animals with macrocytic red cells.

4.3.5   WHITE CELLS OF ARTIODACTYLA

The fact that the normal total white cell count is unusually low in some groups of animals in this order is important in the interpretation of results, particularly in sick animals. Counts of less than $3 \times 10^9/l$ are normally found in many species of Cervidae, Bovinae and Caprinae (Fig. 4.3). In domestic artiodactyls the total count is influenced by age (Holman 1955), breed (Ryan 1971b), pregnancy and parturition (Holman 1955, Moberg 1955) but these factors have not been studied in non-domesticated members of the group. In eland and impala, certain anaesthetic drug combinations have been shown to lower the white cell count (Drevemo & Karstad 1974). In cattle, sheep, pigs and goats and in most but not all wild artiodactyls, lymphocytes are the predominant white cells in the circulating blood. A reversed neutrophil/lymphocyte ratio is found in newborn animals of some species. Monocytes are present in expected numbers. Eosinophils are rare at birth but increase with age, probably in association with parasitic infestation. Basophils are generally rare but individuals may show up to 4 per cent of these cells.

On Romanowsky-stained blood films the degree of granulation of the neutrophil cytoplasm shows marked species differences. In some species, granulation is virtually absent (e.g. yak, gnu, reindeer) while in others, heavy basophilic granulation is apparent (e.g. llama, nilgai, moose). There is also species variation in the neutrophil nuclei; in many species the lobes are poorly defined. The eosinophils have small, well staining spherical or oval granules which usually do not fill the colourless or greyish-blue cytoplasm. The basophils show species differences in shape, size and staining characteristics of the granules. Of the lymphocytes, large forms generally predominate and in some species, cytoplasmic granules are prominent. Monocytes have no unusual features. Histochemical reactions of the white cells have not been studied in wild animals of this order.

In domestic artiodactyls the response of the white cells to bacterial infections is less than in primates and carnivores and the same may be true for wild members of the order. In a large series of captive wild artiodactyls studied, the total white count in animals with bacterial infections was usually between $15–25 \times 10^9/l$; counts of greater than $30 \times 10^9/l$ were extremely rare. The leucocytosis is due to neutrophilia with a shift to the left. In camels Döhle bodies are sometimes seen. A similar white cell picture has been recorded in association with malignant disease but some species show neutropenia in response to trauma. Marked eosinophilia is relatively common in individuals and groups of animals with intestinal parasites.

Lymphatic leukaemia is relatively common in domestic cattle but has not been described in wild Artiodactyla.

4.3.6   NORMAL WHITE CELLS OF OTHER MAMMALS

For a number of mammalian orders, white cells have been studied in normal animals although little is known about their pathological variations. In the following section, normal white cell counts and morphology in captive animals of some of these orders is described briefly to provide base-line information for further studies.

4.3.6.1   Pinnipedia

In seals and sea lions the total white cell count is normally between 4 and $12 \times 10^9/l$ and neutrophils outnumber lymphocytes. The neutrophils are poorly granular; their nuclei have an average of 4 well-defined lobes. In wild caught seals, eosinophils are relatively common, sometimes in association with the presence of microfilaria in the circulating blood. These cells have small, regular spherical granules which do not completely fill the blue-staining cytoplasm. Basophils are rare. The lymphocytes are usually small and monocytes are without unusual features.

4.3.6.2   Cetacea

In cetacean blood the total white count normally ranges from 4 to $12 \times 10^9/l$ and neutrophils are the predominant cell type. In the neutrophils, nuclear lobulation is only moderately distinct and the average number of lobes is 4. The cytoplasm of these cells contains sparse pink-staining granules. Nuclear drumstick appendages are prominent in female animals. In the bottle-nosed dolphin, neutrophilia occurs in response to bacterial infection and although a shift to the left is not always apparent, Döhle bodies are usually present in infected animals. The eosinophil count is usually relatively high in normal animals, often without evidence of parasitic infestation or other cause. These cells have well-staining spherical granules and blue cytoplasm. Eosinophils disappear from the circulating blood in stressed animals and in bottle-nosed dolphins a low eosinophil count has been found to be a reliable indicator of the presence of stress or disease. Basophils are rare. Most lymphocytes are of the large variety and the monocytes often contain reddish cytoplasmic granules.

4.3.6.3 Proboscidea

In both African and Indian elephants the total white count is normally relatively high; in captive animals ranging between 7 and $14 \times 10^9/l$. In captive adult African elephants neutrophils outnumber lymphocytes while in wild adult African elephants and in all adult Indian elephants and juveniles of both species, the neutrophil/lymphocyte ratio is reversed. In both species a significant proportion of large cells with clear blue cytoplasm and distinctly bilobed nuclei occur. These cells have been variously classified as lymphocytes (Nirmalan *et al* 1967) or monocytes (Schalm *et al* 1975). No clinical significance has been attributed to their presence.

The neutrophils of elephants show sparse pink cytoplasmic granulation. Their nuclei normally have 2–4 lobes. The eosinophil granules are small and spherical, barely filling the colourless cytoplasm. Basophils are rare. The majority of the lymphocytes are of the large variety and monocytes are without unusual features.

4.3.6.4 Rodentia

The white cells of those rodents commonly used as experimental animals are mentioned elsewhere in this book. Some comments on comparative differences in white cells of rodents as a whole, derived from studies of less common species, are however of interest. There is apparently much species and individual variation in the total white count of animals in this order. In some species (e.g. grey squirrels, casiraguas, cuis) the count is often less than $3 \times 10^9/l$. In most but not all species, lymphocytes outnumber neutrophils in normal individuals. In those rodents classified in the sub-order Myomorpha (rats, mice, hamsters, etc.) the neutrophil nuclei are often without obvious lobulation and take the form of horseshoes, twisted sausages or rings. In contrast, in hystricomorph rodents (guinea pigs, cuis, capybara, coypu, casiraguas, etc.) and in the few Sciuromorpha (squirrels) examined the neutrophil nuclei have distinct lobes, often showing a shift to the right compared with man. The neutrophil cytoplasm of hystricomorph but not of other rodents contains well-marked eosinophilic granules, similar to those found in rabbits (Hawkey 1975) and responsible for the classification of these cells as 'pseudoeosinophils'. The most extreme example of this phenomenon occurs in capybaras, but even in this species the size and distribution of the granules in pseudoeosinophils does not lead to confusion of the cells with true eosinophils. In the neutrophils of wild-trapped grey squirrels, parasites, probably haemogregarines, are sometimes present.

Guinea pig lymphocytes are of interest for the occasional presence of cytoplasmic inclusion bodies known as Kurloff bodies (Schermer 1967). These inclusions have not been observed in cells of the cuis (wild guinea pig) or any other rodent species studied (Watson & Hawkey 1976).

4.3.6.5   Marsupialia

In animals of this order there is species variation in the total white cell count and neutrophil/lymphocyte ratio. The neutrophil cytoplasm generally contains distinct basophilic granules. The nucleus may be hyperlobulated but in some species lobulation is indistinct. Eosinophil granules are small and spherical, and do not fill the greyish-blue cytoplasm. Basophils are rare and lymphocytes and monocytes are without unusual features. In the Bennetts wallaby, the neutrophil/lymphocyte ratio is reversed in immature animals.

4.4   BLOOD PLATELETS

4.4.1   GENERAL CONSIDERATIONS

Platelets are found in the blood of all mammals as anuclear cytoplasmic fragments. The platelet count varies from around $100 \times 10^9/l$ in some dolphins to greater than $600 \times 10^9/l$ in elephants and some carnivores and rodents. Species differences in the size of platelets have been observed but not quantitated. In carefully collected blood samples, the platelets normally appear disc-shaped with occasional dendritic pseudopodia. An interesting shape variation has been noted in the platelets of spiny anteaters, primitive mammals in which two populations of platelets are apparently present. In 3 species of spiny anteater (*Tachyglossus setosus*, *T. aculeatus* and *Zaglossus bruijni*) about 50 per cent of the platelets appear in wet preparations and on stained films as elongated structures without spreading tendencies in contrast to the remaining platelets which are similar to normal mammalian platelets (Hawkey 1975) (Fig. 4.10).

Although it is evident that platelets carry out the same haemostatic functions in all mammals, the results of published studies on platelet structure and reactivity in common laboratory animals and amongst different primate species indicate that there are marked species differences in response to aggregating agents (Mason & Read 1967, Sinakos & Caen 1967, Hawkey & Symons 1968, Mills 1970, Tschopp 1970, Loeb & Makey 1973, Hawkey 1975) and in inhibition of aggregation (Hawkey & Symons 1968, Mills 1970, Donner & Houskova 1972). The relative amounts of adenine nucleotides

(Mills & Thomas 1969, Mills 1970), 5-hydroxytryptamine and histamine (Humphrey & Toh 1954, Baumgartner & Born 1968) vary with species and species differences in platelet surface glycoproteins have been demonstrated (Nurden 1974, 1976). Limited results of platelet function tests on representative wild species are given in Table 4.3 and Fig. 4.4, but it must be emphasized that within a related group of animals, species differences in the results of standard platelet function tests are likely to be encountered. This may render diagnosis of functional platelet defects in a given individual difficult unless

Table 4.3 Platelet characteristics of mammals

Order	Count × 10⁹/l	Adhesive index %	Clot retraction %	Platelet factor 3 total	release
Primates	260	44	64	107	65
(non-human)	(147–468)	(27–75)	(52–71)	(80–133)	(58–81)
Carnivora	319	46	63	82	64
	(150–634)	(26–69)	(55–70)	(74–89)	(55–80)
Perissodactyla	266	58	50	77	57
	(154–634)		(46–65)	(73–83)	(56–68)
Artiodactyla	317	81	61	109	63
	(140–512)		(50–78)	(84–152)	(42–85)
Rodentia	320		62	106	64
	(192–459)		(61–65)	(89–124)	(58–70)
Pinnipedia	456			86	63
Cetacea	410				
Proboscidea	540			75	72
	(455–677)				
Marsupialia	258				
	(148–427)				
Monotremata	215				
	(195–235)				
Normal human	210	30	63	104	79
values	(140–342)	(24–36)	(57–68)	(100–120)	(71–90)

a normal representative of the same species is tested at the same time. Species variation can also lead to interpretation problems when animal models are used to further the understanding of human platelet function.

Thrombocytopenia is encountered only rarely in wild animals in captivity. Cases studied include thrombocytopenia in association with diffuse intravascular coagulation in a Baikal seal with haemolytic anaemia of unknown origin and in Aotus monkeys experimentally infected with malaria (Voller *et al* 1969). A reduction in platelet count is one of the first abnormalities evident in experimental folate deficiency in baboons (Siddons 1974a).

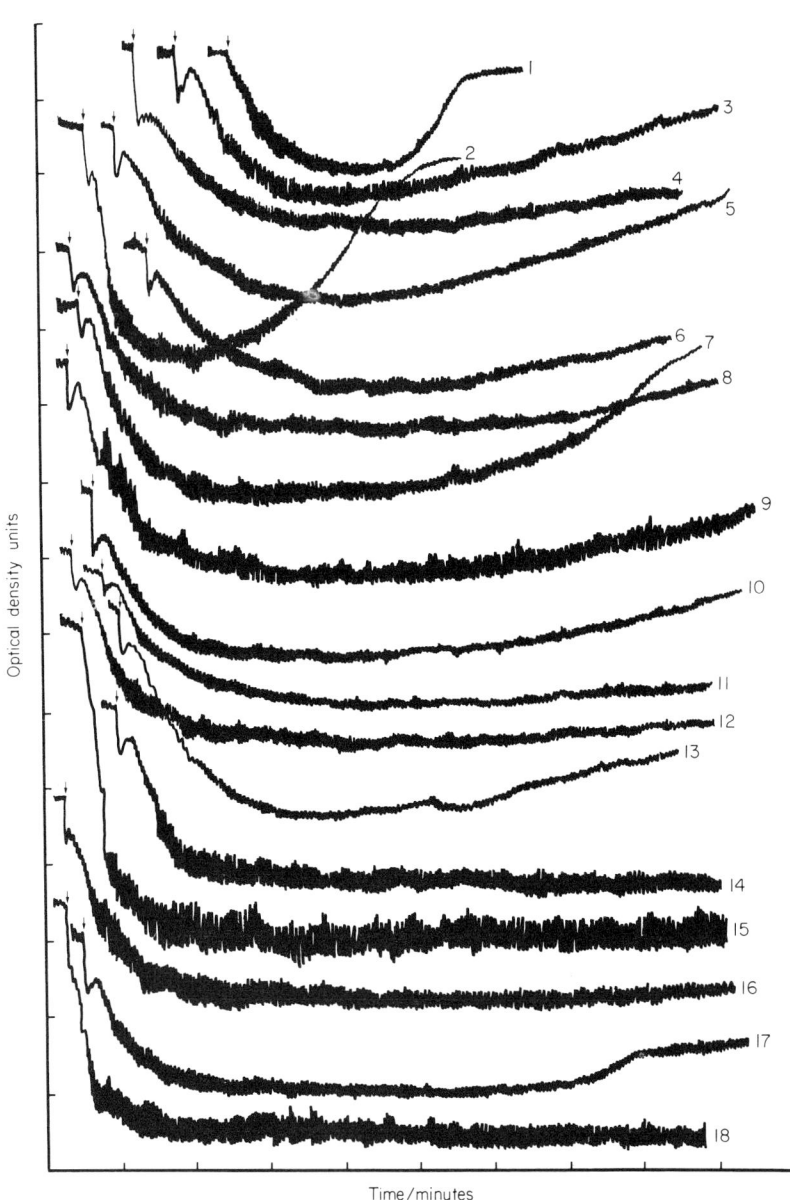

Fig. 4.4 ADP-induced platelet aggregation in normal Primates. ADP at a final concentration of 30 μM added to platelet-rich plasma adjusted to contain 400×10^9 platelets/l. Arrows indicate point of addition of ADP.

Key: 1. Chimpanzee (*Pan troglodytes*). 2. Yellow baboon (*Papio cynocephalus*). 3. Diana monkey (*Cercopithecus diana*). 4. Sacred baboon (*Papio hamadryas*).

Thrombocytopenia together with neutropenia and reduced erythropoiesis has also been recorded in Aotus monkeys receiving intravenous BCG vaccine (Voller & Hawkey 1976).

Functional platelet defects have not been reported in non-laboratory species. Congenital varieties of these conditions are unlikely to be found for reasons to be discussed later. It should be borne in mind that the platelet abnormality described in human patients with scurvy (Hardisty, 1969) and in scorbutic guinea pigs (Born & Wright 1968) could probably arise in other mammalian species (all primates, fruit bats) which do not synthesize their own vitamin C.

4.5 BLOOD COAGULATION

4.5.1 GENERAL CONSIDERATIONS

Comparative studies on blood coagulation in mammals have almost always taken the human coagulation mechanism as the theoretical starting point and have used human methodology to demonstrate species similarities and differences throughout the group. This approach has led to a useful understanding of the coagulation process in mammals in general and, although there are considerable difficulties in interpreting the results of some standard tests employing human reagents, it can be shown that, with certain specific exceptions, the same plasma clotting factors are present in the blood of all normal mammals. There may, however, be marked differences in the measurable activity of these factors. Both congenital and acquired coagulation defects similar to those found in human patients have been identified in some other mammalian species. It is of interest that the congenital defects reported have been confined to domesticated animals such as dogs, horses and cattle (see Chapters 10, 5 and 6). This may be because larger numbers of individuals of these species have been available for examination but it is also unlikely that wild animals with defective blood coagulation would survive the processes of natural selection in their natural habitat. Acquired coagulation deficiencies are not common in captive wild animals but they are occasionally found and it is probable that the same aetiological factors operate in all species. Provided that species variation in clotting factor activity and methodological

---

5. Rhesus monkey (*Macaca mulatta*). 6. Gelada baboon (*Theropithecus gelada*).
7. Patas monkey (*Erythrocebus patas*). 8. Hoolock gibbon (*Hylobates hoolock*).
9. Sooty mangabey (*Cercocebus torquatus*). 10. Black ape (*Cynopithecus niger*).
11. Mona monkey (*Cercopithecus mona*). 12. Pig-tailed monkey (*Macaca nemestrina*). 13. Crab-eating monkey (*Macaca irus*). 14. Stump-tailed monkey (*Macaca speciosa*). 15. Assamese macaque (*Macaca assamensis*). 16. Man (*Homo sapiens*). 17. Moor monkey (*Macaca maurus*). 18. Brown capuchin (*Cebus apella*).

Table 4.4 Acquired haemorrhagic defects in exotic mammals requiring further investigation

Species	Symptoms	Abnormal laboratory tests	Presumptive diagnosis	Aetiology
Aotus monkeys	Subcutaneous and intramuscular haemorrhage. Blood in faeces	Prolonged prothrombin time, corrected by injection of vitamin K_1. Severe normocytic anaemia	Vitamin K deficiency	Unknown
Cebus monkeys	Subcutaneous haemorrhage of scalp	None	Vitamin C deficiency	Dietary insufficiency
Tree shrew	Cerebral and/ or subcutaneous haemorrhage. Yellow discoloration of tissues	Prolonged prothrombin time or thrombotest. Severe anaemia	Vitamin K deficiency associated with hypervitaminosis A.	Vitamin A enriched diet
Baboon	Prolonged bleeding from puncture wounds	Reduced fibrinogen. Low platelet count. Severe normocytic anaemia	Diffuse intravascular coagulation	Haemorrhagic shock associated with experimental bleeding.

difficulties are taken into account, it should be possible to diagnose these conditions by the same criteria as used for human studies. Occasionally, however, spontaneous haemorrhagic conditions are encountered in captive wild animals where practical problems prevent complete characterization of the defect. Some examples of these are given in Table 4.4.

In the following sections, methodological problems and species similarities and differences in clotting factor levels in normal mammals are discussed in order to provide a basis for clinical diagnosis. As before, closely related animals are considered together and it is evident that species of the same order or family generally show a similar pattern of coagulation activity. Acquired coagulation abnormalities are described in the few species where they have been encountered.

4.5.2 METHODOLOGICAL PROBLEMS IN COMPARATIVE CLOTTING FACTOR ASSAYS

Apart from fibrinogen, clotting factors are trace proteins and cannot at the present time be measured in plasma in absolute amounts. In human blood, prothrombin and factors V, VII, VIII, IX, X, XI and XII are assayed by the ability of test plasma to correct the clotting time of substrate plasma specifically deficient in the factor in question and the results are expressed as a percentage of the mean activity present in normal human plasma (Hardisty & Ingram 1965). For clotting factor measurements on plasma from other species, this approach raises several problems.

Substrate plasmas for clotting factor assays are usually obtained from human patients with severe congenital coagulation defects—for example factor VIII is measured by the degree of correction by test plasma of the clotting time of plasma containing less than 1 per cent factor VIII obtained from a human patient with severe haemophilia. For some factors (e.g. factor V) (Stefanini 1951, Wolf 1953) substrate plasma can be artificially prepared but the starting material is usually human plasma and the methods of preparation have not been standardized for plasma from other species. Apart from some domesticated species in which severe congenital coagulation defects have been found, species-specific substrate plasmas are generally not available. It is known that for many of the inter-protein reactions involved in the coagulation process, reactivity is not optimal between factors of different species. The most obvious example of this phenomenon, which is usually termed 'species specificity', is in the reaction between tissue factor and factors VII and X where the problem has been most extensively studied (Mann & Hurn 1952, Hawkey & Stafford 1961, Irsigler *et al* 1965). For many factors, however, the potential influence of minor differences in molecular structure and function of clotting factors on their reaction in heterologous test mixtures is not known. It must, therefore, be clearly understood that in any clotting test in which a mixture of plasma from animals of different species is used to assess the coagulation process, the measured activity may be less than the true value, and the results obtained may be of no relevance to physiological haemostasis in the animal being tested. In practice it is usual to accept results as valid if the animal plasma shows as much as or more than the normal human level of activity. Low levels of activity recorded in heterologous test systems are, however, very difficult to interpret and the problem becomes worse the less closely related to man the test animal is. The difficulty can be illustrated by an example from a non-mammalian vertebrate. An apparent lack of factor VIII activity has been demonstrated in blood of the clawed toad (*Xenopus laevis*) by failure of toad plasma to correct the clotting time of blood from a human haemophiliac. However, it is also possible to show that this animal has a short whole blood clotting time and that prothrombin activation by an intrinsic activation pathway takes place as rapidly in toad plasma as in normal human plasma (Anstall & Huntsman 1960). These findings could mean that the intrinsic coagulation pathway in toads does not require the presence of factor VIII but the possibility that toad factor VIII does not react with human factor IX can by no means be ruled out. The net result of the difficulty is that although positive answers in coagulation assays may be valid, negative answers cannot be interpreted at present. This should be borne in mind when assessing the results of all comparative studies of the coagulation mechanism including those reported in this chapter.

A second problem stems from the practice of expressing the activity of plasma clotting factors as a percentage of the activity present in normal human plasma (Hardisty & Ingram 1965). When clotting factors from other mammals are measured in human assay systems and their activity is expressed in terms of the normal human value it can be shown that the activity of some factors, particularly factor VIII, is as much as 10 times the value found in man. The question then posed is what does this mean in terms of physiological haemostasis in individual animals? Is it justifiable to interpret these results to mean that the coagulation process is more efficient in, for example, a Malay tapir with 850 per cent factor VIII than in a human individual with only 100 per cent factor VIII? This problem in interpretation arises on 2 scores, the first of which is that the results have been obtained in heterologous test systems and possibly if tapir factor VIII was assayed in a tapir system it would be found that the factor VIII activity was limited by a low level of some other factor. This particular question can be answered to some extent by carrying out whole blood clotting times on a comparative basis. In this test the time taken for native blood to clot under standard conditions is measured; there is no addition of any biological or chemical reagents. When the whole blood clotting times of mammals are measured by thrombelastography, generally speaking they are shorter than the average normal human value (Hawkey 1975). This finding supports the conclusion that high levels of some clotting factors give rise to an increased coagulation potential *in vitro*, but the relevance of this to physiological haemostasis is not known. It is, however, interesting to speculate that wild animals, both predators and prey, may need a more efficient haemostatic mechanism than civilized man in his protected natural environment.

4.5.3 SPECIES SPECIFICITY

Tissue factor, which brings about rapid clotting of recalcified, citrated human plasma via the extrinsic pathway of factor X activation can be extracted from most organs and tissues of the body. Brain, lung and placenta are particularly

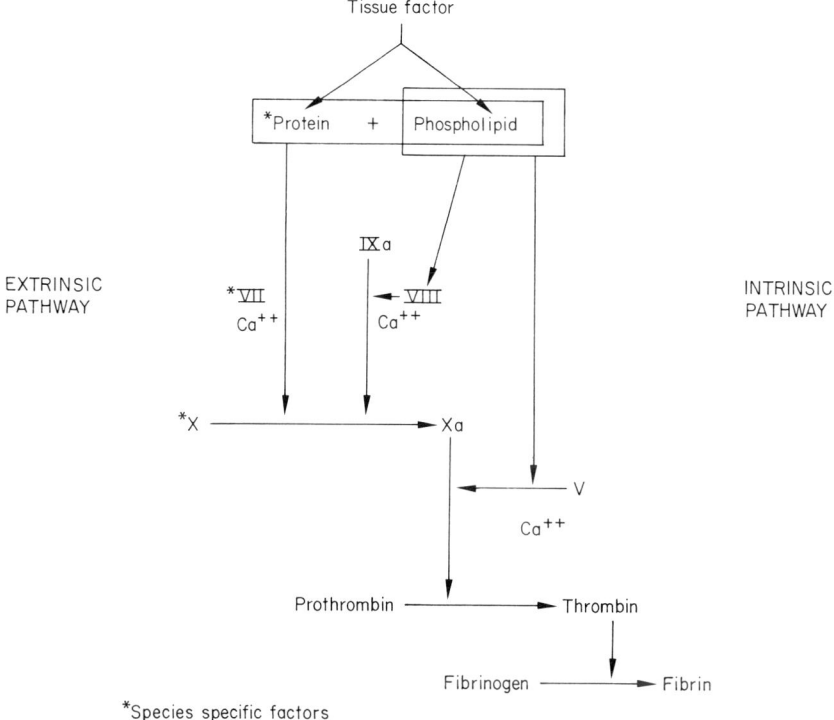

Fig. 4.5 The part played by tissue factor in human blood coagulation.

active in this respect (Quick 1935, Biggs & Macfarlane 1962). It has been shown that human tissue factor is made up of two components, a phospholipid fraction and a protein fraction (Chargaff *et al* 1944). In combination these activate factor X in a reaction accelerated by factor VII (Esnouf 1972). The phospholipid fraction also takes part in the reaction by which prothrombin is converted to thrombin by factor Xa and in the reaction of factor VIII with factors IXa and X (Biggs 1972). These reactions are shown in

Fig. 4.5. Phospholipid from tissue of any mammalian species reacts equally well with factors V and VIII from any other, thus species specificity does not affect the intrinsic pathway of prothrombin activation (Fig. 4.5). The protein component, however, does not always react optimally with heterologous factors VII and X (Mann & Hurn 1952, Hawkey & Stafford 1961) and is responsible for the problem of 'species specificity'. Thus, in the one-stage prothrombin test and in clotting factor assays depending on modifications of this method, combinations of tissue thromboplastin and plasma from different species may indicate spuriously low levels of clotting activity.

Table 4.5 Cross reactivity of tissue factor and plasma of mammals

Plasma from	Clotting time (secs) with brain thromboplastin from							
	Human	Rhesus monkey	Moor monkey	Patus monkey	Cebus monkey	Dingo	Lion	Rabbit
Human	14	15	15	14	14	28	23	13
Rhesus monkey	15	14	14	14	14			13
Moor monkey	15	14	14	15	14			14
Patas monkey	14	14	14	14	14	20		14
Cebus monkey	14	14	14	14	14			13
Dingo	9	10	9	10		7	10	
Mongoose	15	15	16	15			14	
Lynx	13			14			12	
Bear	9			9			9	
Rabbit	15	14	15	14				
Zebra	49			40				
White rhino	18			20				
Blesbok	16			20				
Mouse	11			10				
Porcupine	26	25	30	30				
Wallaby	80	75	83	76				
Echidna	44			49				

In fact, the term 'species specificity' is apparently a misnomer since tissue factor from a given mammal will cross-react normally with plasma from other species in the same zoological order. In addition there is often apparently normal cross-reactivity between mammals of different orders. Standardized human tissue factor gives normal one-stage prothrombin times with plasma from other primates, carnivores, Suidae, Caprinae, rabbits, myomorph rodents, cetaceans, seals and elephants but not with Perissodactyla (horses, zebra, rhinoceroces, tapirs), Camelidae, some Bovidae, some hystricomorph rodents, marsupials or monotremes (Hawkey 1975). Plasma from non-mammalian vertebrates never reacts optimally with human tissue factor.

It appears that, in general terms, the less closely related the species from which the tissue factor and plasma are obtained the less well the factors react together. In clinical and experimental terms this means that test reagents designed for use on human blood, employed to measure the one-stage prothrombin time in other species, may not provide a true assessment of their clotting status; prolonged clotting times may be due to lack of cross-reactivity.

Table 4.6

Standard laboratory tests which should give results in all mammals not influenced by 'species specificity':
Whole blood clotting time
Thrombelastography
Partial thromboplastin time
Activated partial thromboplastin time
Recalcification time
Thromboplastin generation test
Thrombin generation test
Thrombin clotting time
Fibrinogen measured as clottable protein
One-stage prothrombin test using homologous tissue factor
Clotting time with Russell's viper venom
Factor V assay (using human substrate plasma)
Factor VIII assay (using human substrate plasma)
Factor IX assay (using human substrate plasma)
Factor XI assay (using human substrate plasma)
Factor XII assay (using human substrate plasma)
Factor II assay using Taipan snake venom
Factor X assay using Russell's viper venom
Contact activation test

Standard laboratory tests influenced by species specificity of the reactants unless homologous reagents are used:
One-stage prothrombin time
Prothrombin consumption test
Two-stage prothrombin test
Factor VII assay
Thrombotest

It has been shown, however, that using plasma and tissue factor from the same species, one-stage prothrombin times comparable to those found in homologous normal human test systems can be obtained (Table 4.5). Thus, for any species the coagulation pathway depending on activation by its own tissue factor will be effective in haemostasis. In all mammals, with the possible exception of marsupials, this reaction apparently involves the activation of factor X.

The case for marsupials must be considered separately because in these animals factor X has not been detected in tests involving activation by Russell's viper venom (Hawkey 1975). There are 2 possible reasons for this. Either the molecular structure of marsupial factor X is different in a way which prevents its activation by the venom or factor X really is missing. If the second possibility proves to be correct, marsupials may represent an early stage in the evolution of the mammalian coagulation mechanism.

For the sake of convenience, coagulation tests which are not influenced by the problem of species specificity and those in which the reactants should be homologous are given in Table 4.6.

Table 4.7   Fibrinogen levels in mammals

Order	*Fibrinogen, mg/100 ml (mean and range)	No. of species tested
Primates (non-human)	399 (211–608)	35
Carnivora	347 (128–621)	25
Perissodactyla	514 (377–632)	7
Artiodactyla	300 (187–624)	24
Rodentia	639 (525–865)	3
Lagomorpha	317	1
Cetacea	385	1
Pinnipedia	439 (392–486)	2
Proboscidea	768 (641–876)	2
Marsupialia	799 (353–1270)	5
Monotremata	206	1
Normal human values	302 (194–408)	No. of individuals = 55

* Measured as clottable protein by the method of Ratnoff & Menzie (1951)

4.5.4   THE THROMBIN–FIBRINOGEN REACTION

The clottable protein, fibrinogen, is present in the blood of all mammals, often in quantities considerably greater than normally found in man (Table 4.7). Reduced fibrinogen levels have been found in non-human primates and in a Baikal seal in association with diffuse intravascular coagulation. Significant increase in the fibrinogen level is apparently a useful non-specific indicator of disease which warrants further investigation on a comparative basis. There are no marked species differences in the rate of conversion of fibrinogen to fibrin by standardized human or bovine thrombin and the thrombin clotting test should have the same diagnostic value in other mammals as in man. Factor XIII is present in all mammalian species which have

Table 4.8 Antithrombin levels in mammals

Order	Antithrombin units/ml of plasma (mean and range)	No. of species tested
Primates (non-human)	445 (143–625)*	16
Carnivora	514 (300–670)	9
Perissodactyla	1280 (1160–1200)	2
Artiodactyla	339 (230–515)	9
Rodentia	415	1
Lagomorpha	312	1
Normal human values	329 (200–560)	No. of individuals = 37

* Mean and range excludes high values (1426, 1290–1610) found in 12 owl monkeys (*Aotus trivirgatus*).

been tested (Hawkey 1975). High plasma antithrombin levels have been found in the Aotus monkey and in some perissodactyls; in other species the ability of the plasma to neutralize thrombin is within the normal human range (Table 4.8).

4.5.5 PROTHROMBIN (FACTOR II)

Prothrombin is the inactive precursor of thrombin present in the blood of all mammals. Human patients with congenital prothrombin deficiency characterized by relatively mild haemorrhagic symptoms have been described (Pool *et al* 1962). Congenital defects have not been reported in other mammals although in a few marsupials examined the prothrombin level is apparently very low (Hawkey 1975). A possible reason for this is discussed later in this section.

Prothrombin can be assayed in human plasma by a modification of the one-stage prothrombin test using human tissue factor as the activator, an artificially prepared prothrombin-free substrate mixture containing $BaSO_4$-adsorbed bovine plasma as the source of fibrinogen and factor V and human serum as the source of factors VII and X (Pechet 1964). For use in comparative studies this method is complicated by the existence of species specificity between the reactants and should be modified by substitution of homologous tissue factor and serum for the human counterparts. Lack of appreciation of this problem could explain the low levels of prothrombin sometimes recorded in comparative studies and may account for the very low levels reported in marsupials. An alternative assay method makes use of the fact that venom from the Taipan viper directly activates prothrombin to thrombin

Table 4.9 Prothrombin (factor II) levels in normal mammals expressed as a percentage of the normal human value.

Order	Prothrombin % (mean and range)	No. of species tested
Primates (non-human)	87 (40–270)	27
Carnivora	132 (20–470)	24
Perissodactyla	90 (16–230)	6
Artiodactyla	38 (11–135)	19
Rodentia	47 (15–92)	4
Lagomorpha	30	1
Cetacea	88	1
Pinnipedia	190	1
Proboscidea	150	1
Marsupialia	23 (12–33)	2
Monotremata	37	1
Normal human values	94 (70–125)	No. of individuals = 35

Table 4.10 Factor V levels in mammals expressed as a percentage of the normal human value.

Order	Factor V % (mean and range)*	No. of species with values > 1000%	No. of species tested
Primates (non-human)	292 (57–800)	0	26
Carnivora	780 (290–1000)	8	23
Perissodactyla	313 (160–510)	1	5
Artiodactyla	367 (86–900)	4	20
Rodentia	348 (100–590)	0	4
Lagomorpha		1	1
Cetacea	469	0	1
Pinnipedia	450	0	1
Proboscidea	360 (270 450)	0	2
Marsupialia	860	3	4
Monotremata	760	0	1
Normal human values	107 (83–140)	0	No. of individuals = 33

* Means and ranges exclude values of more than 1000%.

without the participation of plasma cofactors (Denson *et al* 1971). This method should therefore be applicable to other species although it should be borne in mind that species differences in the structure of the prothrombin molecule may prevent or reduce its susceptibility to the venom. This fact is perhaps suggested by the comparatively low levels shown in Table 4.9, but would appear unlikely for teleological reasons.

The normal human range for prothrombin measured by Taipan snake venom activation is 70–125 per cent (Table 4.9). The level in man is reduced in liver disease, vitamin K deficiency and by treatment with coumarin drugs (see Hardisty & Ingram 1965); these conditions are likely to apply to other mammals.

Prothrombin has been measured in other mammalian species by the Taipan venom method. The results shown in Table 4.9 suggest that, compared with man, the level in other species is sometimes low. The animals studied had no clinical or biochemical evidence of liver disease and did not respond to injection of vitamin K. Their one-stage prothrombin times with homologous tissue factor and their clotting times via the intrinsic pathway of activation (partial thromboplastin times) were normal (see Table 4.9). There was no evidence of an increased tendency to bleed. It is possible that high levels of factor V (Table 4.10) found in these animals could compensate for the apparent lack of prothrombin.

4.5.6 FACTOR V

Factor V was discovered as the cause of a rare congenital haemorrhagic state in man (Owren 1947). Congenital deficiency of this factor has not been described in any other mammalian species.

Factor V can be assayed by a modification of the one-stage prothrombin test using substrate plasma from which factor V is removed by adsorption with $Al(OH)_3$ followed by incubation at 37°C (Stefanini 1951, Wolf 1953). In man the normal range is 83–140 per cent (Table 4.10). The level is reduced in cyanotic heart disease (van Crevald 1958), during defibrination (Hardisty & Ingram 1965) and sometimes in liver disease (Owren 1959a). Increases have been recorded during pregnancy (Davidson & Tomlin 1963). It is normal in vitamin K deficiency and is not affected by coumarin drugs (Hardisty & Ingram 1965). In other mammals similar findings would be expected.

Factor V activity has been measured in other mammals using artificially prepared human substrate plasma (Wolf 1953) and human tissue factor (Hawkey 1975). Species specificity would not be expected to affect this reaction (see Fig. 4.5). Compared with man the level in other mammals is high. This may compensate for low levels of prothrombin also recorded (Table 4.10).

4.5.7 FACTOR VII

Factor VII is the most difficult clotting factor to study on a comparative basis because it is affected by species specificity but, unlike other species specific factors, cannot be directly activated by any known snake venom. In man, factor VII deficiency is identified by various modifications of the one-stage prothrombin test. Plasma from patients with factor VII deficiency shows a prolongation of the clotting time with this test but standard tests, depending on the intrinsic coagulation pathway, are normal. The clotting time with Russell's viper venom is also normal (Hardisty & Ingram 1965). Similar results have been reported for factor VII deficient dogs (Capel-Edwards & Hall 1968). In comparative studies, however, it is essential to use homologous tissue factor in order to obtain valid information about factor VII in the one-stage prothrombin test. Canine and rat factor VII has been measured by a modification of the 'Thrombotest'* (Spurling 1970, Spurling *et al* 1974). This test was originally designed for control of anticoagulant therapy with coumarin drugs in man and measures only the vitamin K dependent clotting factors including factor VII (Owren, 1959b). Other clotting factors are provided by the inclusion of adsorbed normal bovine plasma in the 'Thrombotest' reagent and tissue factor is provided by ox brain extract. Thus, species specificity will affect the reaction between factor VII in the test plasma and bovine tissue factor and factor X and the test cannot be used indiscriminately in comparative studies.

Similar problems beset tests designed for the specific assay of factor VII. For measurement of factor VII activity in human blood, assay procedures are based on the one-stage prothrombin test using factor VII-deficient substrate plasma obtained from human patients with factor VII deficiency (Dische & Benfield 1959) or, because factor VII is the first clotting factor to be depressed by coumarin drugs, from human patients during the initial stages of anticoagulant therapy (Denson 1961). Factor VII-deficient plasma of canine origin can also be used for measuring the human factor (Capel-Edwards & Hall 1968) because, fortuitously, species specificity is not evident between primates and carnivores (Hawkey 1974). It is of great interest that canine substrate plasma is only useful for the human assay if its high initial level of factor V is reduced by pre-incubation at 40°C (Garner *et al* 1967). This underlines the fact that the relative proportions of clotting factors as well as their absolute levels can affect the rate of reaction and offers a possible explanation for lack of haemorrhagic symptoms in factor VII-deficient dogs, since the deficiency may be compensated for by high levels of factor V. A similar compensating function has been proposed for the apparent low levels of prothrombin in many mammalian species.

Neither human nor canine factor VII-deficient substrate plasmas can be

---

* 'Thrombotest' reagent is manufactured by Nyegaard & Co A/S, Oslo.

used to measure factor VII in multi-species comparative surveys. For a given species, substrate plasma can be produced by treating an animal of the species in question with coumarin drugs; this substrate will also be suitable for testing closely related animals. The tissue factor used must always be at least from an animal of the same order (Hawkey 1974). Presumably this could be done for each mammalian order but doubt exists in the author's mind of the validity of then comparing results on different mammalian groups obtained using basically different substrate plasmas and tissue activators. Currently there are no broad spectrum comparative assays of factor VII levels in

Table 4.11 Factor VII levels in primates and carnivores measured by 2 different assay methods and compared with the normal human level

Order	Factor VII % (mean and range)	No. of species tested
*Primates (non-human)	378 (115–1000)	18
**Carnivora	182 (88–330)	4
*Normal human values	112 (70–180)	No. of individuals = 25

* Assayed using human tissue factor and human factor VII deficient substrate plasma (Dische & Benfield 1959).
** Assayed using carnivore tissue factor and factor VII deficient plasma obtained from ferrets (*Putorium furo*) treated with Warfarin Na (Hawkey 1974).

mammals. Results of factor VII assays on primates and carnivores have been reported by the author (Hawkey 1974, 1975) and are discussed later in this section.

Using homologous human test systems the normal human range for factor VII is 70–180 per cent (Table 4.11). The level is reduced in liver disease, in vitamin K deficiency states and by coumarin drugs (Hardisty & Ingram 1965). Similar reductions have been reported in dogs (Hall 1972) and would be expected in other mammalian species. Increased levels have been reported in pregnancy (Pechet & Alexander 1961). The normal range for factor VII in non-human primates, measured in a human test system is given in Table 4.11. In monkeys the factor VII activity is apparently greater than in man. Using carnivore tissue extract and substrate plasma obtained by treating a carnivore, the domestic ferret, with 3-(a-acetonylbenzyl)-4-hydroxycoumarin (Warfarin) (Hawkey, 1974) the factor VII level in 4 carnivoran species is also high (Table 4.11).

4.5.8. FACTOR VIII

Haemophilia is the most common simple inherited coagulation defect in man and has also been found in dogs of at least 15 different breeds (see Hall 1972) and in horses (Archer 1961, Sanger *et al* 1964, Hutchins *et al* 1967) but not in any non-domesticated species. In both dogs and horses the clinical symptoms, mode of inheritance and response to treatment are apparently similar to human haemophilia (Hall 1972, Nossel *et al* 1962). Acquired factor VIII deficiency occurs in association with diffuse intravascular coagulation in human patients and in other primate species (Voller *et al* 1969).

Table 4.12 Factor VIII levels in mammals expressed as a percentage of the normal human value

Order	Factor VIII % (mean and range)*	No. of species with values > 1000%	No. of species tested
Primates (non-human)	604 (180–1000)	0	18
Carnivora	696 (395–1000)	21	28
Perissodactyla	344 (95–850)	2	6
Artiodactyla	478 (130–852)	23	17
Rodentia	438 (120–900)	2	6
Lagomorpha		1	1
Cetacea	438		1
Proboscidea		2	2
Marsupialia		1	1
Monotremata		1	1
Normal human values	102 (64–160)	0	No. of individuals = 45

* Means and ranges exclude values of greater than 1000%

Assay of factor VIII in other mammals using substrate plasma from a severe human haemophiliac (Hawkey 1975) shows that the measurable activity is normally very high in most species; in many it is more than 10 times that found in normal human plasma (Table 4.12). The effect of stress on these animals cannot be assessed; however, most were anaesthetized at the time of obtaining the blood sample (Hawkey 1975) and even in stressed human individuals the factor VIII activity rarely increases to more than 2–3 times the original level. The suggestion that high levels of factor VIII are a possible cause of thrombosis in man (Penick *et al* 1966) is not borne out by these findings since spontaneous thrombosis is extremely uncommon in other mammalian species (Finlayson 1965).

4.5.9 FACTOR IX

Congenital deficiency of factor IX activity in man results in a severe haemorrhagic state (Christmas disease, haemophilia B) with hereditary and clinical characteristics similar to classical haemophilia (Hardisty & Ingram 1965). Congenital factor IX deficiency has also been described in Cairn terriers (Rowsell *et al* 1960, Mustard *et al* 1960, Dodds 1968). Clinical symptoms and mode of inheritance are apparently similar to those of the human disease (Dodds 1968).

Table 4.13 Factor IX levels in mammals expressed as a percentage of the normal human values

Order	Factor IX % (mean and range)*	No. of species with values > 1000%	No. of species tested
Primates (non-human)	104 (42–513)**	0	17
Carnivora	490 (120–900)	6	18
Perissodactyla	81 (78–84)	1	3
Artiodactyla	318 (50–620)	5	16
Rodentia	100	0	1
Lagomorpha	220	0	1
Cetacea	130	0	1
Proboscidea	390 (280–500)	0	2
Marsupialia	22	0	1
Normal human values	96 (60–150)	0	No. of individuals = 30

* Means and ranges exclude values of greater than 1000%.
** Low levels of factor IX activity found in the Cercopithecidae.

Factor IX has been assayed in other groups of mammals using human factor IX-deficient substrate plasma (Hawkey 1975). The level in Pongidae and Cebidae is within the normal human range but low activity has been found in the Cercopithecidae (Table 4.13). These animals do not show any clinical or laboratory evidence of liver disease and the factor IX level is not increased after administration of vitamin K.

4.5.10 FACTOR X

Congenital factor X deficiency was first described in human patients with a haemorrhagic state by Telfer *et al* (1956) and a similar condition has been found in dogs (Dodds 1968) but not in other mammals. Factor X is considered to be a key factor in human blood coagulation since it is activated by both the extrinsic and intrinsic coagulation pathways (Seegers *et al* 1963, Macfarlane & Ash 1964). It is also activated by Russell's viper venom; this reaction provides a means of assaying factor X not involving the use of tissue factor and therefore independent of the problems of species specificity. Factor Xa activates prothrombin in a reaction accelerated by factor V, platelet phospholipid and calcium ions. The reaction with tissue factor is species specific (Hawkey & Stafford, 1961), partly explaining the reason for reduced prothrombin activated and prolonged one-stage prothrombin times in mixtures of plasma and tissue factors from different species (Hawkey 1975).

Table 4.14 Factor X levels in mammals expressed as a percentage of the normal human values

Order	Factor X % (mean and range)	No. of species tested
Primates (non-human)	124 (59–390)	24
Carnivora		
fam. Canidae	288 (150–450)	15
fam. Felidae	62 (20–145)	8
Perissodactyla		
Artiodactyla		
Rodentia	110 (20–250)	6
Lagomorpha	480	1
Cetacea	48	1
Pinnipedia	130	1
Proboscidea	188 (170–205)	2
Marsupialia	<1 (0–1·5)	3
Monotremata	15	1
Normal human values	101 (54–200)	No. of individuals = 24

Russell's viper venom apparently activates factor X in most mammalian species (Hawkey 1966, 1975) although the reaction may be impaired in Marsupialia (Hawkey 1975). The normal human range is 54 to 200 per cent of the mean value (Hawkey 1975). In man and probably in other mammals factor X is reduced in liver disease, vitamin K deficiency (Hardisty & Ingram 1965) and by treatment with coumarin drugs (Douglas 1962). The level increases during pregnancy (Pechet & Alexander 1961).

Factor X has been assayed in other mammalian species using the method based on Russell's viper venom activation of artificially prepared bovine plasma (Denson 1961, Hawkey 1975). The results are shown in Table 4.14. There is an interesting difference between the 2 Carnivore families which have been studied, high levels being found in Canidae and low levels in Felidae. Factor X activity is virtually undetectable in the Marsupialia. It is not known if the factor is missing or if it does not react normally with Russell's viper venom. If the factor really is missing, marsupials may present an example of a stage in evolution of the coagulation mechanism in which the number of plasma factors required for prothrombin activation is reduced since their clotting with homologous tissue factor is normal (Fantl & Ward 1957). However, if the alternative explanation that marsupial factor X is not activated by Russell's viper venom is shown to be the case, this would indicate interesting structural differences in the factor X molecule.

4.5.11 FACTOR XI

Factor XI was discovered in 1953 as a result of study of human patients with a mild congenital haemorrhagic disease (Rosenthal *et al* 1953). Subsequently factor XI deficiency has been described in cattle (Kociba *et al* 1969) and dogs (Dodds 1968) and possibly in the Greater Kudu (Hawkey 1975).

Table 4.15 Factor XI levels in mammals expressed as a percentage of the normal human level

Order	Factor XI % (mean and range)	No. of species with values > 1000%	No. of species tested
Primates (non-human)	201 (120–400)	0	6
Carnivora		18	18
Perissodactyla	123 (30–245)	0	4
Artiodactyla	74 (22–250)*	3	18*
Rodentia	224 (122–325)	0	2
Cetacea	74	0	1
Normal human values	100 (50–150)	0	10

* Excluding results on the Greater Kudu. The three individuals of this species had factor XI levels of less than 1%.

The normal human range for factor XI is from 50 to 185 per cent of the mean (Egeberg 1961). Reduced maternal levels during parturition have been reported and during the neonatal period the level is also low (Nossel *et al* 1966). Low levels have been found in association with diffuse intravascular coagulation and in some patients with liver cirrhosis (Nossel 1972). An increase in the factor after exercise has been described (Ikkala *et al* 1963) but not confirmed (Egeberg 1963). One report exists of an increased level of factor XI induced by ingestion of hydrogenated margarine and vegetable oils (Egeberg 1966).

Factor XI assayed in other mammalian species using human factor XI deficient plasma as substrate (Hawkey 1975) shows high levels of activity in Carnivora (Table 4.15). Values of less than 1 per cent factor XI have been recorded in three *Tragelophas strepsiceros* (Greater Kudu); these animals also have prolonged partial thromboplastin times but show no evidence of abnormal bleeding. It is not yet known if the deficiency is a congenital abnormality present in the group of Greater Kudu available for study or if it is a characteristic of the species, perhaps as an extreme manifestation of the generally low levels found in Bovidae. It is interesting that congenital factor XII deficiency has been found in Holstein cattle (Kociba *et al* 1969). These animals, however, suffer mild haemorrhagic symptoms.

4.5.12   FACTOR XII

Factor XII is activated by contact with foreign surfaces (see Nossel 1972) and this reaction initiates the intrinsic pathway of prothrombin activator production. The coagulant activity of factor XIIa is to convert factor XI to XIa (Yin & Duckert 1961, Nossel 1964). Activated factor XII also plays a part in the

Table 4.16 Factor XII levels in mannals expressed as a percentage of the normal human value

Order	Factor XII % (mean and range)*	No. of species with values > 1000%	No. of species tested
Primates (non-human)	213 (66–487)	0	14
Carnivora	630 (310–1000)	2	18
Perissodactyla	247 (125–540)	0	5
Artiodactyla	417 (98–680)	3**	17
Rodentia	288 (140–420)	0	4
Lagomorpha	430	0	1
Cetacea	0	0	1
Normal human values	100 (50–100)	0	10

* Means and ranges exclude values of greater than 1000%.
** High levels of factor XII in Cervidae (deer).

fibrinolytic and kinin-forming systems. Stimulation of fibrinolysis by factor XIIa has been demonstrated by Niewiarowski and Prou-Wartelle (1959). The reaction is thought to involve activation of plasminogen in the presence of two cofactors (Ogston *et al* 1969). Factor XIIa has been shown to activate kinin release by Margolis (1958), Webster and Ratnoff (1961) and Eisen (1964). It is not yet known if factor XIIa directly converts kallikreinogen to kallikrein (Nagasawa *et al* 1958) or if it activates one or more intermediates in the reaction (Ratnoff & Miles 1964).

Human patients with congenital factor XII deficiency have been identified but rarely suffer from haemorrhagic disorders (Ratnoff 1966). In these patients all laboratory tests depending on the intrinsic pathway of activation are abnormal and the defect is not corrected by contact with glass, silicone or any other activating surface (Ratnoff 1966). Factor XII is assayed using substrate plasma from patients with congenital factor XII deficiency (Nossel 1964). In normal human plasma the range of activity is from 36 to 152 per cent of the mean normal level (Ratnoff 1966). The level is low in neonates (Kurkcuoglu & McElfresh, 1960) and increased levels induced by exercise have been reported (Iatridis & Ferguson 1963, Egeberg 1963). Reduced levels have been found in defibrination states (Nossel *et al* 1966).

In other mammals, factor XII has been measured by its ability to correct the clotting time of factor XII-deficient human plasma (Hawkey 1975). Compared with man, factor XII activity is high in most other groups studied (Table 4.16). An interesting exception reported by Robinson *et al* (1969) and confirmed by Hawkey (1975) is that in members of the Cetacea (whales, dolphins, etc.) factor XII is absent. Like human individuals with congenital factor XII-deficiency these animals do not have an increased tendency to bleed. It has been suggested that activation of factor XII by acidosis during diving is a cause of the diffuse intravascular coagulation in severe decompression sickness (Holland 1969) and that absence of factor XII may, therefore, be advantageous in diving mammals. However, there is no evidence of a similar deficiency in members of the Pinnipedia (seals and sea lions).

In Primates an inverse relationship has been found between factor XII and plasminogen. This is interesting in the light of the fact that factor XIIa is an activator of plasminogen (Iatridis & Ferguson 1963). This relationship does not hold for other groups of mammals examined. In Cetaceans circulating plasminogen activator can be demonstrated in the absence of factor XII.

4.5.13 FLETCHER FACTOR

Fletcher factor was discovered in man as a result of study of a family in which intrinsic prothrombin activation in the blood was not stimulated by contact with activating surfaces (Hathaway *et al* 1965). Results of clotting tests on these patients were similar to those found in factor XII deficiency and, like patients with factor XII deficiency there was no abnormal bleeding tendency. The defect was corrected by addition to the blood of plasma deficient in factor XIIa and by plasmas deficient in all other known clotting factors. Further reports have confirmed the existence of the deficiency (Hattersley & Hayse 1970) and the missing factor has been named 'Fletcher factor' after the original family in which it was studied.

Recently it has been shown that clotting tests on blood deficient in Fletcher factor are corrected by addition of human plasma prekallikrein (Wuepper 1972) and that the defect can be produced in normal human plasma by treatment with specific antibody to a human plasma kallikrien (Saito & Ratnoff 1974). These findings suggest that Fletcher factor is a prekallikrein necessary for normal *in vitro* clotting of human blood and additional studies on the role of the factor in the coagulation process have shown that its action is in the early stages of the intrinsic pathway of prothrombin activation involving surface contact and factors XII and XI (Saito *et al* 1974).

Comparative studies on Fletcher factor have not yet been carried out by the present author but levels of 63 to 206 per cent have been reported for non-human primates by Abildgaard *et al* (1971). Levels in several mammalian species have been reported by Saito *et al* (1974). Compared with man high levels are found in pigs, guinea pigs and a gibbon but virtually no activity is detected in plasma of rabbits, dogs, cats, cetaceans, chickens or ducks. Precipitin lines are obtained in cross reactions between anti-human kallikrein serum and plasma from non-human primates, but not with the other species examined. These results must be interpreted with caution since the substrate plasma used was obtained from a case of human Fletcher factor deficiency and apparent lack of coagulant activity could therefore be due to species specificity between the reactants. Further comparative studies of this factor would be of great interest.

4.5.14   FITZGERALD FACTOR

The existence of a hitherto unrecognized clotting factor in human plasma was proposed as a result of studies on the purification of factor XI by Schiffman and Lee (1974) and an asymptomatic deficiency of this factor has since been described (Waldmann *et al* 1975). In laboratory tests, plasma from this patient was normalized by addition of plasma with every known clotting factor defect including factor XII and Fletcher factor. The defect was not corrected, however, by addition of factor XIIa or Fletcher factor but was normalized by factor XIa. These findings indicate that the deficient factor operates after activation of factor XII and Fletcher factor but before the activation of factor XIa. There is evidence that it also participates in fibrinolysis and kinin generation (Waldmann *et al* 1975).

Fitzgerald factor has not yet been studied in non-human species.

4.5.15   PLATELET PHOSPHOLIPID (PLATELET FACTOR 3) AND PARTIAL THROMBOPLASTIN

It has been shown that in human blood, the reactions between factor IXa, VIII, and X and between Xa and prothrombin are accelerated by the presence of a phospholipid (Biggs 1972). The source of phospholipid during clotting of whole blood without addition of tissue factor is the platelets (Biggs *et al* 1953). Platelet phospholipid is apparently associated mostly with the surface membrane and the cytoplasmic organelles (Born 1972), and is released by mechanical damage, contact with activating surfaces or during the second phase of platelet aggregation (Hardisty & Hutton 1966). The main lipid components are the phospholipids of serine, ethanolamine and inositol, but other lipids are also present in smaller amounts (Born, 1972). It is not known which of these are important in the reaction. It has been suggested that chemical and physical properties such as the size of the suspended phospholipid particles, the charge on their surface, the degree of saturation of fatty acids present and the chemical configuration of the base are more important than the actual phospholipids present (Bangham 1961). Crude brain cephalin (Bell & Alton 1954) or lecithin (Biggs 1972) can be substituted for platelet phospholipid in clotting tests depending on the intrinsic activation of prothrombin.

Platelet phospholipid release is measured in laboratory tests by exposure of platelet-rich plasma to activating surfaces such as kaolin (Hardisty & Hutton 1965) and total platelet phospholipid is measured after mechanical disruption of the platelets. The normal human levels are shown in Table 4.3. Human patients have been described in which the release of platelet phospholipid is impaired. These patients suffer superficial bruising, ecchymoses and increased bleeding after injury (Hardisty 1972). Congenital conditions where this is found include thrombasthenia (Hardisty, 1972) and albinism (Hardisty & Hutton 1967). A similar condition has also been studied in acquired bleeding disorders such as those associated with scurvy (Born & Wright 1968, Hardisty 1969), uraemia (Horowitz *et al* 1967) and after ingestion of aspirin (O'Brien 1968). In other species an inherited condition resembling thrombasthenia is found in dogs (Dodds 1966, 1968) and failure of platelet phospholipid release has been studied experimentally in scorbutic guinea pigs (Born & Wright 1968). The status of albino laboratory rabbits and rodents in this respect is not known, but it appears unlikely that congenital functional platelet defects could have escaped notice in these animals. A haemorrhagic tendency described in albino wallabies (Jones 1976) should, however, be investigated further in the light of the findings in human albinism.

Total platelet factor 3 and the amount released by kaolin has been studied in standardized platelet-rich plasma of some other mammalian species (Hawkey 1975). The results, shown in Table 4.3, suggest that release of phospholipid may be greater from human platelets than from those of other mammalian groups. However, if the total circulating platelet count is taken into consideration this apparent difference in non-human primates and carnivores is eliminated (Hawkey 1974).

It is not yet known if platelet phospholipid is the same as the phospholipid supplied by tissue factor (Esnouf 1972). Apparently neither moiety is species specific amongst mammals; this may be explained by the suggestion that the physico-chemical properties of the complex are more important than the molecular structure of the phospholipids present (Biggs 1972, Esnouf 1972). Crude human brain cephalin (Bell & Alton 1954) will activate coagulation in all mammals tested (Hawkey 1975). In many the clotting time is shorter than the normal human range (Table 4.17) suggesting that the intrinsic pathway of prothrombin activation is potentially more active. These results may be explained by the high levels of factor VIII and other clotting factors also recorded.

Table 4.17 Activation of the clotting time of mammalian plasmas by human brain cephalin in the partial thromboplastin test (PTT).

Order	PTT/secs (means and ranges)	No. of species tested
Primates (non-human)	51 (35–77)	35
Carnivora	38 (34–37)	32
Artiodactyla	38* (26–59*)	
Perissodactyla	73 (30–135)	8
Lagomorpha	53	1
Rodentia	49 (34–85)	8
Cetacea	302**	1
Pinnipedia	68 (63–76)	2
Proboscidea	65 (49–81)	2
Marsupialia	40 (35–53)	5
Monotremata	30	1
Normal human values	71 (48–90)	No. of individuals = 102

* Excludes results on Greater Kudus with factor XI deficiency.
** Factor XII deficiency.

The reaction of human brain with plasma from cetaceans and from the Greater Kudu is prolonged. These findings are explained by lack of factor XII in cetaceans and lack of factor XI in the Greater Kudu.

4.6 FIBRINOLYSIS

The blood fibrinolytic mechanism is the physiological converse of coagulation in that the end product of coagulation, fibrin, is the substrate for the fibrinolytic mechanism, plasmin. Fibrinolysis in man has been reviewed extensively by Fearnley (1965) and Konttinen (1968). The main function of the fibrinolytic mechanism is thought to be to prevent the build-up of fibrin deposits in the blood vessels. It would appear likely, therefore, that in all animals in which a fibrin-forming coagulation mechanism is present, a fibrinolytic process would be necessary and, although there are again some methodological problems in comparative studies on fibrinolysis, there is evidence that the mechanism is present in the blood of all mammals which have so far been studied (Hawkey 1970, 1975).

In man the fibrinolytic enzyme plasmin is not present in the blood under normal circumstances and similarly it has not been detected in other mammals. It is present in the plasma as an inactive beta globulin, plasminogen. Human plasminogen can be measured by exposure of plasma to various

Table 4.18 Plasminogen levels in mammals

Order	Plasminogen units/ml plasma (mean and range)	No. of species tested
Primates (non-human)	5·77 (3·7–8·0)	18
Carnivores	5·42 (3·7–6·9)	11
Perissodactyla	4·77 (2·0–6·9)	5
Artiodactyla	3·74 (1·5–7·6)	11
Rodentia	7·45	1
Cetacea	5·3	1
Marsupialia	6·5	1
Normal human values	2·8 (1·9–4·0)	No. of individuals = 42

activating substances and measuring the proteolytic activity developed (Alkjaersig *et al* 1959). Activators used for this process include urokinase, extracted from normal human urine (Williams 1951) and streptokinase produced by certain strains of *β-haemolytic streptococci* (Tillett & Garner 1933). Comparative studies on other mammals show that proteolytic activity can be induced by exposure of the plasma to human urokinase. In some groups similar activity is generated by streptokinase; in others it is necessary to activate the streptokinase with a small amount of human serum to obtain a result (Clifton & Cannamela 1951, Hawkey 1970, 1975). However, in all mammalian species which have been studied, the results of such tests demonstrate the presence in the plasma of a plasminogen-like fibrinolytic precursor. Quantitative measurements of plasminogen in mammals suggest that most species have a higher plasminogen level than is normally found in man (Table 4.18). This may offset their apparently greater coagulation potential.

Physiological fibrinolysis in man occurs as a result of release into the plasma of a plasminogen activator from the vascular endothelial cells (Todd

1964). Small amounts of this activator can be detected in normal human blood providing the inhibitors of fibrinolysis are first removed (Fearnley *et al* 1957); the level increases rapidly in response to mental or physical stress (Biggs *et al* 1947, Müllertz 1953). In other mammals it is difficult to assess the degree of stress engendered by taking a blood sample; however, demonstration of circulating plasminogen activator under any circumstances is evidence

Table 4.19 Plasminogen activator levels in mammals

Order	Plasminogen activator units (mean and range)*	No. of species with < 1 unit	No. of species tested
Primates (non-human)	12·4 (1·6–120·0**)	0	37
Carnivora	5·8 (2·4–10·2)	0	16
Perissodactyla	3·6 (1·7–13·0)	0	6
Artiodactyla	2·1 (1·0–10·0)	6	15
Rodentia	5·0 (2·0–8·3)	0	6
Lagomorpha	3·9	0	1
Cetacea	3·0	0	1
Proboscidea		2	2
Marsupialia	2·5 (1·3–5·0)	0	3
Monotremata		1	1

* Means and ranges exclude values of less than 1 unit.
** High levels found in Cebidae.

Table 4.20 Inhibitors of fibrinolysis in mammals expressed as a percentage of the normal human value

Order	Fibrinolytic inhibitor %	No. of species tested
Primates (non-human)	103 (50–150)	9
Carnivora	115 (90–140)	6
Normal human values	100 (90–125)	No. of individuals = 25

of a mechanism similar to that found in man. Measurement of circulating plasminogen activator in captive wild mammals by the euglobulin lysis test (Buckell 1958) shows that activity is present in primates, carnivores, perissodactyls, rodents, lagomorphs, cetaceans and marsupials. In elephants, a monotreme and some artiodactyls, however, the activity is very low or apparently absent (Table 4.19). The negative findings may be due to failure to adapt a method designed for use on human blood to take account of unknown differences in other species. Further study of the methodology for measuring circulating plasminogen activator in other species is required.

The other important components of the blood fibrinolytic mechanism are the inhibitors. These comprise antiplasmins, at least 2 of which are present in normal human plasma (Norman 1958), and an antiactivator which may be enhanced by activating surfaces (Flute 1959). Comparative studies on total plasma fibrinolytic inhibitors in a small number of human and non-human primates and carnivores fail to reveal any basic differences (Table 4.20).

In human patients haemorrhage due to primary or secondary hyper-fibrinolysis sometimes occurs. In other mammalian species although occasionally individuals are found with exceptionally high levels of circulating activator, haemorrhagic symptoms have not been evident.

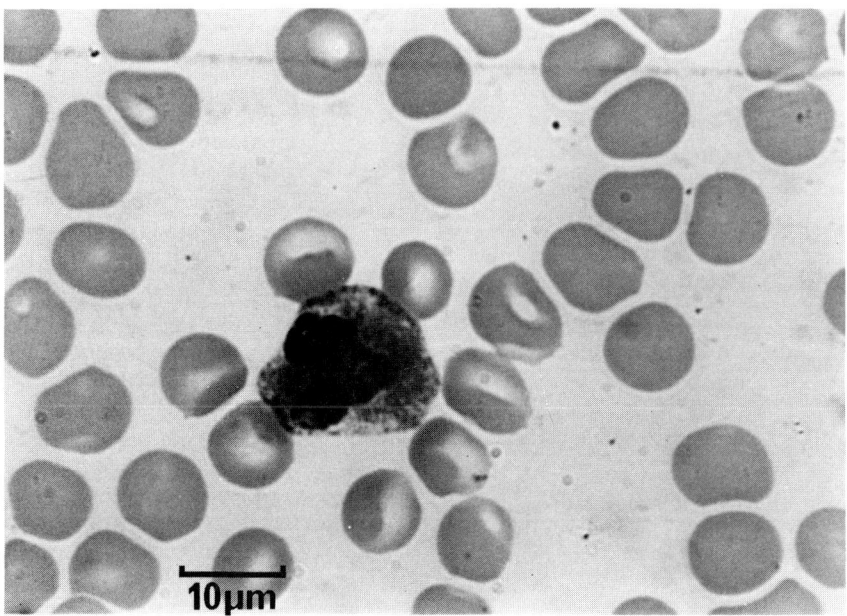

Fig. 4.6 Granular neutrophil in a normal gorilla. (Figs 4.6–4.10 stained with May-Grunwald Giemsa)

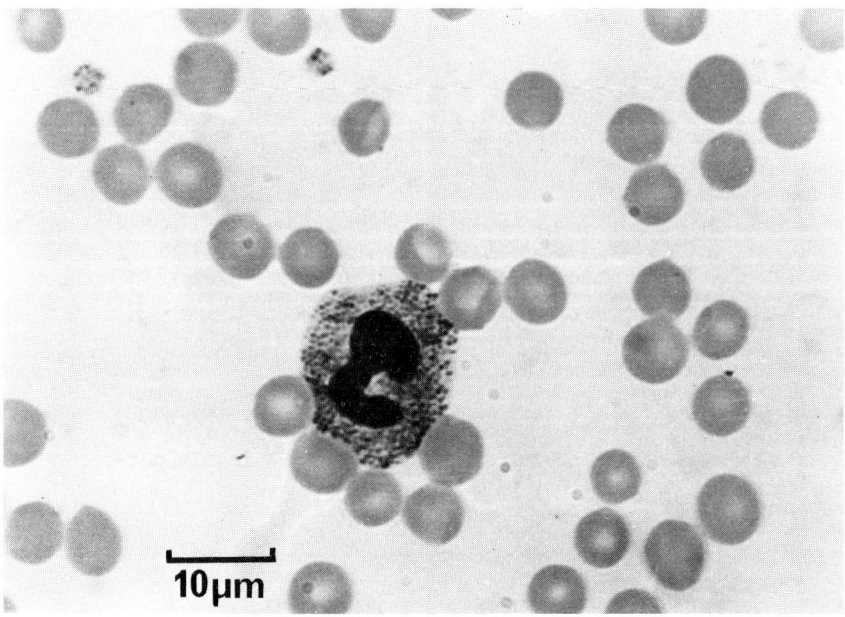

Fig. 4.7   Neutrophil showing basophilic 'peppering'. Normal nilgai.

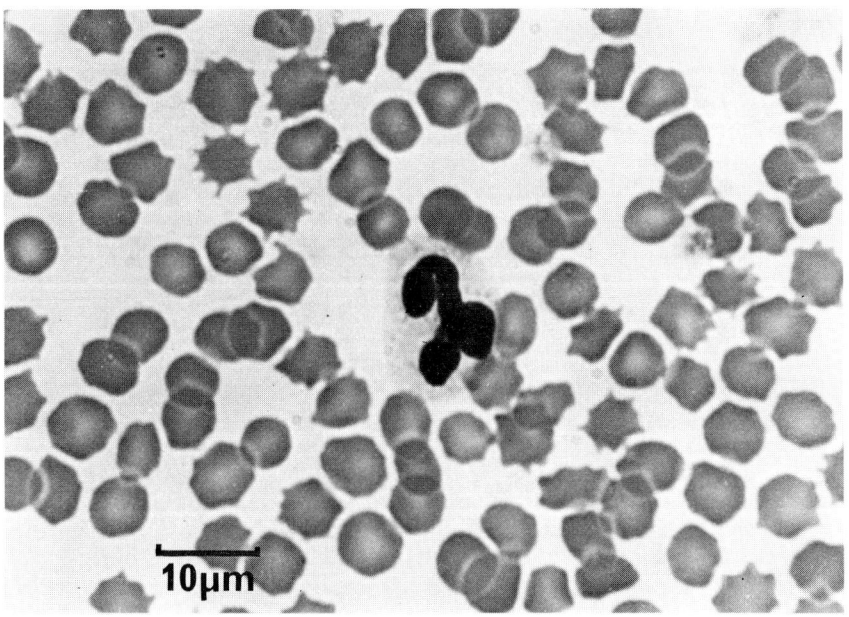

Fig. 4.8   Agranular neutrophil. Normal lion.

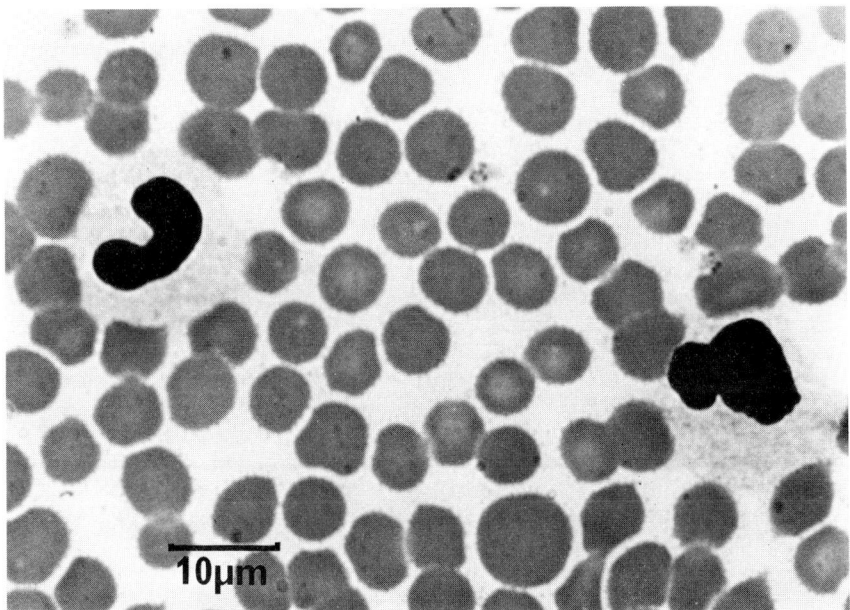

Fig. 4.9 Neutrophils showing 'shift to the left'. Normal in white rhinoceros.

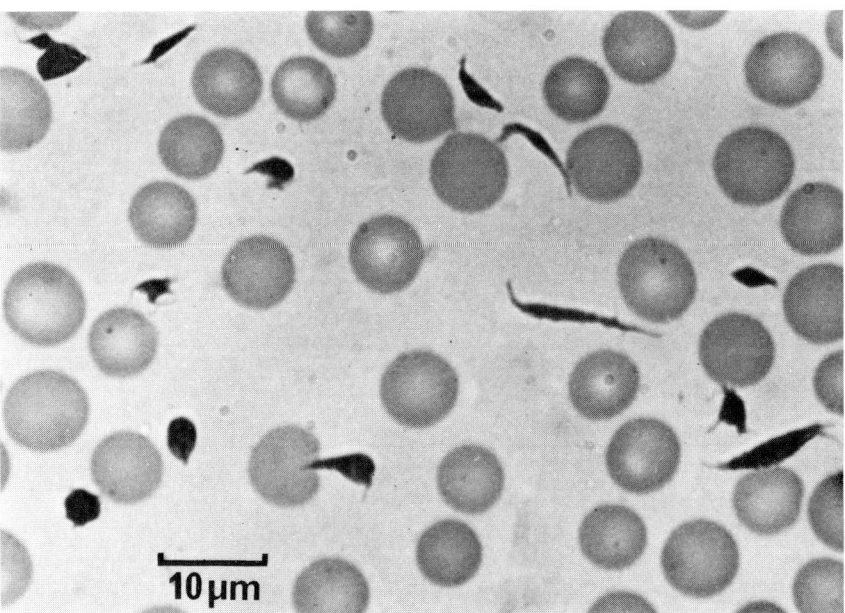

Fig. 4.10 Atypical platelets in echidna (spiny anteater).

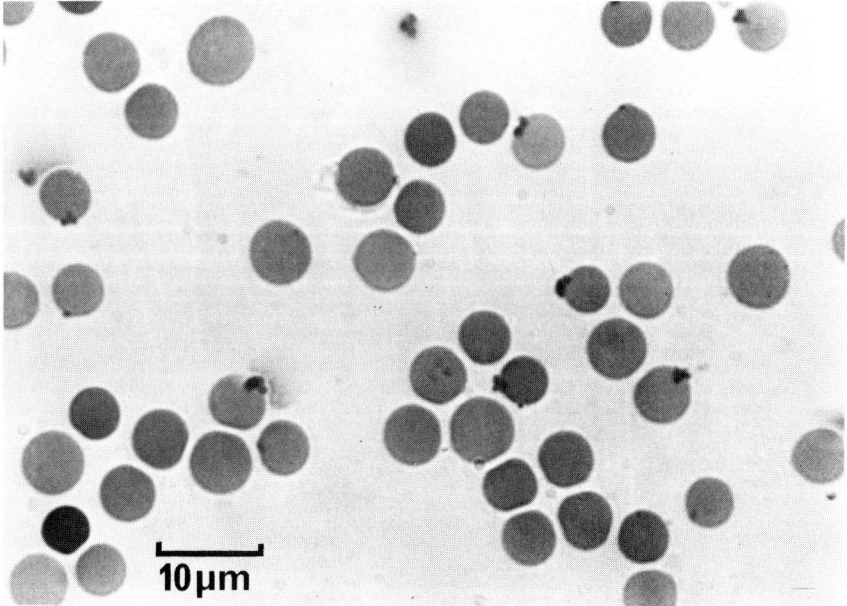

Fig. 4.11   Red cell inclusion bodies resembling Heinz bodies in a normal white rhinoceros. Stained with new methylene blue.

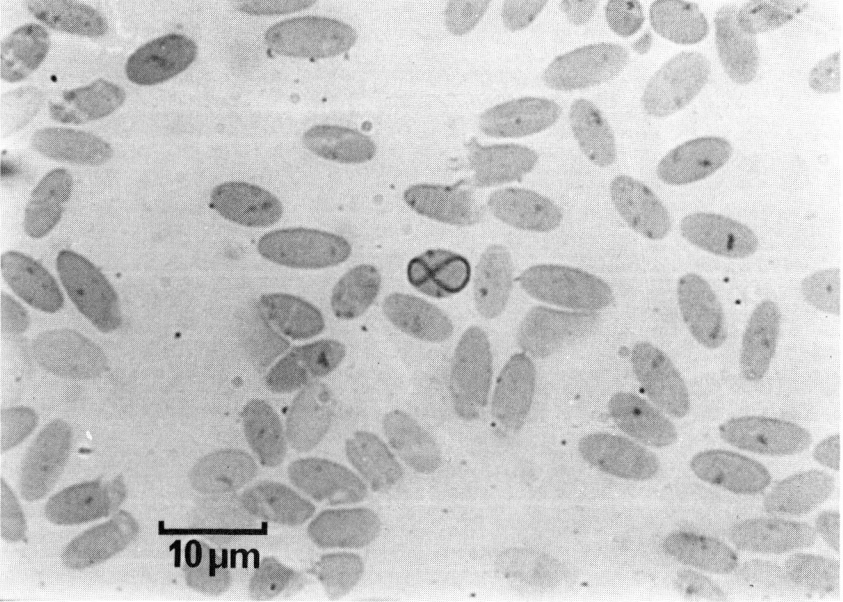

Fig. 4.12   Llama red cells showing Cabot's ring. Stained with new methylene blue.

5

CLINICAL HAEMATOLOGY OF THE HORSE

L. B. JEFFCOTT

5.1 INTRODUCTION

Clinical haematology in the horse has wide application in veterinary practice not only in the valuable racing Thoroughbred but in all other breeds and types (Table 5.1). As well as being employed as a diagnostic aid, attempts have been made to use the haematological profile as an assessment for fitness and performance potential in the racehorse (Archer 1974a, Jeffcott 1974, Stewart & Steel 1974, Schalm, Jain & Carroll 1975). Perhaps because of their economic value and the ever increasing popularity of the horse in recent years, a considerable amount of research and investigation has been done in this field in the last 20 years or so. In this review I will not attempt to cover all the published material available but will select and discuss the more practical points which may be pertinent in equine medicine. Since writing this chapter, the proceedings of an international symposium on equine haematology has been published (American Association of Equine Practitioners, 1975).

There is considerable variation noted in the blood picture (haemogram) of different breeds, ages and sexes of horses, and a number of useful publications on the interpretation of the equine haemogram exist (Archer & Miller 1959, Cosgrove 1969, Seckington 1969, Schalm *et al* 1975, Ricketts & Rossdale 1975). Perhaps some of the variations noted between different authors are associated with different techniques and methods of quality control. However, with the introduction of electronic particle counters (see Chapter 14) and modern quality-controlled haematological methods (*International Symposium on Standardization of Haematological Methods*, 1968) far more accurate and reliable results should now be obtainable.

5.2 NORMAL VALUES

5.2.1 ERYTHROCYTES

5.2.1.1 Red cell morphology and numbers according to breed, sex and age

As with other mammals, the erythrocytes of the horse are non-nucleated biconcave discs 5–6 μm in diameter (Fig. 5.1) with a mean cell volume (MCV) of approximately 40–45 fl. Their development takes place in the bone marrow and they have a life span in the circulation of about 140–150 days (Cornelius *et al* 1960a, Marcilese *et al* 1966).

An unusual characteristic of equine erythrocytes is their propensity to rouleaux formation in non-circulating blood so that blood samples left to stand for a few minutes show a rapid separation of the cells and plasma. This property, which will be discussed more fully later on, can be of considerable value as a quick diagnostic aid in such conditions as jaundice, haemolytic anaemia and haemoconcentration.

Table 5.1 References to equine haematological values in various breeds, age and sex

Source	Date	Country	No. of animals	Breed and type of horse examined
Foals				
Aldous	1971	Canada	89	TB
Allen & Archer	1973	UK	153	*TB 1 month–9 months
Hansen et al	1950b	USA	70	TB weanlings
Jeffcott	1971	UK	8	Pony birth–12 months
Ricketts & Rossdale	1975	UK	NR	Breed not specified—birth–12 months
Rossdale	1966	UK	29	TB birth–36 hrs
Schalm, Jain & Carroll	1975	USA		TB and Quarterhorse
Todd et al	1951	USA	28	TB birth–26 wks
Adults				
Allen & Archer	1973	UK	1201	*TB M, F and G—1–4 y.o.
Archer	1959	UK	132	TB all ages and types
Azzie	1973	S. Africa	761	TB in training
Hansen et al	1950a c d 1951	USA	205	TB barren, pregnant, lactating and non-lactating mares and stallions
Hansen & Todd	1951	USA		Arab M, F and G
Knill et al	1969	USA	50	Arab M, F and G
Krzywanek & Witt	1970	Germany		TB
Littlejohn	1968	UK	42	*TB non-TB, M, F and G
Obara & Nakajima	1961	Japan	NR	TB non-TB
Ricketts & Rossdale	1975	UK		TB in training, at stud
Schalm, Jain & Carroll	1975	USA	146	TB Quarterhorse, Standardbred, Appaloosa and Arab, M, F and G
Stewart, Clarkson & Steel	1970	Australia	329	TB 2–3 y.o., M, F and G
Stewart & Holman	1940	UK	36	Clydesdale
Sykes	1966	Australia	11	TB in training—2–4 y.o. M, F and G
Trum	1952	USA	23	Percherons, adults M and F
				TB

* Red cell figures only given.

TB = Thoroughbred; M = male; F = female; G = gelding; NR = not recorded.

The usual haemogram carried out on horse blood involves determination of total red cells (RBC), packed cell volume (PCV), haemoglobin (Hb), the red cell indices (MCV, MCH and MCHC), total white cells (WBC) and a differential white cell count. In addition the erythrocyte sedimentation rate (ESR) or plasma viscosity (PV) is performed. There are many references to the haemograms of different breeds, ages, sexes and types of use (Table 5.1). For the reasons already stated on quality control between laboratories, particularly in the older articles, there seems little point in quoting all these

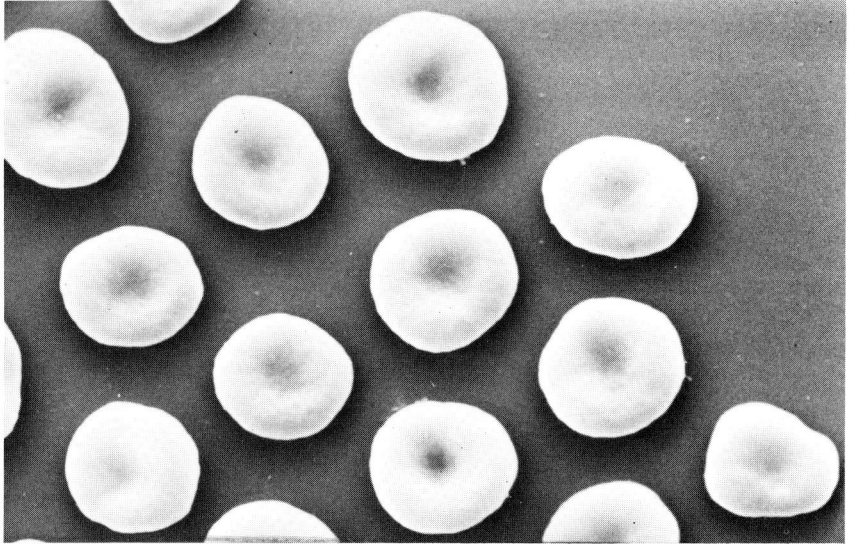

Fig. 5.1 Scanning electron micrograph of equine erythrocytes (prepared by K. W. Thurley and J. G. Matthews, B.Vet.Med., MRCVS).

figures. Those interested should refer to the particular reference given. As far as possible normal figures quoted in this chapter have been obtained from the Haematology Department of the Equine Research Station, Newmarket.

Breed Considerable differences in the red cell parameters of the different breeds exist although as a species there are 2 broad divisions. The so-called 'hot blooded' breeds (e.g. Thoroughbred, Quarterhorse, Standardbred and Arab) have significantly higher red cell figures than the 'cold-blooded' types (e.g. Percheron, Clydesdale, and pony breeds).

Most attention has naturally been paid to the Thoroughbred and it was over 50 years ago (Neser 1923) that the PCV was shown to be noticeably higher than in other breeds. Neser also observed an increase in the red cell

Table 5.2 Normal red cell values in Thoroughbred horses*

Age of Thoroughbred (number examined)	Hb g/dl ±SD	RBC ×10¹²/l ±SD	PCV l/l ±SD	MCV fl ±SD	MCH pg ±SD	MCHC g/dl ±SD
<1 month (78)	13·6±1·90	9·85±1·31	0·378±0·05	38·5±2·49	13·8±1·07	36·1±1·62
1–9 months (75)	12·7±1·55	10·33±1·24	0·353±0·0440	34·3±2·92	12·3±1·23	36·1±2·25
Yearling (100)	13·7±1·44	9·91±1·11	0·375±0·0389	37·9±1·90	13·8±0·68	36·6±1·36
2 years (308)	14·6±1·44	9·86±0·98	0·399±0·0399	40·6±2·53	14·7±0·87	36·2±1·02
3 years (353)	15·1±1·52	9·71±1·06	0·414±0·0418	42·7±2·54	15·6±0·83	36·5±1·07
4 years (138)	15·0±1·65	9·28±0·98	0·408±0·0465	44·3±2·43	16·7±0·86	36·5±1·30
Over 4 years (302)	14·6±1·61	8·80±1·09	0·398±0·0470	45·5±2·56	16·6±0·96	36·5±1·36

* From Allen & Archer (1973)

Table 5.3 Normal values for red cell figures of ponies, donkeys and exotic equidae

Type of animal (number examined)*	Hb g/dl ±SD	RBC×10¹²/l ±SD	PCV l/l ±SD	MCV fl ±SD	MCH pg ±SD	MCHC g/dl ±SD
Adult ponies (27)	12·81±1·65	7·39±1·07	0·320±0·11	48·2 ±4·0	17·4 ±1·3	36·2±1·1
Crossbred ponies from one stud (22)	12·17±1·02	7·65±0·75	0·301±0·10	44·8 ±4·3	16·0 ±1·7	34·7±1·9
Adult donkeys (16)	12·8 ±1·91	6·4 ±1·04	0·369±0·06	57·8 ±3·0	20·1 ±0·9	34·9±1·3
Donkey foals (6–12 mth) (6)	11·9 ±0·24	7·05±0·15	0·339±0·013	47·98±3·9	16·95±1·4	35·3±1·3
Przewalski* (9)	16·3	8·4	0·447	54·4	19·7	35·9
Onager* (3)	17·7	6·9	0·483	71·7	26·2	37·0
Common zebra* (11)	14·8	8·8	0·406	46·9	17·0	36·3
Mountain zebra* (11)	13·9	8·9	0·397	44·7	15·7	35·1

* Figures abstracted from Jones (1976).

figures in response to training although this fact has not been confirmed by other workers (MacLeod *et al* 1947, Archer 1959). The normal red cell figures for the Thoroughbred are given in Table 5.2. These samples were collected at rest from foals and horses in-training on the flat. The results are comparable with other published figures for horses in training at an altitude only just above sea level. Normal values for other hot-blooded breeds are similar but have somewhat lower RBC, PCV and Hb (Schalm *et al* 1975).

The normal levels recorded for clinically healthy ponies and donkeys are given in Table 5.3. The most obvious difference in the donkey is the noticeable increase in the size of the erythrocytes compared to the horse.

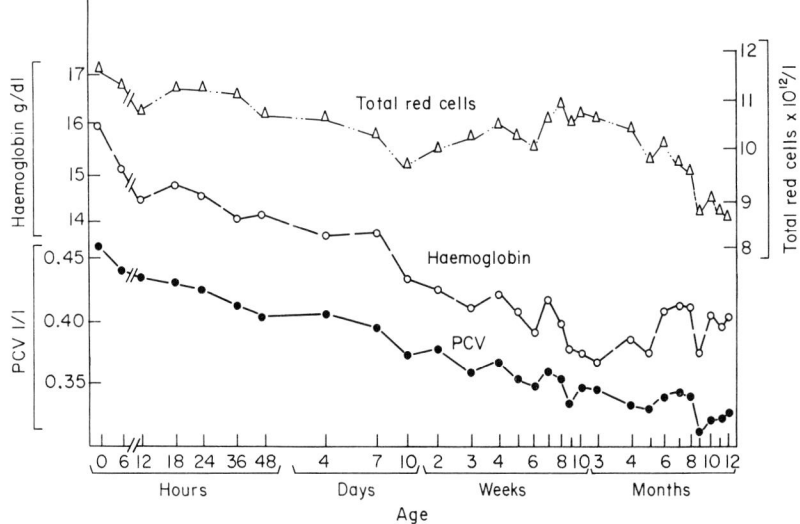

Fig. 5.2 Mean values for RBC, Hb and PCV in 8 pony foals from birth to 1 year (from Jeffcott 1971).

The figures for wild horses (Przewalski, onager and zebra) are quoted from a recent paper by Jones (1976).

Sex The RBC, Hb and PCV of female Thoroughbreds and Quarterhorses are reported to be somewhat higher than in males (Schalm *et al* 1975). On the other hand the concentration of haemoglobin in the red cells of males was greater than the females (i.e. higher MCH and MCHC).

Age The blood picture of 5 normal equine fetuses have been examined by Schalm *et al* (1975). Apart from the red cell size no obvious morphological or structural differences between adult and fetal erythrocytes were seen. The mean MCV in these fetuses (242–303 days' gestation) was 53·8 fl. At term the MCV will usually be 40–45 fl.

In a study of a group of pony foals in 1971, I reported on the changes in the red cell series up to 12 months of age. At the time of birth a degree of haemoconcentration was present but the RBC, Hb and PCV all fell fairly dramatically over the first 12 hours of life (Fig. 5.2). The red cell count rose slightly at 24 hours and then showed a gradual decline to 10 days of age. This was followed by a rise to a peak of 2 months and then a gradual fall to a mean $8.63 \times 10^{12}/l$ at one year old. The Hb content of the blood decreased steadily over the first 3 months, from 16.0 g/dl at 0 hours to 11.2 g/dl at 12 weeks. The level then rose to just over 12.0 g/dl and remained fairly steady to the end of

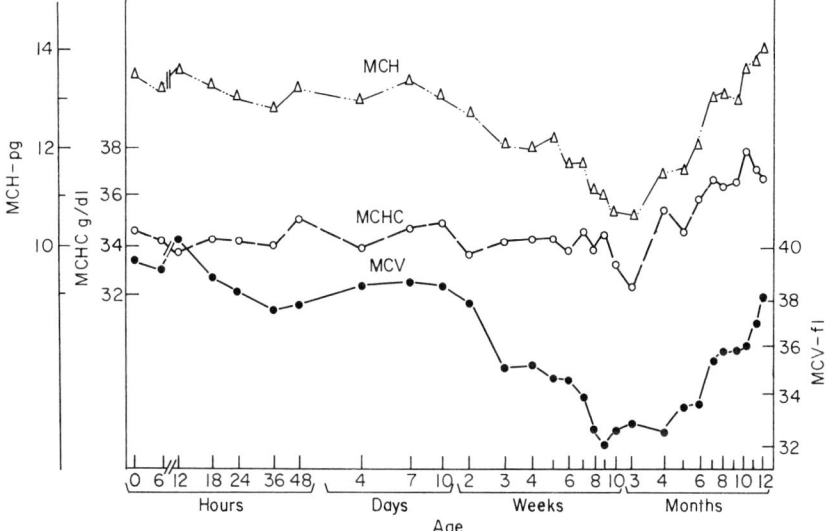

Fig. 5.3 Mean values for erythrocyte standard ratios in 8 pony foals from birth to 1 year (from Jeffcott 1971).

the year. The haematocrit fell nearly 0.06 l/l in the first 48 hours of life and continued to fall to a lowest recorded mean value at 9 months of 0.31 l/l. This was followed by a small rise in the next 3 months.

The most dramatic changes noted were associated with alteration of erythrocyte size in the first year of life (Fig. 5.3). The MCV dropped a little after birth but remained fairly steady until 2 weeks of age. At 9 weeks there was a marked decrease in red cell size noted from 37.8 to 31.9 fl. The level remained low until 4 months and finally rose again to 38.0 fl at one year. The MCH showed a similar picture to the MCV but the drop occurred from 7 days of age and appeared more gradual. The MCHC remained fairly constant during the first 2 months ($33.6–35.2$ g/dl). The lowest recorded level was at 3 months,

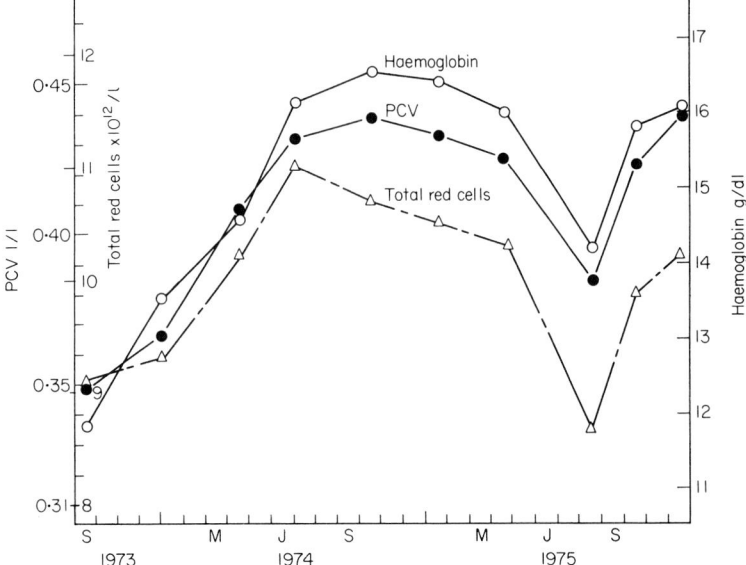

Fig. 5.4 Mean values from RBC, Hb and PCV in 8 Thoroughbreds from the onset of training at 20 months to the end of the 3rd year (derived from data supplied by Catling 1976).

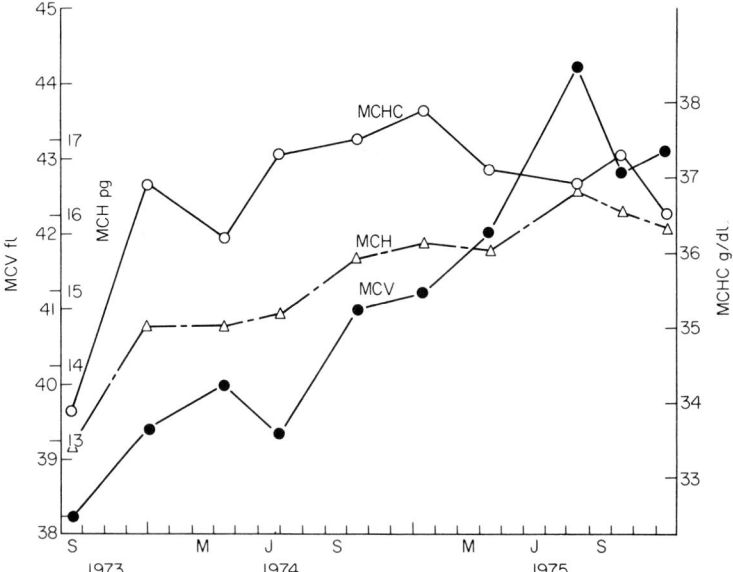

Fig. 5.5 Mean values for erythrocyte standard ratios in 8 Thoroughbreds from the onset of training at 20 months to the end of the 3rd year (derived from data supplied by Catling 1976).

after which it rose to a peak of 37·9 g/dl at 10 months, dropping slightly at 12 months.

A similar trend has been reported in other breeds in the first year of life, (Allen & Archer 1973, Schalm *et al* 1975). The exact significance of the decrease in red cell size in the first few months of life is equivocal. However, from the practical point of view it should not be interpreted as evidence of a microcytic anaemia.

The red cell picture continues to change over the next 2 years of life. A recent study by Catling (1975) shows an increase of the red cell parameters during the early stages of training. The levels plateau by 3 to 4 years of age (Figs. 5.4 & 5.5). An unexpected fall in values during the hot summer of 1975 was seen which was possibly attributable to some expansion of plasma volume leading to a relative haemodilution. No untoward clinical signs were

Table 5.4 The effect of increasing age on the erythrocyte parameters of horses racing under National Hunt rules*

Age of horses (number examined)	Hb g/dl ± SD	RBC × 10¹²/l ± SD	PCV l/l ± SD	MCV fl ± SD
4 and 5 years (94)	13·62 ± 1·33	8·40 ± 1·01	0·376 ± 0·036	44·9 ± 2·90
9 years and over (56)	13·89 ± 1·35	8·29 ± 0·94	0·385 ± 0·038	46·5 ± 2·72

* From Allen & Archer (1976).

noted during this period. The effects of training and exertion will be discussed more fully later (5.5.2).

Allen and Archer (1976) have shown that horses in training under National Hunt (NH) rules do not appear to have lower red cell figures as they grow older, although there is a tendency for the MCV to increase slightly (Table 5.4). These horses did have significantly lower figures than racehorses of similar age but trained on the flat. In general the influence of age is to reduce the red cell figures and there is a concomitant increase in the red cell indices. In ponies and hunters I have seen a notable increase in MCV in aged animals (50–57 fl).

5.2.1.2 Haemoglobin and red cell metabolism

Haemoglobin is the respiratory protein of the red blood cells which carries oxygen from the lungs to the tissues and facilitates the return transport of carbon dioxide. This important molecule, whose structure was first elucidated in the horse (Perutz *et al* 1960), is a conjugated protein (mol wt 64,500) composed of a metalloporphyrin, *haem*, bound to a protein moiety, *globin*. It contains 2 pairs of polypeptide chains, α and β chains, each of which is combined with one haem (Fig. 5.6). In contrast to many other mammals the haemoglobin components in the fetal horse are structurally identical to those of the adult (Stockwell *et al* 1961) and so no distinct *fetal haemoglobin* exists.

There are 2 types of haemoglobin found in all horses and these differ

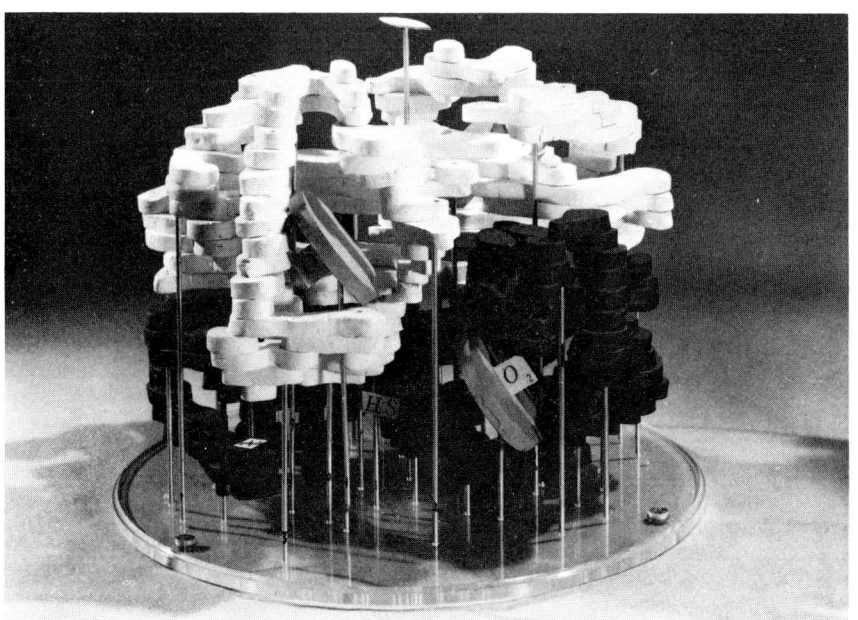

Fig. 5.6   Structural arrangement of the equine haemoglobin molecule (reproduced by kind permission of Dr M. F. Perutz, Cambridge).

only in respect of the polypeptide chains. These 2 haemoglobins are genetically controlled and currently proving of considerable importance in equine blood typing (Braend 1973). Only a single haemoglobin exists in the donkey but the mule has 3 components; one identical to those of the horse.

In addition to containing haemoglobin the erythrocytes also provide a compartment for a number of specific enzymes involved in maintaining the integrity of the haemoglobin and the cell itself. The levels of many of these enzymes and metabolites in normal ponies has been reported by Smith and Agar (1976) (see Table 5.5).

The delivery of oxygen to the tissue depends on the ability of the haemoglobin to take up oxygen from the lungs and release it to the tissues. The

Table 5.5   Red cell metabolites in four ponies*

Metabolite	Mean ± SE m moles/g Hb
Adenosine-5-triphosphate	812·0 ± 29·60
Adenosine-5-diphosphate	46·4 ± 1·80
Adenosine-5-monophosphate	6·54 ± 0·81
Glucose-6-phosphate	26·0 ± 1·49
Fructose-6-phosphate	10·1 ± 0·81
Fructose-1,6-diphosphate	11·4 ± 1·06
Glyceraldehyde-3-phosphate	5·26 ± 0·69
Dihydroxyacetone phosphate	22·2 ± 2·63
2,3-diphosphoglycerate	19·0 ± 0·44
3 phosphoglyceric acid	64·1 ± 4·24
2 phosphoglyceric acid	6·98 ± 3·22
Phosphoenol pyruvate	15·2 ± 0·85

* From Smith & Agar (1976).

organic phosphate (2,3-diphosphoglycerate or 2,3-DPG) significantly reduces the affinity of haemoglobin for oxygen and is, therefore, important in modulating oxygen transport from the lungs to the tissues. In the horse the levels of erythrocyte 2,3-DPG have been reported by Harkness *et al* (1969) and Lewis & McLean (1975). There was some variation with sex as mares had higher levels than stallions or geldings. A decrease in values was noted as a result of training although this was associated with an increase of whole blood haemoglobin levels. There was no demonstrable effect on enzyme levels with age or exercise.

Although no fetal haemoglobin can be demonstrated there is a significantly higher affinity of fetal blood for oxygen saturation than maternal blood (Kitchen & Bunn 1975). This increased affinity appears to be due to a lower content of 2,3-DPG in the fetal erythrocytes.

	Concentration of erythrocyte 2,3-DPG mmol/l RBC (± SD)
Non-pregnant and non-parous mares	6·4 ± 0·85
Foaling mares	6·8 ± 0·89
Newborn foals	4·36 ± 0·98
5 month fetuses	4·13

(from Kitchen & Bunn 1975)

5.2.1.3 Reticulocytes

Reticulocytes or polychromatophilic erythrocytes are seldom found in the peripheral blood of the horse. In most species they are released into the circulation following a haemolytic crisis or hypoxic stimulus. Their number in the blood can therefore be used as a measure of erythropoiesis but this may be misleading because of uneven or atypical responses. It is well known that adult horses even under severe haemolytic stress do not show a circulating reticulocytosis (Kitchen & Bunn 1971, Smith & Agar 1976). However, occasional reticulocytes can be found in newborn foals recovering from haemolytic disease (5.5.3.2).

In the bone marrow of horses reticulocytes may be found as larger cells than mature erythrocytes which have not yet attained the typical biconcave shape.

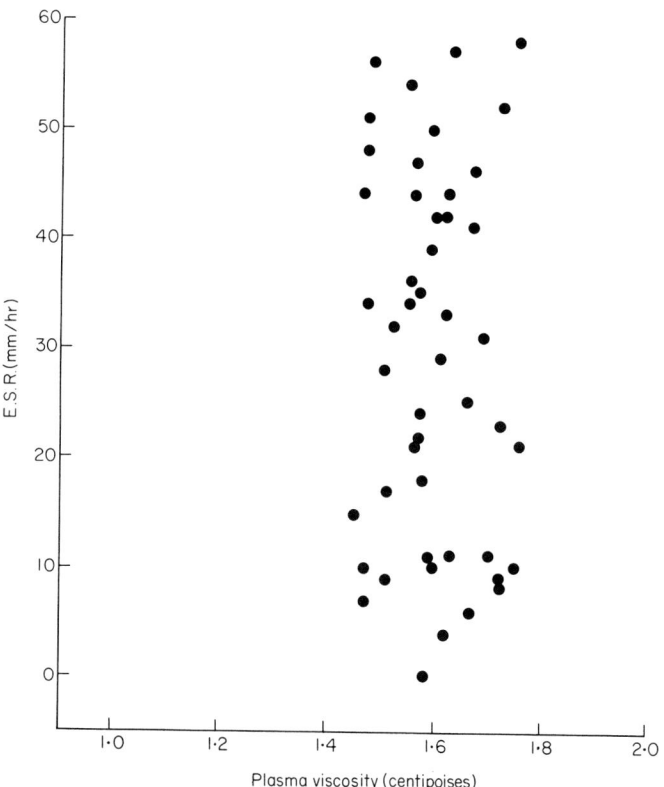

Fig. 5.7 Comparison of the results of estimation of erythrocyte sedimentation rate and plasma viscosity in blood samples from normal Thoroughbred horses (redrawn from Archer & Allen 1970).

5.2.1.4 Erythrocyte sedimentation rate and plasma viscosity

For many years the haemogram of the horse has included the measurement of ESR. The test was probably used because of its wide application in human medicine as a non-specific test of organic disease. It has also been employed as a screening test for horses (Table 5.6). However, sedimentation is always rapid since the red blood cells are small (i.e. MCV 40–45 fl) and tend to form rouleaux. This latter property is associated with the extreme flexibility of equine erythrocytes. They have a mean packing rate of approximately 25 per cent/min as compared with 6 per cent/min for man (Sirs, 1975). The ESR of horse red blood cells remains high even when mixed with sheep or dog plasma (Osbaldiston 1971). It is difficult, therefore, to measure increases in ESR accurately. Seckington (1969) finds that the ESR does give a broad guide to certain obscure, nonspecific conditions if samples are examined almost immediately after collection.

The ESR is not a satisfactorily reproducible test when performed on specimens more than a few hours old and therefore, for laboratories that receive the majority of their blood samples by post, this technique is very unreliable. There are also widely differing effects produced by different anticoagulants. Archer and Allen (1970) compared the results of ESR and plasma viscosity measurements (PV) in 60 normal Thoroughbreds and demonstrated the wide variation in results obtained by ESR compared to that of PV (Fig. 5.7).

At the Equine Research Station the ESR has been superseded by the measurement of PV (Archer & Allen 1970). This test is simple to perform (Chapter 14), reproducible and gives clear-cut abnormal figures in horses suffering from organic disease. Increases above 1·8 centipoises are certainly clinically significant (Table 5.6) and often indicate abnormal plasma protein levels. Chronic inflammatory or parasitic infections, some neoplastic conditions and paraproteinaemias show raised PV.

5.2.1.5 Erythropoiesis

Erythropoiesis commences in the yolk sac of the fetus and is characterized by the production of nucleated red blood cells. As development progresses the site of erythropoiesis shifts from the yolk sac to the liver. The fetal erythrocytes no longer have nuclei and are morphologically similar to adult red cells. Towards the end of gestation there is a second change, this time to the myeloid tissue of the bone marrow.

A recent comprehensive account of erythrocyte formation and development in the adult from fixed and stained films is given by Tschudi, Archer and Gerber (1975). The most primitive haemoglobin-free precursors of erythrocytes are called proerythroblasts or pronormoblasts. The diameter of

Table 5.6 Normal values for erythrocyte sedimentation rate and plasma viscosity for the Thoroughbred

	ESR (mm/h)				PV (centipoises)	
	No. examined	Mean ± SD	Range		No. examined	Mean ± SD
Foal (0–6 months)	38	32·0 ± 18·5	1–61	Foal < 1 month	78	1·48 ± 0·10
2 y.o.	36	45·0 ± 13·1	22–57	1 y.o.	100	1·59 ± 0·09
> 2 y.o. geldings	34	50·8 ± 10·4	19–66	2 y.o.	308	1·50 ± 0·08
				3 y.o.	353	1·51 ± 0·08
> 2 y.o. mares	24	34·5 ± 20·9	0–59	4 y.o.	138	1·53 ± 0·08
				> 4 y.o.	302	1·55 ± 0·10

these cells varies from 16 to 20μ. There is characteristic dark basophilic stippling of the cytoplasm which usually contains a brighter area (hoff) near the nucleus. The nucleus shows a dense, short-meshed and particularly clumped chromatin network. As a rule 1 to 4 nucleoli, surrounded by a rim of chromatin, may be seen. The least differentiated proerythroblasts contain a single sausage-shaped nucleolus. The nuclear–cytoplasmic ratio is wide in the pronormoblast. This ratio decreases progressively as the cell matures, up to the stage of haemoglobinized normoblast.

The basophilic pronormoblast develops into the basophilic normoblast or normoblast A with decreasing size, loss of nucleoli and developing a

Table 5.7 Approximate normal values for differential cell count of equine marrow

Myeloid		per cent	Erythroid		per cent
Polymorphs	Neutrophil	20–45	Normoblasts	C	13–26
	Eosinophil	0–3		B	6–18
	Basophil	0–0·5		A	1·5–8
Metamyelocytes	Neutrophil	10–40	Proerythroblasts		0·5–4
	Eosinophil	0–2·5	Haemocytoblasts		0–11
	Basophil	0–1			
Myelocytes	Neutrophil	8–30			
	Eosinophil	0–1	Lymphocytes		2–8
Promyelocytes	Neutrophil	0–3·	Plasma cells		0–3·5
	Eosinophil	0–0·5	Monocytes		0–2
Myeloblasts		0–1·5			
Megakaryocytes per 10,000 nucleated cells		0–2	Mitotic figures per 1,000 nucleated cells		2–2
Total cellularity per cu mm		20,000	M/E Ratio :1		1–3

coarser and denser chromatin structure. The nucleus is often surrounded by a pale, narrow and ring-like rim in normoblasts A and B corresponding to the hoff of the proerythroblast. The cytoplasm forms a rather narrow intensely blue staining ring around the nucleus. The cell diameter is now only 12 to 13 μ.

With beginning of haemoglobin formation, there is less basophilia and the cell becomes progressively more oxyphilic. A cell with a polychromatic cytoplasm is called a normoblast B or intermediate normoblast. Its diameter reaches 8 to 10 μ. With panoptic staining the cytoplasm is purple-grey or bluish-red. The round nucleus has a coarse chromatin structure.

Table 5.8 Normal values for white cell counts and differentials in various types of equidae

Type of animals	(No)	Total white cell count ×10⁹/l	Neutrophils ×10⁹/l			Eosinophils ×10⁹/l	Basophils ×10⁹/l	Lymphocytes ×10⁹/l	Monocytes ×10⁹/l
			Juv.	Stabs.	Segs.				
Thoroughbreds in training	(611)	9·54±1·83	—	—	—	—	—	—	—
Adult ponies	(27)	8·44±1·46	0·027	0·025	4·37±1·40	0·272±0·206	0·022	3·96±1·30	0·013
Crossbred ponies from one stud	(22)	10·34±1·53	0·002	0·018	4·89±1·42	0·541±0·362	0·026	4·95±0·94	0·076
Adult donkeys	(16)	10·90±1·46	0·008	0·081	4·97±1·18	0·544±0·281	0·006	5·15±1·80	0·088
Donkey foals (6–12 months)	(6)	14·77±3·12	0·036	0·072	4·84±1·74	0·310±0·262	0·047	10·26±2·40	0·102
Przewalski	*(9)	9·20	0	0	4·23	0·24	0	4·88	0·1
Onager	*(3)	10·60	0	0	6·63	0·11	0	3·76	0·16
Common zebra	*(11)	11·70	0	0	6·93	0·12	0·29	4·04	0·23
Mountain zebra	*(11)	10·30	0	0	4·22	0·31	0	5·56	0·15

* Figures abstracted from Jones (1976).

The intermediate normoblast changes into the orthochromatic normo-blast by completely losing cytoplasmic basophilia. At this stage the nuclear chromatin is so heavily clumped that little structure can be discerned on panoptic staining. By expulsion of the nucleus the reticulocyte is formed. This contains a loose reticulum of basophilic threads demonstrable in the cytoplasm only by supravital staining (e.g. brilliant cresyl blue). The develop-ment is completed at the mature stage of the normocyte which is free both of nuclear remnants and of reticular threads except in certain pathological states. The normal figures for bone marrow differential cell counts are given in Table 5.7.

5.2.2 LEUCOCYTES AND PLATELETS

5.2.2.1 Morphology and numbers

There is a wide range of normal differential leucocyte counts in the horse not only as a result of age, type and environment but also some individual variation probably exists. In general terms the total white count for adult horses is about $8 \cdot 0 \times 10^9/l$ (ranging from 6·0 to 12·0). Levels tend to be on the higher side of this figure in ponies and animals kept out at pasture (Table 5.8).

The normal neutrophil/lymphocyte ratio in the adult is about 60:40; approximate values for the other cells are as follows:

Neutrophils	
Juvenile	$0–0\cdot01 \times 10^9/l$
Stab	$0\cdot01–0\cdot50$
Segmented	$2\cdot0–6\cdot0$
Eosinophils	$0\cdot1–0\cdot35$
Basophils	$0–0\cdot10$
Lymphocytes	$1\cdot5–4\cdot0$
Monocytes	$0\cdot01–0\cdot50$

Detailed accounts of the morphology of the leucocytes of the horse are given by Archer (1960a) and Schalm *et al* (1975). The neutrophil has a multilobular nucleus and cytoplasm which contains dustlike pinkish granules. The majority of lymphocytes are small with darkly staining nuclei and limited cytoplasm. The monocyte usually has a broad kidney-shaped nucleus placed to one side of the cell. The cytoplasm is blue-grey and granular. The eosinophils are easily recognized by their numerous, large, tightly packed granules which almost completely fill the cytoplasm and may even obscure the nucleus. Basophils are rarely seen in equine blood smears. They have irregularly sized purplish granules in an uneven pattern throughout the cytoplasm.

There are considerable variations in the normal white cell picture with age. Jeffcott (1971) and Medeiros *et al* (1973) reported gradually increasing white counts during the first 12 months of life in ponies and Thoroughbreds respectively. There was a noticeable alteration in the neutrophil/lymphocyte ratio due to falling numbers of neutrophils and increasing numbers of lymphocytes (Fig. 5.8). The lymphocytes rose from 8 weeks of age to peak values at 7 months. This was considered useful evidence of onset of active immunity as immune responses are not evolved before the appearance of small lymphocytes in the circulation (Miller 1966). By 18 months to 2 years this situation has reverted to the previous 60:40 neutrophil/lymphocyte ratio. Horses in

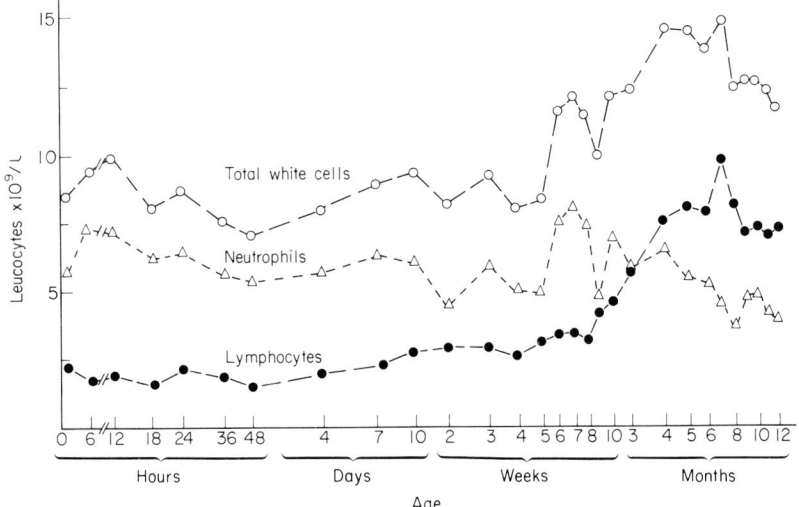

Fig. 5.8 Mean values for total white cells, neutrophils and lymphocytes in 8 pony foals from birth to 1 year (from Jeffcott 1971).

training show a gradual but slight decrease in total leucocyte count with age (Fig. 5.9).

Eosinophils were only occasionally seen before 7 days of age and numbers were usually less than $0.1 \times 10^9/l$ until 5 weeks of age (Fig. 5.10). In both ponies and Thoroughbreds a peak was reached at the 5–6 months stage; values returning to about $0.30 \times 10^9/l$ thereafter. Monocytes showed considerable variation in the first year of life but no obvious pattern was noted.

5.2.2.2 Platelets

Platelets (thrombocytes) in the horse are about 1–2 μ in diameter and numbers are usually lower than other domestic species. There are a number of reports of platelet counts in various types of horse (Table 5.9). The stem cell of the platelet is the megakaryoblast. The protoplasm of this cell is middle blue, stippled, but not granulated. The nucleus is either diploid or

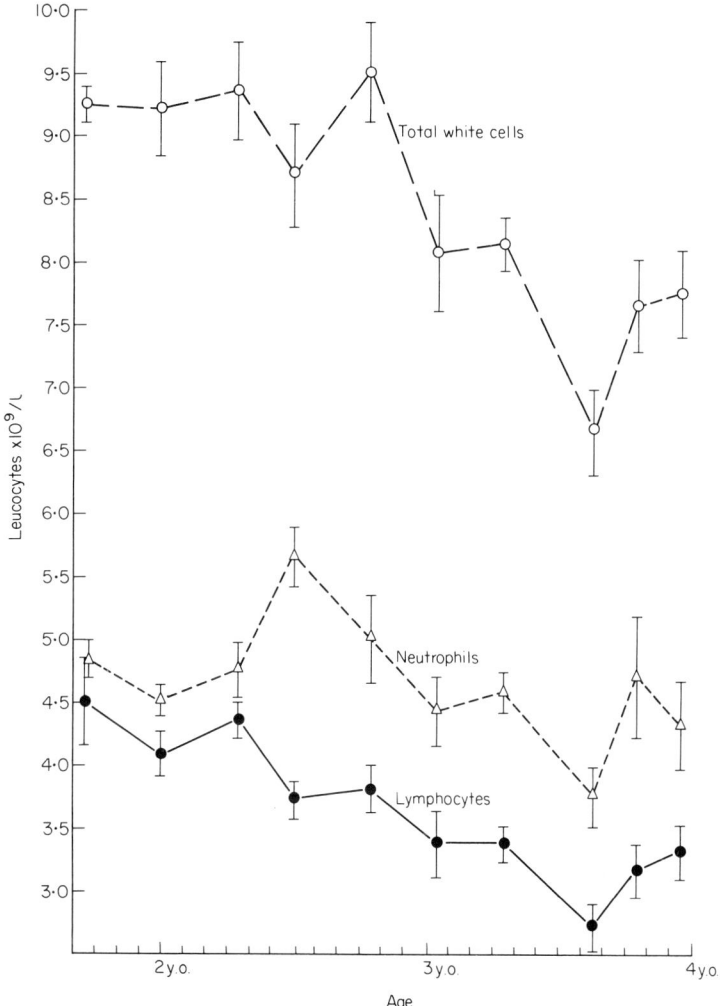

Fig. 5.9 Mean values of total white cells, neutrophils and lymphocytes during training of 8 Thoroughbreds (derived from data supplied by Catling 1976).

polyploid depending on the stage of mitosis (Tschudi *et al* 1975). Usually mitosis results in 2, 4 or more nuclei, but after endomitosis there is only one big, lobulated nucleus within the cell. The chromatin structure is fine meshed and rather dense. Nucleoli are only seen with difficulty.

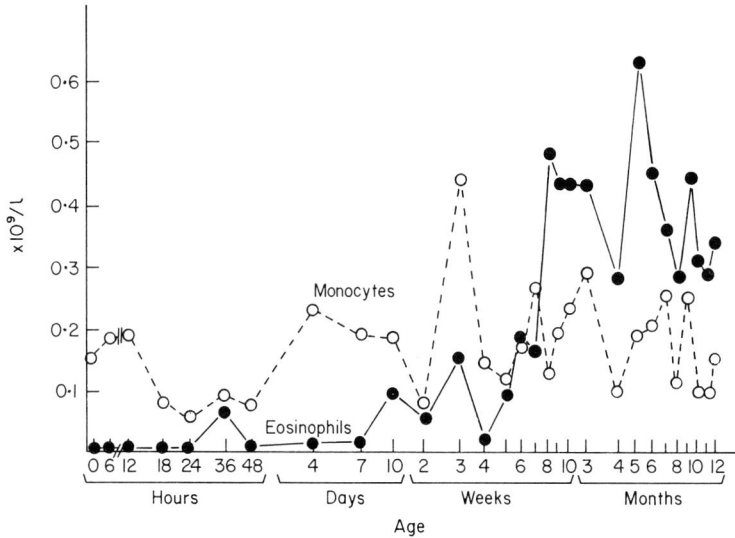

Fig. 5.10 Mean values for eosinophils and monocytes in 8 pony foals from birth to 1 year (from Jeffcott 1971).

Table 5.9 Platelet counts in the horse

Source	No. of animals	Type	Platelets × 10⁹/l Mean	Range
Stewart & Holman (1940)	36	Clydesdale	210	90–410
Bell *et al* (1955)	7	Thoroughbred	—	132–226
	3	Pony	—	223–276
Barkhan *et al* (1957)	8	Thoroughbred	—	114–168
	4	Pony	—	184–312
Stolpe (1970)	46	German Trotters	138	98–199
Finocchio *et al* (1970)	42	Quarterhorses	248·4	130–325·5
	26	Thoroughbred	200·7	92·5–327·5
	11	Shetland ponies	252·5	197·5–347·5
	14	Other breeds	244·7	122·5–377·5

The megakaryocytes are the largest blood-forming cells in the bone marrow, with diameters of 60 μ or more. The large lobulated nucleus contains a mesh of fine chromatin. The cytoplasm appears cloudy and polychromatic because there is a fine acidophilic granulation upon the basophilic background. The cytoplasm is seen to bud off from the borders to form the platelets. These have some azurophilic granules in a basophilic cytoplasm.

5.2.2.3 Leucopoiesis

The following account of leucopoiesis is taken from Tschudi, Archer and Gerber (1975).

(A) GRANULOPOIESIS

The myeloblast is considered to be the stem cell of all granulocytes, its diameter is about 17 μ. The cytoplasm is moderately basophilic, sometimes showing slightly uneven staining but there is no granulation. The nucleus has a characteristic, fine meshed chromatin structure in contrast with the coarse and dense clumping found in the nuclei of proerythroblasts. In the nuclei of myeloblasts there may be 4 nucleoli, or occasionally as many as 6 may be clearly visible by the chromatin rings which surround them.

The formation of azurophilic granules in the cytoplasm of myeloblasts is characteristic of the development of the cell to the next stage, the promyelocyte. These are the largest cells of granulopoiesis and having a diameter of 20 μ or more are larger than any cells of the erythropoietic series. The cytoplasm of the younger cells is basophilic but becomes paler as the cell matures. The brightening process always starts in the bay-shaped convex region of the nucleus. This region often stays free of any granules. The azurophilic granules are quite distinct from the specific eosinophilic, basophilic or neutrophilic granules which latter are also peroxidase positive and sudanophilic. With some further development of promyelocytes can be seen. Those with specific eosinophilic granules show very small and numerous specific granules as compared with the mature eosinophil.

Myelocytes develop from promyelocytes which have lost the azurophilic granules, show decreasing cytoplasm basophilia but increasing clumping of the nuclear chromatin. In the cytoplasm a typical, fine neutrophilic or somewhat coarse eosinophilic or basophilic granulation may be seen. The diameter of myelocytes reaches about 13 to 15 μ. From such cells the metamyelocytes develop, showing increased indentation of the nucleus and a denser chromatin structure. No nucleoli are visible. The cytoplasm is similar to that of the myelocytes.

As the nucleus becomes slimmer and chromatin clumps coarser the stab or staff form of granulocyte is developed. The nucleus often takes the form of an 'S' or a 'U'. When the nucleus is indented so much that the bridges between segments become slimmer than about a third of the neighbouring segments, the cells are called segmented granulocytes. All stages are, of course, further characterized according to their specific granulation in the cytoplasm (eosinophilic, basophilic or neutrophilic). It is usual to talk of eosinophils, basophils or neutrophils as soon as the cells become mature.

(B) MONOCYTES

A differentiation between promonocytes and monocytes on the one hand

and of myeloblasts and promyelocytes on the other hand is usually impossible without the application of special histochemical techniques. The monocytes are very polymorphous and their diameter varies from 12 to 18 μ. The nucleus is seldom round, more often kidney-shaped and more or less lobulated. The nucleus shows regions which are strongly stained and others which are quite pale. The colour of the cytoplasm is usually blue-grey by panoptic stains, often very much like the colour of lymphocyte cytoplasm, but the monocyte cytoplasm often contains extremely fine azurophilic granules.

(C) LYMPHOCYTES

There are few lymphatic follicles with germination centres in the bone marrow and it is best to obtain lymphatic cells directly from lymph nodes. The lymphoblast has a round or oval shape and measures 20–25 μ in diameter. The wide cytoplasm is basophilic but the colouring intensity varies considerably. It sometimes shows a mottling of the basophilia, limited to an area close to the nucleus whereas the periphery is homogeneous. The nucleus has a wide meshed, lumpy chromatin structure and there is a single large nucleolus with a distinct ring around it.

More mature lymphoblasts are small, with a diameter of less than 20 μ; they have a slender, homogeneous cytoplasm and a coarsely lumped nucleus without nucleoli. The fully mature lymphocyte has a diameter of 7 to 12 μ and is characterized by a very narrow band of basophilic cytoplasm usually only on one side of the nucleus. There are occasionally single, coarse azurophilic granules in the cytoplasm.

5.2.3   PLASMA

In this section some comments on the constituents of plasma as they relate to clinical haematology will be briefly considered. The application of plasma viscosity as a nonspecific test for organic disease has already been mentioned (5.2.1.4).

5.2.3.1   Serum and plasma proteins

The major proteins of the plasma comprise albumin, the globulins and fibrinogen. The normal levels of the serum proteins in healthy Thoroughbreds from foalhood to maturity are given in Table 5.10. The site of synthesis of albumin, α and β_1 globulin is the liver. The immune proteins (β_2 and γ globulin) are produced by plasma cells and lymphocytes of the reticuloendothelial system.

In foals, there is a very low total protein at birth but the level rapidly increases after colostrum ingestion. In the neonatal period there is a fall of passive γ globulin and to a less extent of the albumin. The low albumin levels during foalhood may be associated with the great demands for tissue protein during the peak period of growth. There is a steady rise from 2 weeks of age of adulthood at 4 to 6 years of age and an accompanying increase in the total protein.

As immunological competence increases there are rises in the α_2, β and γ globulins of the foals. Nevertheless, the pattern alters from the time the animals go into training as yearlings. The α_2 globulin, which rises steadily from birth, levels off at one year and falls a little over the next 2 to 3 years.

Table 5.10 Serum protein levels in normal Thoroughbreds*

Age	No. of animals	Total protein (g/l)	Albumin (g/l)	Globulins (g/l)			
				α_1	α_2	β	γ
0 h	16	42·5	28·7	1·9	5·9	6·3	0
24 h	17	52·4	29·5	1·8	3·6	9·8	7·6
7 d	19	51·2	26·5	2·6	5·6	10·4	6·3
14 d	19	49·7	24·4	2·6	5·4	12·1	5·4
28 d	18	50·3	24·6	2·9	6·4	12·5	4·3
2 mth	16	53·4	24·5	2·9	8·1	13·4	4·5
3 mth	8	58·1	27·4	2·2	9·1	14·0	5·2
6–9 mth	32	58·8	28·1	2·7	10·3	12·5	5·3
1 yr	23	58·2	29·6	2·1	9·6	12·5	4·2
2 yr	9	59·8	29·9	3·1	8·8	11·6	5·3
3 yr	27	60·7	34·5	2·9	7·1	10·3	6·1
4–6 yr	10	64·6	37·4	2·7	6·6	11·1	7·0

* From Jeffcott (1974).

The β globulin follows a similar pattern but shows a more pronounced drop with age. The γ globulin, which begins with a steady rise from 2 months, declines temporarily at 1 year and then increases gradually. Levels remain below that recorded after birth, the latter resulting from colostrum ingestion. The α_1 globulin shows no significant alteration at any time from birth to adulthood. A very different picture is seen in ponies kept out at grass; these 3 fractions continue to rise in the second year, particularly the β globulins.

The progressive reduction of values in globulin seen in 1, 2 and 3 year old Thoroughbreds may be associated with the rather protected environment of a training establishment and the absence of significant parasitic infection.

FIBRINOGEN

The normal plasma fibrinogen concentration in adult horses is $2·58 \pm 0·072$ g/l (Schalm *et al* 1975). There is no apparent influence of age or breed. The fibrinogen level can be expected to increase in inflammatory, neoplastic and traumatic disorders as it does in other species.

The haptoglobins are normal constituents of serum which migrate with α_2 globulin fraction on electrophoresis (mol wt 100,000). Their function is to conserve iron within the body by binding free haemoglobin into a hapto-globin–haemoglobin complex. Levels in normal Thoroughbreds and ponies have been estimated by Allen and Archer (1971):

	No. examined	Haptoglobin Mean ($\pm$SD) (g/dl)	Range
Thoroughbred and Thoroughbred crosses	77	88 ± 31	47–180
Crossbred ponies	30	69 ± 20	45–107

Similar values were recorded in late fetuses and foals, which is contrary to the situation in man. Allen & Archer found the use of serum haptoglobin level a sensitive and rapid indication of haemolysis.

5.2.3.2 Bilirubin and other serum constituents

The plasma of the horse is an unusually yellow colour. This is due to the amounts of carotenoids and xanthophylls present in the diet and to a partic-ularly high concentration of bilirubin compared to other domestic species. Total serum bilirubin is about 2·7 mg/100 ml (Cornelius *et al* 1960b) and the major portion of this is present as conjugated or 'direct reacting' bilirubin. The level of free or 'indirect reacting' bilirubin is about 0·1 mg/100 ml with a range of 0–0·4 mg/100 ml.

The serum bilirubin content of horses does vary considerably and, in some clinically normal animals, levels may be 5–8 mg/100 ml. Ramsay (1946) noted that starvation for 48 hours produced a considerable increase in plasma bilirubin values. Moderately high levels are sometimes seen in other-wise normal pregnant and barren Thoroughbred mares out at grass during late summer. It is perhaps worth noting that donkeys have a much lower serum bilirubin content ($<0·4$ mg/100 ml) and this is also true for the Przewalski and zebra (Jones 1976). The horse is apparently able to tolerate very high bilirubin concentration in such conditions as haemolytic anaemia and severe liver disease without exhibiting signs of kernicterus or other irreversible damage.

Other serum constituents that prove of diagnostic value in equine clinical haematology are listed in Table 5.11.

Table 5.11 Normal serum constituents in 650 Thoroughbreds

	All ages	Foals <1 year	1 year	2 years	3 years	4 years	>4 years
Enzymes (iu/l at 25°C)							
AAT—aspartate amino transferase	107±20	—	122±20	171±62	143±19	158±52	95±25
CPK—creatine kinase	37±19	—	—	—	—	—	—
SDH—sorbitol dehydrogenase	0·62±0·5	—	—	—	—	—	—
AP—alkaline phosphatase	—	150±355	106±20	92±20	86±12	82±10	80±12
Inorganic constituents							
Ca—calcium (m mol/l)	—	3·19±0·1	3·14±0·08	2·97±0·08	2·97±0·08	2·94±0·08	2·95±0·08
PO$_4$—phosphate	—	1·9±0·13	1·6±0·1	1·45±0·2	1·36±0·13	1·3±0·2	1·25±0·2
Mg—magnesium	0·79±0·08	—	—	—	—	—	—
Na—sodium	144±5	—	—	—	—	—	—
K—potassium	4·2±0·6	—	—	—	—	—	—
Cl—chloride	96±3	—	94·7±3	96·4±3	96·0±2	96·0±3	99·0±3
Hydrogen ion (10^{-PH})	36–47·5	—	—	—	—	—	—
Organic constituents							
Urea (m mol/l)	4·48±0·83	—	—	—	—	—	—
Cholesterol (mg/100 ml)	122±18	—	—	—	—	—	—
Bilirubin (mg/100 ml)	1·62±0·5	—	—	—	—	—	—

5.3 BLOOD TYPING IN HORSES

5.3.1 RED CELL GROUPING AND SERUM PROTEIN POLYMORPHISMS

The term *blood group* dates back to Landsteiner's (1901) original work in which he showed that the antigenic properties of the red cells of man varied, permitting a simple classification or 'ABO' system. *Blood group* describes only the antigens on the red cell surface; the term *blood type* is generally used to include the red cell groups and the polymorphic serum proteins (i.e. those proteins in serum which can exist in several genetically determined forms).

The fundamental research into equine blood groups was initiated after Landsteiner's original publications and was later stimulated by the discovery that haemolytic disease of the newborn foal (iso-erythrolysis) was caused by isosensitization (Coombs *et al* 1948). A number of reports concerning the existence of an ABO system in the horse were reviewed by Podliachouk (1957). There was however no strict reciprocal relationship between agglutinins in the serum and agglutinogens on the red cell. In addition, the reactions of these naturally occurring antibodies were invariably very weak, which explains why it is possible initially to transfuse the blood of one horse into another without fear of harmful reactions.

The various blood typing systems are all completely independent of one another and they are all inherited in a direct manner (i.e. there is no recessive transmission of genes). It follows that blood typing can be broadly divided into red cell grouping, which uses the classical serological methods of agglutination and lysis, and protein polymorphism typing, which employs the more recent techniques of electrophoresis and sophisticated staining procedures. The various alleles which may be used in equine blood typing are listed in Table 5.12. Detailed reviews on this subject have been presented by Braend (1973) and Scott (1973, 1975).

Haemolytic disease in the horse is a natural manifestation of the existence of individual differences amongst the red cell groups. The disease is analogous to rhesus haemolytic disease of humans. The mare is thought to be iso-immunized by transplacental passage of fetal red cell antigens, which are inherited from the stallion. The foals are not affected *in utero* and in most cases the colostrum contains anti-A_1, or anti-Q antibodies. Some of the cases of the disease are due to anti-R and anti-S, and rarely anti-E_2 or anti-U (Scott 1973).

The main application of blood typing is in specification of parentage and identification of the individual (Scott 1975). All parentage tests are based on the principle of genetic exclusion (i.e. by showing that a certain animal could not be the parent of the foal in question). The most common

Table 5.12 The different alleles involved at the various red cell antigen and protein polymorphism loci*

Red cell antigen		Protein polymorphisms	
Locus	Alleles	Locus	Alleles
A	a^{A1}, $a^{A'}$, a^{AH}, a^{H}, a	Albumin	Al^F, Al^S
C	c^C, c	Transferrin	Tf^D, Tf^F, Tf^G, Tf^H, Tf^M, Tf^O, Tf^R
D	d^{E1E2}, d^{E2}, $d^{E'}$ $d^{D2E'}$, d^{D2EY}, d^{EY}, $d^{D1E'}$	Esterase	Es^F, Es^G, Es^H, Es^I, Es^S
		Prealbumin	Pr^F, Pr^I, Pr^L, Pr^N, Pr^S, Pr^U, Pr^W
K	k^K, k	Haemoglobin	Hb^A, Hb^a
P	p^{P1}, $p^{P'}$, o	Carbonic anhydrase	CA^F, CA^I, CA^L, CA^S
Q	q^Q, q^{QR}, q^R, q^{RS}, q^S, q	6-phosphogluconate dehydrogenase	PGD^D, PGD^F, PGD^S
		Phosphoglucomutase	PGM^F, PGM^S, PGM^V
U	u^U, u	Phosphohexose isomerase	PHI^F, PHI^I, PHI^S
X	x^X, x	Acid phosphatase	AcP^F, AcP^S

* From Scott (1975).

situation is the case where there are 2 possible sires for a foal. The 4 animals (both stallions, the dam and the foal) are blood typed and the results evaluated. The factors present in the foal that are absent in the dam, must have been inherited from the true sire. The stallion which does not have these factors can then be excluded as the parent. The total probability of solving a parentage case is approximately 94 per cent and the chance of randomly finding 2 horses with the same blood type is about 1 in 13,600.

5.3.2   BLOOD TRANSFUSION IN EQUINE PRACTICE

Routine blood transfusion for horses is not in common use at present, although, with the recent advances in equine surgery, its application could well be increased, particularly in the larger practices and veterinary schools. It is generally employed as a life-saving measure and if performed with care, the risks are minimal. Haemolytic disease of the newborn is a rather special case and acutely ill foals may require an exchange transfusion. The clinical details, diagnosis and treatment of this condition will be dealt with in more detail later (5.5.3.2).

A single transfusion of blood without crossmatching is considered safe provided the recipient has never before received a transfusion. Repeated transfusion of the same blood is safe if it is given within 24 hours of the first transfusion. It may also be repeated at intervals of not more than a day for about 7 days.

The major indications for transfusion are:

(1) Acute and severe haemorrhage
  (a) Trauma or accident
  (b) During or after surgery
  (c) At parturition following rupture of the uterine artery
  (d) Haemophilia
(2) Haemolytic disease of the newborn foal
(3) Chronic or haemolytic anaemias
(4) Haemodilution and anaemia due to chronic intestinal damage (e.g. protein-losing enteropathy).

A possible contraindication for blood transfusion is in surgical shock, as this may tend to overload an already failing circulatory system.

5.3.2.1   The selection of a donor and the relation to blood groups

It is not considered essential to cross match the blood of the donor and recipient. However, this would be required if the recipient had already received one or two more transfusions or the donor or recipient were isosensitized mares. The usual method for cross matching is by the Coombs' indirect antiglobulin test (Coombs *et al* 1946). It is unwise to do a simple direct agglutination test because of the tendency for the red cells to form rouleaux giving a false positive result.

An intimate knowledge of equine blood typing is not necessary for a practical blood transfusion service. However, if laboratory facilities are available and typing can be performed then the most suitable donors are those animals with A_1 and Q negative cells. These two red cell types are the most antigenic and, therefore, more likely to cause a transfusion reaction.

5.3.2.2 Method of collection and storage

Blood should be collected aseptically into sterile transfusion bottles or plastic containers with acid citrate dextrose (ACD) as anticoagulant. The volume that may be collected from the donor will vary according to the body weight and clinical condition. It is usually quite safe to take 5–8 litres from a 600 kg animal.

Once collected the blood should be transfused as soon as possible. There is little information relating to the effects of storage on the survival of transfused red blood cells in the horse. If the blood is to be stored for more than 2 or 3 hours it should be kept at 4°C. It must not, of course, be frozen or gross haemolysis will occur. Under these conditions blood that is more than about 7 days old should be discarded.

5.3.2.3 Technique of transfusion

The transfused blood should always be administered via a sterile giving-set. As a precaution against untoward reactions, it is wise initially to give a small quantity of blood, halt the transfusion for a few minutes and check the pulse and respiration before continuing. It is important to give the blood slowly, at about one litre per 15 to 20 minutes. This will enable the heart and circulation to accommodate the increased volume without undue embarrassment.

The volume of blood given to a patient will depend on the degree of anaemia and clinical state of the patient. The clinical improvement seen after transfusion of a few litres of donor blood is often surprising even if there has been little demonstrable improvement in the red cell picture. Very occasionally blood transfusions fail to give a beneficial response and this may be due to an excessive amount of anticoagulant in the donor blood so that the recipient is deprived of calcium and bleeding ensues (Archer & Franks 1961).

Transfusion of incompatible blood may result in a harmful reaction or alternatively the donor cells will be rapidly removed from the recipient's circulation. In the conscious horse the first sign of a transfusion reaction is shifting of weight on the hindlimbs, accompanied by flaring of the nostrils and increased respiratory rate. The animal appears lethargic, may yawn and has rapid shallow breathing and tachycardia. In severe reactions defaecation and micturition will occur and the horse may become unsteady and fall down (Archer & Franks 1961).

5.4 CLINICAL HAEMODYNAMICS OF THE HORSE BLOOD

It has been known for a long time that physical exertion of horses leads to an increase in the erythrocyte count. The horse has a very large blood-cell reservoir (Persson 1967) which can be mobilized with great rapidity and efficiency. This may well be associated with the horse's natural tendency to

Table 5.13 Factors affecting the resting haemogram of the horse

Haemoconcentration (rise in PCV)	*Haemodilution (fall in PCV)*
Excitement	Haemorrhage or acute blood loss
Handling	General anaesthesia
Adrenalin injection	Tranquillization
Exertion	Administration of hypotensive drug (e.g. acetyl promazine)
Diuresis	
Disease (e.g. septicaemia, toxaemia etc.)	

'fright and flight' resulting in a sudden alteration in the cell/plasma ratio of the peripheral blood with an associated shift of intravascular to extravascular fluid.

A variety of factors may significantly alter the resting blood picture (Table 5.13). The effect of excitation and exertion (Fig. 5.11) on the PCV has been described by Archer and Clabby (1965) and it is striking how rapidly the red cells are mobilized, within a matter of seconds in most instances. The resting PCV of fit racehorses is about 0·40 l/l while under exertion this will rise by 0·1–0·2 l/l, thereby greatly improving gaseous exchange and tissue oxygenation. There is, of course, a concomitant rise in blood viscosity at this time (Fig. 5.12) which results partly from increased red cell mass and partly from a fluid shift out of the peripheral circulation.

Persson (1967) observed that under the influence of excitement or injection of adrenalin the plasma volume (PV) was reduced suggesting a shift of body water across capillary walls. This has recently been confirmed by Catling (1975). The plasma proteins increase slightly with increasing PCV suggesting that water leaves the vascular system in partial compensation for the sudden increase in circulating blood volume (Schalm *et al* 1975).

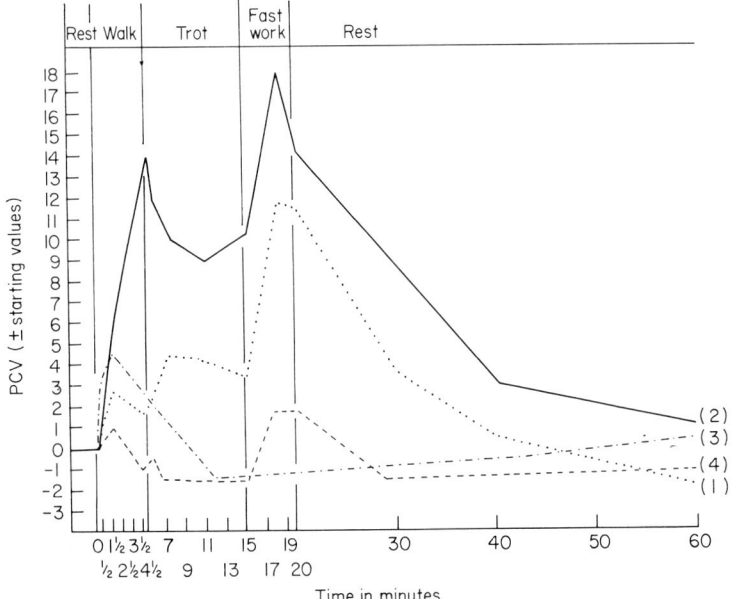

Fig. 5.11 The effect of excitation and exertion on the PCV (from Archer & Clabby, 1965). The PCVs are recorded as deviations from the starting level for each experiment: thus a change of from 40 to 45 would be recorded as '+5'. Curve (1): a pony exerted according to the schedule marked at the top of the figure. Curve (2): a Thoroughbred mare similarly exerted. Curve (3): a pony twitched from 0 to 1½ minutes. Curve (4): a pony watching another pony, the latter being exerted as in Curve (1).

The ability of horses to call on their reserves of erythrocytes by rapid haemoconcentration can easily be reversed. A hypotensive drug such as acetyl promazine can produce a significant drop in the blood picture (Jeffcott 1974). This is accompanied by very little change in the plasma viscosity or the serum proteins although there is probably some increase in intravascular fluid.

The return to normal red cell values after exertion takes some hours and levels may fall temporarily below the usual resting state in a transitory 'rebound effect'. A similar situation may also be seen following administration of a hypotensive drug.

The red cell reservoir in the horse is apparently confined to the spleen (Torten & Schalm 1964, Persson *et al* 1973a b, Catling & Jeffcott 1975). The size of the spleen varies very considerably and large increases can be expected after administration of some drugs (e.g. barbiturates). The effect

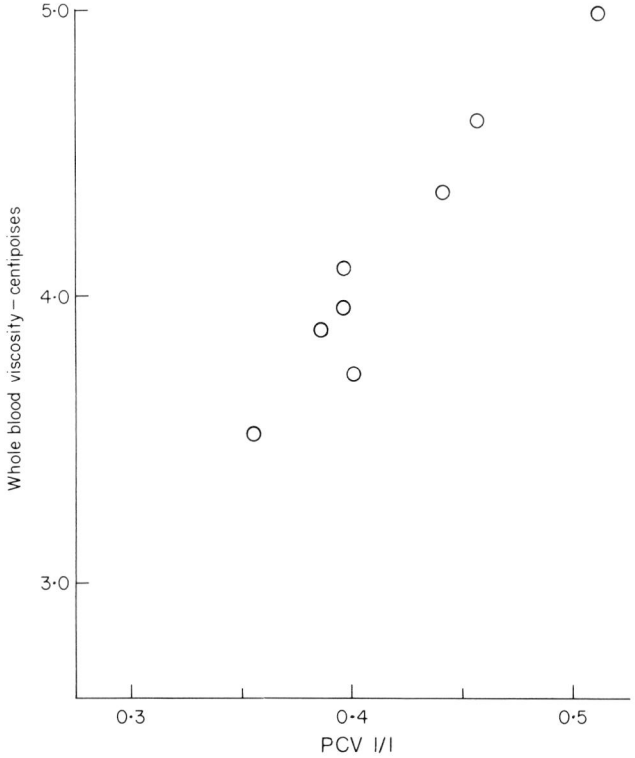

Fig. 5.12 The increase of PCV and blood viscosity with exercise (from Catling 1976).

of splenectomy is to abolish the ability to significantly haemoconcentrate or haemodilute the peripheral blood picture. Persson *et al* (1973a) reported that in splenectomized animals the resting PCV was intermediate between the resting and exercise values prior to splenectomy. However, in 2 ponies Catling and Jeffcott (1975) showed that there was a somewhat higher red cell picture immediately after splenectomy but that levels gradually fell to a little below the values prior to splenectomy. A substantial and persistent increase in the platelet count was seen after splenectomy. There was no indication that any other organ took over the spleen's function up to a year after surgery. The spleen was found in 2 horses (Torten & Schalm 1964) to be capable of supplying red cell volume equal to approximately 33 per cent of the circulating red cell mass. No clinical effects following splenectomy have been reported, although the effects on performance post-splenectomy are currently being investigated (Catling 1976).

5.5   ALTERATIONS IN THE HAEMOGRAM

5.5.1   EFFECTS DUE TO MANAGEMENT, ENVIRONMENT AND ALTITUDE

There seem to be only minor alterations in the blood picture associated with management, unless, of course, there are gross deficiencies in nutrition. Some owners and trainers advocate the regular administration of haematinic medication to their horses, although their effects on improving the red cell figures has been disappointing (Kirkham *et al* 1971, Laufenstein-Duffy 1971). One other possible effect of management relates to upset in fluid balance and temporary alteration of plasma volume. This may be associated with hot weather or abnormal fluid intake and can result in either haemo-concentration or haemodilution.

It is surprising, in view of the extent of horse travel today, that there is so little published material on haematological data during transit to race-meetings and other equine events. Azzie (1973) in South Africa reports that prolonged journeys by train can cause mild dehydration due to sweating but blood figures return to normal within 48 hours.

There are no obvious differences in the haemograms of horses kept at high altitude (Trum 1952). However a marked change in altitude may have some effect and animals require a few weeks to acclimatize to their new conditions (Azzie 1973). Much of this is probably due to sweating, although other sources of water loss (e.g. in urine, faeces and from the lungs) may be involved. Horses taken from low to high altitudes showed a temporary rise in PCV and the reverse situation occurs with some increase in MCHC and MCV after transit to sea level from high altitude.

5.5.2   EFFECTS DUE TO FITNESS AND TRAINING

Neser (1923) endeavoured to show that the blood count of the horse depended to a large extent on its physical condition. In his results he showed stabled horses to have RBCs of $3.9–7.0 \times 10^{12}/l$. However, it is now clear that these differences were mainly accounted for by the type and breed of the animal rather than the state of fitness.

A steady increase in red cell parameters is seen during early training of young racehorses (Fig. 5.4). This is chiefly attributed to maturity rather than the stage of training or the condition of the animal (Kitchen *et al* 1965). The figures level off as a 2 year old and remain fairly steady thereafter. Irvine (1958) found a slight drop in erythrocyte parameters with increased fitness of horses in training but Archer (1959) noticed no appreciable difference either way. Stewart *et al* (1970) showed some fall in the blood counts of racehorses after a period of rest from training.

It is not possible to assess performance potential accurately by examination of the haemogram. However, haematological analysis may be of use in assessing the health status of the animal and in conjunction with biochemical tests may be of some value in assessing fitness. It may, therefore, be possible to predict that a horse will *not* perform to its expected potential on a particular occasion (Jeffcott 1974). The effect of training improves the haemodynamics of the peripheral circulation (i.e. by allowing for a greater and more sustained rise of PCV during exertion) but does not significantly alter the resting haemogram.

5.5.3 ANAEMIA

Anaemia is defined as a reduction in the number of the erythrocytes and/or the haemoglobin concentration in the blood. It is a relatively uncommon condition in Thoroughbreds but when it does occur it is usually associated with haemorrhage or is secondary to a number of chronic debilitating conditions. Anaemia is more often seen in hunters and ponies where, again, it is often associated with chronic cachexia or parasitism.

Many reports on normal values of red cell parameters of the horse have been published (Table 5.1) but few specific papers on the causes of anaemia are available (Archer & Poynter 1957, McGuire & Henson 1968, Dixon & Archer 1975, Schalm *et al* 1975). There are 3 major causes of equine anaemia (Table 5.14). Firstly there is anaemia due to loss of erythrocytes from haemorrhage; secondly that associated with accelerated red cell destruction or haemolysis and thirdly that due to reduced or defective production of erythrocytes by the bone marrow. The morphological classification of anaemia in horses is much less easily defined although most types are normocytic and normochromic. No evidence of such conditions as pernicious or sickle cell anaemia has been found in the horse. Haemolytic disease of the newborn does occur as a natural manifestation of isosensitization of the dam and is analogous to Rhesus haemolytic disease of man.

The diagnosis of anaemia in the horse is complicated by the rather unstable haemodynamic state of horse blood (see p. 190). There are a number of factors which tend to increase the erythrocyte reservoir in the spleen which may therefore produce an apparent 'anaemia'. A possible cause of this in

Table 5.14 Causes of anaemia in the horse

Direct Blood Loss	*Haemorrhage from trauma and surgery* *Epistaxis* *Defective coagulation*: 　Haemophilia 　Warfarin poisoning 　Primary idiopathic thrombocytopenic purpura
Haemolysis	*Haemolytic disease of newborn* *Infections*: 　Equine infectious anaemia (EIA) 　Babesiosis 　Ehrlichiosis 　Trypanosomiasis 　Leptospirosis *Poisons and toxic chemicals*: 　Lead 　Phenothiazine 　Onion poisoning *Autoimmune haemolytic anaemia* *Idiopathic haemolytic anaemia*
Dyserythropoiesis	*Primary*: 　Nutritional—iron and folate deficiency 　Idiopathic hypoplastic anaemia *Secondary*: 　Parasitic infestation 　Chronic inflammatory disease and debility 　Purpura haemorrhagica 　Malignant neoplasia 　Aplastic anaemia

equine practice is collection of blood samples following acetyl promazine tranquillization. Red cell figures may decrease by some 25 per cent following usual therapeutic doses (0·005 mg/kg acetyl promazine) (Jeffcott 1974). On the other hand a degree of anaemia may be temporarily masked due to excitement by the rapid mobilization of the red cell reserves from the spleen. One other condition that must not be misinterpreted as a microcytic anaemia is in weanling to yearling foals, when the erythrocytes are normally of small size (Fig. 5.3).

5.5.3.1 Anaemia from direct blood loss

HAEMORRHAGE

Acute or chronic blood loss constitutes a major cause of anaemia. Direct trauma is the most common precipitating factor but rupture of damaged blood vessels or defective coagulation may also result in severe bouts of haemorrhage. In cases of guttural pouch mycosis there is rupture of the internal carotid artery (Cook 1968) and in old brood mares there may be rupture of a small aneurysm on the uterine artery. Severe haemorrhage may also result following accidental damage to major blood vessels or as a consequence of certain surgical procedures.

The amount of blood lost before any clinical signs are evident may be up to one-third of the total red cell mass. It is perhaps surprising how profound an anaemia can exist in horses (e.g. RBC 4.0×10^{12}/l; Hb 3.0 g/dl; PCV 0.15 l/l) without showing the expected clinical effects. The type of anaemia in acute blood loss is normochromic and normocytic. Immediately after a serious haemorrhage there is an increase in the platelet count and this is followed by some leucocytosis, often with a slight shift to the left. In the ensuing days some anisocytosis of the erythrocytes may be seen but no punctate basophilia occurs and as already mentioned little release of reticulocytes from the marrow takes place. There is however an increase in some of the red cell metabolites (Smith & Agar, 1976) particularly adenosine-5-triphosphate (ATP) for about a week following blood loss. Smith and Agar also showed experimentally that after reducing the PCV to approximately 0.15 l/l by phlebotomy that there is a linear increase in PCV over the next 2 weeks of 0.007 l/l per day.

Severe haemorrhage will provoke some erythroid hyperplasia with increased number of reticulocytes detectable in the bone marrow. These changes may be associated with some secondary myeloid hyperplasia during the recovery stage.

EPISTAXIS

The incidence of epistaxis in racehorses, often referred to as 'bleeders', is quite high (Cook 1974). Many of these animals have some pre-existing pulmonary disease which provokes haemorrhage from the lungs. The condition is usually seen after exercise or racing and is colloquially known as 'breaking a blood vessel'. It often occurs on more than one occasion, but the haemorrhages produced are not usually very serious and so the animals do not often become anaemic. The exact aetiology is, in many cases, obscure and a large number of empirical treatments have been tried. It has been suggested that epistaxis may be due to formation of defective fibrinogen or to a thrombocytopenia (Loeb 1972). Vitamin K therapy has been quite extensively used in practice although in the majority of cases there is no evidence of defective blood coagulation.

More serious haemorrhages with secondary anaemia sometimes occur in such conditions as mycosis of the guttural pouch (Cook 1968) and progressive ethmoidal haematoma (Cook & Littlewort 1974).

DEFECTIVE COAGULATION

Haemophilia Disorders of coagulation in the horse appear to be rare. True haemophilia (Haemophilia A) has been reported in the Thoroughbred (Archer 1961, Hutchins *et al* 1964) and in the Standardbred (Sanger *et al* 1964). It is an inherited defect in the blood clotting mechanism due to a deficiency of factor VIII or antihaemophilic globulin (AHG). The condition is probably similar to the human counterpart (Archer & Allen 1972); the character for haemophilia occurring as a sex linked recessive on the X chromosome.

The clinical picture is one of extensive subcutaneous bleeding. Foals are apparently normal at birth, but within a few days show a number of small subcutaneous haematomata along the back or where the mare may nibble the coat. A little later larger swellings over the hindquarters and hocks appear and a secondary normocytic anaemia develops. The prognosis is grave and foals are usually euthanased before the age of 6 months. Treatment with bovine and porcine AHG has been shown to be beneficial but only on a temporary basis (Nossel *et al* 1962). The diagnosis is based on the clinical and haematological pictures and demonstrations of Factor VIII deficiency.

Factor IX (Christmas factor) deficiency has not been recorded in horses although Sjølin (1965) and Gardikas *et al* (1965) concluded that normal horses had less Factor IX in the blood than man.

Warfarin is a dicoumarol-like agent and in cases of poisoning produces clinical signs of petechiation of the visible mucosae and haemorrhages. There may be a fall in the red cell parameters and retinal haemorrhages may also be seen. There is usually a delay of about 2 days before the 1-stage prothrombin test shows any significant diminution of factor VII. For treatment the administration of vitamin K_1 is beneficial.

A useful and practical screening test for detection of warfarin poisoning in blood samples transported by post can be carried out by the commercially available Normotest system (Allen & Archer 1972).

In the horse warfarin has 2 distinct effects upon the coagulation system. In the first place a reduction of the ability of the plasma to react to contact with a foreign surface occurs within about 24 hours. The effect is more pronounced after 48 hours but thereafter disappears. The second effect is a deficiency of factor VII which cannot be demonstrated by 1-stage techniques until at least 48 hours after warfarin dosing and the effect is not demonstrable with viper venom as a thromboplastic source (Archer 1960b).

Primary idiopathic thrombocytopenic purpura Only one case of this condition has been reported in the horse (Sorenson 1972), although it is not unduly rare in the dog, pig and man. The animal presented with thrombocytopenia, petechiation of the mucosal surfaces, oedema of the ventral abdomen and haemorrhage of the skin and intestinal tract. The low platelet count was regarded as the cause of haemorrhage but the exact aetiology was not ascertained. In man the condition is usually regarded as an autoimmune disease (Harrington *et al* 1953). In Sorenson's case there was no anaemia initially but platelets were only $33 \cdot 0 \times 10^9/l$ and there was a neutrophilia. Other haematological and biochemical parameters were normal. The haemoglobin level dropped over the ensuing few days as a result of intestinal bleeding. Treatment with cortisone administration for 10 days was successful, the platelet count returned to normal and no further bleeding took place.

Purpura haemorrhagica is not associated with a thrombocytopenia or any other coagulation defect and will be considered later (see p. 207).

5.5.3.2   Haemolytic anaemia

Haemolytic anaemias in the horse may be caused by iso-sensitization, protozoan parasites, viral or bacterial micro-organisms, poisons or toxic chemicals and, rarely, by autoimmune diseases. When the anaemia is severe and sudden in onset there are usually associated signs of jaundice and haemoglobinuria. There will also be a fall in the circulating haptoglobin levels due to their rapid saturation with free haemoglobin to form a haptoglobin/ haemoglobin complex which can be eliminated by the reticuloendothelial systems.

HAEMOLYTIC DISEASE OF THE FOAL

This condition is caused in newly born foals by the absorption of haemolysins and haemagglutinins from the colostrum of a sensitized mare. The mare is thought to be iso-immunized by transplacental passage of fetal red cell antigens which are inherited from the stallion. The fetus is not affected *in utero*, perhaps because there is a barrier for transfer of antibody across the mare's placenta. Iso-immunization does not occur in every incompatible pregnancy. *Clinical signs*   On the basis of symptomatology the disease may be divided into peracute, or subacute types. The severity of the disease in a foal is related to the antibody titre of the colostrum, the volume of colostrum ingested and probably to the type of antibody present (Jeffcott 1969).

The foals appear healthy at birth and remain so for some hours. From 8 hours to 5 days they show progressive lethargy and weakness, pallor and jaundice of the mucous membranes. Suckling is infrequent and then only for short periods, though the appetite is not usually affected till much later in the course of the disease. The condition is essentially afebrile. Clinical signs of acute and severe anaemia due to intravascular haemolysis are evident.

The cardiac sounds are increased in amplitude and area of audibility. The peripheral arterial pulse is imperceptible but a marked jugular pulse is sometimes noted. The respirations are normal except where severe anaemia is present. Clinical evidence of kernicterus has not been recorded in the literature. In acute and severe cases, haemoglobinuria is sometimes seen, and this is often the first clinical sign observed. Foals under 3 days old are usually more severely affected and die within 24–36 hours, while older foals tend to show milder symptoms and sometimes recover with good management alone. Sudden death in mild cases over 4 days of age does occasionally occur and is apparently the result of undue stress or exhaustion superimposed on the anaemic state.

Seventy-eight per cent of first haemolytic foals are produced in the fourth to seventh pregnancies (Franks 1962). Cronin (1955) suggested that insufficient antibody is stimulated during an 'incompatible' first pregnancy to produce a dangerous concentration of antibody in the colostrum at foaling time. Cases of the disease occurring in the first pregnancy are very rare. Brion (1949) and Cronin (1955) each cited a case, but there is always the possibility that these mares were initially sensitized at an earlier pregnancy which terminated unnoticed in abortion.

Haematological picture In the acute cases a profound anaemia rapidly develops and the red cell figures may fall as low as RBC $2·0 \times 10^{12}/l$, Hb $2·0$ g/dl and PCV $0·05$ l/l. There is usually free haemoglobin in the plasma (up to 600 mg/100 ml) and quite large numbers of ghost cells may be seen in the spun sample. Very high levels of serum bilirubin can occur (up to 40 mg/ml) depending on the severity of the haemolytic process. There is usually a degree of haemoglobinuria.

In foals less severely affected clinically, the red cell figures may be almost as depressed as in the acute cases but the levels fall more slowly. The plasma oxyhaemoglobin levels, bilirubin and ghost cells are usually less obvious. There is invariably an accompanying neutrophilia. In untreated foals that survive, the red cell figures gradually increase over 2–3 months and the bilirubin and white counts return to normal.

Diagnosis Diagnosis on clinical grounds can be made with a fair degree of certainty as there are few other diseases of the newborn which present a similar clinical picture. Physiological icterus of the newborn may occur occasionally but is rarely associated with clinical illness. Jaundice is sometimes seen with neonatal septicaemia, but haematological examination usually reveals a haemoconcentration, not anaemia. In South Africa the condition has been confused with neonatal babesiosis (Erbsloh 1975).

A very useful and simple technique as an aid to diagnosis is the examination of the foal's PCV by the microhaematocrit method. In addition to indicating whether or not there is a low PCV or obvious anaemia, an idea of the extent of the haemolysis and of discoloration attributable to the presence of bilirubin may also be seen in the plasma. A layer of 'ghost' cells will also be detectable in some cases. These features, if noted, as well as confirming the diagnosis will assist in making a more accurate prognosis of the case.

The serological diagnosis of haemolytic disease in the foal is dependent on the demonstration of maternal iso-antibodies on the foal's erythrocytes. Titration of the mare's serum or colostrum will usually reveal a high titre of antibody. There is no strict relationship between the level of the titre in the mare's blood and the severity of onset of clinical signs in the foal.

Detection of sensitization in mares is based on an adaptation of the indirect antiglobulin technique employed by Coombs *et al* (1945) for use in man. This method employed anti-horse globulin, produced in rabbits, to demonstrate the 'incomplete' agglutinins on available test erythrocytes sensitized by sera or colostra under investigation. The direct antiglobin test, originally developed for use in babies (Coombs *et al* 1946), is also used where possible to demonstrate iso-sensitization of the red cells of foals. The antigens most frequently encountered are anti-A_1 and anti-Q, although anti-R, anti-S, anti-E_2 and anti-U have been encountered (Scott 1973). The most acute and severe cases of haemolytic disease are usually associated with anti-A_1; perhaps because this is by far the most antigenic of the red cell groups.

The means by which the fetal antigens traverse the epitheliochorionic placental barrier has not been determined although it is assumed to be attributable to placental passage of fetal erythrocytes. An increase of iso-antibody titre in the sera of sensitized mares towards the end of pregnancy occurs. The mare's iso-antibody titre usually falls rapidly after parturition. An active foal reduces these antibodies in the colostrum to insignificant levels by 15 hours after birth. Franks (1962) suggested that a substantial trans-placental haemorrhage might produce primary immunization in the mare, whereas a small amount of fetal tissue, perhaps not even in the form of intact red cells, could produce a secondary response in subsequent pregnancies. Although it is rare for a mare to become iso-immunized this may explain why once having done so, she may continue to produce haemolytic foals. The first cases of the disease with some mares are mild and subclinical but further immunization during subsequent pregnancy results in a more severely affected foal.

Pathology   At postmortem examination few macroscopic lesions are to be found, except for anaemia and jaundice. The icteric discoloration of the tissues and internal organs varies with the length of time that the foal survives. In foals which die within 24 hours of birth very little icterus, or possibly none, is seen but pallor of the tissues is pronounced. The colour of the urine varies from light yellow to deep red brown. Splenomegaly occurs in foals dying under 48 hours old.

The severity and extent of the degenerative and necrotic changes in the liver are dependent on the duration and intensity of the haemolytic process and tissue anoxia. The hepatic damage results from the effects of prolonged anaemia and from the toxic effects of the jaundice itself. Foals which die within 24 hours often show no pathological changes, although some central necrosis and erythrophagocytosis by the Kupffer cells is occasionally observed. After 24–48 hours of icterus, erythrophagocytosis becomes prominent. There is marked diffuse degeneration with vacuolation of hepatic cells and focal necrosis, principally around the central veins, but occasionally dispersed throughout the liver. There is also distension of bile canaliculi by bile pigments, hyperplasia of the Kupffer cells and large deposits of haemosiderin in the organ.

Very little significant histopathological change is seen in the other organs, apart from some cholaemic nephrosis, and no evidence of kernicterus has yet been recorded.

Treatment and prevention   The first exchange transfusions in the Thoroughbred foal were given by the method of Farrelly, Belonje and Cronin (1950) with polythene catheters placed in the tibial and femoral veins; one for infusion, one for exsanguination. Cronin (1953) utilized a single intravenous catheter in the jugular vein in conjunction with a three-way tap and a hypodermic syringe as a pump. A much more rapid and simple method using a double intravenous catheter is described by Roberts and Archer (1966). An alternative method of treatment is to use mare's own cells as a source of erythrocytes (Osbaldiston *et al* 1969). About 2 litres of blood are collected into ACD and washed 2 or 3 times with saline. The cells are then packed to 1 litre and given to the foal by slow intravenous transfusion. This technique has now been used at the Equine Research Station even for acute anti-A_1 cases and has proved effective. It is a much simpler method in practical terms; it avoids unnecessary sedation or general anaesthesia of the foal and does not require cross-matching of donor blood.

Once a mare has had a haemolytic foal she need never lose another with this condition. All mares having once produced a haemolytic foal should be tested for rising titres of antibody in the later stages of subsequent pregnancies. If this procedure is not adopted, it is better to assume that the mare will be positive and take the necessary precautions. The mare must foal under supervision and the foal be muzzled immediately after birth, as even a very small quantity of the first colostrum may be sufficient to initiate clinical signs. If the ingestion of colostrum is completely prevented for 24 hours, the disease will not arise. There are now commercially available some mare's milk substitutes (e.g. Equilac, Pegus Ltd; Denkavit, RHM Ltd) for feeding the foal while it is muzzled.

INFECTIOUS HAEMOLYTIC ANAEMIA

Equine infectious anaemia (EIA) or 'swamp fever' is a disease affecting all *equidae* but outbreaks in donkeys and mules are uncommon and wild equines are probably only rarely affected. There is a worldwide distribution of the disease although it is probably most prevalent in the United States (Hyslop

1966). A case has recently been reported in the United Kingdom (Rossdale *et al* 1975) and most other countries in Europe have recorded the disease.

EIA is usually a subacute disease associated with progressive debility, intermittent fever and anaemia (Henson & McGuire 1972). Less frequently it runs an acute course which may be followed by collapse and death. In enzootic areas a high proportion of horses may be symptomless carriers. The disease is caused by a virus which is present in the blood during the periods of fever. The most important vectors are biting arthropods. However, it has been suggested that a foal from an infected mare may be infected at birth or shortly afterwards (Stein & Mott 1942). The virus may persist throughout the life of an infected animal and transmission may therefore be perpetuated by injections, vaccinations or surgical procedures in which instruments or needles may be contaminated with blood.

The virus is present during all stages of the disease but the titre is highest during the febrile phase. The anaemia produced is predominantly haemolytic with both intra- and extra-vascular haemolysis. The PCV and RBC fall during the course of the disease and the rapidity of the decline is related to the clinical signs. The bone marrow is hypofunctional during the episodes of pyrexia (McGuire *et al* 1969). The total white cell count varies but there is often a leucopenia, mainly due to a decrease in activity of the granulocyte series, during the bouts of fever. This may result in an apparent lymphocytosis upon which a superimposed increase in the monocytes is sometimes seen. There is usually bilirubinaemia and a fall of serum haptoblogin levels.

Buffy coat cells from horses with EIA often contain stainable iron. These cells have been called 'siderleucocytes' or 'siderocytes' (Henson *et al* 1967) but they may also be seen in other acute haemolytic anaemias. There is nearly always fairly severe liver damage in EIA and mild depression of serum albumin, often with concomitant increase of the globulin fractions, may be present. In addition there is a change in lactic dehydrogenase (LDH) levels and progressive increase in cholinesterase activity (Osbaldiston *et al* 1970).

The diagnosis of EIA is based on the clinical signs and an agar gel immunodiffusion test (AGID using spleen from) an infected horse as antigen (Coggins *et al* 1972). There is no specific treatment for the disease although supportive therapy may be helpful. There is always the danger of a recovered animal serving as a source of further infection.

Equine babesiosis (piroplasmosis or biliary fever) is a tick-borne protozoan infection characterized by anaemia, jaundice, debility and intermittent fever. The disease occurs in most tropical and subtropical regions of the world although its distribution depends on the terrain and the presence of the appropriate tick vectors. There are 2 species of parasite involved, *Babesia caballi* or *B. equi* and single or mixed infections may occur. A variety of species of ticks are capable of transmitting the parasite but *Dermacentor nitens*, the tropical horse tick, is the commonest (Ristic 1972). Most of the development cycle occurs within the tick vector with asexual multiplication occurring in the erythrocytes of infected horses.

The disease may be acute, subacute or chronic. The parasites invade the erythrocytes of susceptible hosts and divide into 4 daughter forms which eventually separate and escape to penetrate other red blood cells. Horses raised in infected areas acquire a pre-immunity which depends on the continued presence of the causative agent in the blood. Nevertheless a relapse of babesiosis may occur in unfavourable conditions.

The clinical signs are variable but they usually include sluggishness, depression, anorexia, lacrimation, pyrexia and swelling of the eyelids. There is also marked jaundice, anaemia, tachycardia, weakness and oedema of the ventral abdomen and legs. In acute experimental *Babesia caballi* infection there is a decrease in the platelet count which remains low for about 2 weeks. The concentration of plasma fibrinogen increases and fibrin clots may be observed in small blood vessels of various organs (Holbrook *et al* 1973). The PCV decreases rapidly particularly in *B. equi* infection and may fall as low as 0·12 l/l. There is usually an accompanying haemoglobinuria. If the animal survives it becomes a carrier; in the case of *B. caballi* this carrier state may persist for 1–4 years, but with *B. equi* it will persist for the rest of the animal's life unless sufficient doses of babesicides are given.

The disease has been diagnosed in aborted fetuses and newborn foals in South Africa (Erbsloh 1975). The fetus can be infected at various stages of pregnancy presumably by passage of infected erythrocytes across the placental barrier. The mare does not show any overt clinical signs apart from abortion, which may occur at any time during pregnancy. The highest incidence of abortion is between 8 and 10 months. If infected foals are carried to term the clinical picture resembles haemolytic disease except that signs of jaundice may be seen before the ingestion of colostrum. Some foals appear normal at birth but show signs of jaundice, pyrexia and haemoglobinuria after 2 to 3 days and frequently die. Treatment is by blood transfusion and general supportive therapy.

Ehrlichiosis The existence of equine ehrlichiosis in California, USA was recorded by Gribble (1969). In the 5 cases reported there was a mild anaemia, jaundice and thrombocytopenia with associated leucopenia and cytoplasmic inclusion bodies in some of the neutrophils. The clinical signs included oedema of the limbs, increased pulse and respiratory rates, pallid mucous membranes, anorexia and lethargy. Experimental transmission of the disease produced pyrexia for 1–6 days, oedema, anorexia and altered respiratory rate. A transient normocytic, normochromic anaemia developed with the PCV rarely dropping below 0·25 l/l. A leucopenia was seen during the period of pyrexia and the differential count showed both neutropenia and lymphopenia. The levels fairly rapidly returned to normal followed by the development of a degree of lymphocytosis.

Trypanosomiasis Haemolytic anaemia may accompany infection of horses with trypanosomiasis due to *Trypanosoma equiperdum*, *T. equinum* and *T. evansi*. However the haematological changes are usually of secondary importance to the fairly dramatic clinical signs.

Leptospirosis as a cause of infective jaundice has been reported in Russia (Lyubaskenko & Novikova 1947). Affected animals may show anaemia with anisocytosis of erythrocytes, pyrexia, marked jaundice of the mucous membranes and anorexia. A fairly high mortality rate was recorded and the strains of leptospires isolated were identical to those recoverable from foxes and cattle.

POISONS AND TOXIC CHEMICALS

Lead poisoning Chronic lead poisoning in horses causes anorexia, loss of weight, colic, muscular weakness, gradual paralysis including laryngeal hemiplegia and anaemia (Hammond & Aronson, 1964; Knight & Burau, 1973). The haematological changes have not been particularly stressed, but there is evidence of a haemolytic anaemia with basophilic stippling of cells and the presence of circulating late normoblasts (metarubricytes). There is depression of bone marrow activity and a low myeloid/erythroid ratio. Determination of lead levels in blood and urine are the most useful parameters in diagnosis. Successful treatment has been achieved by intravenous administration of Ca EDTA (calcium disodium versenate; dose rate 75 mg/kg daily) to the lead cases not irreversibly damaged by the poison.

Phenothiazine has been used for many years as an anthelmintic for horses although its application has been considerably reduced with the introduction of more efficient and less toxic drugs. Phenothiazine is a derivative of phenylhydrazine and in overdose or in susceptible horses it can cause injury to the erythrocytes, resulting in haemolysis. The way in which this drug exerts its toxic action is not understood. There is some evidence that the metabolites of phenothiazine may be more toxic than the drug itself (Clarke & Clarke 1967).

McSherry *et al* (1966) reported on the haematological changes following a 20 g dose of phenothiazine to 15 horses. Three animals developed varying degrees of haemolytic anaemia with hyperbilirubinaemia and Heinz body formation. The affected animals were unthrifty prior to treatment and it was suggested that this was an important factor in producing the signs of toxicity. Two other animals showed some hyperbilirubinaemia but were not clinically ill or anaemic.

Onion poisoning Acute haemolytic anaemia following ingestion of wild onions was reported in 2 animals and confirmed by experimental feeding of another horse (Pierce *et al* 1972). The PCV gradually decreased and there was a raised MCHC with the presence of Heinz bodies in the damaged red cells. There was haemoglobinuria and jaundice.

Horses do not usually eat onions unless other forage is lacking. However, there is one report of domestic onion poisoning in horses which occurred on an onion farm in Colorado, USA (Thorp & Harshfield 1939).

AUTOIMMUNE HAEMOLYTIC ANAEMIA (AHA)
A 4-year-old Thoroughbred mare suffering from chronic debility and lymphomatosis of the small intestine was reported by Farrelly *et al* (1966). There was a severe haemolytic anaemia with associated leucocytosis, raised serum bilirubin and globulin. There was a positive direct Coombs test. Examination of the bone marrow revealed a myeloid/erythroid ratio of 0·41:1 with evidence of myeloid metaplasia. A diagnosis of AHA was suggested. Farrelly *et al* (1966) recorded 2 further cases of possible AHA, diagnosed by the Coombs test, and both these horses showed clinical signs of purpura haemorrhagica with some degree of anaemia.

IDIOPATHIC HAEMOLYTIC ANAEMIA
Occasional cases of haemolytic anaemia are seen in horses which resemble the haematological pattern of the previously mentioned conditions but are, as yet, without a recognized aetiology.

5.5.3.3 Dyserythropoietic anaemia

PRIMARY NUTRITIONAL DYSERYTHROPOIESIS
In man there are 2 megaloblastic types of macrocytic anaemia associated with vitamin B_{12} and folic acid deficiency. The metabolism of vitamin B_{12} has been studied in the horse by Alexander and Davies (1969) and Davies (1971) and there is no evidence that a deficiency anaemia occurs in *equidae* (McGuire & Henson 1968, Archer 1969). The vitamin is produced along the whole length of the intestine by microorganisms, particularly certain strains of *Escherichia coli*, and this provides an adequate supply of B_{12} to the host.

The situation concerning folic acid deficiency as a cause of anaemia is not completely clear cut and may be partly due to the difficulties in laboratory estimation of folate. There is, however, fairly good circumstantial evidence that folate-deficient diets can produce a mild anaemia with lowered racing performance. There may be some degree of anisocytosis present but macrocytosis is not frequently encountered. The clinical diagnosis of human folic acid deficiency may also be complicated by the fact that serum folate levels will not necessarily give an accurate index of total body folate stores. However, in practice folate assay can prove to be a sensitive index of developing deficiency (Herbert 1965). Stabled horses have been shown to have lower levels of serum folate than grass-fed animals and mares after foaling also tend to have decreased values (Seckington *et al* 1967). Archer (1974b) recognizes an anaemia in horses which have been on low-folate diets for more than 2 months. There is a tendency to macrocytosis in these cases and they respond well to parenteral folate therapy. Oral treatment even with very high doses is not always successful, perhaps because of inactivation by acidity of the stomach.

Iron deficiency resulting in macrocytic anaemia has been considered a clinical entity for many years. However, no conclusive studies to confirm this have been reported. If it does occur the anaemia is mild, normochromic and normocytic. The estimation of serum iron levels has not been of much

Table 5.15 Normal values for vitamin B_{12}, serum folate, iron and total iron binding capacity (TIBC)

Source	Type	Vitamin B_{12} ($\mu\mu g/ml$)	Serum folate $\mu g/ml$	Serum Fe $\mu g/dl$	TIBC $\mu g/dl$
Alexander & Davies (1969)	Pony	6300 ± 370	—	—	—
Seckington *et al* (1967)	TB grass fed	—	11·5	154	800
	TB stabled	—	7·5	144	700
Stewart & Clarkson (1968–69)	TB	—	—	156 ± 37	446 ± 33
Stewart & Clarkson (1968–69)	Standardbred	—	—	167 ± 40	381 ± 28
Allen (1976)	TB in training		$3·8 \pm 1·26$		
	TB out of training	—	$8·0 \pm 2·59$	—	—

TB = Thoroughbred.

practical value because of wide individual variation and the rapid mobilization of large iron stores in the body. Only a small fraction of total body iron is present in serum and it is transported loosely bound to the β globulin protein, transferrin. The total amount of iron that can be taken up by the transferrin is referred to as Total Iron Binding Capacity (TIBC). This parameter is probably useful in the early recognition of iron deficiency in the horse (Stewart & Clarkson 1968–69).

Further evidence against the frequent occurrence of iron deficiency anaemia has been the disappointing results recorded following therapeutic administration of various haematinics (Kirkham *et al* 1971, Laufenstein-Duffy 1971).

The normal values for vitamin B_{12}, serum folate, iron and TIBC are given in Table 5.15.

Idiopathic hypoplastic anaemia A case of hypoplastic anaemia of undetermined aetiology was described by Archer and Miller (1965). This was a 2-year-old Thoroughbred in poor condition for some time which showed a leucocytopenia and hypochromic anaemia. The anaemia gradually worsened, a definite hypoplasia of the bone marrow was noted and there was a normal platelet count. A postmortem examination did not shed any further light on the origin of the anaemia although it was possible to eliminate aplastic anaemia, EIA and aleukaemic lymphocytic leukaemia.

SECONDARY DYSERYTHROPOIESIS

Chronic low-grade anaemia due to faulty haematopoiesis is not an infrequent occurrence in horses although it is usually secondary to some other condition. These anaemias are most often normochromic and normocytic in type.

Anaemia due to chronic parasitic infection must be regarded as one of the most important causes of depressed red cell figures in horses kept at pasture. Archer and Poynter (1957) showed a normochromic, normocytic anaemia and accompanying erythroid hypoplasia of the bone marrow in ponies with mixed strongyle infections. The ponies also showed an eosinophilia of the peripheral blood and bone marrow. Round (1968) confirmed the presence of mild anaemia in animals with chronic parasitic burdens. He also noted a variable leucocytosis and eosinophilia but found the most striking feature to be a marked increase of the serum globulin fractions (Round 1971).

In chronic infections, particularly long-standing inflammatory conditions of the intestines, the red cell figures can fall dramatically over a period. In addition to hypoplasia of the bone marrow much of this may be due to the effects of upset fluid balance resulting in haemodilution and pancytopenia. This type of situation is also seen in cases of purpura haemorrhagica which is a nonthrombocytopenic condition often occurring secondarily to some respiratory infection. The severe form of the disease is characterized by pronounced oedema, involving particularly the face, jowl, anterior pectoral region and lower limbs. There is congestion of the nasal mucosa and the appearance of petechial and ecchymotic haemorrhages on the visible mucous membranes. The oedema may become severe and lead to dyspnoea, pulmonary oedema and in some cases death. Haematologically there is a gradual decrease in the red cell figures. A leucocytosis with neutrophilia is present and total counts of $40–50 \times 10^9/l$ have been recorded (Sorensen 1972).

Bracken (*Pteris aquilina*) poisoning has been reported (Hadwen & Bruce 1933, Evans *et al* 1951) but there are no appreciable changes in the red cell figures. There is an associated thrombocytopenia, leucocytosis and an eosinopenia. The clinical signs are improved by administration of vitamin B_1.

Malignant neoplasia, particularly lymphosarcoma of the intestinal wall, may also give rise to chronic anaemia. However, this is usually associated with a definite neutrophilia with a shift to the left and myeloid hyperplasia in the bone marrow.

Aplastic anaemia has been experimentally induced in horses by feeding trichloroethylene-extracted soya bean oil meal (TCESOM) (Pritchard *et al* 1956c). Haematological changes were typical of aplastic anaemia with the presence of a marked thrombocytopenia before appreciable anaemia or leucopenia. In the latter stages platelets were reduced to levels of the order of $10 \times 10^9/l$. Erythrocytes and leucocytes were similarly reduced, lymphocytes being apparently least affected. In addition three were petechial haemorrhages seen on the visible mucous membranes.

Another cause of aplastic anaemia is whole radiation with exposures in the lethal range (i.e. 100–500 rads over a short period). The effects in the donkey have been reviewed by Wilkins (1962, 1963a b). Clinical signs of apathy and malaise were seen on the 2nd day and death occurred in a few animals. From the 14th day animals were seen to die with an increasingly severe haemorrhagic diathesis due to disturbance in clotting. The changes in the blood were spectacular. Almost immediately following irradiation there was a precipitous fall in lymphocytes which all but disappeared from the peripheral circulation within 48 hours. There was a progressive reduction in all other cellular elements until the 4th week when some animals began to show signs of recovery. Total white cells fell from a mean $16 \times 10^9/l$ to as low as $0.5 \times 10^9/l$. RBC dropped about $11 \times 10^{12}/l$ to as low as $1.0 \times 10^{12}/l$. Death was unpredictable even if there were initial signs of recovery but it always occurred within 45 days.

5.5.4 HAEMOCONCENTRATION AND POLYCYTHAEMIA

The presence of polycythaemia (i.e. an increase of erythrocyte numbers per unit volume of blood) may be relative when it is due to reduction in plasma volume, or absolute when it is due entirely to increased number of cells. Relative polycythaemia is essentially haemoconcentration and is frequently encountered in the horse. Animals under stress, those being exerted or suffering from painful abdominal conditions (e.g. twist, perforation etc.) show a rapid onset of haemoconcentration. The PCV gives a rapid guide to its extent and provides a useful indication of the fluid balance as well as a simple aid to prognosis.

There are no confirmed reports of absolute polycythaemia in the horse. Primary polycythaemia (polycythaemia vera) has been noted in the dog, cat and ox. Secondary polycythaemia resulting from the congenital cardiac anomaly, tetralogy of Fallot, has been noted in most domestic species. One case of this anomaly has been recorded by Prickett *et al* (1973) in a Thoroughbred foal but no evidence of polycythaemia was present.

A number of workers have referred to a clinical condition of fit racehorses which show chronic haemoconcentration or apparent polycythaemia (Sykes 1966, Persson 1967, Cosgrove 1969, Jeffcott 1974). These animals rarely perform well and often 'blow up' in the final stages of a race, finishing well below their expected form. Probably what happens is that with the increasing PCV during exertion, the blood becomes so viscous that there is increased resistance to blood flow in small blood vessels and capillaries which leads to a rapid reduction in oxygenation of the tissues. Sykes (1966) suggests administration of 500 ml of 5 per cent saline and sodium citrate to reduce PCV by temporary transfer of fluids in the blood stream.

Williamson (1974) has seen the same condition in New Zealand and attributed it to an adrenal insufficiency. He suggested that animals which were not allowed sufficient recovery time between stressful experiences (i.e. training and racing) might develop an adrenal exhaustion and therefore hypoaldosteronism. It may be that this condition has similarities with the relative polycythaemia of stress seen in man (Lawrence & Berlin 1952). As well as the high red cell parameters in these horses, there is an elevated serum K^+ with depression of Na^+ and Cl^- levels. Williamson recorded 94 cases of the condition and found a good clinical response to treatment with mineralocorticoids, replacement of Na^+ ions and the provision of bicarbonate, lactate or citrate to correct the acidosis. Aldosterone controls the homeostasis of water, Na^+ and K^+ by preventing loss of water and Na^+ from the renal tubules. The administration of the mineralocorticoid DOCA (desoxy corticosterone acetate) by injection or implant is probably the treatment of choice, as aldosterone itself is expensive and only has a very short period of action. Naturally under the rules of racing in many countries this could not be given to horses prior to racing.

5.5.5 LEUCOPENIA

A reduction in the total white cell count is much less common than the reverse situation of leucocytosis. Leucopenia occurs at the outset of a number of conditions and for this reason may well be missed haematologically. Leucopenia commonly occurs in cases of haemodilution due to upset in the homeostatic mechanisms of fluid balance. This is seen in some chronic intestinal conditions (e.g. malabsorption and protein-losing enteropathy syndromes) where there is leakage of albumin into the intestinal lumen and loss of oncotic pressure.

The classic situation of panleucopenia occurs in horses with acute viral infections. Bryans *et al* (1957) studying experimental equine viral arteritis (EVA) infection noted a generalized leucopenia during the period of fever and for 24–72 hours afterwards. This situation has also occurred with other equine virus infections (e.g. influenza, equid herpes virus EHV 1 infection and EIA).

Horses are sensitive to minute amounts of histamine and endotoxin; challenge by either of these agents produces a dramatic leucopenia. In the case of histamine there is a very rapid fall in the number of circulating eosinophils and clinical signs of anaphylaxis (Archer 1956). Carroll *et al* (1965) administered *Aerobacter aerogenes* endotoxin intraperitoneally to a horse and evoked sudden collapse, dyspnoea, watery diarrhoea and death within 8 hours. There was definite leucopenia from 1 to 5 hours after dosing, followed by a gradual return of leucocytes to circulation. There were a number of similarities in this case with the well recognized clinical condition of 'exhaustion shock' or Colitis 'X' (Rooney *et al* 1966) and it was suggested that this latter condition might also result from an endotoxaemia. Probably for the same reason a panleucopenia is also seen in cases of acute abdominal crisis (e.g. twist, intussusception and perforation).

Other conditions which exhibit a leucopenia are ehrlichiosis and radiation sickness. The administration of ACTH, glucocorticoids and insulin has fairly dramatic effects on the circulatory white cells. Both ACTH and insulin produce an eosinopenia (Alexander & Ash 1955) and Osbaldiston and Johnson (1972) reported an accompanying neutrophilia and lymphopenia. Parenteral injection of the synthetic glucocorticoids, dexamethasone and flumethasone, induced a marked neutrophilia. Dexamethasone had a more pronounced effect with a longer period of lymphopenia and it also produces an eosinopenia. Neither of these compounds of ACTH had any effect on the red cell figures, platelets or monocytes (Osbaldiston & Johnson 1972).

A condition of primary combined immunodeficiency has been recorded in Arabian foals (McGuire *et al* 1974). The disease was diagnosed in 18 foals which died from a variety of infections, especially adenoviral infection. Diagnosis was based on lymphopenia and the absence of one or more serum immunoglobulin classes. At postmortem examination there was thymic hypoplasia, absence of splenic germinal centres and hypogammaglobinaemia.

5.5.6 LEUCOCYTOSIS

The presence of a leucocytosis is probably the most frequent abnormality encountered in equine haematological analysis. However, it is not always easy to detect mild inflammatory responses as the normal white count of the horse can be so variable (5.2.2.1). Unless there is evidence of haemoconcentration, counts of over $12 \times 10^9/l$ are usually diagnostic but values can rise to $40 \times 10^9/l$ in some conditions. The major causes of increased white cell counts are listed in Table 5.16.

Parasitic infections are a constant problem with horses kept at pasture and mixed strongyle infections tend to stimulate a generalized leucocytosis. There is often a eosinophilia and in some cases a neutrophilia (Round 1968). Parasitic infections with *Parascaris equorum*, lungworm, *Oxyuris equi*, tapeworms and bots have little effect on the haematological picture unless there are very severe infestations.

Neutrophilia occurs in many suppurative conditions (e.g. septic arthritis

Table 5.16 Major causes of abnormal white cell counts in the horse

LEUCOPENIA

Generalized leucopenia	Neutropenia	Lymphopenia	Eosinopenia
Haemodilution	Early acute inflammatory response	ACTH and corticosteroid administration	Anaphylaxis
Acute viral infection		Combined immunodeficiency (CID) in Arab foals	Histamine release
Endotoxaemia (exhaustion shock or colitis X)		Radiation sickness	Endotoxin shock
Acute abdominal crisis			ACTH, insulin, adrenalin and corticosteroid administration
Ehrlichiosis			
EIA (during pyrexia)			
Radiation sickness			

LEUCOCYTOSIS

Generalized leucocytosis	Neutrophilia	Lymphocytosis	Eosinophilia	Monocytosis	Basophilia
Haemoconcentration	Inflammatory response	Chronic bacterial infection (e.g. tuberculosis)	Parasitism	Some chronic infections	?
Polycythaemia	Suppurative focus of infection	Leukaemic leucosis	Some allergic conditions	EIA	
Mixed stronglye infections	Septicaemia (plus shift to the left)		Antigen/antibody reactions		
	Haemolytic anaemia				
	Lymphosarcoma				
	Purpura haemorrhagica				
	Glucocorticoid administration				

L. B. Jeffcott

of foals and *Corynebacterium equi* pneumonia) and in septicaemia. This is frequently accompanied by a shift to the left due to the appearance of stab and juvenile neutrophils in the peripheral circulation. There is also some degree of neutrophilia present in cases of haemolytic disease of the newborn, purpura haemorrhagica and lymphosarcoma, in which there is invasion of the bone marrow. Most cases of lymphosarcoma in horses are aleukaemic and show a pronounced neutrophilia.

Monocytosis is much less commonly encountered but is sometimes seen in cases of chronic infection or in some cases of EIA. Increased counts of basophils are rarely seen and the clinical significance of this is unknown.

5.5.7 LYMPHOSARCOMA AND LEUKAEMIA

5.5.7.1 Lymphosarcoma

Lymphosarcoma is the generally accepted term for conditions in the horse variously named lymphocytic leukaemia, malignant lymphoma, leucosis, lymphomatosis and lymphoblastoma. Contrary to some authorities (Moulton 1961, Schalm *et al* 1975) it is probably the commonest cause of malignant neoplasia in the horse and is certainly the most frequently encountered tumour of the haemopoietic system.

The clinical picture varies according to the site of the lesions, but involvement of the alimentary tract, spleen and the associated lymph nodes is seen most frequently (Mettam 1915, Runnels & Benbrook 1944, Reed 1949, Thielen & Fowler 1962). The tumours may arise locally in the alimentary tract with subsequent spread to the lymph nodes, lungs and other abdominal organs, or in other cases they develop multicentrically with generalized lymph node involvement and invasion of parenchymal organs. There is no particular age incidence although it tends to be seen more commonly in older horses. The clinical signs are often quite sudden in onset and there may be even sudden death (Pascoe 1970). Where the small or large intestine is involved there may be chronic diarrhoea, rapid loss of condition with symptoms of malabsorption or intermittent mild colic. In cases involving the viscera and lymph nodes of the abdominal cavity the technique of *paracentesis abdominis* and demonstration of lymphocytes in the peritoneal fluid is a useful diagnostic aid (Bach & Ricketts 1974). Vaughan (1969) reported a case in a 6-year-old gelding which presented with extensive swelling of the pectoral region. At postmortem a large mediastinal tumour was found with metastiasis to the prepectoral, mediastinal and renal lymph nodes. A combination of abdominal lymphosarcoma and invasive melanoma was recorded in an aged grey Arab stallion (Conboy & Powers 1971).

The haemogram in lymphosarcoma usually shows some evidence of anaemia and/or haemodilution, particularly if there is a diffuse lesion involving the wall of the small or large intestine. The majority of cases are aleukaemic but a leukaemic form, with a large number of circulation pleomorphic lymphocytes, is occasionally seen when there is extensive involvement of the bone marrow. Most cases of lymphosarcoma do show a marked leucocytosis due primarily to a neutrophilia. In some horses cell counts of over $30 \times 10^9/l$ can be detected.

5.5.7.2 Multiple myeloma

Multiple myeloma or plasma cell myelomastosis has also been reported in a horse (Cornelius *et al* 1959). The case presented with lameness, oedema and pain over the right forearm. A severe macrocytic normochromic anaemia with anisocytosis of the erythrocytes was also present. There was a variable thrombocytopenia and bone marrow biopsy revealed large numbers of plasma cells with significantly depressed myeloid and erythroid activity. Examination of serum protein profile revealed hypoalbuminaemia and hyperglobulinaemia. The latter was due to the presence of a 'myeloma' glycoprotein. The diagnosis of myelomatosis was confirmed at postmortem examination. A more recent case of a vertebral plasma cell myeloma causing posterior paralysis in a horse was reported by Drew and Greatorex (1974).

Other forms of leucosis have not been recorded in the horse.

HAEMATOLOGY OF THE OX

D. L. DOXEY

6.1 INTRODUCTION

The blood of man undergoes clearly defined and precisely documented cellular changes in a variety of pathological processes but unforunately, from a diagnostic point of view, bovine blood does not follow the same pattern. In addition, the cellular changes which do occur in the bovine are not as clear-cut nor of such magnitude as those of humans, nor do they indicate exactly what type of pathological change is taking place (e.g. it is very difficult to differentiate between acute viral or acute bacterial infections).

There has, however, recently been an increase in the use of haematology as an aid to the diagnosis of diseases of *bovidae* because it is now recognized that selective haematology (bleeding only carefully selected clinical cases and, if possible, using serial samples) can be helpful to diagnosis. In addition, it is clear that cattle in particular are now regarded not just as isolated, individual cases but as a whole herd, and the introduction and use of metabolic profile testing in highly intensive cattle systems has introduced some haematological parameters, such as packed cell volume (PCV), as aids to diagnosis of management malpractice.

Haematology in the ox is used on a herd basis as part of profile testing and, in addition, can still prove useful in individual cases provided these cases are carefully screened prior to sampling.

6.2 NORMAL HAEMATOLOGICAL VALUES IN THE OX

6.2.1 NORMAL FETAL VALUES

Hubbert and Hollen (1971) used a variety of breeds and investigated fetal values from 100 days' gestation to parturition. The trends which emerged were that the erythrocytes, PCV and haemoglobin (Hb) increased as parturition got nearer, while reticulocytes and nucleated red blood cells decreased (e.g. erythrocytes rose from $3·84 \times 10^{12}/l$ at 120 days' gestation to $8·29 \times 10^{12}/l$ at term, while reticulocytes fell from 9 per cent to 0 per cent and nucleated erythrocytes from $6·50 \times 10^{9}/l$ to $0·35 \times 10^{9}/l$ during the same period). Leucocytes rose from 2·10 to $10^{9}/l$ to $6·77 \times 10^{9}/l$ by term and this increase was due primarily to lymphocyte and mature neutrophil numbers increasing. Tennant *et al* (1974) give mean total leucocyte counts in the last month of gestation as $8·50 \pm 2·70 \times 10^{9}/l$. Platelets differed from other cell types and remained static in number during gestation.

6.2.2 NORMAL VALUES—BIRTH TO ONE YEAR

6.2.2.1 Erythrocytes

By the time parturition occurs, normal calves are well able to manufacture their own cells and Valli *et al* (1971a b) considered that the production time of late normoblasts was $3·79 \pm 2·06$ days and that of sequestered granular leucocytes $5·77 \pm 1·43$ days. Another factor which normal calves have in common is fetal Hb. This type of Hb accounts for between 60 and 97 per cent of the calf's total Hb at birth but after parturition it declines in an erratic manner unrelated to age (Tisdall & Crowley 1971) until, 4 weeks after birth, fetal Hb composes 34–62 per cent of total Hb and after 10 weeks is down to 10–22 per cent (Lee *et al* 1971). After 20 weeks of life, fetal Hb composes less than 2 per cent of the total Hb, having been virtually replaced by adult Hb A or Hb B. Scheidegger (1973b) showed very similar results but observed that the disappearance of fetal Hb is slower in anaemic veal calves fed solely on milk (5 per cent fetal Hb left at 110 days of age).

Haematological changes continue in the calf after birth, but can be modified by external factors. Greatorex (1957) recorded high erythrocyte counts, PCV and Hb at birth but he, and a variety of other workers, showed that values declined, although not always steadily, as the animal ages. Holman (1956), using Ayrshires, recorded a fall in RBC between $9·82 \times 10^{12}/l$ at birth and $7·65 \times 10^{12}/l$ at 12 months. PCV and Hb fell during the same period from 0·425 l/l to 0·359 l/l and 12·9 g/dl to 10·4 g/dl respectively. Baars (1971), in conventionally reared calves, demonstrated the same trend with average Hb falling from 11·1 g/dl at birth to 10·0 g/dl at 3 months of age and PCV falling from 0·39 l/l to 0·32 l/l over the same period. Scheidegger (1973a) recorded that RBC did not fall from birth to 4 months of age, but that PCV fell from 0·402 l/l to 0·328 l/l and Hb from 13·1 g/dl to 11·4 g/dl over the same period. Tennant *et al* (1974) noted the same trend from birth to 6 months of age but the fall was much less obvious.

D. L. Doxey

Table 6.1 Calves, birth to one year. Normal erythrocyte values

Age	RBC $10^{12}/l$	PCV l/l	Hb g/dl	MCV fl	MCH pg	MCHC g/dl	Fe μmol/l	*TIBC μmol/l	Retics. %
Normally reared calves									
Birth	8·38	0·430	12·5	51·3	14·9	29·1			0·2
1 week	8·04	0·363	11·1	45·1	13·8	30·5	13·2	73·4	0·05
1 month	8·06	0·337	10·4	41·8	12·9	30·8	13·4	103·8	
3 months	8·36	0·330	10·9	39·4	13·0	33·0	28·1	73·4	0·02
6 months	8·06	0·361	11·7	44·8	14·5	32·4	25·9	69·4	0
12 months	7·57	0·359	9·7	47·4	12·8	27·0	23·2	75·7	0
Veal calves									
Birth	7·68	0·393	12·3	51·2	16·0	31·2	12·6	68·0	
3 months	6·65	0·236	7·4	35·4	11·1	31·3			
4½ months	6·74	0·270	9·0	40·0	13·3	33·3	5·7	143·2	

* TIBC = Total iron binding capacity

In fact, the erythrocyte count and Hb hardly moved and only the PCV fell from 0·348 l/l to 0·317 l/l. There were marked fluctuations from week to week. Greatorex (1954) showed similar fluctuating results but both PCV and Hb did fall noticeably over a 12-month period (PCV from 0·48 l/l to 0·36 l/l and Hb from 13·5 g/dl to 9·5 g/dl) but red blood cell counts do not fall over the same period.

In conjunction with the changes just described, variations in cell size, Hb content, iron and reticulocyte values also occur (Bremner 1966b). Tennant *et al* (1974) showed that reticulocyte percentage rose from birth to the fourth day of life, reaching a maximum level of 0·5 per cent and thereafter it fell to levels of <0·1 per cent where it remained. Mean cell volume (MCV) and mean cell haemoglobin concentration (MCHC) varied from author to author and results are summarized in Table 6.1.

According to Bremner (1966) plasma iron and total iron-binding capacity (TIBC) varied markedly from calf to calf at 1 week of age. The iron values were reasonably static from 2–12 weeks of age but TIBC rose to a maximum at about 4 weeks of age, after which it declined.

Veal calves are reared commercially and work done in Europe indicated that the 'normal' values for such calves, which are fed solely on an anaemia-inducing milk diet, are at variance with those from conventionally reared calves. The pattern shown by Breukink *et al* (1974), Scheidegger (1973a), Baars (1971) and Vermeersch and Vanschoubroek (1974) indicates the same decline in erythrocyte values but at a greatly accelerated rate (Table 6.1).

Möllerberg (1975) showed that mean values for 1-month-old calves purchased in markets were similar to the results shown in Table 6.1, but that up to 35 per cent of calves could be classified as anaemic (Hb values of <10·0 g/dl).

The normal erythrocytic values in calves from birth to 1 year are summarized in Table 6.1 and include data from the authors already mentioned plus Peters *et al* (1973) and Vagher *et al* (1973). Considerable variation in absolute values occurs from one author to another. Parker and Blowey (1974) found value differences between jugular vein and coccygeal vein samples, and Tennant *et al* (1974) found that both Jersey and Friesian calves showed marked individual variations in PCV at 1 day of age (e.g. majority 0·26–0·40 l/l, but extremes of <0·16 to >0·45 l/l occurred). Nevertheless, despite these known variations, the averages in Table 6.1 will illustrate the trends in normally reared calves that are due to age (i.e. falling PCV and Hb, static or erratically declining red blood cells and rising serum iron). In veal calves fed wholly on milk, all values decline rapidly from birth onwards. In animals on this type of managemental regimen haematological values may easily fall into the pathological range within 8–10 weeks of birth. It is difficult to know if such animals can be classified as 'normal', but they appear to be clinically healthy and consequently have been included here.

6.2.2.2   Leucocytes

Leucocytes also show some degree of variation during the first year of life. Most authors record high total leucocyte (WBC) values at birth, followed by some decline in numbers over the first few weeks. Holman (1956), Greatorex (1957), Scheidegger *et al* (1974), Tennant *et al* (1974) and Breukink *et al* (1974) all described this declining pattern but there was some variation between the authors when absolute figures were quoted. Holman (1956) recorded the highest mean WBC value at birth ($12\cdot90 \times 10^9/l$) and the lowest mean value in normally reared 2- to 3-month-old calves is $8\cdot87 \times 10^9/l$ (Vagher *et al* 1973, Peters *et al* 1973). In veal calves the values are lower and drop to between $5\cdot5$ and $6\cdot5 \times 10^9/l$.

Table 6.2   Calves, birth to one year. Normal leucocyte values

Age	WBC $10^9/l$	N $10^9/l$	L $10^9/l$	M $10^9/l$	E $10^9/l$	B $10^9/l$
Birth	9·40	6·20	2·80	0·30	0·09	0
1 week	7·46	3·80	3·40	0·20	0·06	0
3 months	9·30	2·50	6·00	0·60	0·20	0
1 year	9·90	2·50	6·50	0·65	0·25	0

After this initial fall, leucocyte values rise slightly (Table 6.2) but the degree of elevation will depend not only on age but also on environment. O'Kelly (1974) recorded marked variation in leucocyte values between young calves kept in separate areas (i.e. most calves had mean values of between $4\cdot6$ and $6\cdot0 \times 10^9/l$, but in one group they rose to $21\cdot58 \times 10^9/l$).

Age changes in leucocyte values are in the main caused by declining neutrophil numbers from birth and then compensation by increasing numbers of lymphocytes. At birth, neutrophils are the most numerous cell type but after a few weeks lymphocytes become, and remain, the major cell type. This pattern occurs in both veal and normally reared calves although Scheidegger *et al* (1974) found that after the initial decline in numbers veal calves failed to increase their total counts as much as normal calves primarily due to reduced lymphocyte numbers (e.g. normal calves $8\cdot0 \times 10^9/l$, veal calves $6\cdot0 \times 10^9/l$ or less). A summation of this data is given in Table 6.2.

Other normal values for conventionally reared calves are given in Table 6.3.

Red cell fragility varies depending on the animal's age. Young animals show complete haemolysis in weaker sodium chloride solutions than older animals (i.e. 0·36 per cent at 1 week old and 0·50 per cent at 1 year of age,

Table 6.3 Other normal values for conventionally reared calves

	Author	Mean and range or standard deviation
Erythrocyte diameter in 6–12 week calves	Vagher (1973)	4·7 (4·4–5·0) μm
Total mean red cell volume in 7–15 week calves	Haxton *et al* (1974)	37·45 ± 9·77 ml/kg
Total blood volume in 7–15 week calves	Haxton *et al* (1974)	116·0 ± 27·71 ml/kg
Platelets 6–12 week calves	Vagher (1973)	841·00 (480·0–1200·0) × 10^9/l
Fibrinogen 6–12 week calves	Vagher (1973	2·52 (1·91–3·48) g/l
Prothrombin time 6–12 week calves	Vagher (1973)	17·7 (14·0–22·5) s
Total protein 12 week calves	Peters (1973)	64·8 g/l
Clotting time	Holman (1956)	6·0 min
ESR	Greatorex (1954)	1·00–3·00 mm/h

Table 6.4 Adult cattle—normal values

	Mean	Range
RBC (10^{12}/l)	7·0	5·0 – 9·0
PCV (l/l)*	0·32	0·24– 0·40
Hb (g/dl)*	11·0	8·0 –14·0
MCV (fl)	50·0	40·0 –60·0
MCH (pg)	14·0	11·0 –17·0
MCHC (g/dl)	32·0	30·0 –36·0
WBC (10^9/l)	7·0	4·0 –10·0
Segmented neutrophils (10^9/l)	1·9	0·6 – 4·5
Non-segmented neutrophiis (10^9/l)	0·05	0 – 1·0
Lymphocytes (10^9/l)	4·05	1·8 – 7·5
Monocytes (10^9/l)	0·30	0·08– 0·7
Eosinophils (10^9/l)	0·65	0 – 2·0
Basophils (10^9/l)	Rare	
Reticulocytes (per cent)	Nil	
ESR (mm/hour)		0 – 3·0

* Values higher in bulls.

Holman 1956). Greatorex (1954) showed similar results (e.g. 0·35 per cent at 1 month old and 0·45–0·5 per cent at 5 months of age).

6.2.3   NORMAL VALUES—ADULT CATTLE

In adult cattle, cellular values can also be altered by environmental or physio-logical factors but the basic pattern showing means and ranges is something of the order shown in Table 6.4.

6.2.3.1   Erythrocytes

Erythrocyte values appear to decline only slightly as the animal gets older, although anaemia is more likely to develop in the older, high yielding dairy cows (Whitlock *et al* 1974). It is unlikely that anaemia associated with senility will appear in cattle but, in the few instances when very old cattle are kept, anaemia may develop as it does in the old of many other species.

Table 6.5   Adult bulls. Erythrocytic values—changes with age (Penny *et al* 1966).

	2 *years*	8 *years*	> 10 *years*
RBC (10^{12}/l)	6·68	9·08	7·94
PCV (l/l)	0·378	0·459	0·388
Hb (g/dl)	12·2	16·0	13·5
MCV (fl)	58·1	52·6	49·3

N.B. PCV and Hb of bulls is higher than those 'normal values' quoted in Table 6.4.

Wingfield and Tumbleson (1973) found that, in dairy cattle, total ery-throcyte counts declined from the age of 6 months to 2 years and then became more or less steady as the animal aged. For example, in Holsteins, total counts fell from $8·0 \times 10^{12}$/l at 1 year old to $6·5 \times 10^{12}$/l by 2 years and was down to only $6·2 \times 10^{12}$/l at 10 years old. PCV and Hb for the same period were 0·338 l/l, 0·359 l/l, 0·359 l/l, and 11·7 g/dl, 12·6 g/dl, 12·4 g/dl respectively. Although total counts fell, the other factors did not, due to increased MCV values which reached a maximum of 55 fl at 2 years of age.

Penny *et al* (1966) using Friesian bulls, found that RBC, PCV and Hb tended to rise from 2 to 8 years of age and then the values declined slightly (Table 6.5).

6.2.3.2   Leucocytes

The decline in leucocytes with age is well documented and most authors agree that total counts are highest in animals of 1–2 years old. Moberg (1955) quoted $11\cdot116 \times 10^9/l$ in yearlings and $7\cdot106 \times 10^9/l$ in cows above 6 years old. Chevrier and Gayot (1972) indicated that in Holsteins average total white blood cells fell steadily from around $9\cdot00 \times 10^9/l$ at the age of 18 months to about $5\cdot5 \times 10^9/l$ at 7 years old and above. The most marked fall was between 2 and 5 years old ($8\cdot42$–$5\cdot76 \times 10^9/l$). In this work there was marked count variation between animals of the same age. Wittwer and Böhmwald (1974) recorded very similar findings in Chile. Maximum leucocyte numbers occurred at 1–2 years of age with values of $9\cdot194 \pm 1\cdot401 \times 10^9/l$, while in animals of 6 years of age or over the corresponding values were $7\cdot540 \pm 1\cdot153 \times 10^9/l$. Lymphocytes were at a maximum at about 1 year and so were neutrophils, while monocytes fluctuated and eosinophils increased to a maximum at 4–5 years and then declined (see Table 6.6).

Table 6.6 Adult cattle. Leucocytes—changes with age (Wittwer & Böhmwald, 1974)

Approx. age	*WBC* $(10^9/l)$	*Neutrophils* $(10^9/l)$	*Lymphocytes* $(10^9/l)$	*Monocytes* $(10^9/l)$	*Eosinophils* $(10^9/l)$
1 year	$9\cdot194 \pm 1\cdot401$	$2\cdot889 \pm 0\cdot842$	$5\cdot223 \pm 1\cdot104$	$0\cdot508 \pm 0\cdot221$	$0\cdot574 \pm 0\cdot397$
6 years	$7\cdot540 \pm 1\cdot153$	$2\cdot412 \pm 0\cdot836$	$3\cdot805 \pm 0\cdot8666$	$0\cdot370 \pm 0\cdot167$	$0\cdot953 \pm 0\cdot428$

Penny *et al* (1966) showed that in bulls total leucocytes also declined from $7\cdot28 \times 10^9/l$ at 2 years old to $5\cdot20 \times 10^9/l$ at 8 years old. There was a rise in the 9-year-old values followed by a decline to $4\cdot43 \times 10^9/l$ in animals over 10 years old. These changes were due in the main to a decline in lymphocytes and a partially compensating increase in neutrophils (lymphocytes and neutrophils at 2 years of age $4\cdot00$ and $2\cdot01 \times 10^9/l$ respectively, changing to $1\cdot87$ and $1\cdot99 \times 10^9/l$ at over 10 years of age).

Wingfield and Tumbleson (1973) recorded irregular leucocyte totals in dairy cows from 1 to 5 years old, a peak in values at 5–7 years and then a decline. At 2, 5, 6 and 10 years of age the following mean total leucocyte values were respectively $9\cdot00$, $10\cdot50$, $13\cdot00$ and $6\cdot50 \times 10^9/l$. In a second group of animals, a similar pattern was observed but the total values throughout were lower.

6.2.3.3 Coagulation, fragility, ESR and protein levels

In addition to the normal values in cattle already discussed, there are some additional values which require a mention. The sedimentation rate (ESR) in cattle is very slow ($0\cdot3$ mm/h) and it has been suggested (Olsen 1966) that the test is undertaken at a $45°$ angle to increase sedimentation. In addition, the resultant reading can be corrected in the light of the PCV (low PCV increases ESR).

Red cell fragility for adult cattle is quoted as initial haemolysis 0·60 per cent, complete haemolysis 0·32 per cent (Osbaldiston *et al* 1970) and initial haemolysis 0·50 per cent, complete haemolysis 0·38 per cent (Perk *et al* 1964).

Blood coagulation studies have been undertaken by some workers and normal values are given in Table 6.7.

The concentration of plasma prothrombin is related to the globulin and albumin levels—the higher the globulin, the higher the prothrombin, and the

Table 6.7 Cattle. Coagulation parameters—normal values

	Gentry et al (1975)	*Kociba* et al (1969)	*Osbaldiston* et al (1970)	*Dorner* & *Bass* (1974)	*Schalm* (1972)
Clotting time (Lee & White) (min)	6·0– 20·0	4·0– 15·0	20·5 ± 1·3		
Prothrombin (seconds)	22·0– 28·0	12·0– 14·0	14·3 ± 0·6	11·9	
Platelets (10⁹/l)	200·0–600·0	250·0–500·0	375·0 ± 3·5		200·0–800·0
Prothrombin consumption (seconds)	24·0–102·0		40·0 ± 9·0		
Partial thromboplastin (seconds)	46·0– 52·0	60·0– 70·0	47·0 ± 3·0	49·1	

higher the albumin, the lower the prothrombin (Boiti & Grosso 1972). Prothrombin levels ranged from 0·035 to 0·19 g/l (average 0·1 ± 0·004 g/l) in cattle aged 7 months to 14 years.

Values which are allied to, but not strictly part of haematology, are the various protein contents of plasma or serum. Because of their relative value in herd testing, the normal values are given in Table 6.8.

Tumbleson *et al* (1973) have demonstrated changing protein levels, particularly γ globulins, in association with age and it is clear that total serum proteins are low in calves before colostrum is absorbed. In addition to these variations, Payne *et al* (1973) have shown that there is considerable variation among adult dairy cows from different herds (albumin 34·0 ± 2·5 g/l, globulin 43·0 ± 6·0 g/l), and that these variations are also associated with time of year

Table 6.8 Cattle and buffaloes. Normal serum protein levels

Author	State	Total protein serum g/l	Albumin serum g/l	α Globulin serum g/l	β Globulin serum g/l	γ Globulin serum g/l
Dalton (1967)	Calves*					
	1 week	49·0 (42·0–53·0)				
	2–3 weeks	65·0 (55·0–70·0)				
Tumbleson et al (1973)	Calves*					
	<6 months	76·4±1·4	40·8±0·7	10·1±0·5	9·0±0·3	16·4±1·3
	3 years	89·0±1·0	40·5±0·7	13·0±0·4	8·5±0·2	26·9±1·0
	6 years	94·2±1·4	42·7±1·2	13·0±0·6	8·4±0·4	30·1±1·8
	>10 years	102·0±3·2	39·9±2·6	12·3±1·0	10·3±1·3	39·5±3·9
Irfan (1967)	Adults*	71·6	30·8	7·9	8·6	24·3
Payne et al (1973)	Adults*		34·0±2·5	43·0±6·0		
Vacca et al (1974)	Buffaloes					
	1½–3 years	70·7±8·0	27·9±1·0	12·5±0·6	10·9±0·5	19·3±0·9
	Adults*					
	2–6 years	73·0±7·0	30·4±1·0	9·5±0·4	11·4±0·6	21·6±1·0

* Cattle.

and milk yield. Little (1974) showed that albumin fell sharply after parturition and then rose slowly from 27·1 g/l within 2 weeks of parturition to 33·1 g/l by the end of the lactational period. Balmacida and Bottari (1974) demonstrated variations in γ globulin in different breeds of cattle ranging from 13·9 ± 1·1 g/l in the Charolais to 23·6 ± 7·6 g/l in Holando Argentina, but these variations may be due to herd and environmental factors as well as to breed.

Normal values for fibrinogen vary considerably but are generally higher than in other species. In adults, Schalm (1972) quoted fibrinogen as 4·0 g/l (2·0–7·0 g/l) and the serum protein to fibrinogen ratio as 18:1 (10:1–37:1). See also the values for calves in Table 6.3.

6.2.4 ENVIRONMENTAL AND PHYSIOLOGICAL EFFECTS ON NORMAL VALUES

6.2.4.1 Stress

Apart from the changes due to age, there are other effects which may alter cell counts in cattle. All cellular values may be changed irrespective of the age or country of origin of the cattle if the animals become unduly stressed during blood sampling. Gartner *et al* (1965) found that in beef cattle all red cell values were significantly lower in tranquillized animals at rest, after exercise or after visual stimulation, than in non-tranquillized animals. Considerable changes could occur in the PCV of both groups. In tranquillized animals the PCV at rest was 0·27 l/l and after exercise rose to 0·34 l/l. In the non-tranquillized animals the changes were even greater being 0·29 l/l at rest and 0·39 l/l after exercise. Changes like this could alter the interpretation placed on the results and be most misleading.

6.2.4.2 Breed

This is another factor, although the differences between breeds are not easy to assess. Greatorex (1957) recorded little difference between most breeds but he commented that Jersey and Guernsey cattle are different from the others. Penny *et al* (1966) also recorded lower red blood cell values for Guernsey bulls than for other breeds, but no leucocyte differences. Ryan (1971a b) recorded lower Hb and PCV in Jerseys than other breeds and found the highest values in Charolais cattle. The average leucocyte values vary markedly from breed to breed (e.g. $9·83 \times 10^9$/l in Jersey, $14·47 \times 10^9$/l in Hereford and $13·83 \times 10^9$/l in Charolais cattle), but these variations seem just as likely to be due to environment as to breed. Wingfield and Tumbleson (1973) record marked differences in erythrocyte counts between Holstein and Guernsey cattle, with the Guernsey having markedly lower values. For cattle 2–10 years old, Friesians had values of $6·65 \times 10^{12}/l$ while Guernseys ranged from $4·0–5·0 \times 10^{12}/l$. There was, however, no significant variation in PCV or Hb. Leucocytes varied also with Holsteins having higher total values than Guernseys (e.g. $10·0–13·0 \times 10^9/l$ as against $7·0–10·0 \times 19^9/l$).

It appears that the Jersey and Guernsey cattle do have lower red and white cell totals than many other breeds, and that the Charolais may have high total erythrocyte counts. These exceptions apart, it seems that erythrocyte values show little breed variation and any leucocyte variations are just as likely to be due to environmental factors as to breed variation.

Table 6.9 Cattle. Leucocyte values at parturition (Straub *et al* 1959)

	Average WBC $10^9/l$	Average neutrophils $10^9/l$	Average lymphocytes $10^9/l$	Average monocytes $10^9/l$	Average eosinophils $10^9/l$
Normal	8·00	2·28	4·64	0·320	0·720
Parturition	17·75	9·90	6·38	1·190	0·340
24 hours past parturition	10·00	4·90	3·95	0·833	0·410
48 hours past parturition	10·00	4·08	4·27	1·060	0·575

Some breed variation is also seen in glucose-6-phosphate dehydrogenase and 6-phospho-gluconate dehydrogenase levels in cattle (Steensgaard 1968). G-6-PD varied from 330 ± 43 units per 100 ml PCV in black and white Danish cattle to 315 ± 38 units in Jerseys. 6-P-GD was less affected with $52·8 \pm 12·2$ units per 100 ml PCV in red Danish cattle and $47·1 \pm 9·2$ units in black and white Danish cattle.

Environment and managemental methods can have haematological effects, especially when these are combined with lactational or other stress. An extended consideration of these aspects is given under Metabolic Profiles (6.7.1 & 6.2).

6.2.4.3 Parturition

This has marked but relatively short-lived effects. Erythrocyte counts increase at the time of calving, remain high for 24–48 hours and then decline, often to below normal levels where they may stay for some time. For example, average

Table 6.10 Normal values for exotic cattle

Author	Cattle and origin		RBC × 10¹²/l	PCV l/l	Hb g/dl
Heyns	Afrikander	Cow	8·95		12·64
1971		Calf	12·93		12·54
	Friesland	Cow	6·91		10·14
	(in S. Africa)	Calf	9·41		10·25
Alencar	Dutch red cattle		5·0–8·0	0·24–0·36	5·0–10·0
1971	(Brazil 3–9 years)		(6·5)	(0·28)	(7·9)
Smith	Ankole Longhorn		5·51 ± 0·82	0·307 ± 0·0455	7·7 ± 1·13
1959	cows. Dry season				
	(Uganda)				
Cooper	Twsana and	Cow		0·36 ± 0·042	12·0 ± 1·47
1974	Africander	Calves		0·34 ± 0·044	10·8 ± 3·2
	(Botswana)				
Saror &	Fulani (Zebu)		7·2 ± 0·9	0·366 ± 0·035	12·4 ± 1·1
Coles 1973	Fulani X		6·2 ± 1·0	0·347 ± 0·035	11·5 ± 5·3
	Friesian				
	(dry season 4–8				
	years Nigeria)				
Vohradsky	Friesian (Ghana	Milking	6·44	0·35	13·7
1974	mainly 3 yrs +)		4·7–7·6	0·28–0·42	11·4–15·2
		Dry	6·24	0·37	12·3
			5·0–8·0	0·30–0·45	11·1–15·9
		Heifers	6·38	0·34	12·1
			4·88–7·89	0·28–0·41	9·6–14·0

RBC, PCV and Hb, at parturition, are $7·4 × 10^{12}$/l, 0·40 l/l and 13·2 g/dl, respectively and 2 days later the corresponding values are $6·2 × 10^{12}$/l, 0·37 l/l and 12·6 g/dl (Straub *et al* 1959). Total leucocyte counts showed a marked increase on the day of parturition and an almost equally rapid fall 24–48 hours after calving, with a return to normal in 4–6 days. This upsurge in leucocytes is due mainly to increased numbers of neutrophils with a lesser increase in lymphocytes and monocytes (Straub *et al* 1959) (Table 6.9).

These figures are for animals without retention of fetal membranes. Cattle with persistent ovarian follicles show blood changes rather similar to those described at parturition, with significant neutrophilia and lymphocytosis (Moberg 1965).

6.2.4.4 Exotic cattle

A further complicating factor when studying normal values in cattle is that

MCV fl	MCHC g/dl	WBC ×10⁹/l	N %	L %	M %	E %	B %
		6·3–17·760 11·300	24·4	58·9	3·7	12·3	
55·6±8·9	25·26±3·13						
	33·0±1·97	9·5±3·0	21·0±8·2	67·0±8·2	2·0±1·9	10·0±6·3	
	32·0±3·69	10·0±3·6	19·0±10·0	71·0±9·4	3·0±2·0	7·0±5·0	
51·2±6·8	33·9±1·2	8·9±1·9	25·9±5·4	62·8±7·5	2·6±1·4	8·2±6·8	
57·2±6·4	33·0±0·9	7·4±1·5	28·0±5·9	60·9±6·5	2·8±1·2	8·3±4·1	
54·0	39·0	6·48	19·0	73·0	0·1	8·0	
44·0–73·0	36·0–42·0	3·95–8·55	3·0–40·0	42·0–93·0	0–1·0	1·0–18·0	0
59·0	36·0	7·59	14·0	76·0	0·4	10·0	
50·0–68·0	33·0–42·0	4·7–17·35	4·0–28·0	62·0–90·0	0–2·0	3·0–22·0	
53·0	36·0	7·92	13·0	82·0	0·5	4·0	
42·0–66·0	32·0–38·0	3·50–11·30	4·0–30·3	66·0–94·0	0–1·0	0–14·0	0

the animals live in different countries, are exported to climates for which they are not adapted, or are tropical animals with a different physiological make-up to European and North American cattle. Several studies have been undertaken on such animals and the results are summarized in Table 6.10.

The main change when compared to European breeds is that the dry and wet seasons have an effect. Saror and Coles (1973) showed lower erythrocyte values and higher WBC during the wet season compared with the dry season results shown in the table. Cooper (1974) showed calves as having lower Hb and PCV than adult—possibly a reflection of relatively poor calf nutrition.

Vohradsky (1974) considered the erythrocytic picture to be low in his series, the MCV and MCHC were raised and neutrophils lower than in European counterparts. The Ankole results (Smith 1959) show very low red blood cell counts and Hb, again possibly a reflection of nutrition during the dry season.

Table 6.11　Normal values for buffaloes

Author	Age status	RBC $\times 10^{12}/l$	PCV l/l	Hb g/dl	ESR mm/h	WBC $\times 10^9/l$
Mastran-gelo 1971	<1 year	11·45 ± 0·319		16·8 ± 0·55		
	>1 year	7·12 ± 0·240		13·3 ± 0·50		
Adaval & Gangwar 1972						
Aleyas & Rajamani 1972	4–11 years (female)	5·86 ± 1·03	0·437 ± 0·051	10·50 ± 2·07	40·1 ± 10·9	10·49 ± 2·48
Malik *et al* 1974	9–12 months	5·52 ± 0·52	0·3056 ± 0·007	10·57 ± 0·25		8·57 ± 0·1
Sharma *et al* 1973	Adult	5·13 ± 0·18	0·36 ± 0·018	10·34 ± 0·76	97·6 ± 35·9	11·34 ± 1·32
	Young	6·74 ± 0·44	0·318 ± 0·045	9·99 ± 1·29	80·0 ± 33·0	11·98 ± 0·99
	Calves	7·84 ± 0·31	0·418 ± 0·024	9·94 ± 1·51	50·8 ± 33·3	17·31 ± 0·86
Bokori 1974	Adult 2–9 years	5·8 ± 1·07	0·324 ± 0·031	12·30 ± 1·13	26·0 ± 24·0	8·25 ± 1·84
	Calves 4–11 months	5·50 ± 1·0	0·311 ± 0·038	11·80 ± 2·2	31·0 ± 19·8	12·4 ± 3·66
Vacca *et al* 1974	Adults 2–6 years	6·76 ± 0·34	0·350 ± 0·007	12·0 ± 0·60	70·0 ± 3·0	10·2 ± 0·30

6.2.5　BUFFALO

As well as cattle in foreign countries, we have to consider other ox-like animals, and of these the domesticated buffaloes (*Bubalus bubalis*) are the most important. Normal values will, like those of cattle, tend to alter with management, climate, etc. but for the purposes of this chapter a comparative exercise with values for cattle will suffice. The main differences seen in Table 6.11 are that the ESR in buffaloes is totally different from that in cattle. Cattle erythrocytes sediment 0–3 mm/h, buffaloes vary from 25–95 mm/h. The difference is attributed to the homogenicity of cell size and the greater fibrinogen content of buffalo blood (Vacca *et al* 1972, 1974). These authors reported total serum protein and fibrinogen levels in normal cattle which compare well with those quoted by other authors (e.g. fibrinogen 4·58 ± 0·29 g/l and a mean serum protein to fibrinogen ratio of 16:1). In normal buffaloes, however, the fibrinogen level was 6·88 ± 0·34 g/l and the serum protein to fibrinogen ratio 10·3:1.

% N	% L	% M	% E	% B	Prothrombin time (sec)	Clotting time (min)
					8·0–8·6	
33·1±4·7	61·1±5·4	1·9±1·1	3·7±2·9	0·2±0·4		
28·0±0·9	66·7±0·7	3·29±0·13	1·4±0·11	0·65±0·24		8·0±0·38
33·16±5·7	53·8±9·3	5·6±2·2	5·6±2·8	1·4±0·8		
25·7±3·1	70·0±5·4	1·0±0·7	3·0±1·7	0		
24·0±5·7	70·8±7·6	3·6±2·7	1·2±0·6	0		
40·0±7·4	50·5±5·6	1·0±0·3	8·5±5·7	0·3±0·5		
57·0±8·8	39·0±7·7	1·0	3·0±2·4	0		

Native Asian buffaloes, of which there are many distinct breeds, have slightly lower red cell counts, PCV and Hb, especially as adults, than cattle or the Italian buffaloes examined by Mastrangelo (1971) and Vacca *et al* (1974). The total white blood cells and the distribution of neutrophils and lymphocytes seem at variance between one author and another, and discrepancies are most likely due to the effects of environment and management. As far as can be judged, buffaloes seem to have slightly higher total white blood cell counts than cattle.

6.2.6 BONE MARROW

Bone marrow studies in cattle are not used extensively but can be of diagnostic significance in some diseases. Values will vary somewhat depending on site of biopsy and results depend very much on obtaining good preparations. Poorly smeared and stained preparations are only too easy to obtain, but are very difficult to interpret. Normal values are given in Table 6.12.

D. L. Doxey

Table 6.12 Bone marrow—normal cellular values (cattle)

	Adults Winquist (1954) %	Young adults Wilde (1964) %
Myeloblast	—	0·6– 7·4
Promyelocyte	0·2– 2·0	0·2– 4·0
Neutrophil myelocyte	1·0– 5·0 ⎫	2·8–12·4
Neutrophil metamyelocyte	1·0– 8·0 ⎭	
Neutrophil band form	5·0–12·0	4·4–21·6
Neutrophil	4·0–20·0	1·2–14·0
Eosinophil myelocyte	0 – 2·0 ⎫	0·6–12·2
Eosinophil metamyelocyte	0·5– 4·0 ⎭	
Eosinophil band form ⎫	2·0–10·0	0·6– 7·4
Eosinophil ⎭		0 – 1·0
Basophil	0 – 1·0	0 – 1·0
Total myeloid	20·0–55·0	17·8–58·2
Erythroblast (rubriblast)	0 – 1·0 ⎫	0·8– 7·2
Early normoblast (prorubricyte)	0·5– 2·0 ⎭	
Intermediate normoblast (rubricyte)	15·0–30·0	3·4–12·0
Late normoblast (metarubricyte)	10·0–35·0	24·6–55·2
Total erythroid	30·0–60·0	31·4–64·0
Lymphocyte	5·0–18·0	2·4–17·4
Monocyte	0 – 0·5	0 – 2·0
Plasma cell	0 – 3·0	0 – 1·0
M:E ratio	0·3:1–1·84:1 (Mean 1·7:1)	0·31:1–1·85:1

6.3 THE ERYTHROCYTES IN DISEASE

6.3.1 ERYTHROCYTE REGENERATION

The process of erythrocyte regeneration is basically the same in all species of domestic animals but there are some differences in the way the young erythrocytes are released into the circulation. Under normal circumstances (when erythrocyte regeneration is proceeding at the pace required to keep the body supplied with replacement cells) the normoblasts undergo their period of maturation and loss of nuclear material within the bone marrow. In the ox, only a minute proportion of red cells are released into the circulation containing any evidence of nuclear remnants. These cells can be demonstrated by supravital staining and are known as reticulocytes and, in normal cattle, occupy 0 to 0·02 per cent of the total erythrocytes.

In many species an increased demand for erythrocytes following blood loss results in increased cellular activity within the marrow, and the release of increasing numbers of immature erythrocytes into the circulation. In man, dogs, cats and pigs this rise parallels the demand for new cells but in the ox the situation is not so simple. In many instances, despite quite severe blood loss, the animals fail to release reticulocytes from the marrow even when the marrow has increased red cell production to replace lost cells. In other cases, reticulocytes are released and the factors which govern this appear to be total volume of blood lost, the period of time over which loss occurs and the age of the animal. Bremner (1966a) experimentally bled 4-month-old calves in one day of between 10 and 30 mls of blood per kg body weight. Calves losing 10 ml/kg showed no reticulocyte response, even though their Hb fell from 10·5 g/dl to 8·0 g/dl. Reticulocyte response increased marginally to 0·4 per cent in the 20 ml/kg group and to 1·2 per cent in the 30 ml/kg group. This response appeared 3 days after bleeding and was at its maximum between days 4 and 8. An older group of calves (11 months old), losing 20 ml/kg, showed a greater reticulocyte response with maximum values of 1·6 per cent. In 6-month-old calves, bled daily over a period of 14 days at rates of 2 ml/kg and 4 ml/kg, and in a group of 14-month-old steers bled at 2 ml/kg over the same period, the following occurred. Young animals bled at 2 ml/kg never showed reticulocytes above 0·2 per cent but older animals, losing blood at the same rate, reached maximum values of 0·6 per cent some 14 days after the first bleeding, by which time their Hb had reached 7·5 g/dl. In calves bled at 4 ml/kg Hb fell to 6·0 g/dl at the end of the bleeding period and reticulocyte counts reached 1·6 per cent 4 days before this.

Schnappauf *et al* (1967) removed between 60 and 70 per cent of a calf's red cells over a period of 10 days and reticulocyte counts never reached 0·5 per cent but 30–40 per cent removal over 24 hours elicited a response to 0·5 per cent 3–4 days later. When one-third of the blood volume was removed in 12 hours reticulocytes did appear 2 days later, reached a maximum of between 9 and 14 per cent 5–7 days after bleeding but disappeared 10 days after bleeding. In this case, when reticulocyte response was marked, PCV had been reduced from 0·30–0·34 l/l to 0·12 l/l in only 12 hours. Reticulocytes disappeared when the PCV had risen to between 0·20 and 0·25 l/l and during this period of recovery erythrocyte MCV increased from a mean normal of 35 fl to 50 fl.

Reticulocytes will appear in the circulation of the ox but only when blood loss is massive and very acute, or very prolonged, and is more likely to be obvious in older animals. The number of reticulocytes cannot, however, be used as a reliable means of assessing red cell recovery. In general, animals with erythrocyte life spans in excess of 100 days release reticulocytes infrequently. In cattle, the erythrocyte life span has been variously assessed. Kaneko *et al* (1971), using glycine 2-^{14}C, showed the life span in 3-year-old cows to be in the region of 135 days, while in older cows it was in the region of 162 days. Baker and Douglas (1957), using ^{59}Fe in 3-month-old calves, found the erythrocyte life span to be 55 days.

During active regeneration, variations in cell size and shape and the appearance of polychromatic cells is seen. In addition, basophilic stippling (basophilic granules scattered throughout the erythrocyte) may also occur in ruminants. Heinz bodies may also appear.

6.3.2 INCREASED ERYTHROCYTE VALUES

There are basically 2 methods, apart from the physiological effects of high altitude, by which the red cell total increases, or appears to increase. The first involves loss of fluid (dehydration) and the second derangement of the bone marrow (polycythaemia).

6.3.2.1 Dehydration

This problem is one most often encountered in calves, especially calves less than 1 month old and is, in most instances, precipitated by scouring. It is the commonest cause of death in such cases.

The primary derangement is in osmotic pressure and is brought about by the loss of the electrolytes necessary to maintain this pressure. The haematological changes will not identify the cause of the problem—they are only a guide to the degree of dehydration and hence to the severity of the trouble. (They cannot, however, be regarded as infallible guides because loss of cellular fluid is far advanced before any withdrawal of circulatory fluid starts to occur). Hence, dehydration will be advanced before the PCV starts to change and it must be remembered that PCV varies considerably from calf to calf, and one whose normal PCV is 0·30 l/l may still have values within published normal levels when it dies of dehydration.

Watt (1967) found PCV of 0·47–0·52 l/l in severely dehydrated scouring calves and Dalton (1968) recorded values of 0·42 ± 0·034 l/l and 0·47 ± 0·032 l/l in neonatal and 1-week-old calves deprived of milk for 4 days. Bianca et al (1965), using steers, found PCV increases of between 10 and 20 per cent of the original value when water deprivation occurred and Bianca (1970) noted that water is lost from both the erythrocytes and the plasma and that a transient initial surge in PCV due to excitement and splenic contraction followed access to water in thirsty animals. Tennant et al (1972) recorded PCV in calves with acute scour as being 0·45 ± 0·07 l/l (0·31–0·60 l/l), but Thornton et al (1973) found that the PCV of calves with diarrhoea was only significantly higher than normal in calves with clinically obvious severe dehydration. This latter agrees with the findings of Dalton et al (1965) who found increased PCV in only 10 per cent of diarrhoeic calves.

The PCV is a useful guide to severe dehydration, especially in acutely ill calves but in cases of diarrhoea of several days' duration PCV does not change appreciably and is not related to the clinical severity of the condition.

6.3.2.2 Polycythaemia

This term implies an increase in all blood cell types but in practice its use in cattle is confined to circumstances where RBC, PCV and Hb are increased. Fowler *et al* (1964) described the condition in a steer in which the initial PCV was 0·71 l/l. The value was only kept within reasonable limits by repeated bleedings. It took 3 months after the last bleeding for the animal's PCV to rise from 0·35 l/l to 0·63 l/l. Bone marrow studies indicated rapid erythrocyte regeneration (myeloid/erythroid ratio 0·38:1 on admission and 0·17:1 4 months later), and it was found that erythrocyte life span was normal but erythrocyte mass and total blood volume were increased. No cause was identified.

Tennant *et al* (1967) described 14 primary polycythaemia cases in Jerseys, all offspring of one sire or his son. The condition developed at or after the second month of life and PCV reached 0·60–0·80 l/l, RBC 15·8–$25·5 \times 10^{12}$/l and Hb 19·2–27·2 g/dl. If the animals survived, erythrocyte numbers gradually fell to normal after 12 to 18 months. Myeloid/erythrocyte ratio was 0·19:1 to 0·34:1. Kaneko *et al* (1968) observed that these poly-cythaemic calves had an increased rate of iron transfer from plasma, indicating active erythropoiesis. Serum iron was high and ranged from 25·3 to 145·5 μmol/l, while iron transfer (mg per day) ranged from 100·5 to 180·6 (normal value 14–104, average 73). Tennant *et al* (1969), using the same calves, found Hb saturation to be within normal limits and PCV was shown to rise to a maximum in surviving calves at 6–8 months of age and then decline.

Cases of secondary polycythaemia attributable to cardiac or pulmonary defects are unusual, but the author has seen an Aberdeen Angus steer with a PCV of 0·65 l/l apparently as a result of an intra-ventricular septal defect.

6.3.3 DECREASED ERYTHROCYTE VALUES.

There are basically 3 types of anaemia—dyshaemopoietic (failure of cell production), haemolytic and haemorrhagic. Each type may have a variety of causes and may occur as a primary condition (e.g. babesiosis), or may be discovered as a secondary effect in animals suffering from some other condi-tion (e.g. anaemia during chronic parasitism). Each group will be dealt with separately although in practice the groups are not always as clearly de-marcated as it may appear from the ensuing descriptions.

6.3.3.1 Dyshaemopoietic anaemia

This type of anaemia has 2 distinct basic causes although in both of these bone marrow failure occurs to some degree. In one type, the failure is primary being the main cause of the illness, while in the other the marrow failure is secondary, brought about by some other illness which is not haematological in origin. Dyshaemopoietic anaemia is not necessarily aplastic, can often be cured and may be associated with, and exacerbated by, haemorrhage, especially when platelet counts fall.

Secondary anaemias are difficult to quantitate and depend on the type of primary illness, its duration and severity and the physical condition of the animal. In some, anaemia may be obvious, in others of only minor significance. Any long-standing chronic illness may result in a mild degree of anaemia but the main diseases often associated with anaemia are tumours, protein deficiency due to malnutrition or starvation and severe infestation with non-blood-sucking helminth parasites, such as the trichostrongyles.

BRACKEN FERN POISONING

Classical bracken poisoning occurs after cattle have ingested bracken (*Pteridium aquilinum*) for a period of 1 to 3 months and is associated with bone marrow failure, anorexia, depression and haemorrhage. In addition, bracken is also implicated in a condition of calves in which laryngeal oedema occurs, and in a chronic haematuria syndrome (Austin 1964).

Classical bracken poisoning causes arrested mitosis so that blast cells are not produced by the marrow. This results in a diminution of cells as decreased production fails to keep pace with normal cell loss. If bracken was fed experimentally, Gorišek and Maržan (1965) found that red cell counts started to fall after 30 days and fell precipitously after 60 days. Platelets fell from $900 \times 10^9/l$ to $500 \times 10^9/l$ after 20 days and continued to decline to $10 \cdot 0 \times 10^9/l$ by day 63. Equally dramatic falls in leucocytes occurred ($7 \cdot 00$–$1 \cdot 00 \times 10^9/l$ after 65 days) and both lymphocytes and neutrophils were reduced. Prothrombin levels also fell markedly after 50 days' ingestion of bracken. Evans *et al* (1958) extracted the ethanol-soluble toxic principle and when this was fed to cattle similar haematological changes occurred, the total white cell count falling from $6 \cdot 00 \times 10^9/l$ to $2 \cdot 00 \times 10^9/l$ and platelets from $500 \cdot 0 \times 10^9/l$ to $< 100 \cdot 0 \times 10^9/l$. These changes occurred in 5 weeks whereas the same authors found that it took 6–8 weeks to produce similar effects when bracken was fed. Dalton (1964), investigating naturally occurring cases, found that total leucocyte counts varied from case to case and from one part of the day to another but, in the main, counts varied between $6 \cdot 0$ and $1 \cdot 4 \times 10^9/l$. Animals which died had counts of about $1 \cdot 0 \times 10^9/l$. PCV in affected surviving animals ranged from $0 \cdot 35$ to $0 \cdot 24$ 1/1 but, in animals which died, values fell rapidly a day or two before death to about $0 \cdot 15$ 1/1.

Howell and Evans (1967) demonstrated increased levels of fibrinogen in animals fed bracken for more than 50 days. The toxic principle in bracken is passed into milk and suckling calves can be affected (Evans *et al* 1972). Total leucocyte counts in the calves fell from >8·0 to 4·0×10⁹/l after 70 days and platelets also fell but the PCV remained steady.

Konno *et al* (1971) recorded a condition in Japanese cattle resembling bracken poisoning with evidence of anaemia, total leucocyte counts of 0·80 to 5·40×10⁹/l and severe depletion of granulocytes. The bone marrow revealed a marked reduction in blast cells and immature granulocytes. The exact aetiology was not established but bracken was suspected.

Bracken fed in low doses over long periods can cause chronic cystic haematuria, Stamatovič *et al* (1965) recorded total erythrocyte counts falling over a period of 3 years from 8·70 to 3·36×10¹²/l and over 4 years from 7·14 to 1·92×10¹²/l. Platelets also fell but leucocyte counts remained within normal limits. Smith and Beatson (1970) recorded similar blood loss from chronic haematuria and recorded anaemia in the older cattle affected.

The male fern (*Dryopteris filix-mas*) causes toxic effects in cattle but does not affect the bone marrow (Edgar & Thin 1968).

TRICHLOROETHYLENE-EXTRACTED SOYBEAN OIL MEAL

Haematologically, trichloroethylene-extracted soybean oil meal poisoning resembles bracken poisoning. Animals eating this meal became affected 30 to 230 days after the ration was introduced and showed PCVs of 0·18–0·39 l/l, total red blood cells of 3·2–6·8×10¹²/l, total white blood cells of 0·70–8·60×10⁹/l, gross loss of granulocytes and platelet counts varying from 22·0–73·0×10⁹/l (Pritchard *et al* 1952). The condition was reproduced experimentally (Pritchard *et al* 1956a) and the solvent used during extraction found to be at fault. The effects produced by the toxic feed depended on the amount fed and those animals fed large amounts developed fatal thrombocytopenia after only 6 weeks (Pritchard *et al* 1956b).

DEFICIENCY ANAEMIAS

Deficiencies in the intake of elements essential for the production of haemoglobin or for cell division will lead to dysfunction of the bone marrow. The 3 most often implicated are iron, copper and cobalt.

Iron deficiency will occur in calves raised for veal but unintentional, clinical deficiency is rare. Hibbs *et al* (1963) investigated a problem herd where 30 per cent of calves born had Hb levels of less than 9·0 g/dl. In these calves, Hb ranged from 7·4 to 8·1 g/dl, PCVs from 0·24 to 0·29 l/l and serum Fe levels between 11·9 and 13·9 μmol/l. The dams of affected calves had normal values for all these parameters. By the time affected calves were 8 weeks old and on dry feed, all values had risen to within the normal range. Möllerberg and Jacobsson (1970), describing iron deficiency anaemia, recorded MCV of 46·0±5·0 fl (38·0–68·0 fl) and MCHC of 29·0±2·0 g/dl (25·0–31·0 g/dl) indicating a microcytic hypochromic anaemia. Möllerberg *et al* (1975) and Möllerberg (1975) found that up to 35 per cent of purchased calves had some degree of iron deficiency and that iron injections in veal-type calves prevented the decline of Hb and PCV seen in untreated animals (Hb 9·0 to 5·5 g/dl and PCV 0·30 to 0·18 l/l over a period of 12 weeks). Growth rate in treated calves was improved.

Cobalt deficiency is unusual on its own but has been described in various areas. Kuba *et al* (1963) described the condition in Japan and, in addition to the clinical signs of anorexia and weight loss, showed total erythrocyte counts of 3·0 to 5·0 × 10^{12}/l and Hb of around 6·0 g/dl. Anisocytosis and poikilocytosis were constant features and the red cell diameters were reduced.

Copper deficiency is usually recognized in cattle by the poor growth rates and coat colour changes which occur with any anaemia being of secondary importance. Thornton *et al* (1972) and Howard (1970) have described the beneficial effects of copper in deficient animals and Howard showed that copper and cobalt deficiency can exist together and that material Hb increases in such cases are only obtained when both elements are administered. Field (1957) found little haematological difference between supplemented and unsupplemented cows on copper deficient ground and Todd *et al* (1967) studied copper deficient calves and found that the PCV were normal or only slightly below normal (0·22–0·46 l/l). However, Smith *et al* (1975) showed Hb levels as low as 7·6 g/dl in animals with blood copper levels of 4·7 μmol/l and there were clear haematological differences between deficient and non-deficient animals. Deficient animals showed Heinz bodies in as many as 50 per cent of their red cells, although Heinz bodies were also recorded in copper treated animals.

LEAD POISONING

Lead poisoning is usually an acute condition without haematological changes, although mild haemolytic anaemia has been seen. Hilliard *et al* (1973) describe a normocytic, normochronic anaemia of minor degree associated with impaired erythrogenesis and decreased red blood cell survival time as a result of lead contamination of cattle food. Lead inhibits delta-amino-laevulinic acid dehydrase which is essential for haem synthesis. Uroporphyrin and protoporphyrin changes occurred and Green *et al* (1973) consider that blood prophyrin levels increase in cattle blood following lead poisoning.

MYCOTOXICOSIS

Certain types of fungi produce toxins and, if these toxins are fed to animals, usually as a result of grain or other concentrate feed going mouldy, then changes very similar to those induced by bracken poisoning are seen. This problem is particularly severe in Russia, especially in horses (Forgacs & Carll 1962), but has been seen elsewhere and the author recently had experience of this problem in cattle in Scotland. *Stachybotrys alternans* will affect cattle and produces a three-stage disease. The first stage involves stomatitis, rhinitis and conjunctivitis which may proceed to the second stage, when marked thrombocytopenia occurs, with associated coagulation defects together with leucopenia and agranulocytosis. Stage 3 is a progression of stage 2 with almost total loss of platelets and leucocytes. Forgacs and Carll (1962) record that a calf, force-fed contaminated straw, showed agranulocytosis 9 days later and the total leucocyte count fell from 4.5×10^9/l to 0.15×10^9/l after 15 days. Blood clotting time increased from 9 to 19 minutes. Almost identical signs of panleucopenia are recorded when *Fusarium* spp., especially *F. sporotrichioides*, is ingested by humans eating mouldy grain in Russia and it seems possible that this fungus could affect cattle, although affected grain is not palatable and would probably be refused. Animals affected with thrombocytopenia and agranulocytosis usually die but cases in the earlier stages may recover.

Fungal toxins will, of course, produce other types of disease (e.g. mouldy sweet clover poisoning and mouldy Bermuda grass toxicosis) and these will be mentioned elsewhere. The clinical and haematological signs produced will depend on the toxins elaborated (Harwig & Munro 1975).

DRUGS

Hofmann *et al* (1974) and Hoffmann-Fezer *et al* (1974) describe a bone marrow dysfunction in milk-fed veal calves induced by continuous feeding of 4.0 to 8.5 mg furazolidone/kg body weight. This resulted in a haemorrhagic syndrome associated with thrombocytopenia. In the control veal calves, platelets remained in the normal range, RBC fell from 7.5×10^{12}/l to 5.5×10^{12}/l over 9 weeks and granulocytes were reduced from 4.0×10^9/l to 1.0×10^9/l over the same period. Calves on 8.5 mg furazolidone showed loss of red blood cells only if haemorrhage occurred but in all cases platelets fell to below 100.0×10^9/l after 8 weeks and, in the worse cases, to less than 10.0×10^9/l. Granulocytes fell to virtually nil after only 5–6 weeks in 2 cases. Animals on 6 mg and 4 mg/kg dosages showed similar effects but over a longer period of time. For example, platelets took as long as 20 weeks to fall to less than 50.0×10^9/l but granulocytes were severely affected after 5–10 weeks. Bone marrow studies revealed severe depletion of megakaryocytes 3 weeks after dosing started and subsequent falls in both erythrocyte and granulocyte precursors.

Espinasse *et al* (1973) also describe a haemorrhagic syndrome in veal calves, which is associated with a thrombocytopenia. Calves affected had platelet counts of between 7.5 and 25.0 10^9/l and bone marrow studies revealed an absence of megakaryocytes. The cause was not discovered and no mention is made of furazolidone being fed.

Tartour *et al* (1973) describe the effects on Zebu calves of prolonged feeding with the leaves of *Ipomoea carnea*. A moderate anaemia (red blood cell counts fell from 6·5 to $4·8 \times 10^{12}/l$) of a normocytic hypochromic type developed. Leucocyte numbers tended to fall (lowest value $3·7 \times 10^9/l$) and it may be that these changes result from bone marrow damage. No marrow studies were conducted.

6.3.3.2 Haemolytic anaemia

With the dyshaemopoietic anaemias, classification is not always easy because the resulting anaemia, although primarily due to marrow malfunction, may be exacerbated by bleeding (e.g. in thrombocytopenia). The same applies to haemolytic anaemias for haemolysis may only be one part of a more complex problem.

CONGENITAL PORPHYRIA

This rare condition is inherited as a simple Mendelian recessive (Wass & Hoyt 1965a) and, although classified as haemolytic, arises originally as a defect in the production of Hb. Haemoglobin is derived from the combination of haem and globin and haem is formed from protoporphyrin III plus ferrous iron. The normal process of haem production is complex but involves the formation from prophobilinogen of 2 substances, uroporphyrinogen III and uroporphyrinogen I. Uroporphyrinogen III is processed to form protoporphyrin III and this combines with Fe^{++} to form haem. Uroporphyrinogen I is a waste product which is transformed to uroporphyrin I and coproporphyrin I, both of which are excreted in the urine and faeces. In animals suffering from congenital porphyria, there is an inherent defect in this process and the animals form inadequate amounts of protoporphyrin III and excessive amounts of uroporphyrin I and coproporphyrin I. The end result is deficient haem production and the deposition in bones, teeth and tissues of the waste products which, in turn, gives rise to a photosensitization syndrome, the severity of which is related to the amount of uroporphyrin produced. Kaneko *et al* (1971) demonstrated that erythrocyte survival is reduced in affected animals and that the survival is shortest in animals with high coproporphyrin levels. Normal survival time is 135 to 162 days and in affected animals it is reduced to 35 to 120 days. Engel *et al* (1973) showed that faecal urobilinogen was raised in affected animals (normal 1183 mg/day, porphyric 2071 ± 728 mg/day) and that the percentage of carboxyhaemoglobin was raised in affected animals when compared to normal animals in the same environment (normal $0·43 \pm 0·12$ g/dl, porphyric $0·72 \pm 0·24$ g/dl). These findings suggest a reduced life span and rapid marrow turnover of red cells, hence the classification of haemolytic anaemia. Zinkl and Kaneko (1973) showed that erythrocyte 2,3-diphosphoglycerate (2,3-DPG) was higher in newborn affected calves than in normals and these increased levels could be due to erythrocyte immaturity.

Clinically, the anaemia and rate of red cell destruction is increased with high uroporphyrin levels and if the animals are exposed to sunlight. In housed cattle, the effects are less obvious. Wass and Hoyt (1965b) recorded haematological values in animals protected from and exposed to sunlight and showed marked exacerbation of anaemia after sunlight exposure. Of the examples they gave, 3 animals had mean PCV of 0·26 l/l and mean Hb of 8·4 g/dl prior to exposure to sunlight. After exposure, the mean values had fallen to 0·19 l/l and 6·3 g/dl respectively.

The anaemia was associated with anisocytosis, poikilocytosis, basophilic stippling and many normoblasts indicating active regeneration.

Kaneko and Mills (1970) compared values from birth to 24 days of age in normal and porphyric calves (both housed) showing that in affected calves at birth PCV and Hb were normal and MCV and reticulocytes raised. Normal calves showed little variation in these values between birth and 24 days of age. Affected calves, however, showed declining PCV, Hb and MCV, and the discrepancy between normal and affected calves became more pronounced as the animals grew older.

TOXIC ANAEMIAS

Acute or chronic copper poisoning may induce a haemolytic crisis. In the acute case, this is due to a massive overdose of copper or, in the chronic case, due to a slow build-up of copper in the liver until massive amounts are present which are suddenly released at a time of stress. At the time of haemolytic crisis the copper ions oxidize free Hb to methaemoglobin, but initial haemolysis precedes methaemoglobin formation (Steiner 1973). Mylrea and Byrne (1974) recorded deaths in 44 calves following injection of copper compounds and in later deaths haemoglobinuria and haemorrhages were a feature.

Water intoxication in calves may occur when the animals are deprived of water for long periods and then given sudden access to unlimited supplies. Mortality may reach 25 per cent (Fagan 1965) and bloat and haemoglobinuria are features of the condition. The haemolysis is presumably due to dilution of circulating electrolytes (Hannan 1965). Recovery, when it occurs, takes about 48 hours (Wright 1961).

Plant poisoning by some plants used as animal feeding stuffs has long been known to cause anaemia and there are also toxic effects resulting from the ingestion of plants available on open range grazing. *Lantana camara* is known to cause photosensitization, liver damage and death in a high percentage of cases (Aluja 1970). Haematological studies tended to indicate that slight decreases in erythrocytes occurred (Duivedi *et al* 1971) or that severe dehydration resulted in raised PCV (as high as 59 per cent) (Dhillon *et al* 1970). Hari *et al* (1973) found that the PCV fell after initial dehydration and that some haemolysis occurred. The mild anaemia produced by this plant is of doubtful origin and of only minor significance, the liver damage being far more serious.

Other plants cause anaemia which is of major significance and the principal origin of illness. Plants of the *Brassicae* spp. (i.e. kale, rape, white cabbage and brussels sprouts) may cause illness and, of these, kale is the commonest being widely grown as a feeding crop. Clegg and Evans (1962) describe haemoglobinuria and jaundice, with some deaths, in a dairy herd fed on frosted marrowstem kale. Most cases were in cows within 8 weeks of calving. Red cell counts were as low as $1.65 \times 10^{12}/l$ in cows which recovered, and $0.36 \times 10^{12}/l$ in cows which died. Even cows showing minimal clinical signs had total red blood cell counts of $2.60 \times 10^{12}/l$ and Hb down to 6.0 g/dl. In anaemic cows MCV was raised (59–151 fl) and MCHC was reduced (25–31 g/dl). Heinz bodies appeared in 2 of the cows. Heinz bodies are round or oval, single or multiple inclusions found within red cells. They can be demonstrated only by supravital stains when they appear as blue structures (see p. 585). They are composed of precipitated denatured Hb and are formed by oxidative agents overcoming the normal anti-oxidant system involving reduced glutathione and glucose-6-phosphate dehydrogenase.

Dunbar and Chambers (1963) recorded similar clinical anaemia and haemoglobinuria in dairy cattle fed frosted kale, while Penny *et al* (1964) reproduced the condition by feeding kale over a period of 17 weeks to non-lactating cows. RBC fell to about $4.0 \times 10^{12}/l$ after 6 weeks and then stabilized, while controls fed hay had counts of 6.0 to $8.0 \times 10^{12}/l$. The kale-fed animals had raised MCV of 65–75 fl and exhibited Heinz bodies which reached a maximum of 27 per cent after 5 weeks and then fell to between 5 per cent and 15 per cent over the rest of the period. Reticulocytes rose only to a maximum of 0.8 per cent after 5 weeks. No clinical signs of haemoglobinuria occurred in these animals, nor was there any obvious increase in erythrocyte fragility. Prior to this experiment, Penny *et al* (1961) had already shown that Heinz bodies appeared in up to 27 per cent of red cells in heifers fed kale for periods of 4–8 weeks but after this time the animals appeared to compensate and Heinz body percentages fell.

Grant *et al* (1968) used lactating cows and found that the PCV and Hb values fell in cows fed kale *ad lib*. (Hb 11.06 ± 0.8 g/dl to 9.21 ± 1.1 g/dl and PCV 0.33 ± 0.03 l/l to 0.28 ± 0.03 l/l after 39 days feeding) but values remained normal in cows limited to 10 kg of kale per day. Bäckgren and Jönsson (1969) fed rape to lactating cows and failed to produce anaemia but did find that the bone marrow was affected and that the myeloid/erythroid ratio fell from 1·08:1 to 0·49:1, indicating increased erythropoiesis. Greenhalgh (1969) states that the haematological changes seen in kale poisoning can be simulated by feeding hay, concentrates and 40 mg hydroxylamine hydrochloride per kg body weight, but the exact cause of kale poisoning is unknown. Greenhalgh *et al* (1969) fed different types of kale to steers and found that anaemia could be readily induced after 3 weeks on either thousandhead or marrowstem kale, and that frosted kale had the same effect. He substantiated Penny's earlier ideas that old erythrocytes are more susceptible to lysis than young cells. In animals made anaemic, taken off kale and then returned to the diet, the severe anaemia could not be reproduced a second time.

Both Clegg and Evans (1962) and Penny (1967) have drawn similar conclusions concerning kale poisoning and post parturient haemoglobinuria. In kale anaemia there are obvious signs of rapid red cell regeneration with numerous Heinz bodies. The condition is worse in lactating cows, especially soon after calving, and those with low serum inorganic phosphate levels. Post parturient haemoglobinuria has long been recognized (Cumming 1853). Penny (1956) described 3 cases in which inorganic phosphate levels ranged from 0·45 to 0·58 mmol/l, but the outbreak occurred in severe winter weather in animals being fed on kale. Mullins and Ramsay (1959), in Australia, describe the condition in freshly calved cows in aphosphorosis areas with lameness, haemoglobinuria and anaemia. Red cell counts varied from $1·8 \times 10^{12}/l$ to $3·1 \times 10^{12}/l$ in cows showing haemoglobinuria but were higher in cows showing lameness only. Inorganic phosphate levels varied from less than 0·32 mmol/l to 0·58 mmol/l.

Martinovich and Woodhouse (1971) found cases in 2- to 3-year-old lactating animals and observed marked signs of red cell regeneration, together with Heinz bodies. This case seems to have been precipitated by a change of pasture, and the authors remark on the similarity of this condition to kale poisoning and postulate that low G-6-PD levels would allow a Heinz body anaemia to develop more rapidly.

Seffner (1972) found that 7 out of 10 cows with post parturient haemoglobinuria had some degree of osteomalacic change.

Other plants may produce a haemolytic anaemia in the ox. El-Latif and Awad (1964) describe severe haemoglobinuria, together with anaemia and jaundice, in 4- to 7-month-old pregnant buffaloes fed on barseem (*Tripholium alexandrinum*). Total red cell counts ranged from $2·25 \times 10^{12}/l$ to $3·85 \times 10^{12}/l$ and Hb was 8·0 g/dl or below in 9 out of 10 cases. The serum inorganic phosphate levels ranged from 0·16 mmol/l to 0·64 mmol/l and the authors drew a comparison with post parturient haemoglobinuria. Malik and Gautam (1971) describe an almost identical clinical and haematological situation in 60 buffaloes and considered low phosphate levels to be a precipitating cause.

Tanner grass (*Brachiaria* spp.) is described by Rosenfeld *et al* (1971) and Andrade *et al* (1971, I–III) as the cause of haemoglobinuria and anaemia in cattle. Affected animals showed red blood cell counts as low as $1.9 \times 10^{12}/l$, considerable amounts of methaemoglobin in the plasma (up to 40 per cent of total Hb) and between 1 per cent and 70 per cent of the red cells showed Heinz bodies. Leucocyte counts varied but were often raised (maximum $69.0 \times 10^9/l$) a finding seen in field cases of kale poisoning and attributed to phagocytosis of disrupted cellular material. The cause in this case is the excess amount of nitrate in tanner grass, resulting in nitrate poisoning. Nitrate poisoning may also occur with cornstalk poisoning and alfalfa silage (Case 1957, Winter 1962).

Onions are not normally fed to cattle but, if they obtain access to onions, a haemolytic anaemia can result. Kroger (1956) describes 4 cases ending fatally and Lazarus and Rajamani (1968) describe 2 cases. In the latter instance, Hb levels were only 2.0 to 2.5 g/dl and PCV was 0.10 to 0.11 l/l. Leucocytes appeared reasonably normal but haemoglobinuria was seen. Schalm (1972) shows clearly in 4 cases that onions induce a Heinz body haemolytic anaemia. Red cell counts fell as low as $1.39 \times 10^{12}/l$ and PCV to 0.11 l/l. In severe cases, MCV was increased to 79–91 fl, reticulocytes rose to 10.0–26.0 per cent, normoblasts were present together with other signs of erythrocyte regeneration and many Heinz bodies. The injurious agent in onions which induces the irreversible oxidation of haemoglobin to form Heinz bodies is n-propyl-disulphide.

INFECTIOUS ANAEMIA

Leptospirosis may be due to a variety of serotypes, but *Leptospira pomona* is the commonest in cattle and, in acute cases, may induce anaemia, haemoglobinuria and jaundice, in conjunction with pyrexia. Andreani and Scarano (1973) describe 300 cases in cattle with calves worst affected. Haematological tests may be undertaken but are less useful diagnostically than leptospiral isolation and serological tests.

Bacillary haemoglobinuria is caused, in cattle, by *Clostridium haemolyticum* and, if the animals are alive when seen, they will show pyrexia, haemoglobinuria and jaundice. Erythrocyte counts may be as low as $1.0 \times 10^{12}/l$ and leucocyte numbers are often raised but haematology is of limited diagnostic use as death occurs so rapidly. Post mortem findings are of greater diagnostic value.

BLOOD PARASITES

A considerable variety of blood-borne protozoan parasites occur in the ox, but here only those causing obvious illness and haematological change will be considered.

Of the various *Babesia* species *B. bigemina*, *B. bovis*, *B. divergens* and *B. major* are the ones occurring in cattle, the first being large and the others small *Babesia* (Goldman & Rosenberg 1974, Riek 1968). The blood stage of this tick-transmitted organism causes erythrocyte destruction and the clinical symptoms vary depending on the animal's 'immune' status and the virulence of the *Babesia*. In acute cases in susceptible cattle, severe anaemia and haemoglobinuria are seen due to destruction of erythrocytes by the parasite. Tammemagi (1966) found that 4 infected calves had rapid loss of Hb even before parasitaemia became apparent and that the lowest values occurred 4–8 days after the parasitaemia. Mean Hb values before infection were 10·2 g/dl, on the day of parasitaemia values had fallen to 8·1 g/dl and the lowest values averaged only 3·7 g/dl.

Wright (1973), using splenectomized calves, found that marked falls in red cell indices started 5–6 days after infection and reached their lowest values after 10–16 days (e.g. PCV fell from 0·32 l/l to 0·14 l/l). The MCH rose markedly after this fall occurred and reticulocytes appeared. This coincided with increased osmotic fragility of erythrocytes.

Even in cattle preimmunized against *Babesia* after import to Sri Lanka, very large falls in red blood cells and PCV occurred within 3 days (i.e. PCV fell from 0·38 l/l to 0·20 l/l). The lysis was not directly related to the parasitaemia (Ranatunga & Wanduragala 1972).

Anaplasmosis is caused by the tick-transmitted organism *Anaplasma marginale* and a similar protozoan *Paranaplasma candata*. Kreier *et al* (1964) showed that the organism multiplies in the blood and that the parasitized cells are phagocytosed by the spleen and bone marrow. The PCV declines very markedly (from 0·38 l/l to 0·10 l/l in 7 days) and only at the end of this period is the animal ill. At the time of peak anaemia, up to 22 per cent of red blood cells were infected, but 2 days later none could be found. Only after the peak anaemia did the bone marrow show signs of erythroid regeneration and a shift in the myeloid/erythroid ratio. Jones *et al* (1968) showed that age affected the degree and duration of parasitaemia with calves showing only 11 per cent infected cells and a parasitaemia of 9·8 days, while in old cows the figures were 44 per cent and 22 days respectively. PCV showed the same trend with a decline of 49 per cent in the pre-infection level in calves, while in old cows values declined by 71 per cent. PCV of 0·10 l/l or less may be seen and at this level mortality is high. In all survivors erythrocyte regeneration occurred after anaemia. Williams and Jones (1968) concluded that the red cells of newborn calves and immature red cells are more resistant to *Anaplasma* infection. Schroeder and Ristic (1968) confirmed that serum opsonins sensitized erythrocytes to phagocytosis by the reticulo-endothelial system and Morris *et al* (1971) showed that these opsonins appeared in the blood before the parasites and before the onset of anaemia. Maximum titres occurred at the time of the anaemic crisis, indicating a state of autoimmunity. Total leucocyte values vary greatly from normal to over $30·0 \times 10^9/l$ (mostly neutrophils).

D. L. Doxey

Trypanosomiasis is primarily a disease of parts of Africa and South America. In Africa, *Trypanosoma congolense, T. brucei* and *T. vivax* are the most important. Fiennes (1954) showed that trypanosomiasis is really a chronic disease in cattle extending over many weeks although acute episodes can occur. Red cell counts fell very markedly over the first 4–5 weeks of infection and then stabilized at a low level. He showed red blood cell values falling from $6 \cdot 0 \times 10^{12}/l$ to $3 \cdot 5$ and $2 \cdot 8 \times 10^{12}/l$ over a 5-week period. In chronic cases, the fall was slower but no less severe. The MCV rose when anaemia was present and there was evidence of red blood cell haemolysis. Naylor (1971), using Zebu cattle, showed a marked erythroid decline over an 8-week period from the time of infection and it took many weeks before values approached normal levels again (see Table 6.13).

Table 6.13 Blood picture in trypanosomiasis (Naylor, 1971)

	Start of experiment	After 8 weeks	After 16 weeks	After 24 weeks
RBC $10^{12}/l$	9·3	3·5	4·3	6·5
PCV l/l	0·36	0·18	0·20	0·26
HB g/dl	13·0	6·3	7·0	9·6
MCV fl	38·5	55·0	47·0	41·0

Apart from the raised MCV, there was little obvious evidence of red cell regeneration and some depressive factor seems to affect the marrow. Bilirubin levels rose and the author considered this was due to the haemolysis. Leucocyte counts tended to be low with both neutrophils and lymphocytes reduced.

Roberts and Gray (1973), using various trypanosome infections, found that in single infections erythrocyte declines were moderate (RBC 8·0 to $5 \cdot 5 \times 10^{12}/l$ and PCV 0·36 to 0·27 l/l over an 8-week period) but, when repeated infections took place, deaths occurred and haematological values fell markedly over a 20-week period (RBC from 7·5 to $3 \cdot 0 \times 10^{12}/l$ and PCV from 0·39 to 0·16 l/l). These effects were worse in Zebu than in N'dana cattle.

The organism *Theileria parva*, the cause of East Coast fever in cattle, does not cause haemolytic anaemia. It affects the lymphoid and reticulo-endothelial systems and the toxic effects of the schizonts cause maturation arrest in the bone marrow, resulting in leucopenia. Total white blood cells may fall to below $1 \cdot 0 \times 10^9/l$ and both lymphocytes and granulocytes are affected (Barnett 1968). A high proportion of red blood cells are parasitized but red cell destruction is not a feature of the disease, although anaemia can occur during clinical recovery. Wilde (1966) records mean erythrocyte counts of $6 \cdot 86 \times 10^{12}/l$ prior to death, and mean leucocyte counts of $1 \cdot 55 \times 10^9/l$ at the same time. The lowest blood values were erythrocytes $3 \cdot 75 \times 10^{12}/l$ and leucocytes $0 \cdot 30 \times 10^9/l$. Bone marrow changes indicated that maturation of the granulocytic series was arrested but that red cell precursors were less affected.

ISO-IMMUNE HAEMOLYTIC ANAEMIA

Natural iso-immunization does not seem to occur in calves although cases of haemolytic disease in newborn calves have been recorded after vaccination of the dam against blood parasites. Dennis *et al* (1970) reported anaemia and jaundice in newborn calves born to cows which had been vaccinated against anaplasmosis. The dams' serum contained antibodies which produced lysis of the erythrocytes of the sire and the calf. The erythrocytes of the calf were Coombs positive. In affected animals, there was a mortality rate of up to 24 per cent, the PCV fell precipitously to $0 \cdot 06$ or $0 \cdot 07$ l/l after they had ingested colostrum and there was evidence of massive erythrocyte regeneration by the bone marrow. Langford *et al* (1971) recorded similar findings in calves from a herd vaccinated against babesiosis and reported that repeated vaccination increased the risk of iso-immunization. Bovine autoimmune haemolytic anaemia is not recorded in the literature although a probable case has occurred in an adult Ayrshire cow (McPherson 1975). This animal showed petechial haemorrhages when first seen and extreme anaemia. Blood samples taken over a period of several days prior to treatment showed erythrocyte counts of between $1 \cdot 9$ and $1 \cdot 4 \times 10^{12}/l$ and platelet counts consistently less than $5 \cdot 0 \times 10^9/l$. There was evidence of massive red cell regeneration. All other tests were negative including a direct Coombs test, but the animal was treated with massive doses of cortisone on the assumption that this was a case of autoimmune thrombocytopenia. Within 4 days of treatment starting, platelet counts had risen to $160 \cdot 0 \times 10^9/l$. Five days after this they were $376 \cdot 0 \times 10^9/l$ and the red blood cells were $2 \cdot 95 \times 10^{12}/l$. The animal made an uneventful recovery.

6.3.3.3 Haemorrhagic anaemia

There are several causes of haemorrhagic anaemia in cattle. Some have already been covered (e.g. bracken poisoning) and the others are due to causes unrelated to haematological factors (e.g. trauma and surgical interference). Tumours which have become eroded may bleed as may abomasal or ruminal ulcers. Heavy louse or tick infestations may result in considerable blood loss although, in the latter, the anaemia is not always clinically obvious. In all these cases, signs of red cell regeneration are seen, the degree of anaemia is very variable and responds to treatment of the primary cause.

6.4 COAGULATION DEFECTS

The majority of coagulation failures in the ox have already been mentioned and generally result from platelet deficiency (e.g. bracken poisoning, myco-toxicosis and furazolidone poisoning) but there are at least 2 conditions recorded in the ox in which interference with the actual clotting mechanism occurs.

6.4.1 DICOUMAROL POISONING (SPOILED SWEET CLOVER POISONING)

This is widely recorded and results from coumarin in this fodder crop being converted to dicoumarin when the clover is spoiled by weather and becomes mouldy. Fresh clover is harmless. Dicoumarin causes reductions in factors VII, IX, X and in prothrombin, so adversely affecting coagulation. Wignall *et al* (1961) recorded cases where considerable haemorrhage followed the feeding of hay which subsequently proved to affect rabbits when fed to them. In experiments on cattle using affected hay, the prothrombin activity was greatly reduced (i.e. prothrombin time greatly extended). This test can be rendered normal, and haemorrhage stopped, by therapy with vitamin K_1. Meads *et al* (1964) recorded a very similar picture when mouldy hay was fed to heifers.

White (1970) says that the appearance of the hay is no guide to its toxicity. The macrocytic anaemia, which can be very severe, with red blood cells down to $1 \cdot 0$ to $2 \cdot 0 \times 10^{12}/l$ and in which marked red cell regeneration is seen, is always accompanied by a deficiency of factor VII which can be detected using Quick's one-stage prothrombin time test. In affected cases the prothrombin time will always exceed 25 seconds, in many cases it will be over 40 seconds and often is several minutes long.

Wiesner *et al* (1968) indicated that dicoumarol poisoning can be confused with mycotoxicosis unless haematological tests are undertaken.

6.4.2 THROMBOPLASTIN ANTECEDENT (FACTOR XI) DEFICIENCIES

These are rare in most species and in the bovine almost unheard of. Kociba *et al* (1969) do, however, record factor XI deficiency in a Holstein cow which died of leucosis. The deficiency may have been familial as a half-sister was also affected. The clotting time was 45 minutes (normal 4–15 minutes) and the partial thromboplastin time 432 seconds (normal 60–70 seconds). Factor XI activity in cattle is about 90 per cent of the normal human level but in the deficient animal was only 6 per cent.

Gentry *et al* (1975) also recorded the condition in a Holstein steer. The clotting time in this case was 55 minutes. Prothrombin time was 22 seconds, partial thromboplastin time 308 seconds and factor XI activity only 1 per cent.

6.5 THE LEUCOCYTES IN DISEASE

6.5.1 GENERAL RESPONSES

The normal leucocyte values and physiological variations seen in the ox have been recorded earlier. It is clearly seen that the ox and, in fact, domesticated ruminants in general, all have a greater number of lymphocytes than neutrophils in the circulation, in contrast with the picture in dogs, cats and horses. Valli *et al* (1969, 1971) did comparative work on the ability of calves and dogs to produce granulocytes as a response to granulocyte removal and found that, although the granulocyte reserve in the bone marrow was the same in both species (2×10^9 granulocytes/kg body weight), the calf was not capable of responding to granulocyte leucopenia by neutrophilia as was the dog. In both the dog and the calf Valli *et al* (1969) found that leucopenia of short duration followed granulocyte removal but that this was rapidly overcome as the animal called on its marrow reserves. Before granulocyte depletion, the calf's circulating white blood cell level was 5·5 to $7·2 \times 10^9$/l and 24 hours later 6·3 to $13·0 \times 10^9$/l, whereas the figures for the dog were 13·0 to $17·0 \times 10^9$/l before and 21·0 to $41·0 \times 10^9$/l afterwards. In addition, the calf took 6 days to replenish its depleted marrow reserves (neutrophil production time $5·77 \pm 1·43$ days) while the dog took only 2–3 days.

This species difference is attributed to the relatively larger pool of precursor cells in the marrow of dogs and to the shorter neutrophil regeneration time in that species. Just because the calf fails to produce a neutrophilia does not, however, mean that it fails to make new cells, for it is known that large numbers of granulocytes can move from the marrow to the tissues without a marked circulatory granulocytosis occurring (Craddock *et al* 1963).

This inability of the bovine to respond to inflammation by the rapid production of neutrophilia is a disadvantage from the diagnostic point of view because the total white blood cell and the neutrophil numbers are not clear indicators of either the severity, acuteness or duration of the pathological lesions inducing the blood response. Only by serial sampling can such information be gained.

6.5.1.1 Neutrophil response

In the bovine, situations which result in local tissue neutrophilia are not usually accompanied by a circulatory neutrophilia. In fact, the demand for neutrophils is followed by a circulatory neutropenia. In the days which follow, the total cell numbers will fall again if the body defences are overwhelmed or, as happens in all cases where the animal is fighting the lesion, the total numbers will remain static or slowly rise. At the same time, the neutrophil percentage will increase, and eventually a position is reached when the total counts are normal or raised and the neutrophil percentage is greater than 50 per cent. Thus, in the ox, a normal total white blood cell count does not preclude the possibility of bacterial infection being present and it is almost impossible from one blood sample to distinguish between an early bacterial lesion and a virus-induced neutropenia.

6.5.1.2 Lymphocyte response

The lymphocyte population of the body is engaged mainly in humoral antibody formation and cellular immunity. It is also probable that sensitized lymphocytes can produce toxic factors (e.g. lymphotoxin) which are capable of destroying target cells. The ox can withstand considerable inflammatory lesions, often bacterial in nature, quite satisfactorily without any marked circulatory neutrophilia and it may be that the lymphocytes in this species are more actively engaged in body defence than was previously recognized. Valli *et al* (1971) recorded that calves made anaemic by bleeding and calves treated intravenously with *Salmonella* endotoxin responses with both neutrophilia and lymphocytosis.

Monocytes and eosinophils of the ox do not apparently have differing functions from the comparable cells of other mammals.

6.5.1.3 Fibrinogen response

Because the leucocyte response in cattle is not specific, the use of fibrinogen estimations is a valuable diagnostic aid. The normal level is 2·0–7·0 g/l and in inflammation, trauma and neoplasia the values increase. Age does not affect the normal fibrinogen level (Schalm 1972). The total plasma protein is determined, the amount of fibrinogen is calculated and the difference between these 2 results is the combined albumin and globulin content. The ratio between albumin plus globulin and fibrinogen changes in inflammation. Normally this ratio is 15:1 or more, but in inflammation the ratio falls to 10:1 or less. In normal calves, Schalm (1972) reported ratios of 12–30:1 (average 15·3:1) while in cows the figures were 10–37:1 (average 18:1). These increased levels of fibrinogen fall rapidly once the inflammatory lesion has been overcome (Ek 1972).

Sutton and Hobman (1975) examined several hundred cattle and found that it was often possible to get normal leucocyte counts and raised fibrinogen levels (9 per cent of cases) or raised leucocyte counts and normal fibrinogen

(26 per cent of cases). In addition, plasma protein levels may be low, especially in calves, or dehydration may mask changes in fibrinogen levels. In consequence, they considered that albumin plus globulin:fibrinogen ratios should be 8:1 before they are considered to be abnormal and that values of 8:1 to 10:1 should be interpreted with caution, especially when the fibrinogen level is only about 8·0 g/l.

6.5.2 LEUCOCYTE RESPONSE TO DISEASE IN THE OX

Several conditions in which leucocyte numbers change have already been mentioned (i.e. bracken poisoning and mycotoxicosis) and these will not be covered again.

6.5.2.1 Leucocyte response to corticosteroids

It should be made quite clear that haematological changes simulating those seen in inflammation can be induced by corticosteroids and the blood pictures of animals treated with these drugs are difficult to interpret. Jain and Schalm (1966) showed increased leucocyte counts as a result of ACTH injections in dogs, and cattle respond in the same way. Schalm (1972) showed that when 9-alpha-fluoroprednisolone acetate was injected into cows WBC rose. With 50 mg, WBC rose from $6·2 \times 10^9$/l to $13·35 \times 10^9$/l after 18 hours, with 100 mg they rose from $14·2 \times 10^9$/l to $22·8 \times 10^9$/l after 12 hours and with 500 mg from $8·4 \times 10^9$/l to $14·6 \times 10^9$/l after 48 hours. In all cases, the raised WBC were due almost entirely to raised neutrophil counts. Monocytes also rose but lymphocytes and eosinophils were consistently depressed. Paape *et al* (1974) injected cows with 250 I.U. adrenocorticotropin and found that WBC rose in normal cows from $6·325 \times 10^9$/l to a maximum of $10·128 \times 10^9$/l after 6 hours and in cows with mastitis from $7·885 \times 10^9$/l to $13·231 \times 10^9$/l after 10 hours. In both cases, neutrophils made up the increase and lymphocytes and monocytes remained static.

The degree of neutrophilia induced by corticosteroids and the duration of the response will depend on the drug used, dosage and frequency of administration.

6.5.2.2 Acute inflammation

The typical pattern is leucopenia followed by an increase in neutrophil production, often with a shift to the left, then counts in the normal range, then increasing numbers of mature neutrophils and, finally, normal or raised

D. L. Doxey

total counts with a high percentage of neutrophils. An example is described by Theilen *et al* (1959) for mastitis due to *Escherichia coli* which responded slowly to treatment (Table 6.14).

In very severe cases the early leucopenia may be even more obvious. In some cases leucocyte counts may go much higher (e.g. 15·0 to 20·0 × 10⁹/l) and increased red cell counts may occur as a result of dehydration in some cases.

Table 6.14 Leucocyte response to acute inflammation (Theilen *et al* 1959)

Days from onset	WBC 10⁹/l	Non-lobulated neutrophils %	Segmented neutrophils %	Lymphocytes %	Monocytes %	Eosinophils %
1	2·950	7·0	2·0	75·0	7·0	8·0
2	3·950	12·5	4·0	73·5	8·0	2·0
6	4·450	12·0	39·0	46·0	1·0	2·0
13	9·500	0·5	51·5	34·5	13·5	0
21	8·350	1·5	50·5	23·0	13·0	11·0

Table 6.15 Leucocyte response in overwhelming infections (Theilen *et al* 1959)

Days from onset	WBC 10⁹/l	Non-lobulated neutrophils %	Neutrophils %	Lymphocytes %	Monocytes %	Eosinophils %
1	1·800	1·0	2·0	83·0	12·0	2·0
2	1·350	0	1·0	85·0	6·0	8·0
3	2·850	0	1·0	82·0	8·0	9·0
4	3·250	39·0	0	51·0	7·0	3·0
5	6·300	7·0	0	84·0	9·0	0
7	7·800	35·0	7·0	51·0	7·0	0

In instances where the infection is overwhelming, the recovery pattern does not take place or there is gross overproduction of non-lobulated neutrophils (degenerative shift to the left). Theilen *et al* describes such a case, again with mastitis (Table 6.15). This animal died. Note the early failure of neutrophils to appear and then later the overproduction of immature forms with no mature forms—always a bad sign. Eosinophils usually decline more rapidly in such cases than in this illustration.

The types of response illustrated may occur in any acute inflammatory condition and the inadvisability of relying on one blood sample, rather than a series, for diagnostic purposes is shown by the gross variations noted by Brown *et al* (1959) in cases of reticuloperitonitis. They noted total leucocyte counts ranging from 4·10 to 35·25 × 10⁹/l in the same type of clinical case. The results obtained depend in fact on the severity and duration of the clinical condition.

In acute conditions, Schalm (1972) noted fibrinogen levels as described in Table 6.16. The albumin plus globulin:fibrinogen ratio is not always reflected by the total leucocyte count.

Schalm *et al* (1967) described the effects of acute indigestion in cattle. In 8 cattle, WBC averaged 17·318 × 10⁹/l with 18 per cent of the cells being immature neutrophils, 48 per cent mature neutrophils, 30 per cent

Table 6.16   Changes in fibrinogen during inflammation (Schalm 1972)

Diagnosis	WBC $10^9/l$	Albumin + globulin g/l	Fibrinogen g/l	A + G : F ratio g/l
Acute mastitis	12·10	57·0	11·0	5·2:1
Peritonitis	16·90	106·0	20·0	5·3:1
Fibrinous pneumonia	4·10	75·0	15·0	5·0:1

lymphocytes and almost all of the remainder monocytes. This reaction occurred much more rapidly than the picture seen in acute inflammatory responses and the neutrophilia seen persisted because the cells were not so rapidly removed from the circulation as they were when an inflammatory reaction was present. Results in this type of case vary with severity and duration of the condition.

6.5.2.3   Chronic inflammation

Usually the haematological response involves mature neutrophils with increasing monocyte counts as tissue debris builds up but even in severe infections the total counts may remain within the normal range.

In Johne's disease, Allen *et al* (1967) recorded the following differential percentages in advanced clinical cases—neutrophils 53·4, lymphocytes 40·7, monocytes 4·9 and eosinophils 1·2. Variations will occur depending on type and duration of the disease. In chronic traumatic reticulitis, Brown *et al* (1959) recorded average total leucocytes of 11·5 × 10⁹/l with neutrophils and lymphocytes occupying 50 per cent each of the total, while Van Pelt (1970) found that in calves with septic arthritis the WBC ranged from 5·5 to 20·6 × 10⁹/l (mean 11·5 × 10⁹/l) and the neutrophil component ranged from 15 to 67 per cent. Monocyte numbers were often increased reaching a maximum of 19 per cent. In many chronic infections the percentage of mature neutrophils and of monocytes will be very high but no clear haematological pattern can be laid down for chronic infections. In the majority of cases there is a normal or high WBC and the normal lymphocyte:neutrophil ratio is partially or wholly reversed. Remember that acute phases may occur in chronic disease thus altering the haematological pattern.

Fibrinogen levels are often increased and Schalm (1972) records albumin plus globulin:fibrinogen ratios of 7:1 in endocarditis and 5·5:1 in pyelonephritis.

6.5.2.4   Viral infections

The haematological pattern varies but most virus infections induce leucopenia usually as a result of neutropenia. Welch and Dellars (1973) recorded WBC of $2·5–4·2 \times 10^9/l$ in adenoviral infections in dairy cows. This change may be transient and occur very early in the disease (e.g. viral pneumonia) and be superseded by a bacterially induced neutrophil response. In some cases (e.g. acute mucosal disease) the leucopenia may be more pronounced and of longer duration, although here, too, leucopenia is often followed by a neutrophil response. Only in the more obvious cases is the blood picture useful diagnostically and considerable confusion can occur when trying to distinguish the leucopenia induced by viruses from the leucopenia of acute bacterial infection.

6.5.2.5   Other leucocyte responses

Lymphocyte changes will be discussed under the section on leucosis (6.5.3.1). Eosinophils increase, as in other species, in parasitic or allergic responses but the changes in blood are invariably transient and not always a reliable guide. Only if high eosinophil counts persist can clinical suspicions be confirmed.

The Pelger–Huët anomaly (apparent immaturity of the nucleus of granulocytes) is recorded by Osburn and Glenn (1968) but only for short periods during early neutrophilia as a response to acute infection. These authors recorded 3–52 per cent of such forms in 3 cows but the existence of true Pelger–Huët leucocytes in cattle has not yet been confirmed.

The Chediak–Higashi syndrome is a rare inherited abnormality in which all granulocytes contain abnormally large and numerous granules. Padgett *et al* (1964) and Padgett (1968) described the condition in cattle with granules of up to 5 μ in diameter and up to 100 per cent of cells such as eosinophils affected. Other clinical abnormalities such as albinoism and hepatomegaly also occur in this condition.

6.5.3 NEOPLASIA OF LEUCOCYTES

6.5.3.1 Leucosis

This is the most important type of haemopoietic neoplasia and the one most widely studied in cattle. It involves the lymphocyte exclusively and the condition is also known as lymphosarcoma. Morphologically, there are 2 basic types of lymphocyte, the large and the small but they are also capable of morphological transformation. Some lymphocytes can develop into other cell types (e.g. plasma cells) and this confuses the issue in a neoplastic disease in which morphological change is an integral part. Functionally, there are different types derived from bone marrow (B cells) or thymus (T cells) with different life spans and different functions but the cells act together to produce cellular or humoral immune responses (Craddock *et al* 1971).

Bovine leucosis is a complex disease in the same way as the lymphocyte is a complicated cell—both have different forms and different origins. Leucosis (lymphosarcoma) has 3 distinct forms namely sporadic leucosis, cutaneous leucosis and enzootic leucosis (Markson 1975).

Sporadic leucosis occurs as single isolated cases, affects young cattle (even newborn calves) and there is multicentric symmetrical enlargement of the lymph nodes with infiltration of internal organs. A thymic form is also seen which is sometimes classified separately. Sporadic leucosis is the form most commonly seen in the United Kingdom (the incidence is about 300 cases per annum) but it also occurs in many other parts of the world. It is relatively easy to diagnose clinically owing to the marked enlargement of the thymus gland or palpable lymph nodes.

Cutaneous leucosis is an unusual form but has been seen in most of the countries in which leucosis occurs. Cases usually involve cattle in the $1\frac{1}{2}$- to 3-year age group and it appears as multiple small swellings on the skin, which develop into large lumps and may become encrusted. The skin generally is thickened and the infiltration lymphoreticular in nature. Infiltration of internal organs occurs late in the course of the disease.

Enzootic leucosis is not seen in the United Kingdom but occurs in many Western European countries, the USA and other parts of the world. It differs markedly from the first 2 types because it affects adult cattle and it can occur as multiple cases within a herd. There is strong evidence to show that this form is transmissible. Although clinically affected animals show generalized lymph node enlargement and can, therefore, be detected easily, there are always a few animals in the herd who have the disease, can spread it to others and yet are themselves clinically normal. This form of the disease is a serious problem in several countries, although it is now being brought under control by slaughter policies. For example, in Denmark, an incidence in 1960 of 6 cases per 100,000 cattle was reduced by 1963 to 2·9 cases per

100,000 cattle (Penny 1967). In Belgium in 1971 20 herds were leucotic and 67 suspect out of the 283 herds examined for the disease and Haremski *et al* (1973) reported 25 out of 1000 tuberculosis-free cattle had leucosis in some areas of Poland.

AETIOLOGY

Sporadic leucosis and cutaneous leucosis do not appear to have the same aetiology as enzootic leucosis. The first 2 forms are not apparently transmissible and Hugoson (1967) could find no relationship between sporadic leucosis, herd lymphocytosis or family relationships. No known causal agent has been isolated in either sporadic or cutaneous leucosis and their aetiology is at present unknown.

The aetiological factors of enzootic leucosis are rather better understood and fall into 2 types (i.e. genetic and viral). Genetic factors have been implicated for some time because familial groups appear to be predisposed to a high frequency of the disease. Cypress *et al* (1974) described the family history in a closed Jersey herd where the leucosis death rate was 7·9 per cent but could not prove conclusively that there was a genetic component involved, although the evidence pointed strongly in that direction. Earlier authors have described the presence of the disease in certain families (Wittman 1968, Ritter 1965) and Kostromitinov *et al* (1972) are reported by Abramova *et al* (1974) as saying that inheritance is determined by a recessive gene. Nakhmanson (1973) reported on investigations with 32 bulls and 2,723 daughters showing that leucosis occurred in 10·5 per cent of animals and that this evidence supports the theory of inheritance of susceptibility.

Only in recent years has the viral theory gained strong support and reports of viral isolation have been numerous. Miller *et al* (1969) isolated virus from 5 out of 9 cattle affected and identified the particles as C-type virus. Virus was also isolated from the control animals. Lee *et al* (1970) isolated C-type virus and Kukaine *et al* (1973) obtained C-type oncornovirus from both spontaneous and experimentally induced leucosis. Similar results have been obtained by many other workers including Valikhov *et al* (1974). Olson *et al* (1973) tested 1000 cows in 11 herds for precipitins against bovine C-type virus and found 222 reactors; 10 per cent of cows in non-affected herds reacted and 33 per cent in leucosis-affected herds. Virus was isolated from 100 of 117 reactors. Ferrer and Bhatt (1973) obtained similar results indicating that bovine leucosis virus was widespread but that only certain herds were susceptible.

Transmission studies by Theilen *et al* (1967) indicated that the condition could be spread from the cow to the calf through milk and Olson *et al* (1972) transmitted the condition from cattle to sheep by inoculation of C-type virus. The demonstration of fluorescent antibodies against viral antigen gave positive results in 90 per cent of leukaemic cows and 80 to 100 per cent

of cows with lymphocytosis (Ferrer *et al* 1974). There appears to be a connection between virus leucosis and the lymphocytosis seen in normal cattle
in leucosis herds (Bendixen 1965). IgG immunofluorescent techniques have
indicated that when lymphocyte numbers increase they are probably B lymphocytes and many have surface immunoglobulins (18 per cent in normal
cows and 67 per cent in leucotic cows) (Weiland & Straub 1975). Straub *et al*
(1974) found vertical transmission to be the most important method by which
leucosis was spread.

As enzootic leucosis is almost certainly transmitted from mother to
offspring and because it has such a long latent period, it is of great importance
to make a diagnosis as early as possible when trying to eradicate the disease.

DIAGNOSIS OF LEUCOSIS

Sporadic leucosis by its very nature is not looked for and only when the lymph
node enlargement occurs or the animal becomes ill in the final states of the
disease does the owner seek advice. In about half of all cases no true leukaemia or lymphocytosis is observed, the blood picture showing varying
degrees of anaemia and either a normal leucocyte pattern or one indicating
a neutrophil response to cell necrosis.

In the other half of cases, the leucocyte response is either suspicious or,
occasionally, diagnostic. Most cases have normal total counts and a lymphocyte percentage of 70 to 90 per cent. Careful screening of the blood film may
reveal evidence of immature or bizarre lymphocytes in varying numbers.
This type of picture may occasionally change terminally to one of neutrophilia but in most cases lymphocytes predominate. A typical example was
seen by the author in a Friesian bullock which died the day after the blood
sample was taken. Large atypical lymphocytes were observed in the blood
smear, the PCV was 0·14 l/l, WBC 14·4 × 10⁹/l and the differential count
showed neutrophils 4·5 per cent, lymphocytes 87·5 per cent and monocytes 8·0 per cent. In the few cases which are leukaemic, and this may be in
very young calves, WBC range from 20 to 300 × 10⁹/l, lymphocytes occupy
90 per cent or more of the total cells and a high proportion show bizarre
forms, nucleoli and other evidence of immaturity.

Cutaneous leucosis is very obvious clinically but no significant haematological
changes occur early in the disease. As cellular infiltration of internal organs
occurs, so some neoplastic blood changes may be seen. An illustration of
this late haematological change is a case of an animal where, 7 days
before death, RBC was 5·8 × 10¹²/l, PCV 0·31 l/l and WBC 10·5 × 10⁹/l
(neutrophils 8 per cent, lymphocytes 92 per cent). Three days before death
the RBC had fallen to 3·3 × 10¹²/l and the WBC to 7·5 × 10⁹/l (neutrophils 12 per cent, lymphocytes 88 per cent). On both occasions many
of the lymphocytes were atypical and immature. The erythrocyte fall was

Table 6.17 Haematological keys used to diagnose suspect or positive cases of enzootic leucosis

Author	Age (in years)	Lymphocytes ($10^9/l$)		
		Normal	Suspect	Positive
Bendixen (1960)	0–1	< 10·0	10·0–12·0	> 12·0
	1–2	< 9·0	9·0–11·0	> 11·0
	2–3	< 7·5	7·5– 9·5	> 9·5
	3–4	< 6·5	6·5– 8·5	> 8·5
	> 4	< 5·0	5·0– 7·0	> 7·0
Clague & Granzien (1966)	< 2	< 11·0	11·0–14·0	> 14·0
	> 2	> 9·0	9·0–12·0	> 12·0
		< 4·5	4·5–10·0	> 10·0 { % abnormal lymphocytes
Gotze *et al* (1954)	< 3	< 7·8 (WBC < 12·0)	7·8–13·5 (WBC 12·0–18·0)	> 13·5 (WBC 18·0+)
	> 3	< 6·0 (WBC < 10·0)	6·0–13·5 (WBC 10·0–18·0)	> 13·5 (WBC 18·0+)
Mammerickx (1971a b)	0–1	12·5	12·5–15·5	> 15·5
	1–2	11·5	11·5–14·5	> 14·5
	2–3	9·5	9·5–12·0	> 12·0
	3–6	8·5	8·5–11·0	> 11·0
	> 6	7·5	7·5– 9·5	> 9·5
Perman *et al* (1970)	0–2	< 7·7	7·7– 9·4	> 9·5
	2–3	< 6·6	6·6– 7·7	> 7·8
	3–4	< 6·3	6·3– 7·4	> 7·5
	4–5	< 5·9	5·9– 7·0	> 7·1
	6	< 5·7	5·7– 6·7	> 6·8
	7	< 5·4	5·4– 6·4	> 6·5
	8	< 5·1	5·1– 6·1	> 6·2
	9	< 4·9	4·9– 5·8	> 5·9
	> 10	< 4·7	4·7– 5·5	> 5·6
Tolle (1965)	0–1	< 10·0	10·0–13·0	> 13·0
	1–2	< 9·0	9·1–12·0	> 12·0
	2–3	< 7·5	7·5–10·0	> 10·0
	3–6	< 6·5	6·5– 9·0	> 9·0
	> 6	< 5·5	5·5– 7·5	> 7·5
Theilen *et al* (1964)	1–2	< 11·0		< 11·0
	2–3	< 7·7		> 7·7
	3–4	< 6·9		> 6·9
	4–5	< 6·5		> 6·5
	> 5	< 5·9		> 5·9

Table 6.17 *continued*

Author	Age (in years)	Lymhocytes ($10^9/l$) Normal	Suspect	Positive
Seelemann *et al*	0–1	< 12·0	12·0–13·0	> 13·0
(1963)	1–2	< 10·0	10·0–11·0	> 11·0
	> 2	< 7·5	> 7·5	> 7·5–> 12·0
		(WBC < 10·0)	(WBC < 10·0)	(WBC 10·0–16·0)
		or	or	or
		< 6·0–< 9·6	> 6·0–> 9·6	> 9·6
		(WBC 10·0–16·0)	(WBC 10·0–16·0)	(WBC > 16·0)
			or	
			< 9·6	
			(WBC > 16·0)	

associated with internal haemorrhage. In this animal antibodies against bovine leucosis C-type virus were not detected.

The early diagnosis of *enzootic leucosis* has created a problem for years which is not yet resolved. The number of lymphocytes is normally higher in young animals than in mature adults and this makes haematological diagnosis difficult because it is based on the demonstration of lymphocytosis in affected but clinically normal animals. In Europe, haematological 'keys' were worked out and used as a guide to the detection of suspect cattle. Since then, other keys have been devised in other parts of the world and the various results are given in Table 6.17.

There is some variation in these keys. This is because they were compiled in different countries, with different managemental environments and varying breeds of cattle. Rudolph *et al* (1972) used the Bendixen, Tolle and Theilen keys in Chile and considered Tolle's to be best suited to their conditions. Montemagno *et al* (1972) compared the Bendixen, Gotze and a cytological key and considered Bendixen's the most successful, but Marshak and Abt (1967) found that the Bendixen key did not work satisfactorily in the USA. Some keys (e.g. those of Mammerickx and Gotze) give such high lymphocyte values that their diagnostic application must be limited to the areas in which the keys were compiled. The diagnostic success or failure of all haematological keys depends on there being a close similarity in lymphocyte distribution between the area in which the key was compiled and the area in which it is used for diagnostic purposes.

A further drawback to the successful use of these keys is that there is no way of knowing with certainty that the key is picking out all leucosis cases. Bendixen considers that 90 per cent or more of tumour cases have lymphocytosis some time prior to the onset of clinical signs. Clague and Granzien

(1966) recorded between 4 per cent and 9 per cent of positive cases and between 9 per cent and 25 per cent suspect cases in 3 leucosis herds, and Perman *et al* (1970) recorded 1·7 per cent positive and 2·4 per cent suspect in a normal herd compared to 17·2 per cent positive and 8·6 per cent suspect in a leucosis herd. The keys used picked out some cases and, in all probability, the lymphocytosis was a prelude to true leucosis but none of the authors could claim to have isolated all cases. Albrecht *et al* (1974) found that in a control programme in Saxony 28 per cent of the lymphocytosis cases later became normal, but that only 13 per cent of animals showed a trend in the opposite direction. This has led to a build-up of affected, but aleukaemic, cases which can perpetuate the disease. This view is supported by Simonyan (1974) who found 9 out of 34 proven leucosis cases with total leucocyte counts of less than $10·0 \times 10^9/l$, and by Singh (1970) who reported that 7 out of 36 buffaloes, with lymphocyte counts of less than $8·0 \times 10^9/l$, had lymphosarcoma.

Another diagnostic difficulty is that there is no clear way of knowing whether the lymphocytosis is due entirely to leucosis. Some of the factors previously thought to cause lymphocytosis, such as seasonal variations and mastitis, have been discounted (Chander & Gilman 1974a, Sorvettula & Andersson 1968) but the evidence to show that trypanosomiasis causes lymphocytosis is uncertain with Guillemain *et al* (1975) claiming that lymphocytosis does occur and Chander and Gilman (1975) being unable to establish a connection between lymphocytosis and trypanosomiasis. Rudolph *et al* (1972) considered that brucellosis is capable of stimulating a lymphocytosis and Bernstad *et al* (1971) reported lymphocytosis in up to 5 per cent of normal cattle.

It seems clear that the haematological keys do have a use in picking out probable enzootic leucosis cases but there are considerable disadvantages associated with the procedure and some better diagnostic method is required.

Many attempts have been made to find a diagnostic technique which will detect all cases of leucosis. Chander and Gilman (1974b) and Chander (1972) found that, by using autoradiography following incubation with tritiated thiamidine, they could pick up S phase lymphocytes and DNA synthesizing cells. Correlation of haematological results and autoradiographic results gave better overall diagnostic results, but this technique is not really a practical proposition on a wide scale and the interpretation is still open to doubt.

Several authors, including Weber *et al* (1969) have described the presence of nuclear pockets (evaginations from the nucleus that partially surround portions of cytoplasm). These are detectable on the electron microscope and a correlation was observed between leucosis and the incidence of these pockets. In normal animals, the mean frequency was 4·1 per cent, while in lymphocytosis and leucosis cases the incidence was 38–40 per cent. Weber *et al* (1974) found a similar correlation but it is not yet clear if the technique is better than, or correlates with, the haematological results.

Lima and Mitscherlich (1973) showed by the EAC-rosette technique that T lymphocytes outnumbered B lymphocytes in normal cattle (B lymphocytes maximum 18 per cent) and that in leucosis and lymphocytosis cases both B and T lymphocytes increase.

Rademacher *et al* (1974) used bone marrow as a diagnostic material and found that the lymphocyte counts were increased above normal in pre-clinical and clinical leucosis cases (normal 2 per cent, affected 5 to 25 per cent) but bone marrow biopsy is not an ideal technique for widescale use.

Considerable work has been done on the detection of antibodies to C-type virus by various workers and immunofluorescence studies have also been undertaken. Egorova (1974), Ivanov (1973) and Ryagin and Aptekar (1973) found the immunofluorescence technique useful in positive cases but, un-fortunately, the antisera are not widely available.

Immunoglobulin studies suggest that IgM levels are low in many leucosis cases. Trainin *et al* (1973) found 77 per cent of affected calves deficient in IgM but Frymus (1974) found only 4 out of 14 affected cows to be deficient.

No diagnostic technique has been proven so far to be a specific and reliable means of diagnosing asymptomatic leucosis, although combinations of the techniques already described will help greatly in eradication programmes.

Clinically affected animals show the typical lymph node involvement and blood picture changes do occur late in the disease, in addition to persistent lymphocytosis (10·0 to $20·0 \times 10^9/l$) and lymphocyte abnormalities. Clague and Granzien (1966) recorded rapid terminal transformation in 7 out of 8 cases with blood lymphocyte counts exceeding $50·0 \times 10^9/l$. Bendixen recorded similar lymphocyte figures with values up to $500·0 \times 10^9/l$ terminally. These terminal cases can be positively confirmed histologically (Braço *et al* 1972a b). In fact, all leucosis cases can be confirmed histologically but even the cer-tainty of this technique is not applicable to these early cases which show no symptoms.

6.5.3.2 Monocytic leukaemia

There is only one record of this condition and that is by Miura and Ohshima (1967) in 2 dairy cows. In the first case, loss of weight, cardiac abnormalities and some dyspnoea occurred over a period of 1 month. The initial blood picture showed a WBC of $300·0 \times 10^9/l$, rising 3 days before death to $421·4 \times 10^9/l$. The leucocytes were almost exclusively monocytes (97·8 per cent), most of them immature.

The second case had similar clinical signs over a period of 6–8 weeks. Haematological examination 8 days prior to death revealed a WBC of $200·0 \times 10^9/l$ and an erythrocyte count of $2·03 \times 10^{12}/l$. The percentage of monocytes was never below 98 per cent and most were immature.

6.5.3.3 Myelogenous leukaemia

This is as rare as the monocytic form. Feldman (1932) and Piening (1936) recorded cases designated as myelogenous leukaemia. Hyde *et al* (1958) recorded an instance in a 4-month-old calf, but this animal was dead when seen and a differential count is all that was obtained apart from the post mortem results. The differential showed that 72 per cent of all blood cells were neutrophils and the majority of these were myelocytes or blast forms. There were many normoblasts present as well.

Table 6.18 Blood picture in mast cell leukaemia

	Trautwein & Stober (1965)	*Doxey*
RBC × 10^{12}/l	3·5	0·74
PCV l/l	0·12	0·045
Hb g/dl	3·85	1·6
WBC × 10^9/l	5·2	11·4
Neutrophils (mature) %	52·0	10·5
Neutrophils (immature) %	3·0	3·5
Lymphocytes %	19·0	65·5
Monocytes %	11·0	6·0
Eosinophils %	6·0	0
Basophils %	9·0	14·5

6.5.3.4 Mast cell leukaemia

Mast cell tumours occur in cattle but the presence of basophils in the blood is rare. Groth *et al* (1960) recorded a case in a Hereford cow but no haematology was done apart from the PCV (0·13 l/l). Trautwein and Stobber (1965) recorded the disease in a cow and confirmed their diagnosis at post mortem examination.

I have seen a case in a 2-year-old Ayrshire bullock which was emaciated when first seen and died shortly after the clinical examination. The diagnosis was substantiated at post mortem examination and the invasive nature of the tumour confirmed. The circulating basophils were large, immature and resembled tissue basophils. The blood picture for both cases is shown in Table 6.18.

6.6 BLOOD GROUPS

In the human field the A, B and O red cell blood groups discovered at the turn of the century are still of major importance, especially in the prevention of transfusion incompatibilities. In the ox, blood groups are also important but for wholly different reasons.

It should be made clear that the term 'blood groups' was originally applied to red cells. These cells have a lipid membrane outside which is a layer of protein and carbohydrate and the structure of these proteins and carbohydrates varies from animal to animal. These differences are known as blood groups (Spooner, 1967). Today the term blood group has the same basic meaning but it is now applied not only to red cells but to different types of Hb, lymphocytes, plasma proteins and enzymes.

Table 6.19 Internationally recognized blood groups in cattle (Spooner, 1977)

Genetics System	Antigens
A	A D H Z'
B	B G I_1 I_2 K O_1 O_2 O_3 O_4 P_1 P_2 Q_1 Q_2 T_1 T_2 Y_1 Y_2 A' B' D' E'_1 E'_2 E'_3 F' G' I' J'_1 J'_2 K' O' P' Q' Y' B" G" I"
C	C_1 C_2 E R_1 R_2 W X_1 X_2 C' L'
F/V	F V
J	J
L	L
M	M M'
S	S_1 U_1 U_2 H' U'_1 U'_2 H" S" U"
Z	Z
R'/S'	R' S'
T'	T'

It is impossible to cover these specialized aspects here, so I will confine my remarks to red cell blood groups which, in cattle, are unlike their human counterparts. Instead of the simple A, B and O system, cattle have 11 blood groups, many of which are subdivided into other groups. Stormont (1958) gave a theoretical estimate of the possible blood types in cattle as 'in excess of a thousand million'. Certainly it is true that, out of 1000 Red Danish cattle, only 4 would by chance be expected to have the same red cell factors (Hall 1963). The well-recognized blood groups in cattle are shown in Table 6.19 (Spooner 1967, Bell 1972).

Blood transfusions are undertaken in cattle, usually from adult to calf and, because of the wide variety of blood types and the lack of strong anti-bodies in most cattle, transfusion incompatibilities are very rare. Van der Walt and Osterhoff (1969a b) obtained only 9 reactions out of 22 transfusions using pregnant cows selected so that their blood types were as varied and dissimilar as possible. They found no correlation between the number of haemolysins produced and transfusion reactions. The only risks in practice are those associated with repeated transfusions in the same animal, and Van der Walt and Osterhoff (*loc. cit.*) found that several transfusions can be given in the 5 days following initial transfusion but thereafter the risks increase, especially in high yielding and pregnant cows (e.g. 13 per cent transfusion reaction in young animals and 41 per cent transfusion reaction in pregnant cows). In these cases the recipient elaborates antibody enabling it to destroy the transfused cells. Generally speaking, blood groups in cattle are not important, certainly not in the human sense, in relation to transfusion

Table 6.20 Example 1 of the use of blood groups to identify parentage

Calf	A [B O_1 Q_2 T_2 E'_3 K']	/A C_2 R_2 W [X_2] F/F	[R']
Dam	A	Y_2/A C_2 W	F/F
Sire 1	A [B O_1 Q_2 T_2 E'_3 K']	R_2 W [X_2] F/F Z [R']	
Sire 2	A B O_1 J' O'	C_2 R_2 W	F/F Z

The blood groups in brackets are those which the calf could not have received from the dam or sire 2, but could have received from sire 1, proving sire 2 could not be the father.

Table 6.21 Example 2 of the use of blood groups to identify parentage

			Tf	Hb
Calf	B G K O_1 Y_2 A' E'_3 G' K' O' Y' C_2	W X_2 F/F [S_1 S''] Z	AD_2	AA
Dam	B G K O_1 Y_2 A' E'_3 G' K' O' Y' C_2 R_2 W X_2 F/F	Z R' T' AA		AA
Sire	G Y_2 D' E'_3 G' O' P'	W F/V	AD_2	BB

In this case the blood groups in brackets show that the sire sampled is not the calf's father, as it could not have transmitted S_1 S'' and should have transmitted Hb B (Spooner 1967).

incompatibilities but there is another aspect, which has an ever increasingly important role to play, in the field of paternity.

It is well known that different breeds of cattle have different blood groups (Hall 1959). For example, J blood groups are present in 70 per cent of Welsh Black cattle but in only 12 per cent of South Devons (Hall 1963). As blood group research spreads to other countries and other breeds of cattle, so the incidence of new blood group alleles increases (Singh *et al* 1970, Khanna *et al* 1970). At the same time, studies on water buffalo (*Bubalus bubalis*; *Bos bubalis*) will yield new information. Granciu *et al* (1973) have found only 13 out of 36 of the cattle blood group factors they were equipped to look for in Rumanian buffalo and it is known that Asian strains of the animal have different values again (e.g. factor O is absent in Rumanian buffalo but present in 88 per cent of Indian Murrah buffalo). In addition, individual animals within breeds will have widely differing combinations of blood groups and this makes it possible to identify any bull or cow which is definitely not one of the calf's parents. All the AI bulls in Britain are typed and consequently their offspring can be identified in a case where the cow has received two services from different bulls. Two examples are given by Spooner (1967) (Tables 6.20 and 6.21).

In a similar way, the techniques are used to aid in the detection of twins, freemartins and the mother of a calf when the sire is known (e.g. when 2 cows calve together and there is doubt as to which calf belongs to which cow).

Blood groups in cattle are used for research purposes in many fields but in practical terms the most important uses are in the establishment of paternity and, in this field, they are used extensively to help the farming community.

6.7 METABOLIC PROFILES

The introduction of the metabolic profile test by Payne *et al* (1970) allowed both haematological and biochemical parameters to be used on a herd basis. It meant that instead of sampling an obviously ill animal in the hope of confirming a clinical diagnosis the approach had been changed and the laboratory studies were to be employed on a preventative basis for clinically healthy animals.

The majority of the parameters which were used were biochemical in nature (e.g. urea, glucose, calcium, magnesium, etc.) but 2 haematological parameters were included—Hb and PCV. In addition, it became obvious that quite often there was a link between 2 dissimilar parameters being used in the profile test and one of these links was between the haematological parameters and the levels of protein. In consequence, I will mention here the changes seen in all 3 parameters during metabolic profile testing.

The variations which occur in profile results for dairy cows are basically related to at least 4 different factors, the season of the year, the herd of origin, the milk yield of the animal(s) involved and their nutritional status. These variations are different from those associated with the markedly fluctuating temperatures from day to night which can reduce both the total erythrocyte and leucocyte counts (Paape *et al* 1973).

The changes are also different from the small diurnal and larger circadian variations which occur naturally in cattle (Abt *et al* 1966). It is important to take notice of such natural phenomena and consequently metabolic profile results must be related to time of year and to the time of day (usually a standard time in the morning).

6.7.1 SEASONAL EFFECTS

These have been shown to be of considerable importance in metabolic profile testing. Hewett (1974) bled several hundred Swedish cows and heifers during autumn and spring and obtained the results shown in Table 6.22.

Hb, PCV and serum protein were higher in spring than in autumn or winter but serum iron was significantly lower. Poulsen (1974), using cattle from 5 Swedish dairy herds, also described seasonal variations although these were small. Hb levels were highest in March and June (11·9 g/dl)

Table 6.22 Metabolic profile—seasonal effects (Hewett 1974)

	Winter	Summer	Autumn
Hb (g/dl)	11·7	13·2	11·9
PCV (l/l)	0·305	0·332	0·319
Albumin (g/l)	31·8	31·1	31·2
Globulin (g/l)	43·6	45·5	45·2
Fe (μmol/l)	30·4	36·1	32·7

and lowest in October/January (11·1 g/dl). PCV showed only minimal alterations at different times of the year but total protein levels followed the Hb and were highest in spring and summer (71·0 g/dl) and lowest in winter (68·0 g/dl). The seasonal differences just described were very small but Payne *et al* (1973), using a very much larger sample (75 herds), also detected similar seasonal variations particularly in protein levels. Hb levels were marginally lower in the winter than in the autumn but both albumin and globulin showed considerable variation from season to season and from one year to the next. For example, in the autumn serum albumin was 40·0 g/l and globulin 37·0 g/l but in the winter the ratio had altered to 32·0 g/l albumin and globulin levels of 44·0 g/l.

Rowlands *et al* (1974) used lactating and non-lacting groups to demonstrate that Hb, PCV, serum globulin and serum Fe were all lower in the autumn and winter than in the summer. Albumin showed the opposite trend. In winter Hb was 11·7 g/dl, PCV 0·305 l/l, albumin 31·8 g/l, globulin 43·6 g/l and serum iron 30·4 μmol/l. The corresponding summer values were Hb 13·2 g/dl, PCV 0·33 l/l, albumin 31·0 g/l, globulin 45·5 g/l and serum Fe 36·1 μmol/l.

Although the absolute values given by various authors differ, they do illustrate a common trend with the values under discussion (except for globulin) all being to some extent lower during the winter months than in the spring and summer when environment and feeding are improved.

6.7.2 INTER-HERD EFFECTS

These can be considerable and are nearly always greater than variations within a single herd. Payne *et al* (1973) showed that inter-herd variation was important for all the parameters under discussion here. Poulsen (1974) and Hewett (1974) found much greater differences for PCV and Hb between herds than within herds. These inter-herd variations are due to differing environment, management, lactation stage and feeding regimen.

6.7.3 LACTATIONAL EFFECTS

These have been well studied. In Sweden, Hewett (1974) investigated the lactational effects in 29 herds. He found that overall variations were irregular but that within any one herd a constant trend would emerge although it

Table 6.23 Metabolic profile—lactation effects (Rowlands *et al* 1974)

	WINTER		SUMMER	
	Lactating	*Non-lactating*	*Lactating*	*Non-lactating*
Hb (g/dl)	10·6	11·7	12·0	13·2
PCV (l/l)	0·272	0·305	0·298	0·332
Albumin (g/l)	32·3	31·8	30·7	31·1
Globulin (g/l)	43·5	43·6	44·8	45·5
Fe (μmol/l)	28·4	30·4	31·1	36·1

may not be the same trend as that for another herd. In a single high yielding herd, Hb, PCV and serum globulin all rose irregularly as lactation proceeded but in the overall picture for the 28 other herds, Hb and PCV both fell irregularly as lactation proceeded, while globulin rose marginally but erratically.

Rowlands *et al* (1974) looked at the effects of lactation in relation to season and also found values declining during lactation, and quite clearly, lactating animals have lower Hb, PCV, serum Fe and globulin than non-lactating animals, irrespective of the season (Table 6.23).

Payne *et al* (1973) found that the reduction in values was related to milk yield (i.e. values for Hb and PCV fell as milk yield increased with dry cows having PCV of 0·32 l/l and Hb of 12·7 g/dl). High yielding cows had corresponding values of 0·29 l/l and 11·6 g/dl. These results are at variance with earlier work by Lane and Campbell (1969) who found that pregnancy effects and lactational effects balanced each other in the Guernsey cattle they used. Paape *et al* (1974) related both erythrocytes and leucocytes to the stage of lactation with erythrocytes fluctuating only slightly as lactation proceeded and leucocytes falling. Leucocyte values fell from a mean of $9 \cdot 1 \times 10^9/l$ in cows lactating for less than 20 weeks to $6 \cdot 3 \times 10^9/l$ in animals lactating for over 40 weeks. This fall was due entirely to a decline in neutrophil numbers.

Hewett (1974) also found that overall values tended to change as the number of lactations increased. In the older animals, Hb, PCV and albumin fell while total protein and globulin rose. Values for animals in their first lactation were Hb 10·7 g/dl, PCV 0·32 1/l, albumin 36·0 g/l, globulin 35·0 g/l and total protein 71·0 g/l. In animals having more than 7 lactations the corresponding values were Hb 10·5 g/dl, PCV 0·30 1/l, albumin 34·0 g/l, globulin 44·0 g/l and total protein 80·0 g/l.

The effects of milk yield at different times has been investigated by Whitlock *et al* (1974). They defined anaemia as an Hb value of less than 9·8 g/dl and found that the overall incidence of anaemia was as high as 10·6 per cent of 7075 dairy cows. Further breakdown of the results shows that anaemia is more likely to occur when the milk yield is high and that the problem is worst in the winter months. Low yielding cows (<7 kg milk/day) had an incidence of anaemia of 4·4 per cent, moderate milkers 9·8 per cent and high yielders (>16 kg milk/day) 15·9 per cent. In the winter the incidence in the high yielding group rose to 17·7 per cent and, although no clinically apparent disease may develop, such a high anaemia incidence must surely have an adverse effect on the productive performance of affected cows.

Lactation and pregnancy usually occur together and the pregnancy effects may disturb the lactational ones. Moberg (1955) found that leucocyte counts rose marginally up to the 4th month of pregnancy and then declined, while Bostedt *et al* (1974) recorded falls in PCV and Hb during the later stages of pregnancy and in the majority of cows serum Fe values fall and were at their lowest around calving. Levels of serum copper appeared to be unaffected.

Stevens *et al* (1974), besides advocating the metabolic profile test considered that the Hb and PCV levels were related to management and that declining values indicated poor management. It may be that management has at least some part to play in the declining values described as due to pregnancy or lactation and certainly nutrition has marked effects.

6.7.4 NUTRITIONAL EFFECTS

Blowey *et al* (1973) used a reduced and modified profile test with glucose, urea and albumin as parameters and found that they could adequately check the herd's nutritional status, although slightly less than 50 per cent of nutritional changes actually affected the blood values they were measuring.

Manston *et al* (1975) fed dairy animals on high, medium and low protein ratios for 7 months and found that the PCV, Hb and albumin were altered considerably. The PCV fell after calving, irrespective of diet but animals on high protein recovered after 4–5 months while those on low protein took 9–10 months. The lowest PCV on a good diet was 0·27 l/l and on a poor diet 0·25 l/l. Hb followed a similar pattern being fairly steady (11·5–12·3 g/dl) in high protein diet animals but falling from calving to 9 months later (12·0–9·0 g/dl), before recovering in the low protein diet animals. Albumin tended to fluctuate but the level was lowest on the low protein diet. A prolongation of this experiment yielded similar but more pronounced results with these animals on continuing low protein diets having much reduced Hb and PCV levels (i.e. PCV as low as 0·22 l/l in mid-lactation). In addition, albumin levels showed considerable reduction, falling as low as 26·0 g/l in the low protein group in comparison to levels of 32·0–34·0 g/l in animals whose diets had been improved.

A low level of nutrition in lactating cows has an adverse effect on Hb and PCV and if the poor feeding is continued for long periods albumin levels will also be affected. These 3 parameters can be used as a method of detecting the long term protein status of lactating dairy cows.

In addition, total and fractionated protein levels can be used, in conjunction with other tests, to detect certain disease states unrelated to management (i.e. chronic wasting diseases or peritonitis (Miclaus *et al* 1973).

7

HAEMATOLOGY OF THE PIG

P. IMLAH AND H. S. McTAGGART

7.1 INTRODUCTION

The following give a general indication of normal values for some primary haematological parameters in the pig.

Red blood cells (RBC $\times 10^{12}$/l)	7·2 (6·0–9·0)
Packed cell volume (PCV l/l)	0·42 (0·37–0·50)
Haemoglobin (Hb g/dl)	14·0 (11·0–17·0)
White blood cells (WBC $\times 10^9$/l)	18·0 (10·0–23·0)
Platelets ($\times 10^9$/l)	400·0 (250·0–700·0)

Any table of normal values which refers to pigs as a whole is of limited value, since what is 'normal' for one category of pigs may not be 'normal' for another and will depend on such factors as age, management and nutrition. This is reflected in the literature where different authors commonly give widely discrepant values for the same parameters. For this reason we have laid particular emphasis on the effects of a variety of influences on the numbers of the various cells found in the peripheral circulation.

The discrepancies in the literature are particularly marked in the case of monocytes. This reflects our own problem of deciding just what constitutes a monocyte in a smear. Typical monocytes present little difficulty, but at one end they blend with large lymphocytes and at the other with early neutrophils so that normal values ranging between virtually zero and, say, 10–12 per cent may be obtained from a single smear, depending on where one draws the line of morphological differentiation. For this reason we have made no attempt to discuss normal values for monocytes nor the changes affecting them.

Erythrocyte sedimentation rates (ESR) are extremely variable in normal pigs, even in the same pig from day to day, so that it is difficult to distinguish physiological from pathological effects. Nonetheless, Raynaud (1961) found the ESR to be a better test for hepatic cirrhosis in pigs than fibrinogen and bilirubin concentrations and thymol turbidity.

7.2 NORMAL HAEMATOLOGICAL VALUES

7.2.1 EFFECT OF AGE

Most haematological parameters are affected to a greater or lesser extent by the age of the animal. Some of these age-related changes are of considerable magnitude in the pig, making it essential to take the animal's age into consideration when assessing the normality or otherwise of a particular measurement.

7.2.1.1 Age-related changes in the red cell picture

The haematology of fetal pigs has been investigated from about 30 days' gestation until birth (ca. 114 days' gestation) by Waddill *et al* (1962), Brooks and Davis (1969) and Upcott *et al* (1973). They found that RBC counts

Table 7.1 The main peaks and troughs in various red cell parameters of pigs during the first year of life. Each age group consisted of between 11 and 758 animals. Piglets received iron-dextran at 3 days old. Males were castrated at 4 weeks. Weaning occurred at 5–6 weeks. Up to 6 months of age each group consisted of approximately equal numbers of males and females; thereafter, females only, which were bred to farrow at one year old. Eleven months = mid to late pregnancy. Twelve months = near farrowing. Abridged by permission from Miller *et al* (1961)

Age	RBC $10^{12}/l$	Reticulocytes % of RBC	PCV l/l	Hb g/dl	MCV fl	MCHC g/dl	MCH pg
Birth	6·20	0·65	0·40	12·6	64·8	31·5	20·5
2 days	—	—	—	—	60·0	—	18·0
3 days	4·57	5·25	0·31	9·3	—	—	20·1
7 days	—	—	—	—	—	28·6	—
10 days	—	—	0·39	10·9	67·2	—	—
3 weeks	—	1·40	—	—	—	—	—
5 weeks	5·98	—	—	—	—	—	15·1
7 weeks	5·26	7·25	0·31	9·1	—	—	—
3 months	—	—	—	—	50·5	—	—
5 months	—	0·15	—	—	—	33·8	—
7 months	7·52	—	0·44	14·2	64·3	31·2	—
8 months	—	—	—	—	—	—	21·8
11 months	7·61	7·4	0·41	14·3	56·9	34·9	18·8
12 months	6·90	6·3	0·39	13·2	56·0	34·2	19·2

— Intermediate figures not reproduced from original.

increased steadily from $0·56 \pm 0·22 \times 10^{12}/l$ at 30 days, to between 4·0 and $6·4 \times 10^{12}/l$ at birth. The PCV ranged from $0·123 \pm 0·0055$ l/l to $0·204 \pm 0·005$ l/l at 30 days, rising to between 0·25 and 0·40 l/l at birth. Hb values were $6·4 \pm 0·4$ g/dl at 51 days, reaching between 8·0 and 12·4 g/dl at birth. Mean cell volume (MCV) decreased from $148 \pm 16·4$ fl at 35–45 days to reach below 70·0 fl at birth. Reticulocyte percentage was low at all ages studied.

Miller *et al* (1961) made a detailed study of the changes in various red cell parameters of post-natal pigs relative to age. Table 7.1 is a simplified version of their data.

It will be seen that the RBC, PCV and Hb were high at birth but fell rapidly during the first few days, the fall being reversed by the administration of iron at 3 days. This was followed by a rapid increase in PCV and Hb due partly to an increase in cell size to a peak at 10 days of age, after which the cells decreased steadily in size to a minimum at 3 months. After administration of iron the RBC increased steadily till bacon weight was reached, apart from a temporary setback following weaning. Falls in RBC were accompanied by appreciable increases in the proportion of reticulocytes which was also high during pregnancy.

MCV was highest at 10 days and lowest at 3 months. At sexual maturity it was similar to that of newborn animals but it was rather lower during pregnancy. Mean cell haemoglobin concentration (MCHC) showed its lowest value at 7 days but otherwise presented little variation, being the least variable of all the red cell indices. Mean cell haemoglobin (MCH) was lowest at 5 weeks (just before weaning) and highest in females of breeding age.

During pregnancy, the RBC, PCV and Hb decrease, this being attributed to a dilution effect due to increased plasma volume so that MCV, MCHC and MCH remain fairly steady.

Since the red cell status of pigs is so dependent on the level of nutrition, in particular the availability of iron, it is to be expected that age-related changes in the red cells may be exaggerated or reduced by nutritional factors.

7.2.1.2 Age-related changes in the leucocyte picture

Upcott *et al* (1973) found that only 2 of 13 samples taken from 35-day fetuses and 1 of 5 samples taken at 40 days had any leucocytes. From 45 days both lymphoid and myeloid cells were seen in most specimens. White cell counts increased from $0.46 \pm 0.25 \times 10^9/l$ at 35–45 days to 4.32 ± 0.29 at 114 days' gestation. During the fetal period, lymphocytes predominated except between days 45 and 60 and again at term and immediately after birth, when a usually dramatic neutrophilia occurred. Brooks and Davis (1969) found a predominance of lymphocytes at 98 days (87·5 per cent), decreasing to 48·5 per cent at birth with a corresponding increase in neutrophils. Waddill *et al* (1962) found about 60 per cent neutrophils at birth.

The leucocyte picture of newborn piglets before ingestion of colostrum resembles that of the late fetus. In a blood sample taken thereafter but within about 12 hours of birth the neutrophils almost invariably outnumber the lymphocytes, averaging about $6.0 \times 10^9/l$ but with a wide range (3·0–$15.0 \times 10^9/l$). The absolute number of lymphocytes increases and the neutrophils decrease, the curves crossing over during the first week or 10 days of life, resulting in a predominantly lymphocytic picture which remains characteristic of the healthy pig for the rest of its life.

McClellan *et al* (1966) draw attention to a lymphocyte peak occurring at 3 months of age in miniature swine but its presence seems to have escaped most other authors whose discussions often centre around changes in WBC or changes in the relative percentages rather than the absolute numbers of lymphocyte and neutrophils.

Our own observations indicate that within 12 hours of birth the lymphocytes usually number between 2·0 and 5·0 × 10^9/l. They increase steadily until, between 9 and 15 weeks of age, they are very significantly higher than in the preceding and subsequent periods (McTaggart 1975). During the high-count period, most pigs show one, or sometimes 2, distinct lymphocyte peaks. These average 15·0 × 10^9/l but may reach as high as 30·0 × 10^9/l and represent over 80 per cent of the total leucocyte count. During these highest peaks, perhaps 20 per cent of the lymphocytes will be very small cells consisting of little more than a densely staining spherical nucleus with little or no visible cytoplasm. Such peaks are transient and decline rapidly, so that they are easily missed.

Other pigs show no obvious lymphocyte peak, the steady increase from birth levelling out at about 10·0 × 10^9/l before declining slowly to the adult level. As yet, there is no explanation of these changes, nor does there appear to be any relationship between the height of a peak and the age at which it occurs.

McClellan *et al* (1966) found a neutrophil peak in miniature pigs which coincided with the lymphocyte peak. The neutrophil count rose from less than 4·0 × 10^9/l at weaning to over 6·0 × 10^9/l at 3 to 6 months, and declined thereafter to an adult level of about 4 ·0 × 10^9/l. We have observed no such neutrophil peak in Large White pigs except in response to some degree of disease challenge. It is possible that the high neutrophil counts encountered soon after birth have a similar aetiology so that neutrophil counts exceeding about 5·0 × 10^9/l may be indicative of a response to some challenge.

Eosinophil counts drop during the first 4 days of life, probably due to post-partum stress (Stegeman 1962). In 41 litters of normal pigs Dvořák (1969) found a steady increase in eosinophils from a low level soon after birth to 0·172 ± 0·111 × 10^9/l at 10 weeks of age.

7.2.1.3. Age-related changes in platelet counts

Lie (1968) found a mean platelet count of 337 ± s.e. 79 × 10^9/l (range 190–575) in over 100 piglets at birth. This dropped to 241 ± 48 (range 175–375) at 2 days old and then rose to a peak of 578 ± 128 × 10^9/l (range 290–775) at 10 days before subsiding to 492 ± 115 (range 300–900) at 15 days.

Linklater (1971) followed the changes in platelet count in 2 litters of pigs

(15 animals in all) from birth (pre-colostral) to 5 weeks of age. At birth, platelet counts for the 2 litters had mean and s.e. of $252 \pm 12 \cdot 5 \times 10^9/l$ and $289 \pm 8 \cdot 7 \times 10^9/l$ respectively. Twenty-four hours later there was a slight drop followed by a gradual rise to 598 ± 25 and $849 \pm 68 \cdot 0 \times 10^9/l$ at 10 days with a subsequent gradual fall to $452 \pm 18 \cdot 7$ and $476 \pm 13 \cdot 6 \times 10^9/l$ at 5 weeks.

Linklater and McTaggart (1972) studied a litter of 5 normal pigs for 7 weeks. These had a mean platelet count of $220 \pm 14 \times 10^9/l$ 2 hours after receiving colostrum. This fell to 165 ± 15 at 24 hours, subsequently rising to about $560 \times 10^9/l$ at 8 and 11 days then levelling off thereafter at about $400 \times 10^9/l$ apart from a transient rise to $623 \pm 53 \times 10^9/l$ at 3 weeks.

McClellan *et al* (1966) observed values of just over $600 \times 10^9/l$ in miniature pigs at weaning, falling to 200–$500 \times 10^9/l$ at 9 months and remaining static thereafter.

7.2.2 EFFECT OF MANAGEMENT

The effects of different types of management were illustrated in a study by McTaggart and Rowntree (1969) in which the haematology of Large White pigs kept under minimal disease (MD) conditions and bled when they reached

Table 7.2 Comparisons of erythrocyte measurements of MD and conventional bacon pigs. Abridged by permission from McTaggart and Rowntree (1969)

	MD pigs 25 animals Mean ± s.e.	Conventional pigs 34 animals Mean ± s.e.	Significance p <
RBC ($10^{12}/l$)	$7 \cdot 93 \pm 0 \cdot 08$	$6 \cdot 88 \pm 0 \cdot 09$	$0 \cdot 001$
PCV (l/l)	$0 \cdot 4602 \pm 0 \cdot 0047$	$0 \cdot 4144 \pm 0 \cdot 0046$	$0 \cdot 001$
Hb (g/dl)	$15 \cdot 19 \pm 0 \cdot 20$	$13 \cdot 40 \pm 0 \cdot 17$	$0 \cdot 001$
MCV (fl)	$59 \cdot 19 \pm 0 \cdot 60$	$60 \cdot 34 \pm 0 \cdot 59$	$0 \cdot 05$
MCHC (g/dl)	$33 \cdot 03 \pm 0 \cdot 29$	$32 \cdot 34 \pm 0 \cdot 28$	n.s.
MCH (pg)	$19 \cdot 20 \pm 0 \cdot 18$	$19 \cdot 49 \pm 0 \cdot 19$	n.s.

bacon weight (90 kg) was compared with that of genetically related pigs kept under similar conditions but without MD restrictions. The differences between the red and white cell pictures of the 2 groups are summarized in Tables 7.2 and 7.3 respectively. It will be seen (Table 7.2) that the red cell counts, PCV and Hb were all very significantly higher in the MD pigs than in the conventional group. Of the derived indices only the MCVs showed any significant difference, the cells being somewhat smaller in the MD group. These results indicated that the differences between the groups were attributable essentially to greater erythrocyte numbers in the MD group.

More spectacular differences were found in the leucocyte pictures (Table 7.3). The mean WBC was about 25 per cent higher in the conventional than in the MD pigs. A similar difference was found between farm pigs and pigs kept in metabolic cages by Šlesingr (1967). It will be seen from Table 7.3 that the lymphocyte counts of McTaggart and Rowntree's 2 groups were virtually the same and that the difference in WBC was attributable essentially to the granulocytes, the neutrophils, eosinophils and basophils each being about twice as numerous in the conventional pigs as in the MD pigs. These differences were interpreted as reflecting the higher exposure to disease

Table 7.3 Comparison of absolute leucocyte counts of MD and conventional bacon pigs. Abridged by permission from McTaggart and Rowntree (1969)

	MD pigs *25 animals* *Mean ± s.e.*	*Conventional pigs* *34 animals* *Mean ± s.e.*	*Significance* *p <*
WBC × 10^9/l	15·95 ± 0·43	19·63 ± 0·84	0·001
Neutrophils	3·06 ± 0·18	6·31 ± 0·56	0·001
Eosinophils	0·58 ± 0·04	0·98 ± 0·08	0·001
Basophils	0·07 ± 0·01	0·13 ± 0·01	0·001
Monocytes	0·95 ± 0·06	1·25 ± 0·77	0·01
Lymphocytes	11·02 ± 0·34	10·57 ± 0·39	n.s.

challenge in conventional pigs. Subsequent studies have indicated that a rise in the absolute neutrophil count is a sensitive indication of a breakdown in the MD protection even before the appearance of clinical disease.

7.2.3 BREED DIFFERENCES

There is little reliable evidence of differences in haematological parameters specifically associated with breed. In particular, we have not been able in our experience to demonstrate any consistent differences between miniature swine and other breeds. Pond *et al* (1968) found no differences in the Hb of 11 Pitman-Moore miniature pigs and 26 Hampshire and Hampshire/Yorkshire cross conventional pigs followed from birth to 20 weeks of age, although they did find transiently significant differences in some biochemical parameters. Milicevic *et al* (1960) found that Landrace and Poland/China boars and sows had significantly higher WBC counts than Durocs and Hampshires (p < 0·01) and Morgan *et al* (1966) showed that administration of iron-dextran to Hampshire piglets produced a rise in platelet count whereas in Durocs it produced a fall.

7.2.4 SEX DIFFERENCES

Gábriš (1973) found no significant differences between the sexes in Hb, RBC and WBC levels. Crookshank *et al* (1975), however, bled 14 males and 11 females every 4 weeks for 12 months commencing at 4 to 67 months of age and found that males had significantly higher RBC and percentage of segmented neutrophils, while females had significantly higher MCV, MCH and percentage of lymphocytes. MCHC, PCV, Hb, ESR, WBC and percentages of non-lobulated neutrophils, eosinophils, basophils and monocytes showed no sex differences.

Stegeman (1962) found significantly higher eosinophil counts in male pigs than in females from weaning onwards but Rossi (1953) found that castrated or spayed Large White pigs had just over 1 per cent eosinophils, whereas entire males and females had about 5 per cent.

7.2.5 DIURNAL VARIATIONS

Rottmann (1969) reported that RBC counts in pigs were highest at 06.00 h and 18.00 h with lower values at other times of the day and night. Hb and PCV values were highest at 06.00 h. WBC counts were lowest in the early morning, rose till about mid-day, then fell slightly till 15.00 h, finally rising to a maximum at 20.00 h.

Gabriel *et al* (1965) demonstrated that the pig shows a true 24-hour rhythm in eosinophil counts which can be reversed in 14 days by changing lighting and feeding times. In a normal day the count is minimal at 06.00 h and maximal in the evening (18.00 h to midnight). Karg (1955) and Stegeman (1962) made similar observations. Minimal and maximal values generally bear a 1:2 ratio to each other.

According to Feider (1971) platelet counts are at their lowest ($361 \pm 8 \cdot 2 \times 10^9/l$) at 02.00 h, rising during the day to reach a maximum ($531 \pm 11 \cdot 8 \times 10^9/l$) at 14.00 h.

7.2.6 BONE MARROW

The bone marrow of the normal young pig has been described in detail by Köhler (1956). An electron microscopic study was carried out by Nafstad and Nafstad (1968). In our opinion, smears made from aspiration biopsy samples from whatever site give much less useful information than core biopsy samples subjected to histological techniques. We have found such samples taken from the wing of the ilium of young pigs with a Jamshidi needle (Kormed Inc.) to be the most satisfactory.

7.3 HAEMATOLOGICAL CHANGES IN DISEASE

7.3.1 RED CELLS

The most important disease affecting the red cells of the pig is piglet anaemia. This is an iron deficiency disease resulting in a microcytic normochromic anaemia later becoming hypochromic. It is associated with other clinical manifestations and develops between one and 4 weeks of age. The extensive literature on this subject has been reviewed by Seamer (1956) and Hannan (1971). The economic importance of the disease has decreased considerably since the introduction of effective iron injections.

A severe hypochromic anaemia attributed to copper deficiency has been described in young pigs (Brooksbank 1954). The anaemia was associated with a neutropenia and a lack of reticulocyte and nucleated red cell response. It did not respond to iron therapy.

Anaemia has been described in association with deficiency of a number of factors of the vitamin B complex. Little detailed haematological information is available but it seems unlikely that such deficiencies are important under field conditions (Whitehair 1970).

Aplastic anaemia due to destruction or replacement of haemopoietic bone marrow is commonly normocytic and normochromic with a notable absence of regenerative forms. It is not of frequent occurrence in pigs and only arises in chronic haemorrhage, ionizing radiation (Case & Simon 1972), rare tumours of the reticuloendothelial system or metastases from other tumours invading the bone marrow. Lymphosarcoma is the commonest such metastasizing tumour of pigs. Head *et al* (1974) described a progressive macrocytic, sometimes hypochromic anaemia, which may show periods of remission, in the hereditary form of the disease. Normoblasts were not much more numerous than in normal pigs of the same age.

Haemorrhagic anaemia is characterized by a reduction in RBC, Hb and PCV. If the haemorrhage is relatively slight the morphology of the cells remains normal apart from some increase in regenerative forms. As the haemorrhage becomes more severe the cells remain normochromic but become macrocytic with numerous regenerative forms. In very severe cases the cells become hypochromic and microcytic. Haemorrhagic anaemia may result from acute blood loss following injury or chronic blood loss associated with blood-sucking helminths (e.g. *Hyostrongylus rubidus*), haemorrhagic diseases such as coal tar poisoning (Davis & Libke 1968), and coagulation defects including thrombocytopenic purpura, warfarin poisoning and mouldy corn poisoning. High nucleated red cell counts (70 per 100 leucocytes) have been reported in blood loss anaemia associated with atrophic rhinitis (Reichel 1963).

Haemolytic anaemia results from excessive intravascular destruction of erythrocytes. In the early stages it is normochromic and macrocytic, later becoming hypochromic and microcytic. In the pig it may be caused by isoimmune antibodies in the colostrum resulting from sensitization of the sow with blood-group antigens contained in swine fever vaccine and giving rise to haemolytic disease of the newborn (see 7.6). It may also arise in association with protozoan parasites such as Eperythrozoon. *Eperythrozoon suis* is a small anaplasma-like parasite of the red cells, capable of causing anaemia and jaundice in young pigs under field conditions in the United States (Splitter 1950). The parasites, which are about 1 μm in diameter, are commonly ring-shaped and are found free or in numbers on the surface of the red cells. *E. parvum* is a similar but smaller organism occurring in Great Britain. It causes a similar disease in splenectomized but not in normal pigs (Jennings & Seamer 1956).

Hypochromic anaemia may develop in yellow fat disease due to feeding fish scraps to pigs (Gorham *et al* 1951). The red cell count is normal but the Hb level is low in severely affected animals.

7.3.2 WHITE CELLS

In general the development of a leucocytosis is *per se* of little diagnostic significance in the pig. It is often encountered in exceptionally severe outbreaks of enzootic pneumonia and infectious rhinitis, in local or generalized pyogenic infections including meningitis and serositis and also in salmonellosis, uraemia, NaCl poisoning and blood-loss anaemia. Reichel (1963) found that about 70 per cent of such cases had total white counts between 20 and 35×10^9/l, the highest value encountered being 96×10^9/l in a purulent bronchopneumonia. Such leucocytoses are all attributable to neutrophilic reactions and are commonly associated with a shift to the left and an absolute reduction in lymphocytes and eosinophils.

The blood cytological changes reported to occur in acute erysipelas are rather confusing and in some respects uncharacteristic of the changes usually seen in acute bacterial infections. In the first 12–35 hours after acute or sub-acute infection there is a leucocytosis with a marked increase in immature neutrophils. The initial leucocytosis is followed by a leucopenia within 60–80 hours after infection (Dougherty *et al* 1965).

Neutrophilia also results from stress due to transportation, restraint, blood sampling, psychological factors, etc. (Palmer 1917, Ludwig 1956, Milicevic 1960; Eikmeier & Mayer 1965). The neutrophils commonly double in number. The increase is not immediate so that the handling of an animal to take a blood sample does not affect the neutrophil content of that sample. However, the changes are detectable within 30 minutes and reach a maximum in 3 to 5 hours after the stress was applied, subsiding to normal during the next few hours. It is therefore necessary to leave a gap of at least 8 hours between serial samples if a blood sample is not to be affected by the taking of a previous one.

Parturition has a similar effect. Fraser (1938) bled a parturient sow at 5 and 3 days pre-partum and at 8 and 24 hours post partum. At 8 hours post partum there was a marked neutrophilia $(42 \times 10^9/l)$ and lymphopenia $(1·8 \times 10^9/l)$. At this time the eosinophils were at a low level $(0·09 \times 10^9/l)$ having been at their highest $(0·748 \times 10^9/l)$ 3 days pre-partum.

Luke (1953a) found a similar neutrophilia and lymphopenia in parturient sows. This usually appeared 6 to 30 hours prior to farrowing, exceptionally as early as 9 days before farrowing or delayed until farrowing commenced. This effect persisted one or 2 days after farrowing by which time the lymphocytes again exceeded the neutrophils. Luke later demonstrated (1953b) that adrenocorticotrophic hormone and adrenal cortical extract produce a comparable effect within 2 hours of injection. Mutsumi (1974) found a statistically significant neutrophilia but no change in lymphocyte count when pigs were injected with 1·0 i.u. ACTH per kg body weight.

An increased WBC may occasionally be attributable to lymphocytosis such as may occur in lymphosarcoma. Most cases of this disease in the pig have been diagnosed only after death but Reichel (1962) described the haematology of 2 cases and Head *et al* (1974) investigated 53 live cases of the hereditary form of the disease. Leukaemia with a WBC as high as $100 \times 10^9/l$ is only rarely encountered in hereditary lymphosarcoma. More commonly the total leucocyte count is at the upper end of the normal range for pigs of comparable age, being commonly between 20 and $30 \times 10^9/l$. Frequently there is a predominance of large lymphoblastic cells, some of which may have bizarre shaped nuclei and show nuclear and/or cytoplasmic vacuolation. Other cells may be difficult to differentiate from monocytes so that it is probably less misleading to classify all non-granulocytes together as mononuclear cells. These commonly constitute over 80 per cent (occasionally almost 100 per cent) of the differential count but from time to time in a single pig the differential count and even the cell morphology may be relatively normal.

A reduction in the WBC occurs in a variety of conditions. Reichel (1963) reported the common occurrence of leucopenia in sucking pigs up to 3 weeks of age suffering from enteritis and diarrhoea, iron and protein deficiencies and inanition associated with agalactia of the sow. The lowest values in two piglets with diarrhoea were 0·2 and $0·4 \times 10^9/l$. In older pigs he commonly encountered leucopenia in typical acute cases of oedema disease. Of 40 such leucopenic pigs 30 had counts ranging from 8·0 down to $1·7 \times 10^9/l$. In breeding pigs Reichel found leucopenia sporadically in a variety of puerperal conditions including intestinal obstruction, pelvic inflammation and toxaemia. The most marked example was a sow with eclampsia which had a WBC count of $2·6 \times 10^9/l$.

Leucopenia commonly occurs during the viraemic phase of acute viral infections such as swine influenza (Shope 1964) and Aujeszky's disease (Sippel 1952). Its chief importance, however, is in swine fever in which it has long been recognized (King & Wilson 1910) as a useful aid to the diagnosis of outbreaks. Lewis and Shope (1929) claimed that if total leucocyte counts of less than $8 \times 10^9/l$ were found in several animals in a suspect herd then this was clear evidence of swine fever.

On the basis of subsequent work by Dunne (1961, 1963) and others, it can be concluded that WBC of less than $10 \times 10^9/l$ should be regarded as leucopenic for pigs over 5 weeks old and that counts of 10 to $13 \times 10^9/l$ should be considered suspicious but that leucopenia is diagnostic of swine fever only when associated with appropriate signs or lesions. Similar changes occur in African swine fever (de Tray & Scott 1957). Where bacterial infections become superimposed on viral infections the initial leucopenia may become masked by a secondary neutrophilia giving rise to a WBC which is within the normal range so that the abnormality is only recognized by carrying out a differential count.

Case and Simon (1972) exposed new-born Yorkshire piglets to 150–450 R of ^{60}Co γ radiation. Lymphopenia developed within 24 hours. In 10 to 14 days neutropenia and anaemia resulted from bone marrow damage. When the dose was lethal the RBC and WBC counts decreased progressively until death occurred. Low white cell counts in adult pigs with heavy *Hyostrongylus rudibus* infestations were found to be due chiefly to lymphopenia with values as low as 0.74×10^9 lymphocytes/l (Maclean 1968). Ketz *et al* (1956) studied the effect of 4 days' starvation on four 30–40 kg pigs. This produced a marked fall in WBC due to neutropenia. Recommencement of feeding resulted in a leucocytosis due to an increase in lymphocytes, and, to a lesser extent, neutrophils. Linklater *et al* (1973) reported a neutropenia at 11–15 days of age in a litter of pigs with simultaneous thrombocytopenic purpura and haemolytic disease of the newborn. In 3 pigs which died the decline in neutrophils was spectacular, one of them having no neutrophils at all in its differential count at 11 days of age.

Eosinophilia commonly occurs in association with helminth infestations, particularly during somatic migrations as in ascariasis (Moncol & Batte 1967), trichinosis (Strafuss & Zimmermann 1967) and lungworms (Mackenzie 1959). The eosinophil count rises to a peak at 2 to 3 weeks after infection, the magnitude and duration of the eosinophilia being related to the weight of infestation. On occasions the eosinophil count may exceed that of the neutrophils.

A reduction in the eosinophil count occurs in association with stress. Karg (1955) transported pigs over a distance of 6 km and found that 3 hours later their eosinophil levels were reduced to between 10 and 50 per cent of the initial value. A similar effect was produced in 4 hours by injection of 400,000 i.u. aqueous penicillin i.m. or 10 to 20 i.u. ACTH subcutaneously. By con-

trast, untreated pigs sampled at 4 hourly intervals showed increases in eosinophil counts of up to 133 per cent above the initial value. Dvořák (1969) found
no eosinophil response typical of stress at weaning. In acute shock there
is a marked but transient drop in eosinophils. In pigs bled daily we have noted
occasions when the eosinophil counts (based on the differential count of
several hundred cells) of a particular pig have dropped from 2 or 3 per cent to
zero in 24 hours. A day later the count has risen to 5 or 6 per cent before
subsiding to the original level thereafter. We assume that such reactions are
attributable to shock arising from some unascertained cause.

7.3.3 PLATELETS

A reduction in the number of circulating platelets occurs in a variety of conditions including viral and neoplastic diseases. Sorensen *et al* (1961) suggested
that thrombocytopenia is a more constant feature of swine fever than is
leucopenia, normal values of several hundred being reduced to between 50
and $5 \times 10^9/l$.

The progressive thrombocytopenia found by Head *et al* (1974) in hereditary lymphosarcoma is presumably due to metastatic invasion of bone marrow. Very few megakaryocytes are seen in bone marrow smears from such
pigs.

Stress results in a temporary thrombocytosis. Feider (1971) found that
physical exertion lasting 20 minutes produced an increase from $425 \pm 12 \cdot 8 \times 10^9/l$ to a maximum of $568 \pm 17 \cdot 6$ 15 minutes after exercise ceased. Psychological stress produced by restraining pigs by the upper jaw for 5 minutes had
a similar effect.

7.4 CYTOGENETICS

In the field of human medicine the study of cytogenetics has been considerably developed and has revealed amongst other things that various clinical
syndromes such as mongolism and Klinefelter's syndrome are associated with
chromosome defects. The pig lends itself to cytogenetic techniques better
than most domesticated animals because its chromosomes are relatively few
and readily grouped and some are even individually identifiable while many
of the techniques used for human chromosome analysis have been found to
work well in the pig with only minor modification. The literature on pig cytogenetics was reviewed up to 1965 by McFeely and Hare (1966).

CHROMOSOME ANALYSIS
Cells have to be obtained in the process of division so that the chromosomes
can be observed in detail. Cells from various body tissues have been used but

peripheral blood leucocytes are convenient and can be cultured by a modification of the method of Moorehead *et al* (1960) such as that described for pig blood by Harvey (1968).

NORMAL KARYOTYPE

It is now generally agreed that the diploid chromosome number of the domestic pig is 38 although that of the wild pig is 36. The female and male sex chromosomes are universally referred to as X and Y respectively. The 18 pairs of autosomes may be arranged and identified in a variety of ways, two of

Table 7.4 Normal karyotype of the domestic pig

| | Classification | | Description |
	McFeely & Hare (1966)	Denver Report (1960)	
Autosomes	A	1	Large subtelocentric
	$B_{1, 2, 3}$	2, 3, 4	Large telocentric
	$C_{1, 2}$	5, 6	Medium subtelocentric
	$D_{1 \text{ to } 7}$	7 to 13	Medium submetacentric
	$E_{1, 2}$	14, 15	Small metacentric
	$F_{1, 2, 3}$	16, 17, 18	Small telocentric
Sex chromosomes			
Female	X	X	Medium submetacentric. Not readily distinguishable from D group.
Male	Y	Y	Smallest metacentric. Paired with an X.

which are indicated in Table 7.4. The terms used to describe their morphology are defined as follows:

Telocentric or acrocentric	Chromatids united terminally. Short arms not measurable.
Subtelocentric	Chromatids united near one end. Short arms less than half the length of the long arms.
Submetacentric	Chromatids united near middle. Short arms more than half the length of the long arms.
Metacentric	Chromatids united at centre. Arms of equal length.

ABNORMAL KARYOTYPES

So far, few chromosome aberrations have been described in the pig. Most pig intersexes are genetically female with the normal 38,XX complement of female chromosomes in all cells, regardless of the degree of masculinization of the reproductive tract (Melander *et al* 1971, Miyake 1973). This observation is supported by the fact that if these intersexes are regarded as female the normal sex ratio is obtained (Breeuwsma 1970). A few may be freemartins which are XX/XY mosaics (McFee *et al* 1966, Bruere *et al* 1968, Breeuwsma 1970). Breeuwsma (1968) described an intersex pig with XXY sex chromosome constitution. Henricson and Bäckström (1964) found an autosomal translocation in a boar with reduced fertility.

Harvey (1968) described a sex chromosome mosaicism, 39,XXY/40,XXXY in a castrated male pig with hereditary lymphosarcoma but subsequent observations by Bain and McTaggart (1974) on 16 cases of the disease (9 females and 7 males, 2 castrated) from the same source as Harvey's case, showed all to be normal karyotypes for their respective anatomical sexes. There appears therefore to be no essential causal relationship between sex chromosome mosaicism and hereditary lymphosarcoma of the pig although such a relationship has been suggested for other species including man.

7.5 BLOOD CHEMISTRY

Although standard values have been recorded in normal animals kept under experimental conditions, little information exists on changes occurring due to disease. From the clinical point of view certain diseases may lead to inappetence and lack of water intake and may consequently make the blood chemistry picture more difficult to interpret. According to Baetz and Mengeling (1971) they consider that inappetence or starvation in pigs can lead to certain changes. The changes are only slight with regard to glucose, calcium, creatine kinase (CPK), bilirubin, phosphorus and magnesium levels. Greater changes may possibly occur in urea nitrogen, chloride, alkaline phosphatase (AP), α and β lipoproteins, total and individual protein fractions, cholesterol, phospholipid, triglycerides and free fatty acids. In their opinion, however, any changes in sodium, potassium, AAT, Al-At and OCT could be interpreted as due to a disease agent or metabolic disturbance, because their levels in the blood are unaffected by starvation.

The lack of information on the blood chemistry of pigs in relation to disease may be partly due to the reluctance of practitioners to take blood samples but is probably due to the fact that the widespread use of balanced rations, creep feeding and supplementation with minerals and vitamins has made deficiency diseases rare. Consequently, the need has never arisen to make extensive use of blood chemical tests as diagnostic aids. Many blood constituents have been measured in the pig and normal values for some are available (Table 7.5). Their use as diagnostic aids has yet to be demonstrated but it should be remembered that a population of normal animals show a wide

Table 7.5 Normal values for chemical constituents of blood

	Age	Whole blood levels Mean±s.d. or s.e.	Serum levels Mean±s.d. or s.e.	Reference
Total protein (g/dl)	3 months	—	7·16±0·91	Haaranen (1960)
	3 months	—	5·87±0·44	McTaggart (1976)
	6 months	—	7·19±0·04	Haaranen (1960)
	Adult	—	6·8 ±0·5	Squibb *et al* (1953)
	Adult	—	7·68±1·11	Haaranen (1960)
	Adult	—	7·3	Baetz & Mengeling (1971)
Albumin (g/dl)	8 weeks	—	2·49±0·04	Tumbleson & Kalish (1972)
	3 months	—	2·93±0·58	McTaggart (1976)
	Adult	—	3·3	Baetz & Mengeling (1971)
α Globulin (g/dl)	8 weeks	—	1·43±0·03	Tumbleson & Kalish (1972)
	Adult	—	1·32	Baetz & Mengeling (1971)
β Globulin (g/dl)	8 weeks	—	1·07±0·03	Tumbleson & Kalish (1972)
	Adult	—	1·62	Baetz & Mengeling (1971)
γ Globulin (g/dl)	8 weeks	—	0·68±0·04	Tumbleson & Kalish (1972)
	Adult	—	1·09	Baetz & Mengeling (1971)
Blood urea (mmol/l)	8 weeks	—	2·81±0·09	Tumbleson & Kalish (1972)
	Adult	2·15±0·56	—	Tegeris *et al* (1966)
	Adult	—	1·25	Baetz & Mengeling (1971)
Creatinine N (μmol/l)	Adult	58·3	—	Hewitt (1932)
Glucose (mmol/l)	New born	3·5	—	Goodwin (1956)
	Adult	5·7 ±1·2	—	Tegeris *et al* (1966)
Calcium (mmol/l)	8 weeks	—	2·9 ±0·025	Tumbleson & Kalish (1972)
	3 months	—	2·77±0·15	McTaggart (1976)
	Adult	—	3·09	Tegeris *et al* (1966)
	Adult	—	2·75	Baetz & Mengeling (1971)
Magnesium (mmol/l)	3 months	—	0·91±0·08	McTaggart (1976)
	Adult	2·6 ±0·3	1·3 ±0·2	Eveleth (1937)
	Adult	—	0·85	Baetz & Mengeling (1971)
Inorganic (mmol/l) phosphorus	3 months	—	2·51±0·28	McTaggart (1976)
	Adult	—	2·34	Hewitt (1932)
	Adult	—	2·5	Baetz & Mengeling (1971)
Sodium (mEq/l)	11 weeks	90·9 ±7·9	—	Imlah (1963)
	12 weeks	—	148·9 ±5·0	McTaggart (1976)
	Adult	—	144·0 ±4·7	Widdowson & McCance (1956)
	Adult	—	131·0	Baetz & Mengeling (1971)
Potassium (mEq/l)	11 weeks	61·4 ±3·7	—	Imlah (1963)
	12 weeks	—	5·5 ±0·5	McTaggart (1976)
	Adult	—	6·0 ±0·6	Widdowson & McCance (1956)
	Adult	—	4·5	Baetz & Mengeling (1971)
Chloride (mEq/l)	12 weeks	—	94·8 ±3·1	McTaggart (1976)
	Adult	—	106·0 ±4·0	Widdowson & McCance (1956)
	Adult	—	105·0	Baetz & Mengeling (1971)
Iron (μmol/l)	Adult	—	22·0	Furugouri (1971)
Copper (μmol/l)	12 weeks	21·7 ±2·4	29·2 ±2·4	Lahey *et al* (1952)
Iodine (μmol/l)	6 months	—	0·12	Gawienowski *et al* (1955)
Zinc (μmol/l)	16 weeks	—	8·8 ±0·5	Hoekstra *et al* (1956)
Cholesterol (mmol/l)	3 weeks	—	4·07	Mouwen *et al* (1972)
	8 weeks	—	3·04±0·06	Tumbleson & Kalish (1972)
	Adult	—	2·07	Baetz & Mengeling (1971)
	Adult	—	2·75	Gupta (1973)
Bilirubin (μmol/l)	Adult	—	5·8	Baetz & Mengeling (1971)
Alkaline phosphatase (KA units/l)	New born	—	738–3230	Imlah (1970b)
	Adult	—	96 ±36	Tegeris *et al* (1966)

Table 7.5 *continued*

AAT (Karmen U/ml)	8 weeks	—	42·8 ±1·5	Tumbleson & Kalish (1972)
	Adult	—	23 ±7·3	Tegeris *et al* (1966)
Al-AT (Karmen U/ml)	Adult	—	25 ±6·7	Tegeris *et al* (1966)
OCT (iu/l)	Adult	—	0·7 ±0·6	Tegeris *et al* (1966)
LDH (Wacker units)	8 weeks	—	320·2 ±7·3	Tumbleson & Kalish (1972)

NOTE: To comply with the new International System of Units, the above values taken from the original publication have been converted to the new SI Units. Original values can be obtained from the appropriate publication listed.

range of values for any one constituent. These values are often related to age, sex, genotype and nutritional state. Nevertheless there are certain constituents of blood which can be usefully estimated. The more important of these are discussed here as follows.

7.5.1 SERUM PROTEINS

At birth prior to colostrum the piglet serum contains albumin, lipoproteins, α globulins and a small amount of β globulins. Immediately after the uptake of colostrum the γ globulins appear and β globulins increase. In normal growing pigs the serum protein profile becomes immunologically adult-like at 3 to 4 weeks of age (Brummerstedt-Hansen 1967).

Changes in serum proteins due to disease have been reported but few of the changes are characteristic of a specific disease. Cartwright *et al* (1948) reported increases in γ globulins in pigs which had been starved and Campbell (1957) demonstrated an increase in α globulin in acute disease and β and γ globulins in chronic disease. We have found significant alteration in the albumin/globulin ratios occurring in hereditary lymphosarcoma of pigs. This alteration is mainly due to a marked increase in the immunoglobulin factor IgG.

In experimental arthritis caused by *Erysipelothrix insidiosa*, Papp and Sikes (1964) found significant decreases in the level of albumin, β_1 and α_2 globulins compared with non-affected controls. Dougherty *et al* (1965) also found a decrease in albumin, but an increase in α globulin with no effect on β or γ globulin in erysipelas infection.

Conflicting reports have been presented about the effect of aflatoxin in groundnut meal. Annau *et al* (1964) reported a reduction in albumin, α and β globulins with an increase in γ globulins. These findings were not confirmed in the report by Barber *et al* (1968).

7.5.2 OTHER SERUM CONSTITUENTS AND ENZYMES

7.5.2.1 Non-protein nitrogen

Uraemia is a feature of acute mercurial poisoning, which can occur when grain treated with mercurial compounds is fed. Loosmore *et al* (1967) described 2 outbreaks of mercury poisoning in pigs, in which death resulted from extensive renal tubular damage.

Dougherty *et al* (1965) found significant increases in blood creatinine in animals dying due to acute erysipelas infection and significant increases in urea in acute and sub-acute infection. Osweiler (1968) found an increase in creatinine and urea in pigs showing signs of perirenal oedema due to poisoning with redroot pigweed.

Jeffcott *et al.* (1967) on investigating the presence of protein in the urine of two sows found an increase in blood urea of 55 to 80 mg/100 ml, which was found to be due to a mild chronic interstitial nephritis. Not all infections involving the kidney necessarily affect the blood urea, because Michna and Campbell (1969) could find no evidence of an increase in blood urea in pigs infected with leptospirosis.

In a survey of 90 clinically normal pigs at slaughter Wilson *et al* (1972) found some evidence of mild liver and kidney damage. This damage was unrelated to the level of serum proteins and serum urea.

7.5.2.2 Glucose

New-born piglets deprived of milk rapidly develop hypoglycaemia and blood glucose levels can fall to less than 1·4 mmol/l (Graham *et al* 1941). Goodwin 1957) demonstrated that newborn piglets had levels of 3·4 mmol/l at birth which rose to 5·6 mmol/l at 4–6 hours and fell to 0·6 mmol/l at 30 hours when deprived of colostrum.

It has been shown by Sampson *et al* (1942) that normal pigs reaching 5–6 days of age are able to withstand starvation. Swiatek *et al* (1968) have also shown that by 10 days of age, piglets can withstand a 21 day fast without developing hypoglycaemia.

7.5.2.3 Major elements

Eveleth and Schwarte (1939) and Eveleth *et al* (1941) studied the chemical changes found in the blood of pigs experimentally infected with swine fever. Slight increases in serum potassium and blood glucose were found with a decrease in serum calcium and sodium. There was also an appreciable increase in cell lipid phosphorus. The authors considered that these changes could be due to an adrenal insufficiency.

In a study of piglets of 4 weeks of age showing signs of diarrhoea, Johnson and Tumbleson (1970–71) found that mean levels for calcium, inorganic phosphorus and potassium were lower than normal and the Ca/P ratio was elevated.

Calcium and phosphorus Although large amounts of calcium are secreted in the milk of sows, eclampsia (Reichel 1963) and osteomalacia (Kernkamp 1941) are rare conditions in the sow. There are few documented cases where blood samples were taken to confirm the diagnosis of these conditions. One would expect a reduction in serum calcium levels in eclampsia and osteomalacia, whereas in rickets low inorganic phosphorus with slightly reduced levels of serum calcium are encountered. An excess of calcium in the diet may interfere with the uptake of other minerals such as zinc and iron.

Sodium and chloride Blood levels are increased in salt poisoning. If the blood sample is taken before pigs go off their food, then serum sodium levels can reach 200 mmol/l and chloride 140 mmol/l in this condition. Experimental salt poisoning of pigs has been studied by Ek (1965).

7.5.2.4 Trace elements

Iron and copper Blood levels of these elements are not normally measured in iron deficiency anaemia. The clinical symptoms and presence of low Hb levels along with a microcytic hypochromic anaemia are sufficient diagnostic features.

Copper deficiency in pigs has been reported by McGavin *et al* (1962), but cases were confirmed by liver levels of copper.

Under experimental conditions of protein deficiency plasma levels of copper and iron dropped to 139 and 115 μg/100 ml respectively, and in iron deficiency the copper levels remained normal at 207 μg/100 ml, whereas iron dropped to 31 μg/100 ml (Cartwright & Wintrobe 1948).

Iodine and zinc Blood levels of iodine may only be important in areas where iodine deficiency is known to occur but no information is available to substantiate the importance of blood levels as a diagnostic aid in this case. Protein bound iodine levels are used in man to detect hyper- and hypothyroidism.

Although zinc deficiency is associated with parakeratosis in pigs there is little information on blood levels in the clinical condition. Only the experimental work of Hoekstra *et al* (1956) has shown that the zinc content of erythrocytes is not affected in parakeratosis but zinc plasma levels can fall from 57 μg/100 ml to 12 μg/100 ml. This level was also affected by incorporating bone meal in the basal deficient diet and could be lowered to 11 μg/100 ml. The feeding of supplemental zinc increased the plasma level to 61 μg/100 ml.

It has been shown by Leibetseder *et al* (1972) that erythrocytes carry 61 per cent of blood zinc, whereas plasma contains 33 per cent and leucocytes 6 per cent. The zinc present in erythrocytes is in the form of carbonic anhydrase (Hove *et al* 1940).

Dietary zinc also appears to affect serum AP. It was shown by Luecke *et al* (1957) that pigs most severely affected with parakeratosis had low serum AP levels. Zinc therapy increased these levels.

7.5.2.5 Fats

It has been shown by Mouwen *et al* (1972) that total fat and free fatty acid levels in the serum of 3 week old piglets with white scour are not affected, but neutral fat is increased and phospholipid and cholesterol are lowered.

7.5.2.6 Bilirubin

In certain pathological conditions such as gastro-enteritis, cirrhosis of the liver, salmonellosis and swine fever, Hojovcová (1971) found hyperbili-rubinaemia. He found that increases of 100–200 per cent in the serum levels were predominantly associated with disturbance in the liver.

7.5.2.7 Enzymes

Transaminases are used extensively in the differential diagnosis of conditions affecting the liver, heart and muscles.

Orstadius *et al* (1959) measured AAT, Al-AT and OCT to try to differentiate between liver and muscle dystrophy in pigs. They found that OCT was mainly increased in liver dystrophy, but AAT and Al-AT were both increased in liver and muscular dystrophy. In carbon tetrachloride poisoning in pigs, AAT levels are increased 300-fold (Cornelius *et al* 1959). Serum OCT can also be increased in this condition (Wretlind *et al* 1959).

Hyldgaard-Jensen *et al* (1969) have shown that plasma glutamate dehydrogenase (GD), AAT and LDH are all increased to peak levels 12–36 hours after carbon tetrachloride administration. All of these enzymes were considered useful in the diagnosis of liver damage, but AP was found not to be useful. *Miniature pigs* Pond *et al* (1968) compared 11 miniature Pitman-Moore pigs with 26 conventional pigs over a 20-week period for serum AP, serum cholesterol, serum proteins, Hb and urea. On the basis of the values obtained for these parameters the authors concluded that there was no appreciable difference between miniature and conventional pigs. The only deviation was in AP and cholesterol levels during the first 6 and 4 weeks respectively. Alkaline phosphatase dropped more rapidly in miniature pigs during the first 6 weeks. Serum cholesterol was lower during the suckling period in miniature pigs. The blood urea was slightly lower in miniature pigs from week 10 to 20 and serum proteins remained slightly higher in miniature pigs throughout the period of study.

7.6 HAEMOSTASIS IN HEALTH AND DISEASE

Until quite recently very little was known about haemostasis in the pig. With the exception of a few clinical entities haemostatic defects have not been studied in detail. There are many diseases involving haemorrhagic conditions which appear to be associated with microbial infections in the pig (Penny 1975). Very few of these diseases, apart from swine fever (Heene *et al* 1971), have been studied from the haemostatic point of view. Most of the information has been obtained from studies of a von Willebrand-type disease, which is an autosomal recessive condition in the pig (Hogan *et al* 1941, Bogart & Muhrer 1942, Cornell & Muhrer 1964, Bowie *et al* 1973, and Owen *et al* 1974). Apart from certain haemorrhagic diseases such as haemolytic disease of the new-born and purpura haemorrhagica, which are discussed in the section on blood groups (7.7), very little information exists about other diseases in the pig. It is apparent that there is an urgent need to acquire information on the haemostatic state of pigs, especially when there have been various reports of haemorrhagic disorders occurring in the field (Osweiler *et al* 1970, Blevins *et al* 1969, Fritschen *et al* 1970).

7.6.1 TECHNIQUES TO ASSESS HAEMOSTASIS IN THE PIG

Most of the tests which can be applied to measure haemostasis are based on techniques developed in man and sometimes involve human factor deficient substrates. Defects in haemostasis usually arise from some abnormality affecting either thromboplastin as an extrinsic or intrinsic factor; or blood vessels; or blood cells; or the composition of the plasma. The tests which can be applied are designed to look at platelet function, coagulation and fibrinolysis. Only the generally more useful tests are discussed with normal and abnormal values for the pig given where known.

7.6.1.1 Coagulation Tests

Platelets A reduction in the number of circulating platelets occurs in various viral and bacterial diseases; idiopathic thrombocytopenia due to drug sensitization; thrombocytopenic purpura of the new-born (Lie 1968) and lymphosarcoma (Linklater & McTaggart 1971).

Bleeding time A number of techniques have been applied in the pig, Duke's method (1910), which involves a deep skin puncture, has been applied by Muhrer *et al* (1942) and Mertz (1942). An average time of 2·9 minutes was recorded for normal pigs. Both investigators found this method to be ineffective in detecting pseudo-haemophilia (von Willebrand's disease). Muhrer *et al* (1942) found that by inserting a 19 gauge needle coated with soft paraffin wax into a marginal ear vein the blood clotted within the needle in less than 5 minutes in normal pigs. Mertz (1942) adopted the saline bleeding time of Doettl and Ripke as modified by Copley and Lalich (1941) and found that in normal pigs the bleeding time was less than 100 seconds, whereas in pseudo-haemophiliac pigs it was more than 10 minutes.

Whole blood clotting time Clotting time can vary considerably with the temperature and technique used. Muhrer *et al* (1942) carried out the test with 5 ml of whole blood in paraffin-coated tubes in an ice-bath and recorded times of up to 40 minutes in normal pigs, whereas haemophilic pigs had a clotting time of 50 minutes or more. Link (1970) stated that markedly increased clotting times may occur in warfarin poisoning.

Clot retraction If there is an absence of retraction, then this may indicate a high fibrinogen level as seen in obstructive jaundice, or a low platelet count. The degree of retraction may be increased by a low PCV.

Bowie *et al* (1973) estimated the mean retraction in 6 normal pigs to be grade 3·3, whereas in three pigs affected with von Willebrand's disease the average was grade 4.

Stypven time (Russell's viper venom time) Besides measuring platelet activity this test can also give a measure of prothrombin and plasma factors V (accelerator globulin) and X (Stuart-Prower factor). Bowie *et al* (1973) estimated the average time in normal pigs to be 11·8 seconds with a range of 9·8 to 14·1 seconds. There is no appreciable increase in von Willebrand's disease.

Platelet retention This test is similar to that described for man in which platelet rich plasma is passed through a column containing small glass beads. Platelet counts are taken before and after and the percentage retention of platelets calculated (Owen *et al* 1973).

Normal pigs have an average retention of 89 per cent (range of 65–98 per cent) with haemophilic pigs giving a low retention of 19 per cent (range of 2–53 per cent).

Defects in the coagulation process can occur through impairment of thromboplastin formation which can be shown by the prothrombin consumption test or the partial thromboplastin time. If there is an interference in thromboplastin formation and prothrombin conversion to thrombin, this can be shown by the one-stage prothrombin time.

Partial thromboplastin time This test is often referred to as the activated partial thromboplastin time because it includes a phospholipid which activates thromboplastin. The test involves mixing 0·1 ml of plasma with 0·1 ml of kaolin-activated cephalin and incubating at 37°C for 10 minutes. As in previous tests 0·1 ml of calcium chloride is added and the time taken for clot formation to take place. Bowie *et al* (1973) found a time of 23·2 seconds (18·4–27·7 seconds) in normal pigs.

Other tests which can be applied to measure intrinsic defects are the thrombin time and assays for specific plasma clotting factors such as factors V, VIII, IX, X, XI and XII. All of these factors have been expressed in terms of normal human standards and estimates calculated for normal pigs by Bowie *et al* (1973). Low levels of factor VIII (antihaemophilic factor) are found in haemophilic pigs.

One-stage prothrombin time (*Quick* 1935)   In normal pigs the time for clot formation ranges from 10 to 15·5 seconds (Blecher & Gunstone 1969).

The most common cause of a prolonged prothrombin time is vitamin K deficiency, which occurs in warfarin poisoning, or advanced liver disease. Rowntree (1968) found an increased prothrombin time in the condition of navel bleeding first described by Shanks (1968). Plasma clotting factors which are also sensitive to vitamin K deficiency are factors VII, IX and X. Percentage levels of these factors in normal pigs are also described in the paper by Bowie *et al* (1973).

7.6.1.2   Fibrinolysis

The fibrinolytic system is believed to be involved in dissolving intravascular thrombi and also for reliquefying blood after death. Excessive activity may lead to a haemorrhagic condition in which lysis of fibrin or fibrinogen may occur. Various bacterial enzymes such as streptokinase and staphylokinase, and pyrogens can cause an increase in fibrinolytic activity. The activator of the fibrinolytic process is plasmin which has a precursor called plasminogen. It is the latter which is stimulated in the first instance to initiate the fibrinolytic process. An excess of plasmin can inactivate other clotting factors. Routinely, this activity should always be investigated in any haemorrhagic disorder. The methods used are the clot lysis time, euglobulin lysis time and plasminogen assay.

Although a fibrinogenaemia does not appear to have been recorded in pigs, an increase in fibrinogen levels can occur in septicaemias. A fibrinogen assay method was developed by Blecher and Gunstone (1969) for pigs based on the gravimetric method of Brown Jaquard (Hardisty & Ingram 1965). Normal values for 13 pigs ranged from 200 to 400 mg/100 ml. Bowie *et al* (1973) have also recorded levels of 250 to 534 mg/100 ml for normal pigs.

7.7   BLOOD GROUPS

Blood grouping may be defined as the identification of genetically controlled differences which exist in the blood of any species. These differences are manifested in various forms. They can be found as distinct antigenic components on the surface membrane of erythrocytes, leucocytes and thrombocytes, also on the polypeptide chains of certain serum proteins. Other differences are found in the form of qualitative and quantitative variations in the proteins, enzymes and ions in the cell fluids and serum. All genetically controlled differences are determined at the time of conception. Some develop during fetal life and others become established shortly after birth. All genetically controlled differences once established remain stable and detectable throughout an animal's life. All blood group factors are inherited in a simple Mendelian manner.

7.7.1 TECHNIQUES FOR THE IDENTIFICATION OF THE VARIOUS BLOOD GROUPS

In pig blood grouping the techniques used for identifying blood group factors have followed the same pattern as those established in man and other animals. Basically, the methods adopted involve immunological, serological and biochemical techniques. Depending upon the material and the type of genetic differences involved the methods used can be described under three sections, that is, immunohaematology, immunodiffusion and immuno-electrophoresis, and zone electrophoresis.

7.7.1.1 Immunohaematology

The identification of genetically determined antigenic factors on the erythrocytes of pigs can be achieved by using naturally occurring isoagglutinins or immune antibodies. Immune antibodies are produced artificially mainly by isoimmunization and very occasionally by heteroimmunization methods. Both natural and isoimmune antibodies can occur as haemagglutinins. Some may occur as haemolysins when rabbit serum which has previously been absorbed with pig erythrocytes is used as a source of complement. The haemagglutinins can be direct or indirect in their reaction with erythrocytes suspended in phosphate buffered saline (pH 7·2). Indirect haemagglutinins are demonstrated by the antiglobulin test (Coombs' test) using rabbit anti-pig globulin. Several indirect agglutinins however can act directly when the suspension medium is replaced with 20 per cent bovine albumin or 5 per cent dextrose, or after the erythrocytes have been previously treated with various proteolytic enzymes such as trypsin, papain, bromelin and ficin. Most of the blood typing reagent antibodies used for detecting antigenic factors on pig erythrocytes are of the indirect isoantibody type. For further details on serological methods the reader is referred to the publications by Andresen (1963) and Hardy (1970).

For lymphocytes the main serological technique used for detecting antigenic factors using isoantibodies is the lymphocyte cytotoxicity test (Vaiman *et al* 1970). Thrombocyte isoantibodies can be used in a direct agglutination test using a 1/10 volume of 2 per cent Triton* in normal saline as a suspension medium for thrombocytes with 1/10 volume of 2 per cent EDTA added to the antiserum (Lundevall 1958, Lie 1966). Recent work has shown that the anti-

* Triton, W.R.—1339—Rugar Chemical Co. Inc, Irvington on Hudson, New York.

globulin consumption test may be used as a method for demonstrating iso-antibodies to thrombocytes (Linklater & Imlah 1974).

7.7.1.2 Immunodiffusion and immunoelectrophoresis

Serum proteins which show different antigenic specificities for different individuals within a species are called allotypes. The first allotypes to be described were found in rabbits by Oudin (1960). Two methods for detecting allotypes in the serum proteins of pigs have been described. The first was reported by Rasmusen (1965). He used the haemagglutination-inhibition method, which was modelled on similar methods used to identify Gm and Inv groups in man. The other more popular method involves the double immunodiffusion of antigen and isoantibody in agar gel. A further refinement of this method can be carried out by immunoelectrophoresis. The technique of immunoelectrophoresis of pig serum has been fully described by Brummerstedt-Hansen (1967). Allotype variations have been described in pigs by Rapacz *et al* (1968, 1970, 1974) and by Lang (1968) using the immunoelectrophoresis method.

7.7.1.3 Zone electrophoresis

The discrete separation of various blood proteins and enzymes by electrophoresis using starch gel as a support medium has provided a wealth of different polymorphic systems in the pig. Starch gel electrophoresis was first described by Smithies (1955). By this technique charged particles on proteins and enzymes in the serum and cell fluids can be separated in an electric field, while at the same time being supported and subjected to molecular sieving in a starch gel medium. The separated components in the gel can then be stained and fixed with a protein-sensitive dye in a methanol–acetic-acid solution. Application of different histochemical and enzyme staining methods has also helped to establish many new systems which cannot be revealed by direct protein staining.

Zone electrophoresis using acrylamide gel as a support medium can also be applied for detecting genetic variations in the blood proteins and enzymes of pigs (Akroyd 1967, 1968). Ansay (1973) has also used cellogel strips as a support medium for resolution of isozymes in pigs.

7.7.2 BLOOD GROUP SYSTEMS AND FACTORS

Blood group systems of pigs can be conveniently divided into red cell and serum protein systems, because most of the established blood group factors have been discovered in these systems. This division is not completely satisfactory, however, because it does not give recognition to factors found on other blood cells, or more recently discovered polymorphisms seen in tissue cell fluids. A more rational approach would be to categorize systems under the 2 main divisions of antigenic and biochemical systems.

7.7.2.1 Antigenic systems

In this division the current knowledge of blood groups can be described under the separate headings of red cell, thrombocyte, lymphocyte and allotype systems and factors.

Table 7.6 Red cell systems and factors

Systems	Factors	Gene symbols or alleles
A	Aa (Ac, Ap), Ao	A^A, A^O, A^- or "i".
B	Ba, Bb	B^a, B^b
C	Ca	C^a, C^-
D	Da, Db	D^a, D^b
E	Ea, Eb, Ed, Ee, Ef	$E^{bdgkmp}(E^1)$; $E^{deghkmnp}(E^2)$;
	Eg, Eh, Ei, Ej, Ek	$E^{aegln}(E^3)$; $E^{defhkmnp}(E^4)$;
	El, Em, En, Eo, Ep	$E^{bdfkmp}(E^5)$; $E^{aefln}(E^6)$;
	Er	$E^{degkln}(E^7)$; $E^{aegil}(E^8)$;
		$E^{deghjmn}(E^9)$; $E^{abgkl}(E^{10})$;
		$E^{abgkm(p)}(E^{11})$; $E^{aegmnop}(E^{12})$;
		$E^{bdgkl}(E^{13})$; $E^{deghjmnr}(E^{14})$;
		$E^{abgmnop}(E^{15})$
F	Fa, Fb, Fc, Fd	F^a, F^{ac}, F^b, F^{bd}
G	Ga, Gb	G^a, G^b
H	Ha, Hb, Hc, Hd, He	H^a, H^b, H^{ab}, H^{cd}, H^{bd}, H^{be}, H^-
I	Ia, Ib	I^a, I^b
J	Ja, Jb	J^a, J^b, J^-
K	Ka, Kb, Kc, Kd, Ke	K^{ac}, K^{ace}, K^{ade}, K^b, K^-
L	La, Lb, Lc, Ld, Lf, Lg	L^{adhi}, L^{adhjk}, L^{adhjl}
	Lh, Li, Lj, Lk, Ll, Lm	L^{agim}, L^{begi}, L^{bdfi}
M	Ma, Mb, Mc, Md, Me, Mf	M^a, M^{ab}, M^{ae}, M^b, M^{bc},
		M^c, M^{cd}, M^d, M^{ef}, M^-
N	Na, Nb, Nc	N^a, N^b, N^{bc}
O	Oa, Ob	O^a, O^b.

Red cell systems and factors   Discrete antigens referred to as blood group factors on the red cells can be defined by the use of monospecific reagents. These reagents are obtained by absorption procedures from immune antibodies. Each factor is controlled by a single gene which is dominant to its absence. This means that a pig can only inherit a factor or factors which are present in either one or both parents. Blood group factors controlled by genes at one site or locus on a chromosome constitute a blood group system. Factors controlled by genes at loci on different chromosomes segregate independently of one another. Some systems may be found to exist on the same chromosome but at different loci. If these loci are sufficiently far apart the genes which they control will still segregate independently but if the loci are close together on the same chromosome, then the genes which they control will be found to be genetically linked. At the moment approximately 66 blood group factors belonging to 15 systems are categorized. The systems and factors are summarized in Table 7.6.

The only system which is a natural antibody system is the A system. In this system A-type cells are demonstrated by naturally occurring pig anti-A serum. The A factor occurs on the red cell and as a soluble substance in the serum of A-type pigs. It is related to the human A, cattle J and sheep R factors. Anti-A serum is found in those pigs in which the A factor is absent. Pigs with anti-A serum may carry an A factor on their red cells which reacts with a cattle anti-O_c (Stormont 1951) or goat anti-O. If the A and O factors are both absent, then a further type known as 'i' has been postulated (Rasmusen 1964). The factors in this system are believed to be controlled by another locus called S, which has an interacting or epistatic effect on the phenotypic expression of the A or O factors. This makes the A-O system unsuitable for parentage determination because A and O offspring can arise from a mating between 'i' parents. Recent observations by Rasmusen (1972) and Hojny (1974) confirm that the H system may be equivalent to the S system postulated, because H blood group genotypes appear to affect the expression of A and O antigens.

The other red cell systems are defined by reagents obtained from immune antisera. Some are simple two factor closed systems controlled by contrasting allelic genes as seen in the B, D, G, I and O systems. In these systems the genotype of the animal is apparent from the phenotype reaction, which in the case of the G system is expressed as shown below

Phenotype reaction		*Genotype*
Ga	Gb	
+	−	Ga/Ga
+	+	Ga/Gb
−	+	Gb/Gb

In closed systems of this type a double negative genotype has not been observed. Where systems show a negative allele as seen in the C, H, J, K and M systems in particular, they are then classified as open systems. Also where several alleles are inherited as a group as seen in the E and L systems they are referred to as multiple allelic systems. They are made up of a series of contrasting alleles, which may be very closely linked in a linear manner on a chromosome.

Thrombocyte factors Four antisera called anti-A, -B, -C and -D have been reported defining four antigenic factors (Lie 1966).

Lymphocyte factors The lymphocytic antigenic system appears to be a histo-incompatibility system similar to the mouse H-2 system and the HLA system in man. It is complex and specific antibodies have not been isolated. The system has been called the SL-A system and compatibility between siblings at this system does not induce lymphocytotoxic antibodies (Vaiman *et al* 1970). White *et al* (1973) have demonstrated that the SL-A (or MHL—major histo-compatibility locus) segregates independently of the A-O, E, I, K, L and M red cell systems and is linked to a locus controlling mixed lymphocyte culture stimulation (MLC). Hruban *et al* (1974), however, demonstrated that survival of skin grafts in semi-inbred pigs appeared to be influenced by differences in the E red cell system. In a previous report Hruban *et al* (1972) showed that certain red cell antigens Ea, Ed, Ef, El and Gb were common on pig lymphocytes as well. Schmid and Otto (1971a b) and Schmid and Cwik (1972) have identified over 30 lymphocyte and 23 granulocyte-associated antigens by cytoagglutination and cytotoxicity tests. In addition, Schmid and Cwik (1972) found a PV receptor site common to lymphocytes and granulocytes by using a water soluble bean extract of *Phaseolus vulgaris* in an agglutination test. Their study on cell receptors also revealed soluble antigens in the serum of pigs which could inhibit the cytoagglutination and cytotoxicity activity of lymphocyte and granulocyte antibodies. A factor called Ll detected by monospecific lymphocyte antibody has been shown by Simon and Hruban (1971) in family studies to be controlled by a dominant gene.

Allotype systems and factors Rapacz and Hasler (1968) reported on the differentiation of at least 11 isoantigens in pigs using isoprecipitins. Subsequently, Rapacz *et al* (1970) described two β lipoprotein allotypes called LDL pp-1 and LDL pp-2, which are determined by allelic genes. It has been suggested by Lang (1968) that some antigenic factors may be common to α, β, and γ globulin components of serum.

7.7.2.2 Biochemical systems

The polymorphic systems mentioned in this section can conveniently be subdivided into serum proteins, serum enzymes and red cell fluid enzymes.

1. SERUM PROTEINS

Transferrins Genetic variation in the iron-binding β globulins has been reported by Ashton (1960) Kristjansson (1960), Imlah (1965), Schröffel (1966) and Baker (1968). The currently recognized types are controlled by 5 alleles designated Tf^A, Tf^B, Tf^C, Tf^D and Tf^E giving 15 possible phenotypes or genotypes. In all the systems determined by zone electrophoresis the genes are expressed in a co-dominant manner, which allows for direct genotyping of an animal for each system examined.

Haemopexins First reported under the name of haptoglobins (haemoglobin-binding) by Kristjansson (1961) and by Hesselholt (1963) and then shown by Imlah (1965) to be haem-binding instead of haemoglobin-binding. The true description of these β globulins has now been universally accepted as haemopexins. It was demonstrated by Imlah (1963) that the true haptoglobins of pigs did not show genetic variation apart from the occasional anhaptoglobinaemic type but that they could vary according to their degree of saturation with the haemoglobin molecule. The haemopexins are the most complex of all the biochemical systems being controlled by at least 6 alleles called Hp^0, Hp^{1F}, Hp^1, Hp^2, Hp^{3F} and Hp^3 giving 21 possible genotypes.

Caeruloplasmins Copper-binding α_2 globulins were shown to be polymorphic by Imlah (1964). Two alleles designated Cp^A and Cp^B control the 3 genotypes which can occur. As caeruloplasmin possesses oxidase activity it can be classified as an enzyme.

Pre-albumins It has been shown by Kristjansson (1963), on zone electrophoresis in starch gel, that certain proteins migrating in front of the albumin can show polymorphism. He described a system which was controlled by 2 genes called Pa^A and Pa^B giving 3 genotypes in all.

Slow α_2 globulins Schröffel (1965) was able to show that the slow α_2 globulins were also capable of showing variation. He established that at least 3 allelic genes called $S\alpha_2^A$, $S\alpha_2^B$ and $S\alpha_2^C$ controlled 6 possible genotypes in this system.

Albumin In addition to pre-albumins the albumin of pig blood can also be seen to vary particularly in an acid gel buffer of pH 6–6·2. Kristjansson (1966) described such a variation and proposed that there were 3 genes called Alb^A, Alb^B and Alb^O controlling the types demonstrated.

Post-albumins At least two alleles called Psta I^A and Psta I^B have been described by Kubek (1968a) to control variation in an unknown protein migrating behind the albumin region.

2. SERUM ENZYMES (SERUM ISOZYMES)

Amylase The first blood enzyme to be shown to behave in a polymorphic manner by electrophoresis was serum amylase and was first described by Imlah (1963, 1965). This enzyme was later found by Ashton (1965) to be identical to the 'thread proteins' he reported in 1960. At least four allelic genes have been found in this system with possibly rarer alleles existing in certain breeds. The system has been given the designation prefix of Am and the currently recognized alleles are Am^1, Am^{2F}, Am^2 and Am^3.

Esterase This was the first serum enzyme found to show genetic variation in pigs and was reported by Augustinsson and Olsson (1961). They classified the enzyme as arylesterase and postulated control by 5 alleles at 1 locus. The 5 alleles were based on enzyme activity and were classified and given a value according to the strength of that activity as follows: allele a—no activity; A_1—25; A_2—50; A_3—75 and A_4—100. Inheritance of these alleles was confirmed by work carried out by Gahne (1970) but he was unable to detect any migratory differences between these types when subjected to starch gel electrophoresis. Kubek (1968b), however, found that the middle region of esterase activity between transferrins and post albumins as demonstrated by zone electrophoresis in starch gel could show variation. The differences he found were controlled by 2 codominant alleles Es^A and Es^B. A further system has since been described by Grunder and Kristjansson (1974) to which they ascribe the symbol EsII. Apparently this system is only seen in post-suckling day-old pigs. Three alleles $EsII^o$, $EsII^E$, and $EsII^F$ controlling 6 phenotypes are described. The exact relationship between arylesterase, Es and EsII systems is not known.

Alkaline phosphatase   Dinklage (1970) in a short communication states that pigs of the German Improved Landrace and Göttingen Miniature pigs showed genetic variation of serum alkaline phosphatase. Five alleles Akp^A, Akp^B, Akp^C, Akp^D, and Akp^E are postulated. Observations by other workers in other breeds have not confirmed this report.

3. RED CELL FLUID ENZYMES (RED CELL ISOZYMES)

6-Phosphogluconic dehydrogenase (6-PGD)   Three variants controlled by 2 alleles called $6\text{-}PGD^A$ and $6\text{-}PGD^B$ have been described by Saison (1968). The heterozygote type forms a hybrid zone not present in the homozygotes.

Glucose 6-phosphate isomerase (phosphohexose isomerase)   First described in pigs by Saison (1968) and subsequently verified by Saison and O'Reilly (1971), this enzyme was originally called phosphohexose isomerase and given the symbol PHI to signify the system. Subsequently, this enzyme has been given the name glucose 6-phosphate isomerase with the symbol GPI. Two alleles GPI^A and GPI^B controlling 3 phenotypes have been found.

Carbonic anhydrase   Two areas of carbonic anhydrase activity can be detected on zymograms. These areas are identified as CaI and CaII. Genetic variation in Danish Black and White pigs has been described by Kloster *et al* (1970) for the CaII area. Two alleles $CaII^A$ and $CaII^B$ controlling 3 phenotypes were found.

High (CaII) and low (CaI) activity carbonic anhydrase has also been detected in pig erythrocytes (Tanis *et al* 1970). The 2 isozymes differ in their properties and chemical composition.

Catalase   The enzymes mentioned above have been found to be polymorphic, mainly by the starch gel electrophoresis technique. This enzyme has been found to be polymorphic in pig haemolysates by the immunoelectrophoresis method. Phenotypically, 3 arcs are distinguishable, 1 fast and 1 slow with the presumed heterozygote giving an extended arc between the other 2. Two co-dominant alleles appear to control the phenotypes described (Baranov 1970).

Phosphoglucomutase Three regions of phosphoglucomutase activity can be detected on zymograms. These areas are referred to as PGM-1, PGM-2, and PGM-3. Region PGM-3 migrates nearest to the cathode. Two alleles have been found in the middle region and were reported by Safarova *et al* (1972). The alleles were found in the Danish Landrace breed and are called PGM-2^A and PGM-2^B. Similar types can also be detected in pig leucolysates (Widar *et al* 1975).

Acid phosphatase Meyer and Verhorst (1973) have described 3 phenotypes called A, AB and B controlled by 2 alleles AEP^A and AEP^B in haemolysates from German Landrace boars. The A allele has the highest frequency.

Peptidases Haemolysates from pigs appear to have peptidase components A, B, C, D and E as in man. The degree of activity varies with B having the strongest activity but only C showing genetic variation. Two alleles called Pep C^{FO} and Pep C^{FS} have been identified with the O allele indicating a lack of slow band and S allele representing the presence of a slow band. All of this work has been carried out by Saison (1973).

Glucose-6-phosphate dehydrogenase Verhorst (1973) has described 2 areas of G-6-PD activity in starch gels. Haemolysates from German Large White pigs show a fast component which is very weak, but also shows polymorphism, and a slow component which is strong but not polymorphic. Two alleles G-6-PD^A and G-6-PD^B are described with an A allele occurring at very low frequency. McDermid *et al* (1975) in a review of red cell enzyme systems suggests that galactose 6-phosphate may be the specific enzyme involved.

Adenosine deaminase First described in pigs by Ananthakrishnan and Walter (1973) who found 3 phenotypes ADA 1-1, ADA 2-2 and ADA 2-1. In a report by Widar *et al* (1974) 5 phenotypes were found in Belgian Landrace and Pietrain pigs called A, AB, BB, BO and O. They found a silent allele ADA^0 which was not expressed in red cells, but was found in white cells and other tissues (Widar & Ansay 1975).

7.7.3 APPLICATION OF BLOOD GROUPS

From the practical point of view blood grouping has the following applications

Identification of animals and use in parentage dispute Blood group factors are an accurate means of identifying individual animals. They are also of universal use in solving problems of parentage dispute particularly where accurate pedigree records are required and in circumstances where more than one parent or offspring is known to be in dispute. Such problems can be resolved on the basis of exclusion. Jamieson (1966) has shown on a theoretical basis the degree of exclusion which may be achieved on the number of blood group loci examined. Exclusion rates of over 95 per cent are possible with the number of blood group loci known in pigs.

Heterospermic inseminations   Widdowson and Newton (1965) have shown the use of blood group loci in identifying offspring from heterospermic inseminations, so that the performance of different genotypes may be examined in the same maternal and external environment. This technique has also been applied by Crossman *et al* (1973) in comparing the viability of offspring from different boars.

Linkage studies   Evidence for linkage between blood group loci has been presented by various authors (Andresen & Baker 1964, Imlah 1965. Hessel-holt *et al* 1966, Andresen 1970a b). Five close linkages have been established involving the blood group systems C and J; Hpx and K; Am and I; PHI and H and PGD and H. Recently, Imlah (1970a, 1972) has shown that linkage between the Tf locus and an early lethal factor exists in a strain of pigs.

Association between blood group loci and factors of economic importance Several studies have been made in the application of blood group loci in determining close association with factors of economic importance such as production characters and reproductive performance. Jensen *et al* (1968) have shown that 0 to 12 per cent of the variation in reproductive traits in Duroc and Hampshire pigs can be accounted for by several blood group loci with the H-locus appearing to have a distinct advantage. More recently Imlah (1972, 1974) has shown that sows of Tf^B/Tf^B genotype have a 5–15 per cent advantage in litter size at birth and at three weeks of age over sows of Tf^A/Tf^A genotype. Rasmusen and Christian (1976) have made the observation that certain genotypes of the H system may indicate susceptibility to the porcine stress syndrome (PSS). These are very recent observations which obviously could have a significant effect on selection of animals in the future.

Blood groups and disease   Haemolytic disease of the new-born can occur artificially when pregnant sows are vaccinated against swine fever with vaccine made from blood of infected animals. This was shown by Goodwin *et al* (1956) when crystal violet swine fever vaccine was used. Several red blood cell antigens were found to be involved in the disease as a result of vaccination (Joysey *et al* 1959a b). Andresen and Baker (1963) have shown the involve-ment of one specific factor called Ba in a field case of haemolytic disease following vaccination. The natural occurrence of haemolytic disease was first reported by Szabo *et al* (1956). It has also been shown by Linklater (1968) that sensitization of sows to their own piglets' red cell antigens may occur naturally. Further evidence for the natural occurrence of haemolytic disease has been provided by Hall *et al* (1972) and Linklater *et al* (1973). Iso-immunization as a cause of disease has also been implicated in thrombocytopenic purpura. (Stormorken *et al* 1963; Saunders *et al* 1966). This condition is similar in pathogenesis to that of haemolytic disease but involves platelets and megakaryocytes (Nordstoga 1965, Saunders & Kinch 1968, Anderson & Nielsen 1973). Lie (1966) has been able to detect 4 antigenic factors on thrombocytes which may be involved in sensitization of sows. Other antigenic factors on neutrophils and erythrocytes may also be involved and may contribute to the condition (Linklater *et al* 1973). After ingestion of colostrum circulating platelets of piglets are reduced to levels below $50 \times 10^9/l$. Haemorrhages and purpura are present at 12–48 hours of age with occasional death, but the majority of piglets survive to 11–14 days and then succumb. At this stage haemorrhages and purpura are due to a lack of megakaryocytes and circulating platelets. Infections may also occur due to a neutropenia.

8

HAEMATOLOGY OF THE SHEEP AND GOAT

BRIAN GREENWOOD

(a) THE SHEEP

8a.1   BLOOD VOLUME

Turner and Hodgetts (1959) showed that as much as one-seventh of the blood volume of the adult sheep can be found in the spleen. In response to excitement, or the injection of adrenaline, a part or all of this may be ejected.

Hodgetts (1961), using red cell labelling with ^{51}Cr, and plasma labelling with T1824 dye, studied total blood volume in Merino sheep and found this to be $66\cdot4\pm5\cdot4$ ml/kg body weight. The ^{51}Cr cell volume was $19\cdot7\pm2\cdot8$ ml/kg. The T1824 plasma volume was $46\cdot7\pm3\cdot6$ ml/kg.

Pipkin and Kirkpatrick (1973) studying the blood volumes of fetal and newborn sheep, showed that the relationship to body weight in the new-born was $80\cdot8\pm2\cdot8$ ml/kg.

8a.2 THE ERYTHROCYTE

8a.2.1 DIAMETER

As with so many other species the cell is a biconcave disc, relatively small, and frequently of a diameter obviously different from that of its neighbour. Anisocytosis is marked in some individuals, and absent in others. It is particularly marked in animals recovering from anaemia or blood loss.

The mean diameter lies between 4 and 5 μm, and values as low as 3 μm and as high as 8 μm are occasionally seen in living preparations. Most of the available measurements have been made upon fixed and stained films. Winter (1966a) described the use of an automatic counting technique to prepare Price-Jones curves based, not upon erythrocyte diameter, but upon cell volume, a certain skewness in the curves being attributed to a population of younger cells with a larger volume being added to the normal distribution of mature erythrocytes. The peak of numerous sheep curves lay at 32 fl (while the similarly determined human curves peaked at 86 fl).

Average cell diameters in lambs are similar to those in adults.

8a.2.2 NUMBER

The number of erythrocytes in different sheep breeds has been an almost unlimited source of research. However, as with its leucocyte count, the sheep shows a degree of variation which leaves much to be desired in establishing normal values. Part of the problem lies in the ability of the sheep spleen to store erythrocytes, and an agitated sheep will force such cells out into the circulation. Turner and Hodgetts (1959) showed that the spleen may contain up to one-quarter of the total red cell mass. Clearly, unless an individual sheep is at peace when bled, the erythrocyte count and PCV may have very limited usefulness. Consequently, studies of red cell numbers and PCVs in a large series of constantly changing sheep may be far less reliable than those upon a small number of sheep which are handled and bled frequently by the same gentle workers.

This note of caution is essential before discussing red cell values, not to afford criticism of those workers who have looked at different breeds at different ages, but to warn the aspiring sheep haematologist to be wary of results from a sheep caught from the flock and unaccustomed to being handled. A low haematocrit will still have its value, and a very high one may be reassuring. Of course, these strictures about handling must apply to haemoglobin measurements also.

Without attempting to confuse standard figures further, or surveying the field of individual studies unnecessarily, one may take the values of Schalm *et al* (1975) for the erythrocyte count: an average of $12 \times 10^{12}/l$, with a range of $9–15 \times 10^{12}/l$.

8a.2.3 PCV

Of much more frequent determination, because of speed since the advent of the microhaematocrit centrifuge, is the PCV. This again has been studied by numerous workers, and, once more, a wide variation is common, even amongst tame sheep living indoors with a minimum worm burden. Individual workers in any one department will entertain views of what is normal almost as numerous as the values exhibited by individual sheep. A mean value derived from numerous authors, and covering many breeds in many countries, is 0·37 l/l. This would be regarded as a high mean in this Institute, although individual animals with values over 0·40 l/l are by no means uncommon. Most of us would regard 0·29 l/l as being a low normal, that value being from a sheep which is accustomed to being bled. Beal (1975) (personal communication) has shown that arterial and jugular venous PCVs show no measurable difference, but the PCV of jugular venous blood taken from an anaesthetized sheep is usually lower than that from the same animal when conscious, probably because of relaxation of the splenic musculature. When sequential samples are taken at short intervals from the jugular vein of a conscious and tame sheep, the PCV will fall as much as 0·03 l/l after the first determination and then remain steady. However, if the sheep has been previously splenectomized, the initial higher PCV in the conscious sheep is not encountered, and all the determinations are similar.

These observations have research interest, but, for clinical purposes, the PCV provides a rapid screening technique for seeking anaemia, or looking at the plasma for haemolysis or icterus.

The PCV of venous blood increases rapidly after feeding begins. This is due to a fall in plasma volume, associated, no doubt, with increased secretion, and there is evidence that red cells are moved from the spleen into the circulating blood partially restoring the blood volume.

8a.2.4 FRAGILITY

Haemolysis may begin in 0·8 per cent saline, or, more frequently below this concentration. It is usually complete by 0·6 to 0·45 per cent saline.

8a.2.5 RED CELL LIFE SPAN

Tucker (1963) used both serological and radioactive tracer techniques on adult sheep. As ^{51}Cr is rapidly eluted from sheep erythrocytes, it was replaced in these studies by ^{59}Fe. There was good correlation between the results obtained by serological and tracer methods, although, of course, in the former the study was of survival of donor cells in a recipient. The ^{59}Fe method has the disadvantage that when cells containing the isotope are broken down the ^{59}Fe can be used again for haemoglobin synthesis, a disadvantage which can be reduced by administering large doses of non-radioactive iron to provide an excess source for synthesis. Potential red cell life span for adult sheep was about 150 days but both methods showed that the average life span of the cells was between 70 and 153 days, indicating that many cells were being lost from the circulation for unknown reasons. This random loss varied between individual sheep, and bore no relation to the degree of worm infestation of those individuals. Nor did it appear to have any obvious correlation with the potential life span of the cells of that animal. Eadie *et al* (1960) had noted that random loss of cells might occur in an individual sheep which had previously shown no random loss. They had suggested that this change was related to infestation by parasites.

Tucker (1963) also remarked that there appeared to be a seasonal factor in the length of potential life span, the means for autumn being $155 \cdot 5 \pm 10 \cdot 6$ days, and for spring $137 \cdot 5 \pm 5 \cdot 6$ days. However, the relationship to seasonal temperature was by no means obvious.

For lambs, the potential life span was about 75 days, with an average life span of 15–36 days. The survival curve, however, showed a tail, suggesting that some of the lambs' cells had a life span similar to that of an adult. As the lamb cells were all studied by the serological method in which they were injected into an adult sheep, the short survival may reflect abnormal survival of lamb cells in an adult animal. Subsequently Tucker (1966) showed that the life span was independent of the type of haemoglobin within the cell. There is evidence that, following a severe blood loss, the red cells exhibit a shorter average life span, although the potential life span remains unchanged.

There was no difference between the life spans of HK and LK type erythrocytes in adult sheep, but sheep red cells with an inherited glutathione deficiency have a shortened life span (Tucker 1974).

8a.2.6 HAEMOGLOBIN

Two main types of haemoglobin exist in adult sheep, HbA and HbB. An animal may have either or both of these types, the genes controlling each type being co-dominant.

Individuals of types HbA or HbAB can produce another haemoglobin,

HbC. This can be detected in the blood of HbA and HbAB lambs between 2 weeks and 3 months of age, or in HbA and HbAB adults when they are severely anaemic.

The type of haemoglobin does not affect the duration of cell life (Tucker 1966). HbC appears 7 days after the cessation of a haemorrhage which has been sufficient to make the animal anaemic, being found in the youngest cells, and replacing the A component. Thereafter it can be detected in the blood of the sheep for 140–150 days, the normal red cell life of the sheep. HbA type cells are less dense than HbB cells (on centrifugal layering) and young erythrocytes are lighter than old (Tucker 1966). As well as their lower specific gravity, HbA cells have a higher water content than HbB cells. Fetal haemoglobin (HbF) can be detected in lambs for 40–50 days after birth by using alkali denaturation or other techniques.

HbA blood has a higher oxygen affinity than HbB blood. Kernohan (1961) ascribed this to differences in the dissociation rates, and the subsequent work of Sirs (1966) confirmed this while prompting him to observe that his own results could suggest the existence of 2 forms of HbB. The differences in oxygen affinity of HbA and HbB remain when the haemoglobin is removed from its intracellular environment.

HbA has also been associated with higher haemoglobin levels and PCVs (Evans & Whitlock 1964).

HbS does not occur in sheep, nor does sickling occur in vivo. Sickling can, however, be induced in vitro in sheep red blood cells containing HbA and HbAB.

The normal haemoglobin content of sheep blood lies between 8 and 16 g/dl, with a mean of 12 g/dl. The Mean Corpuscular Haemoglobin (MCH) has a range from 8 to 12 pg, while the Mean Corpuscular Haemoglobin Concentration (MCHC) has a range from 31 to 38 g/dl.

8a.2.7 SEDIMENTATION

Sheep blood sediments very slowly indeed, a contrast with blood from the horse and the pig. Comparison with the horse shows that this is unlikely to be a function of cell size, which has sometimes been assumed. However, a marked and obvious difference between the two bloods is the rapid gross aggregation of horse erythrocytes, and the rarity of any aggregation of sheep cells. A useful comparative study of aggregation tendency was carried out by Richter (1966) who showed that there is generally a positive correlation between the ESR and the degree of aggregation (an exception being the rabbit).

Osbaldiston (1971) neatly showed that a major reason for poor sedimentation in the sheep could lie with the cell itself, rather than the plasma, although there is much evidence from human studies that plasma factors play a part.

Sirs (1975) has investigated both sheep and horse erythrocytes, and, having shown that rouleau formation depends in part upon the flexibility of the erythrocyte and its ability to adapt its contours to those of its neighbours, has demonstrated that the horse red cell is much more flexible than that of the human, while the sheep cell is very much less. This is a major factor additional to those which exist in the plasma, such as fibrinogen, and are known to play a part in sedimentation.

Sedimentation is much increased by setting the tubes, or glass surfaces, at an angle to the vertical but, carried out with vertical tubes in the conventional fashion, it is of little use as a non-specific test for disease in sheep.

This disinclination of sheep red cells to aggregate has played a part in bringing them to such favour in the eyes of immunologists as an indicator system.

8a.2.8   BLOOD GROUPS

Sheep blood groups have been very fully studied, chiefly on account of their genetic rather than their clinical significance. The major naturally occurring red cell system is the R-O, defined by antiseral lysis in the presence of rabbit or guinea pig complement. The antisera are anti-R and anti-O. Those red cells which are lysed by anti-R serum are described as group R, and those which are lysed by anti-O serum are classed as group O. Red cells which are not lysed by either of these antisera are known as group i.

Anti-R occurs in the sera of group O sheep, and the titres are highest in summer and lowest in winter. It is also present in the sera of some group i sheep. Anti-O is found only rarely, in some group i sheep. It is usually obtained from goat or cattle sera, in which it is uncommon.

The group R gene is dominant to that for group O, so that heterozygous individuals are serologically indistinguishable from homozygous group R animals.

In new-born lambs the erythrocytes have neither R nor O blood group substances, R substance appearing at 1–2 weeks of age, and O substance at 3–4 weeks. Because adult group i sheep erythrocytes can be made to react with anti-R or anti-O sera after the cells have been incubated in group R or group O sera respectively, it has been assumed that the blood group substances can be passively acquired by the erythrocytes from the plasma. This is, no doubt, how lamb erythrocytes acquire their substances.

Sheep erythrocytes have also been characterized by their potassium content, which is subject to genetic regulation. An individual animal may have erythrocytes which have a high potassium and a low sodium concentration (HK) or a low potassium and a high sodium concentration (LK). There are no plasma potassium and sodium differences between these 2 groups of sheep, and the reticulocytes of both HK and LK sheep have high potassium concentrations. The erythrocytes of all young lambs have a high potassium concentration, irrespective of their eventual adult type, the latter being achieved by the sixth or seventh post-natal week. There is evidence to indicate that HK cells are more fragile than LK cells but fetal cells with high potassium levels are least fragile.

8a.2.9 RED CELL CHANGES WITH GROWTH

During the early part of fetal life the erythrocytes are large, but after the 60th day of gestation another population of smaller cells becomes evident, these latter cells resembling those of the adult animal (Karvonen 1954). Work by Perk *et al* (1964) on Awasi sheep and lambs indicated that 2 erythrocyte populations appeared to be present at birth because there were 2 fragility peaks. One peak rose, and one fell in size as the lamb grew. Both cell populations appeared to contain both fetal and adult haemoglobins.

The changes in red cell characteristics from birth to adulthood have been followed by Ullrey *et al* (1965) and Upcott *et al* (1971). Red cell numbers, PCV and haemoglobin fell after birth for a period of 14–18 days. Thereafter there was recovery. MCH also fell, but MCHC, which was low at birth, rose from this date throughout the first year. Both groups noted that a peak of reticulocytes was present in the peripheral blood during or at the end of the second week after birth, this peak being roughly related to the period of low erythrocyte numbers.

The MCV, which was greatest at birth, fell over the subsequent 5 months.

Reticulocytes are not found in the blood of normal adult sheep, but they do occur during the recovery from anaemia.

8a.3 LEUCOCYTES

Sheep show wide variations between individuals in their total leucocyte counts. One sheep followed throughout its adult life will show a consistency of total leucocyte count which is remarkable, and within that count it will maintain percentages of cell types at levels which may seem grossly abnormal.

The range for the leucocyte count is $4-12 \times 10^9/1$ with a mean value of $8 \times 10^9/1$.

The predominant leucocyte in the adult is the lymphocyte (about 60–65 per cent) with the neutrophil comprising about 30 per cent of the leucocytes. Eosinophils constitute 2–12 per cent, and monocytes from 2–8 per cent. Basophils are rarely seen, but when one is seen in a blood film, another is usually found within 2 microscope fields. This has been a consistent and unexplained finding in our experience.

B. Greenwood

8a.3.1 LYMPHOCYTES

Small lymphocytes (8–10 μm) and large lymphocytes (12–16 μm) differ little in appearance from the lymphocytes of other species. Large lymphocytes are few in number, about 4–5 per cent of the total leucocytes. The presence of one, two, or even more azurophil granules in many of the small lymphocytes is not an uncommon finding in an individual animal. With Romanowsky staining these granules take on a darker, but otherwise similar colour to the nucleus. They often appear angular, as though barrel shaped. Lymphocytes with 2 nuclear lobes, with a thin communicating strand occasionally clearly visible, are less uncommon than the literature has sometimes suggested. They are also found in the peripheral lymph. Lymphocytes with very bright sky blue cytoplasm are sometimes seen, and it may be that these are lymphocytes undergoing transformation to plasma cells despite the absence of change in nuclear detail.

Sheep lymphocytes can be separated from other leucocytes by removing the red cells and then allowing the granulocytes and monocytes to stick to glass, while retaining the lymphocytes in suspension. Erythrocytes can be removed by haemolysis or centrifugation. Dextran has proved useless for producing rapid initial sedimentation of sheep red cells, but Kerry (1976) has used hydroxyethylcellulose for producing erythrocyte sedimentation as a first step in sheep leucocyte separation.

By electron microscopy Yamada and Sonoda (1972a) describe the sheep lymphocyte as having no apparent nucleoli in the nucleus, and as many as 5 mitochondria in the cytoplasm. Small round or oval dense bodies, about 0·2–0·5 μm in diameter were seen, and it was suggested that these might be the azurophil granules. Of course, it is difficult to be certain of this by electron microscopy since the granules are defined by their staining characteristics. Facing a similar problem, the authors wondered if those lymphocytes which they observed to have a little rough-surfaced endoplasmic reticulum could be the ones which they had noted as having bright blue staining cytoplasm at the light microscopy level.

8a.3.2 NEUTROPHIL GRANULOCYTES

Despite what sometimes appears to be an alarmingly low number of neutrophils, the sheep mounts a remarkable neutrophil response to any inflammatory lesion and has a truly tremendous ability to deal with sepsis.

Sheep neutrophils are the same size as those of other species, move in the same manner, and have very small granules, much smaller than those of the human neutrophil. These granules can be seen clearly by phase-contrast microscopy but they stain poorly by Romanowsky techniques. Winter (1965) attempted, by changing pH and using different stains, to overcome this problem, unsuccessfully. The cytoplasm and granules of sheep neutrophils he regarded as virtually unstainable. However, he did describe (1964a) the lipid reaction to Sudan Black B of the granules in both neutrophils and eosinophils. He also used the peroxidase reaction successfully, the major purpose of his staining attempts being to show that, in sheep, the specific granules are present in all developmental stages of the neutrophil series. Indeed, he showed that the granules could be identified with certainty in cells as young as myelocytes. The nucleus commonly has 3–5 lobes.

Electron microscopic appearances: In the nucleus no nucleoli have been seen (Yamada & Sonoda 1970a). The cytoplasm contains small amounts of smooth and rough-surfaced endoplasmic reticulum, a small number of mito-chondria measuring 0·3–0·7 μm, and some structures thought to be phago-somes containing platelets. Two kinds of specific granules have been des-cribed, a very dense granule, round, rod, or spindle shaped, with a short axis of about 0·2 μm, and a long axis of about 0·5 μm; and a less dense granule, round or oval, with a diameter of 0·4 μm. Both types of granule have distinct unit membranes, and most of them have a homogeneous interior. However, some granules display what appears to be an intercalated plate-like structure, while others have circular defects, and spaces between the membrane and the matrix of the granules.

8a.3.3 EOSINOPHIL GRANULOCYTES

The number of eosinophils, whether absolutely or as a percentage, varies considerably between individual animals. While one would like to be able to ascribe this to the degree of parasitism it is an irritating fact that in careful studies of parasitic infestation the sheep often appears to have a casual indifference to relating its eosinophil count to the known infestation, let alone to the degree of that infestation. A sheep will often have a known experi-mentally induced infestation, but a completely normal eosinophil count. In our experience it is relatively rare to encounter a substantial eosinophilia in a sheep.

Eosinophils are always easy to find in blood films, stain well, and have smaller eosinophilic granules than most species. Indeed a human neutrophil looks not unlike a sheep eosinophil when studied by phase-contrast micro-scopy, so comparable appear the granule sizes at first glance. These small eosinophil granules are very numerous indeed, and there is less staining of the cytoplasm in Romanowski preparations than in human eosinophils.

The cell, given the opportunity, is extremely motile (Greenwood 1968, 1969a) often exceeding the neutrophil in the speed with which it moves. It is usual for the eosinophil to have 2 or 3 nuclear lobes. The function and life cycle of the cell are unknown, but occasional dead eosinophils are observed in the peripheral lymph of the sheep.

By electron microscopy Yamada and Sonoda (1970b) described 6 types of granule, all with unit membranes. The most common of these was the sandwich type in which a dense middle plate lay symmetrically in the long axis of a less dense ground substance. Other granules were homogeneous or contained a fine reticulated structure in their ground substance. A laminated form of granule with an appearance resembling myelin and having a diameter of 0·4–1·0 μm was also described by Yamada and Sonoda. Similar granules have been studied by Wooding (personal communication, 1973) and resemble those described by other authors in cats, dogs, cattle and mink.

8a.3.4 BASOPHIL GRANULOCYTES

These are relatively rare cells in the sheep, appearing in blood films as some-what angular cells with 2 or 3 angular lobes to their nuclei. The granules are larger than those of the sheep eosinophil, and far fewer in number so that each may be seen individually, surrounded by cytoplasm. The granules stain a deep blue violet colour. They have not been recognized by us in living preparations nor by electron microscopy. However, Yamada and Sonoda (1972b) have described them from Corriedale sheep. The specific granules had a unit membrane and were 0·4–1·0 μm in diameter. Some granules were dense and homogeneous, some had a dense, coarsely granular network within them, and some, less dense, had a finely granular network. Mitochondria were few and the Golgi apparatus was poorly developed. A little rough-surfaced endoplasmic reticulum was present.

8a.3.5 MONOCYTES

Having a diameter between 12 and 18 μm in fixed preparations, the monocyte can be mistaken for a large lymphocyte. However, in its most characteristic form, this is far less easy. When observed by phase-contrast microscopy in the living state on a warm microscope stage it is difficult to confuse it with any other cell commonly seen in circulating blood.

It is a much less granular cell in the sheep than in the human. The blue ground-glass appearance of the cytoplasm of the human monocyte, or the appearance which resembles that of numerous minute glass beads within the central cytoplasm, is far more characteristic of the human than the sheep monocyte. The faint basophilic flecking, seen in human monocytes, is also less common in sheep monocytes. Phase-contrast observation of living cells, as well as electron microscopy, confirm this lack of granularity.

The nucleus of the cell is frequently kidney shaped in fixed and stained preparations, but in the living cell extended upon glass, it is almost invariably horse-shoe shaped.

The monocyte accumulates in chronic inflammatory lesions, and its capacity for phagocytosis in such a situation has been shown by putting diluted carbon ink particles into such a lesion in a sheep. If blood monocytes from sheep are cultured in autologous plasma they grow in size to resemble tissue macrophages, and they begin, after about 4 days, to divide by mitosis, giving rise, not to monocytes, but to macrophages (Greenwood 1969b, 1973). There is every likelihood that monocytes do this in vivo in the sheep as they appear to do during chronic inflammation in rodents. The majority of sheep monocytes, when cultured, replicate their DNA and so prepare for mitosis (Campbell 1972). Sheep plasma has been shown to contain a relatively low molecular weight substance which will promote the mitosis of cultured monocytes (Greenwood 1972), and, after 3 or 4 days of mild chronic inflammation the plasma of a sheep develops further the ability to promote the mitosis of autologous cultured monocytes (Greenwood 1971). It is not known if this is due to the production of some new promoter substance, or an increased concentration of the one already present. This indicates the mechanism by which blood monocytes proliferate in an inflammatory lesion.

For many decades it has been the belief of a minority that the blood monocyte could become converted into a fibroblast in damaged tissue. Exhaustive experimental work upon sheep monocytes has failed to provide any evidence of this conversion.

The majority of sheep blood monocytes when observed in vitro show continuous cytoplasmic movement about their margins, but very little movement from place to place. Occasionally a more than usually motile monocyte is encountered, which, attaching itself to glass, moves around quite swiftly.

Yamada and Sonoda (1972a) used electron microscopy to describe abundant smooth-surfaced endoplasmic reticulum with large numbers of free ribosomes and polysomes in the cytoplasm. High density granules which were round or oval and bounded by a unit membrane, were also present. They were very variable in size, moderate in number, and smaller than the mitochondria, which themselves are visible by light microscopy. There were fine filamentous strands around the nucleus of the kind described in the monocytes of the guinea pig and man.

8a.3.6 LEUCOCYTE CHANGES WITH GROWTH

There have been few observations of lamb leucocyte values immediately after birth. Ullrey *et al* (1965) showed that the number of leucocytes doubled between birth and 12 hours, declined in the period between 12 and 48 hours, and subsequently rose once more to a peak at 3 months. However, Upcott *et al* (1971) taking their first sample one day after birth (and quoting the timing in days post conception) noted that there were no significant shifts in total leucocyte numbers during the first month or so of life.

If one looks within the leucocyte series, Ullrey *et al* (1965) observed a neutrophil rise from 34 per cent at birth to 52 per cent at 12 hours. After one month only 29 per cent of the leucocytes were neutrophils. Upcott *et al* (1971) found similar figures.

Upcott *et al* (1971) also pointed out that the absolute mature neutrophil numbers fell significantly between the day after birth and some 3–8 days later (150 days post conception). There was no apparent shift to the left in the neutrophils but there was a significant rise in the mean population of intravascular neutrophil precursors at this time.

Fraser (1929–30) also gave values for the first day of life. At birth, the neutrophil percentage was 58·2 per cent falling to 51·2 per cent at one day old. If there are differences at birth between Fraser's percentage and Ullrey's, all found about 50 per cent at 12–24 hours of life.

There is general agreement that eosinophil numbers are lower in lambs than in adult sheep.

Ullrey *et al* (1965) also studied leucocyte counts in ewes during gestation and lactation. The neutrophil percentage rose during gestation to 60 per cent at the time of parturition, falling to 45 per cent by the 14th day of lactation. At parturition there were 0·8 per cent band neutrophils in ewe blood, followed by a fall to 0·4 per cent at the 14th day of lactation.

8a.4 MARROW STUDIES

The marrow can be studied in the sheep either by sternal puncture or by puncture of the iliac crest. The former has been far more commonly practised, with sheep fully conscious. For iliac crest puncture it is convenient to anaesthetize the sheep briefly with an intravenous anaesthetic. Of course, excellent marrow smears can be made post mortem from the epiphyses of the long bones so long as the preparations are made within about 15 minutes of death.

Both Grunsell (1951, 1955a b) and Winter (1964b, 1965c) have contributed fully to the English literature on this subject, using the sternal marrow. Depelchin (1956) has described his technique and findings in French, and Schulze and Schützler (1958) have dealt with the normal sternal marrow in German. Winter (1965c) refers to other German authors who have dealt with marrow pictures in disease, and his own small monograph has numerous colour photomicrographs.

It is not necessary here to deal at length with haemopoiesis save in those aspects which may be regarded as peculiar to the sheep. There are no complications to obtaining marrow samples, and the examination of crushed flecks of marrow is simple.

Romanowski staining is adequate, but, as might be expected from the previous comments about neutrophils, it is less distinctive than in human preparations. Winter (1964b, 1965c) has shown that the granules of neutrophils can be seen in the marrow series as early as the myelocyte using Sudan black B staining or the peroxidase reaction. As cells of the neutrophil series mature the cytoplasm becomes increasingly chromophobic.

The erythrocyte series comprises cells which are smaller than those of the human, due to a smaller amount of cytoplasm as a rim about the nucleus. The basophilia of the cytoplasm remains to a greater extent than in man, and young denucleated erythrocytes still retain a blue coloration. The sheep red cell, even when mature, is never as acidophilic as its human equivalent.

It is inevitable that marrow studies have been reported from a limited number of sheep, of different breeds, different states of nutrition, medication, and at different seasons. Winter (1964b) took care to maintain his sheep under conditions where the parasite burden would be minimal, and avoided treating them with anthelminthics. The findings of all the authors are not invalidated by these several factors in so far as basic scientific knowledge is accumulated, but the clinician who wishes to use marrow puncture as a diagnostic tool must appreciate that the conjunction of several 'normal' factors in the life of a sheep on pasture may provide a somewhat different baseline to that which we observe in experimental animals living indoors.

There are considerable differences in the findings of those who have investigated the myeloid erythroid ratio in the marrow. The lowest value is 0·59:1 (Winter 1964b). Grunsell (1951) determined a figure of 1·1:1 while that of Depelchin (1956) is 0·83:1. At this stage it should be pointed out that a considerable part of the marrow is devoted to the production of eosinophils. Grunsell (1951) found that the mean percentage of nucleated cells which comprised the eosinophil series was 18·5 per cent. The neutrophil series equivalent was 29·9 per cent. Winter found the eosinophil series to form 8·76 per cent (the upper limit of his range was 25·4 per cent) while neutrophils and precursors comprised 22·88 per cent of the nucleated cells.

Grunsell suggested that this large eosinophil component of the marrow is an inevitable concomitant of the parasitic infestation of sheep, but Winter has suggested that this distribution may be a characteristic of an individual. Under those circumstances it might be wise to speak of neutrophil/erythrocyte and eosinophil/erythrocyte ratios, rather than of a granulocyte/erythrocyte ratio, his argument being that the special pathology of the sheep might modify one or both granulocyte species independently. This could be disguised by a granulocyte/erythrocyte ratio. Wintrobe *et al* (1974) agree that the eosinophils and basophils should be excluded from the myeloid/erythroid ratio. In these terms the human myeloid/erythroid ratio has a mean value of 2·3:1. (Wintrobe *et al* 1974). Already this ratio, without eosinophils, is far greater than those for sheep quoted above, despite the large eosinophil component which is included. One should bear in mind that the granulocyte is not the predominating leucocyte in the blood of sheep, but of perhaps greater importance in understanding the high proportion of marrow given over to

red cell production, is the remarkable capacity the sheep shows in dealing
with anaemia. The most common anaemias encountered in sheep are those
associated with actual blood loss or red cell destruction. These anaemias are
commonly normocytic and normochromic. Given the opportunity for recovery, the sheep usually takes rapid and full advantage of it. Although it
would be interesting to know when marrow depression does occur in specific
sheep anaemias, the evidence suggests that this is not common. However, one
should perhaps look at the marrow not only from the point of view of the
pathology to which it may be exposed, but from that of the physiology to
which it is continuously exposed.

8a.5 PLATELETS AND COAGULATION

Schermer (1967) commented upon the size of individual platelets, describing
a longitudinal diameter of as much as 5 μm. This would be extremely large
in our experience.

The electron microscope has revealed two kinds of granules in sheep
platelets. Some are homogeneous, while others contain a denser inclusion
with a regular substructure (Wooding personal communication, 1975).

There have been a few determinations of platelet numbers in sheep.

	Range	*Mean*
Schermer (1967)	263–598	$403 \times 10^9/l$
Albritton (1952)	284–659	$441 \times 10^9/l$
Fraser (1929–30)	250–750	$490 \times 10^9/l$
Gajewski (1971)	260–740	$457 \times 10^9/l$

In lambs Fraser (1929–30) found the range to be 540–700 with a mean of
$620 \times 10^9/l$.

The high numbers, when compared with human values, have led Gajewski
(1971) to invoke this as one of several factors which contribute to the ease
with which bleeding can usually be controlled during sheep surgery. Other
factors could be the high platelet adhesiveness and the very low fibrinolytic
activity. In this latter respect there is a significantly lower concentration of
plasminogen in sheep blood than in human blood. The fibrinogen concentration is similar to that in human blood but Fantl and Ward (1960) showed that
factor V is always higher in the sheep than in man, while the prothrombin
level is approximately 70 per cent of the human level. Gajewski's findings for
prothrombin level were even lower (10·5–40·0 as a percentage of the human
control), but the prothrombin time was similar to the human value, and he
comments that, while the levels of factors II (prothrombin), V, VII, and X
were generally different from those in human controls, it is uncertain if there

is any significant physiological difference. Factor VIII is higher in ovine than in human blood.

8a.6 SPECIFIC GRAVITY OF WHOLE BLOOD

Holman (1944) gave 1·052 as a mean value, while Hudson & Osborn (1954) obtained a mean of 1·050, the range being 1·038–1·065. In our laboratory the mean has been determined as 1·052 with a range of 1·049–1·065.

8a.7 PLASMA PROTEINS

There have been a number of studies of serum and plasma proteins in the sheep, to some of which, in the European literature, Schermer (1967) refers. Stubbs and Boyer (1954) did numerous determinations of proteins on rather heavily bled animals. These appear to be plasma values but no description is available as to the technique of determination, or the breeds. The mean value for total proteins was 68 g/l. As each sheep was bled between 36 and 71 times there is a range of mean values for each sheep, this being 64–75 g/l.

In our laboratory a series of 6 Clun Forest sheep (5 wethers and 1 ewe) were used for the collection of a very small daily blood sample, from which 80 values for total plasma proteins were determined by the micro-Kjeldahl method. The mean was 70 g/l with a range of means for the 6 sheep of 63–77 g/l, and an overall range for the 80 determinations of 59–81 g/l.

The identification of plasma protein components in sheep has been based upon comparison with human electrophoretic separation, a system which is open to criticism but which has its convenience. The albumin may show more than one component, depending on the breed, while several globulin components are present. Perk and Lobl (1960) using chiefly Awasi sheep found an increase in total plasma proteins as the lamb matured and became adult. At the same time there was a change in the albumin/globulin ratio: values above unity becoming less than unity as the globulins increased. With increasing immunological experience one would expect the globulins to increase but in Clun Forest sheep studied in this laboratory values in excess of unity have occurred in sheep of 2 years old, and values less than unity in 1-year-old sheep.

The plasma proteins of sheep provide the main plasma lipid transport, as high density lipoproteins (77 per cent) and low density lipoprotein (19 per cent). Very low density lipoproteins are a minor component (4 per cent). The high density lipoproteins move on cellulose acetate with α mobility, while the low density lipoproteins move with β mobility. Suckling lambs have yet another, additional, high density lipoprotein, which disappears at weaning (Kubasek *et al* 1974).

8a.8   ERYTHROCYTE DISEASES

The sheep rarely suffers from primary blood disorders but the blood picture often affords a clue to other diseases.

Most anaemias are parasitic in origin; some are haemolytic due to the toxicity of food factors. Nutritional deficits may be a primary cause, as in cobalt deficiency, but usually they contribute to anaemia from another cause. Haemolysis as the result of immunological phenomena has been inadequately studied.

Leucocyte changes are usually the result of infections or infestations by parasites. They are not usually specific enough to be of much use diagnostically. Leucosis occurs in sheep but it is rare and outside the experience of most veterinarians.

8a.8.1   ANAEMIAS

Normocytic and macrocytic anaemias occur but Holman (1945) pointed out that microcytic anaemias are not seen. However, in a study of post-haemorrhagic anaemia he found anisocytosis in which macrocytes were balanced in numbers by microcytes. Such an anaemia is, by overall quantitative standards, normocytic.

Several authors have studied the effect of gross haemorrhage upon the blood picture, the common finding being the presence of an increasing number of macrocytes. These exhibit punctate basophilia. With recovery of the PCV the macrocytosis diminishes and the Price-Jones curve returns to normal.

Winter (1966b) bled 5 sheep progressively over a period of 9 days and found that the MCV rose, as did the MCH but to a lesser extent. The MCHC fell. These changes became apparent about the fifth day after bleeding began. Volume distribution curves of erythrocytes made throughout the experiment showed the increased number of macrocytes, most of which were basophilic, many showing punctate basophilia. Cells with these characteristics became visible a few days after bleeding began, and were then to be found at all subsequent times during bleeding.

Such an experiment indicates the ability of the sheep to deal with a simple progressive blood loss. It is a common observation that sheep can be repetitively bled and made markedly anaemic without impairing their recovery potential. However, it is reasonable to point out the high nutritional status of most experimental sheep, and the negligible parasite burden which many of them bear. Where parasitism does produce marked anaemia, possibly associated with death, the indications will often be that the blood loss has been great and so long lasting that iron reserves and amino acid supplies have become inadequate. Contributing to this will probably be nutritional inadequacy and inappetence. There must also be awareness of other pathological mechanisms militating against erythropoiesis or red cell survival, as Holmes and Dargie (1975) have discussed when writing on the mechanisms of ovine anaemia. Because morphological changes do not provide a good system for classifying sheep anaemias, they have, as Holman (1945a) did, chosen to classify in terms of aetiology. In this way one can relate anaemias to:

1. Gross nutritional inadequacy, a cause which is almost invariably contributory to other aetiological factors.
2. Inadequate dietary intake of specific nutritional factors (e.g. cobalt).
3. Toxic anaemias due to the ingestion of poisons (e.g. rape)
4. Parasitic anaemias.

This last group, often coupled to group 1, is the largest overall cause of anaemia in sheep. It has been placed last only because it is due to a specific aetiological factor unrelated immediately to food.

It is not necessary to discuss the first group as a separate entity, and one can pass on, therefore, to the second.

8a.8.2 SPECIFIC NUTRITIONAL DEFICIENCIES

Cobalt deficiency has been observed in many countries and gives rise to the condition known as 'pine' in sheep in Scotland. Ruminants synthesize vitamin B_{12} from cobalt in the rumen, and cobalt deficient soil gives rise to a normocytic normochromic anaemia. Sheep plasma B_{12} levels become greatly reduced when the cobalt deficiency has been prolonged. The faecal level also falls. With the decrease in appetite which accompanies the disorder, the diarrhoea and the extreme lacrimation which may occur, there is sometimes a degree of haemoconcentration which serves to support the PCV, haemoglobin and erythrocyte levels. Nevertheless the haemoglobin is often low. Cobalt deficient animals are said to be more susceptible to parasitism and this, in turn, may complicate the picture of anaemia. High levels of iron are found in the liver and spleen which suggests that there is a failure in either iron transport or utilization. The part played in this by cobalt and B_{12} in the sheep is not clear. There is no evidence to show that the red cell life span is diminished as in the human with B_{12} deficiency. The effects of cobalt lack can be countered by the administration of B_{12} alone, as has been shown by Hoekstra *et al* (1952) who measured the changes in haemoglobin concentration as well as observing the sheep clinically.

Copper deficiency may give rise to anaemia in both ewes and lambs (Bennetts & Chapman 1937) but anaemia is a less marked component of the deficiency syndrome in lambs than the obvious neurological signs (swayback, enzootic ataxia). Bennetts and Chapman described the ewes' anaemia as being characterized by a fall in erythrocytes and haemoglobin, a rise in MCV and hyperchromia. Calculations from their figures do not support this last assessment, each MCHC being below those of the normal controls, while the recalculated values for MCH lie within normal limits despite macrocytosis.

Other authors have described the copper deficiency anaemia as macrocytic and hypochromic. Anaemia seen in lambs with severe neurological signs is said to be hypochromic. Treatment with small doses of copper produces a flood of reticulocytes into the circulation and the high haemosiderin content of the spleen, liver and kidney points to defective utilization in erythropoiesis. The few observations that Bennetts and Chapman (1937) made of the marrow showed no erythroid hyperplasia.

Copper appears to be necessary both for the absorption of iron from the bowel and for its incorporation into haemoglobin. This would account for the incapacity to use the iron found in such quantities in the liver, kidney and spleen as haemosiderin. The normal ruminant has a high liver copper content and, as will be discussed later, it can become involved in another disastrous anaemia as a result of chronic copper poisoning. The erythrocyte contains a measurable quantity of copper, but the concentration of the element in sheep erythrocytes is less than that in human erythrocytes.

Iron deficiency due to inadequate intake is said to occur rarely in young lambs whose overall nutrition is poor.

8a.8.3 TOXIC ANAEMIAS

COPPER POISONING

This usually occurs as an acute catastrophe following the persistent ingestion of low levels of excess copper. It is commonly called 'chronic' copper poisoning, though the chronicity relates more to the ingestion and to the inapparent liver damage, than to the clinical condition of acute illness and collapse which usually ends in death. The animal obtains the copper from sprayed pasture, plants which accumulate copper, or from salt licks containing copper. *Heliotropum europaeum* is a plant containing a hepatotoxic alkaloid which interferes with normal copper metabolism and may cause copper poisoning.

The clinical picture is a sudden haemolytic crisis, in which there is massive haemolysis, and during this crisis, or shortly after it, the animal dies. Experimentally, sheep may survive 2 or 3 crises, and Marston (1952) commented on the survival of his Merinos when compared with the English sheep subjected to the same copper feeding but this is unusual in clinical practice.

The condition has been well studied and the sequence of events is probably as follows: copper is accumulated in the liver and there is early evidence of mildly damaged liver function. Plasma and red cell copper remain low, but the plasma bilirubin level may begin to rise slightly. At some point there is a sudden shift of copper to the red cells, and a measurable rise in blood copper. The haematocrit rapidly increases and bilirubin may then be obvious in the spun plasma. The sheep will probably have dirtily jaundiced sclera. The haematocrit rise is accompanied by a red cell and haemoglobin rise, though it has been suggested that cellular swelling is also involved in the PCV rise. Red cell reduced glutathione falls, and haemolysis follows this with haemoglobinaemia and a neutrophilia. The haematocrit falls rapidly to low levels. The sheep becomes prostrate, may occasionally show nervous system signs and usually dies within 1–2 days. The liver and kidney contain large amounts of copper at post mortem.

The repeated episodes of haemolysis which were observed by Ishmael *et al* (1972) were each associated with a raised blood copper. We have followed one ewe which has been shown to have a high liver copper content (biopsied twice) and who has passed through a raised blood copper episode without haemolysis.

The main outstanding points of this intriguing condition appear to be the early functional liver damage associated with the excess copper in the diet (Todd & Thompson 1963, Ishmael *et al* 1972); the shift of copper to the red cells at some stage, possible associated with a critical level of liver damage, for there appears to be a sharp increase in the evidence of liver damage; the fall in reduced glutathione (Todd & Thompson 1963); and the unknown mechanism of haemolysis. Glutathione is known as an agent whose absence from the red cell is coupled with a tendency to haemolysis (glutathione synthetase deficiency in humans). Glutathione deficient red cells in Finnish Landrace sheep have a shortened life span (Tucker 1974). That the glutathione fall apparently precedes haemolysis may be significant in understanding the gross cellular breakdown. The increase in methaemoglobin at the time of the haemolytic crisis may be a reflection of the glutathione fall.

If the sheep survives haemolysis it replaces its red cell population with markedly anisocytotic and poikilocytotic red cells.

The precipitating event which provokes a haemolytic crisis is often described as stress but there has been no apparent stress situation in our own affected sheep, and the ewe with a high liver copper level, referred to above, has undergone two surgical biopsies without haemolysis.

Ammonium molybdate has been used successfully in flocks where instances of copper poisoning have occurred, to prevent further episodes. Molybdenum acts by limiting copper storage by the liver (Dick 1953) and consequently its presence in the soil must have some influence upon the incidence of copper poisoning. We have used D-penicillamine (a chelating agent) orally and by intravenous injection in acutely ill sheep. While in one instance it may have helped to prolong life for a fortnight, it has not been adequately studied experimentally in animals known to be accumulating copper and it is too expensive for flock use. Transfusion with compatible packed red cells, which has restored the haematocrit, has done little to improve the condition of a sheep acutely ill following haemolysis.

Sodium chlorate, which is used as a weedkiller, has caused poisoning in sheep by converting haemoglobin to methaemoglobin. It has been studied by several workers, and while there is no doubt that, once the methaemoglobin level has reached values of 80–90 per cent of the total pigment content, the animal will collapse and subsequently die, the work of both McCulloch and Murer (1939) and Frank (1948) has shown, surprisingly and convincingly, that sheep fed solely upon sprayed herbage for many days exhibit no signs of illness, and in one sheep there was no appreciable amount of methaemoglobin in the blood. Sheep enjoy chlorate sprayed plants and it is not clear if dilution, or the conversion of chlorate to chloride before or after entering the rumen, is responsible for the absence of toxicity in these realistic experiments.

Methaemoglobin formation is also characteristic of *nitrate poisoning*, which occurs in sheep fed upon plants with a high nitrate content. *Salvia reflexa*, the wild mint, or mint weed of Australia, is one such poisonous plant. Fortunately, with a choice of food, sheep avoid plants which contain a large amount of inorganic nitrate. The nitrate is converted, at some stage, to nitrite, possibly by plant enzymes released on maceration, possibly by rumen enzymes, or possibly by reduction in the liver. The plant material itself is free of the nitrite which is responsible for the conversion of haemoglobin to methaemoglobin. With this conversion taking place on a great enough scale the blood of the animal begins to appear brown and, eventually, the animal collapses. There is no haemolysis, even at death, which may be delayed for only 8 hours if sufficient nitrate has been ingested. Bradley *et al* (1940) showed the efficacy of intravenous methylene blue as an antidote in cattle, and an excellent demonstration of the revival of a sheep acutely poisoned by a large oral dose of nitrite was described by Scott (1941). The oxygen capacity of the blood had fallen from 14·6 to 5·1 ml/dl over 5 hours, and the anoxic sheep had collapsed. It was then injected with 0·6 per cent methylene blue in normal saline. After 30 minutes the sheep had recovered, and, at 1 hour, the oxygen capacity of the blood was restored to 11·6 ml/dl.

KALE POISONING
Ingestion of plants of the Brassica family, including rape and kale, produce a variety of signs in sheep, notably a haemolytic anaemia of which haemo-globinuria and jaundice may be the outward clinical signs. The anaemia can-not be related to any deficiency, but appears to be due to some toxic factor which is destroyed by dry heat and by ensilage. Sheep which are fed kale develop a relatively mild anaemia (Greenhalgh *et al* 1969, recorded a lowest haemoglobin of 7·3 g/dl). Some animals begin to recover from this anaemia while still eating kale but recovery takes longer than the recovery of kale fed cattle from a more severe anaemia. Penny *et al* (1964) bled a single animal and allowed it to recover before feeding it kale alongside an unbled animal. The latter became anaemic, while the previously bled animal did not. The increase

in the number of cells bearing Heinz bodies is characteristic of kale poisoning but these hardly increased in the pre-bled sheep, while in the normal kale fed sheep they increased to 37 per cent. Eventually they increased in the pre-bled sheep, an animal which, at the beginning of kale feeding, had a large number of young red cells in its circulation after its recovery from bleeding. If these young cells are less susceptible to haemolysis by the toxic factor in kale and less prone to Heinz body formation than older cells, the freedom of the pre-bled sheep from kale-induced anaemia would be explained. Kale feeding produced no significant change in erythrocyte osmotic fragility.

The toxic factor in kale has been sought by Smith *et al* (1974) who showed that both S-methyl cysteine sulphoxide and S-methyl cysteine are present in the haemolytic fraction from kale. Both substances give rise to methanethiol and dimethyl disulphide in the rumen, and these authors noted the resemblance of these compounds to the disulphides which Gruhzit (1931b) had shown to cause fatal haemolytic anaemia in dogs.

ONION POISONING

Sheep fed upon wild onion are said to develop a haemolytic anaemia, as do cattle. However this is neither a common food nor a common problem. Dogs which are fed fresh or boiled spanish onions are very rapidly afflicted with haemolytic anaemia as Gruhzit (1931a) showed. Unable to obtain allyl propyl disulphide, a constituent of oil of onions, Gruhzit went on to select similar compounds having -S-S- linkages and found that both n-propyl disulphide and di-p-tolyl disulphide, neither of which compounds occur in onions, could produce a fatal haemolytic anaemia. Nor did the animals develop towards these compounds the tolerance which they eventually developed towards onions (Gruhzit 1931b). It is only fair to this author to stress that he was not using the compound found in onions and which he suspected of being responsible for the anaemia and that he commented upon being able to produce a similar fatal anaemia with phenylhydrazine which is structurally unrelated to his thiol compounds. The chemical which causes haemolysis in onion poisoning of sheep remains unknown.

BRACKEN POISONING

This is much less of a problem in sheep than in cattle. Sheep will not readily eat bracken if other food is available. Moreover, a very large quantity has to be eaten over a long period of time to produce symptoms of poisoning. Anaemia is only a small component of the haematological misfortune which then overtakes the sheep. There is a marked fall in the number of platelets accompanied by a fall in leucocytes, notably granulocytes. The depression of marrow activity extends to the erythrocytes, although the fall in their numbers is late in appearance. Bleeding occurs at several sites, especially the stomach, lungs, heart, spleen and small intestine (Parker & McCrea 1965) and bacterial infection with *Pasteurella* may occur. This bleeding must contribute, however little, to the anaemia. The extent of the bleeding may be apparent by the quantity of blood in the faeces. The clinical evidence suggests the existence of a bone marrow depressant as the toxic factor in bracken.

8a.8.4 PARASITIC ANAEMIAS

These comprise the greatest single group of sheep anaemias, less well studied, perhaps, than their bovine equivalents but more accessible to study and diagnosis post mortem. As blood disorders they are usually incidental find-ings in an ailing sheep, providing a clue to the cause of the illness. They may be contributory causes of death. Treatment is by removal of the parasite. The mechanisms by which the anaemias are produced are not always clear, and there may be factors other than the persistent blood loss which is ap-parent in some cases, and by no means obvious in others. Some of these other factors (e.g. suppression of erythropoiesis) have been investigated. Many will undoubtedly remain uninvestigated because of the economic unimportance of this aspect of infestation.

HELMINTHS
The largest group of parasites causing these anaemias are the nematodes.
Haemonchus contortus has a worldwide distribution, providing little clinical problem in low rainfall areas but widespread in its pathogenic effects in the damper parts of the USA and in southern Europe. This nematode attaches itself to the mucosa of the abomasum, sucks blood and then is said to detach itself, leaving a persisting bleeding point. In lambs it can cause death by pro-gressive blood loss. In adults the anaemia may be severe, but death from blood loss *per se* must be rare. Resistance and immunity often develop in older animals, but these are dependent upon good nutrition. There is no doubt about the part played by simple blood loss in this anaemia. If the loss is heavy, macrocytosis and hypochromia are apparent. A lighter infestation will produce less blood loss, and a normocytic normochromic anaemia. Severe infestations lead to depletion of iron stores: PCV is diminished, and eventually the fall in serum iron concentrations shows that the compensatory mechan-isms which had increased erythropoiesis in the marrow are failing.
Trichostrongylus colubriformis, which is found in the small intestine, has been experimentally investigated and is a known cause of anaemia in lambs between 4 and 12 months old. The anaemia produced is seldom severe, the PCV, haemoglobin and red cell numbers falling while the plasma volume remains constant. If the animal survives there is a spontaneous increase in the erythrocyte indices. In one instance (Gallagher 1963) the PCV fell to about 0·17 l/l whatever the larval dose, but by the end of the 4-month experiment the values had risen to 0·25 l/l. Horak *et al* (1968) described severe experimental

infestations in which there was a small rise in PCV and haemoglobin about 14 days after infestation and immediately prior to death. This was not due to a fall in plasma volume. Eosinophil numbers fell progressively in these cases. However, neither Turner (1959) nor Gallagher (1963) had noted a rise in PCV or haemoglobin except when recovery occurred. Gallagher (1963) also studied leucocyte numbers, finding little total change, with no regular eosinophilia, and, in the latter part of his experiment, an increase in neutrophils at the expense of lymphocyte numbers.

The problem posed here is the mechanism of the anaemia, for there can be few who believe that *Trichostrongylus colubriformis* can suck blood. Into a similar problem class must be placed *Ostertagia circumcincta*, *Trichostrongylus axei* (both of which are found in the abomasum), and *Nematodirus*, which is found in the bowel. If the anaemia is not due to haemorrhage and haemolysis cannot be invoked, which would be apparent in the urine and plasma, we are driven back to the hypothetical causes. These include the prevention of absorption of essential nutrients, or their utilization, or the production of some factor which can depress erythropoietic activity (but, in the case of *Trichostrongylus colubriformis*, having no depressive effect upon the leucopoietic activity of the marrow). Moreover we must take into consideration the speed at which anaemia can be produced in lambs following experimental infestation.

Horak *et al* (1968) showed that with *Trichostrongylus colubriformis* in Merinos and Dorpers there was a fall in plasma albumin, not caused by haemodilution, followed by a rise in α, β and γ globulins during recovery. The final total plasma protein concentration was little less than the initial value, despite the depression of the albumin/globulin ratio. The plasma protein loss was further studied by Barker (1973) who showed that Merino lambs lost labelled protein into the gut when showing clinical signs of trichostrongylosis. Cross-bred lambs, even with heavier worm burdens, showed neither signs, nor plasma protein loss.

Cooperia, *Chabertia ovina*, *Oesophagostomum columbianum* and *Strongyloides papillosus* are all intestinal worms which have been implicated in the production of anaemia. About all of them there is doubt regarding the significance, or even occurrence, of direct blood loss, and the contribution made by other mechanisms.

Bunostomum trigonocephalum and *Gaigeria pachyscelis*, found in the intestine, leave no doubt about their blood sucking activities, and whatever other mechanisms may be involved, haemorrhage is certainly a major contributor to this anaemia.

Trichuris ovis may cause mild anaemia by blood sucking in the caecum, and even lungworm (*Dictyocaulus*) has been implicated in anaemia, although it seems likely that the responsible parasite was another worm living in the gut.

Fascioliasis, whether the parasite be *Fasciola hepatica* or *F. gigantica*,

Fascioloides magna (passed from deer and elk to sheep) or *Dicrocoelium dendriticum*, is the major trematode cause of sheep anaemia, having a world-wide occurrence. The anaemia is often severe and its causative mechanisms have produced much speculation, argument, and research. The young flukes, migrating through the liver parenchyma, cause considerable tissue damage and often a heavy loss of blood. If the number of parasites is overwhelming and the liver damage is severe, the so-called acute disease, death may occur at this stage. *Clostridium oedematiens* may play a part in this. More commonly the adult flukes of a more limited infestation then settle in the bile ducts, and, by their blood sucking, cause a considerable blood loss into the intestine via the bile. Several workers have studied aspects of this sequence and one account of it has been given recently by Holmes and Dargie, (1975). Isotopic studies have shown the breakdown products of haemoglobin to pass out of the body in the faeces and not through the kidney, so eliminating intra-vascular haemolysis as a mechanism of cell destruction. The study of the caecal contents of flukes, the presence of blood in the bile, and the clot-covered lesions in the bile duct epithelium where flukes had been attached, all afford substantial evidence for the loss of blood through the biliary tract and the intestine. There is evidence that erythropoiesis, far from being depressed, is increased during the anaemia. Iron deficiency only occurs in sheep that have long-lasting infections. Sinclair (1964) studying the normo-cytic normochromic anaemia of fascioliasis, compared the anaemia developed by fluke infected sheep with that produced by regular bleeding and found well-marked differences. The anaemia produced by bleeding 60 ml of blood each day did not compare in severity with that of the infestation anaemia. It became stable, while the fascioliasis anaemia increased. After 14 days of bleeding there was marked erythroid activity in the marrow, while the increased marrow activity in fascioliasis did not appear until 36 days after the onset of anaemia. Even then the response was less. Sinclair (1964) suggested that disturbances in protein metabolism could play a part. Holmes *et al* (1968), aware of the hypoalbuminaemia of fascioliasis, labelled sheep albumin with ^{131}I and used it to show the shortened half life of the albumin in infected animals compared with the controls. There appeared to be a loss of albumin in the bile followed by degradation in the gut, a not unexpected finding in view of the route of blood loss. Holmes and Dargie (1975) refer to recent work showing terminal extremely low serum iron levels and hypochromia, evidence of the gross depletion of iron reserves.

Confirmation of the diagnosis of this anaemia is the finding of fluke eggs, and the post mortem revelation of flukes. Treatment is that of removing the flukes.

Schistosoma bovis afflicts sheep in southern Europe, Africa and Asia, while *S. mattheei* is an important parasite of sheep in South Africa. It is said that the neutral or alkaline reaction of the rumen and omasum permits the survival of those cercariae which have been ingested. Larvae find their way into the portal blood and, subsequently, into the mesenteric veins. Thereafter they produce eggs, and, at this stage, the disease becomes apparent. Eggs are usually found in the faeces about 6 weeks after experimental infection. Before that, at the 5th week, Preston *et al* (1973a) found no significant differences in PCV between the infected sheep and their controls. The PCV then began to fall and even at that time there was evidence of diminished erythropoiesis (Dargie & Preston 1974). The initial fall in PCV was due solely to haemodilution, there being no fall in red cell mass at this time despite the dyshaemopoiesis. After the appearance of eggs in the faeces, gastro-intestinal bleeding began, with frank blood in the stools. The PCV fell faster, as did the red cell numbers. Usually bleeding was a transient feature over the period of 4–6 weeks following the appearance of eggs and the major change in PCV was during this period, the fall steadying around 0·17 l/l. Changes beyond this were small. The MCV was within normal limits, if somewhat lower than the controls. The anaemia was normocytic and normochromic but, in two sheep which died, there was a terminal macrocytosis in the week prior to death. Mild hypochromia was seen terminally in some cases. No haemolytic activity was observed and it was suggested by Preston and Dargie (1974) that this contrast with schistosomiasis in other species (e.g. mouse) may be associated with the absence of splenomegaly in this condition in the sheep, however long the infestation. The infested animals did not appear able to utilize significant amounts of the iron passing in blood down the intestine. Despite this, frank iron deficiency did not occur, and there was a normal total plasma iron.

Malherbe (1970) commented on the lack of leucocytic changes in experimentally infected sheep, apart from a rise in eosinophils in single isolated determinations. He also remarked the rise in plasma proteins, despite a fall in albumin concentration, and the fall in albumin/globulin ratio. Preston *et al* (1973a) showed that the albumin began to fall about 6 weeks after infection. Labelled albumin studies indicated that this fall was compounded of haemodilution, plasma loss into the gut, and impaired synthesis. The major component of the globulin rise was γ globulin, but there was some rise in α and β globulins also. It is worthy of note that the globulin concentration rose despite the increase in plasma volume, which showed an average rise of 38 per cent by the 8th week. The plasma expansion began about the time of oviposition, possibly even earlier, and sodium and water retention appeared to precede the faecal blood loss (Preston *et al* 1973b).

8a.8.5 ERYTHROCYTE PARASITES

Anaplasmosis is not a very important sheep disease. Widespread in incidence, it gives rise to anaemia, jaundice, and enlargement of the spleen. The literature suggests that the acute disease produces clinical signs. However, in a group of experimentally infected sheep Splitter *et al* (1956) saw no clinical evidence of disease. Splenectomy, however, greatly increases the susceptibility of sheep to infection, and such animals may die.

The causative organism, *Anaplasma ovis*, is classed with the *Bartonellaceae*, and appears in Romanowsky stained films as a dark disc, 0·3–1·0 μm in diameter, overlying and close to the margin of an erythrocyte. Splitter *et al* (1956) found that 0·8 per cent of sheep red cells became infected. The organisms appeared in the blood 12 days after infection, and increased in number for a further 9 days. The anaemia achieved its lowest blood values after the parasites had passed their maximum number. The mean lowest haematocrit value was 0·244 l/l, the haemoglobin descending to 8·0 g/dl. No leucocyte changes occurred.

Sheep were infected with *Anaplasma ovis* by Kreier *et al* (1964) who found a rise in the marrow erythropoietic activity during anaemia. Erythropoietin titres rose before the anaemia became severe and persisted into the recovery period (Jatkar & Kreier 1967). Much of the work upon the anaemia of anaplasmosis (*A. marginale*) has been done upon calves and there is evidence there that phagocytosis of infected erythrocytes occurs in the marrow and in the spleen. There is now much evidence to suggest that phagocytosis is extended to normal red cells and that this is associated with the appearance of an auto-antibody which may coat the cells.

Splitter *et al* (1956) showed that *A. ovis* did not infect or even survive in splenectomized calves, although it produces greater effects in goats than in sheep.

Eperythrozoon ovis is an organism which, like *Anaplasma*, belongs to the *Bartonellaceae*. It has a wide distribution, and is probably disseminated by biting insects. Infection may be accompanied by no obvious clinical signs, and detection of the organism is usually in unthrifty sheep with varying degrees of anaemia. The degree of response to infection may be related to breed susceptibilities, nutrition, and the size of the initial parasite infestation, but it has been suggested that there may be strains of the parasite with differing degrees of virulence. It has defeated attempts to culture it and it can exhibit a startling pleomorphism. It is said to infect goats.

In Romanowsky stained films it usually appears as a purple ring 0·4–0·5 μm in diameter overlying erythrocytes but sometimes free in the plasma. The ring may have up to 3 points on it which are darker staining, or there may be a short rod-like extension on one or on 2 opposite sides. It can exist as a short rod similar in form to *Pasteurella*, and, as the number of organisms in the blood increases, a variety of forms beyond these may appear. Chains of organisms resembling tiny *streptococci*, filaments resembling leptospirae, ovoids, rods, commas, dumb-bells, triangles with rounded angles and even large pale circles, 2 μm in diameter, have been described, the last during the falling phase of parasitaemia. Under phase-contrast microscopy the ring forms appear as spheres. Kreier and Ristic (1963) studied the ultrastructure and commented that, when the parasite lay against the red cell membrane, it appeared to have caused erosion or partial penetration.

After experimental infection there is an incubation period of about a week but ranging from 2 days to a month, and the first appearance of organisms in blood films is usually followed by a rapid increase in number so that they come to exceed the number of red cells by as much as 25–100 times. The number of parasites has been seen to fall or virtually disappear with the onset of anaemia, while in some recorded cases there have been concurrent anaemia and parasitaemia. In mild disease the anaemia is normocytic and normochromic but a severe anaemia is macrocytic and normochromic. There is an increase in the erythroid elements of the marrow at the height of the anaemia.

Øveras (1969) has described the cell morphology in detail. Both anisocytosis and poikilocytosis were seen in heavily infected animals, the former coinciding with high reticulocyte counts, as did the occasional occurrence of late normoblasts in the circulating blood. Heinz bodies, not uncommon in sheep, rose in numbers, so that as many as 50 per cent of the red cells had them during heavy haemolysis and haemoglobinuria.

While in moderate infections the red cell count may change little, heavy infections cause a 40–60 per cent fall in erythrocyte count, associated with a comparable haemoglobin fall, and followed by a plateau and a rise.

In most of Øveras' sheep 75–100 per cent of the red cells showed infection at an early stage. With a high degree of infection 3 animals showed *Eperythrozoon ovis* continuously in the blood with little fluctuation for more than a year. Relapses, with from 2 to 4 distinct periods of parasitaemia, were common in most sheep. Foggie and Nisbet (1964) observed continuous infection for a minimum of six weeks. They also noted that spontaneous infections occurred in summer and autumn.

The mechanism of the anaemia is haemolytic. Other contributory mechanisms have not been described. Erythropoiesis appears to compensate rapidly for the cell destruction. Haemoglobinuria is common in severe infections, and icterus has been described. Littlejohns (1960) who observed large pale erythrocytes in films from infected sheep, suggested that the exogenous enzymes of the parasites could have digested the red cell contents. However, there is nothing more than speculation to reveal the nature of the haemolytic process.

Ferric iron is found as haemosiderin granules in the cytoplasm of kidney convoluted tubule cells, and in the phagocytic cells of the red pulp of the spleen, which is sometimes enlarged. Total plasma proteins fall, and there is a rise in the serum bilirubin level.

Experimental infection has rarely led to death. It is not easy to assess the frequency of eperythrozoon infections. They are not, however, a serious cause of anaemia in sheep, and recovery from infection is the common outcome.

Babesiasis (piroplasmosis) is an infection of erythrocytes with a protozoan, either *Babesia ovis* or *B. motasi*. These organisms belong to the *Haemosporidia*. Babesiasis in sheep has been reported from many countries. The parasites are found in erythrocytes as paired pear-shaped organisms, lying parallel with their pointed ends adjacent. They may however be single, ovoid, or round. The anaemia which they produce is haemolytic, and associated with jaundice and haemoglobinuria. Splenomegaly is not uncommon, and liver degeneration has been reported.

Theileriasis is an infection of the blood with *Theileria ovis* or *T. hirci*. *T. ovis*, commonly found in South Africa, is mildly pathogenic, producing fever and a mild anaemia. *T. hirci* is uncommon in sheep but has clinical importance mainly in tropical regions where it may produce jaundice, anaemia and splenomegaly. *Theileria* in red cells appear either annular, or in the form of rods, and are accompanied by Koch's blue bodies, tiny masses of blue cytoplasm (in Giemsa stained films) which can be found in lymphocytes or free in the plasma. They are 1–2 μm in diameter.

8a.8.6   BACTERIAL AND VIRAL ANAEMIAS

The haemolytic anaemias associated with bacterial infection in sheep are but aspects of a wider and often fatal disease picture. *Clostridium oedematiens* and *Leptospira pomona*, both of which produce disease in sheep, can produce haemolysins. The mechanisms by which red cells are destroyed in vivo by the latter organism has been the subject of a good deal of study and it is still open to proof that immune phenomena contribute to the haemolysis.

Anaemia is not uncommon in caseous lymphadenitis (*Corynebacterium pseudotuberculosis*).

A viral anaemia of sheep and goats was described in Algeria by Donatien and Lestoquard (1926) who observed, amongst many signs, a 50–70 per cent fall in red cells, anisocytosis and poikilocytosis but no punctate basophilia of red cells, which caused them to think that there was no compensation. There was no change in the leucocytes. The blood, bone marrow, and urine were infective, and passage through a filter suggested that the agent must be a virus. While it was possible to transmit the disease to horses, asses and monkeys, it could not be transmitted to dogs, rabbits or chickens. On the other hand, the virus of equine infectious anaemia (it must be assumed from the description in this paper) could not be transmitted to sheep or to monkeys, suggesting a different virus. More recently there has been evidence that equine infectious anaemia can be transmitted to sheep.

8a.9 LEUCOCYTE DISEASES

Sheep have a very low incidence of neoplasia. Of neoplasms which do occur, lymphoma or lymphosarcoma is one of the more common (Cotchin 1960). It is, nevertheless, a rare condition, usually diagnosed post mortem. Migaki (1969) quoted a figure for the incidence of 1 in 200,000 slaughtered animals per year in an American series. Of 17 histologically confirmed lymphomas, 15 were in older animals. All had multiple neoplasms. In all animals the lymph nodes were involved, and the liver, spleen and kidneys were implicated in 40 per cent of cases. The heart, uterus or thymus were not involved in any animal. Of these lymphomas, 10 were described histologically as lymphocytic, and 7 as histiocytic.

Leucosis is to be found more commonly in the German literature. Enke *et al* (1961) described their findings in a single flock of sheep where the incidence was remarkably high. The haematological diagnosis was based upon the total number of leucocytes and the differential count, in a manner which had been applied to the diagnosis of leucosis in cattle. Both the total count and the differential were classified as normal, suspect, or leucotic. There is little about cell types, but the authors recorded some unusually high total and lymphocyte counts, with low numbers of neutrophils. Red cell levels generally remained high. Post mortem findings showed gross lymphocytic infiltration into muscle and organs.

Rudolph and Paulsen (1972) described the ultrastructure of ovine leucosis lymphocytes, from both blood and lymph nodes. The nuclei had granular nucleoli, while within the cytoplasm were many ribosomes, coarse mitochondria, and rough-surfaced endoplasmic reticulum. There were particles in some cells which had no counterpart in control lymphocytes, and which resembled A type virus particles. This finding and the high incidence of leucosis in the flock studied by Enke *et al* (where of 45 sheep the blood picture indicated leucosis in 8 and suspected leucosis in another 12) suggest an infective agent as the cause of leucosis in sheep. Enke *et al* commented that the flock they studied was in a region where bovine leucosis was frequently seen.

It seems likely that ovine leucosis will continue to be recognized more from emaciation with gross lymphatic tumours than by its blood picture and one must hope that it will continue to remain an unfamiliar disorder.

Myelogenous leukaemia has been described as occurring in sheep.

Listeriosis, caused by *Listeria monocytogenes*, does not produce in sheep the mononucleosis which it produces in monogastric animals. This appears to be a distinction of the ruminants, as Gray and Killinger (1966) pointed out. Listeric septicaemia in adult sheep is unusual, its most frequent incidence being in south-eastern Europe and the USSR. Usually the response to infection is a localized encephalitis. Olsen *et al* (1950) described a neutrophil leucocytosis and a fall in the circulating lymphocytes. Immature neutrophils became prominent in the blood.

Tick-borne fever is an infection of sheep by what is thought to be a Rickettsia demonstrable within leucocytes by light microscopy. The infection appears to be carried by ticks, but it can be transmitted by injecting whole blood, serum, or tissues from an infected animal. It is a febrile illness with a rapid rise in temperature, followed by a decline to normal temperatures over a period of several days. The organisms, thought to be *Rickettsia ovina*, or a similar variety, are found in neutrophil, eosinophil and basophil granulocytes, and in monocytes. They appear a few hours before the fever, and persist for 2 or 3 weeks.

In Romanowsky stained films the organisms stain from pale grey to near black, and are found in the cytoplasm singly or in clusters. They exhibit pleomorphism, being round, oval or rod-shaped, with dimensions from 0·5–4·0 μm. Gordon *et al* (1962) illustrated a variety of forms which are encountered. They divided the morphological variations into 3 types. Type I is small, rounded, or rod-shaped, $0·5 \times 0·3$ μm staining deep purple with Giemsa and frequently lying at the cell periphery. Large rounded forms lie deeper in the cytoplasm and measure as much as $2 \times 1·3$ μm, but quite commonly such forms appear to have become fragmented. This is defined as Type II.

A round or oval mass, stained greyish blue or deep purple and containing even deeper staining rounded particles, constitutes Type III inclusion. Such morulae may be up to 4 μm in their greatest diameter. Different types of inclusion may occur within the same cell. Type I is constantly found and is the most frequent, while Type III is the least common. Most of the blood neutrophils may carry inclusions within a short time of an animal being experimentally infected.

Following infection the temperature of the sheep rises and there is a neutrophilia but as the temperature subsides, a neutropenia occurs for a few days before the return of the neutrophil count to normal or slightly raised levels. The parasites decline in numbers and may disappear during the temperature fall and the neutropenic phase. There may be a relapse, with reappearance of the parasites, a month or so after the first attack. The blood remains infective for several months after an attack although no parasites may be apparent.

Death is uncommon as a result of tick-borne fever alone but there appear to be variations in virulence between strains. As it frequently accompanies louping ill, which is also carried by ticks, and probably predisposes the sheep to other diseases, it may contribute considerably to the morbidity within a flock.

Sulphadimidine has been described as suppressing the organism in the blood, but it does not cure the infection.

Table 8a.1   Sheep: normal values

	Mean	*Range*
Erythrocytes	$12 \times 10^{12}/l$	$9–15 \times 10^{12}/l$
PCV	0·33 l/l	0·26–0·42 l/l
Diameter	4·5 μm	3–8 μm
Volume (MCV)	32 fl	28–40 fl
Hb	12g/dl	8–16 g/dl
MCH	10 pg	8–12 pg
MCHC	33 g/dl	31–38 g/dl
Leucocytes	$8 \times 10^9/l$	$4–12 \times 10^9/l$
Lymphocytes %	63	50–75
Neutrophils %	30	10–50
Eosinophils %	4	2–12
Basophils %	<0·5	0–1
Monocytes %	3	2–8
Platelets	$450 \times 10^9/l$	$250–750 \times 10^9/l$

Table 8a.2   Sheep: absolute leucocyte numbers

	Mean absolute numbers
Total	$8·00 \times 10^9/l$
Lymphocytes	$5·00 \times 10^9/l$
Neutrophils	$2·40 \times 10^9/l$
Eosinophils	$0·32 \times 10^9/l$
Basophils	$0·03 \times 10^9/l$
Monocytes	$0·25 \times 10^9/l$

(b) THE GOAT

There is comparatively little haematological literature concerning the goat. Such as there is remains fragmentary and has been collected from several varieties in many parts of the world.

8b.1 BLOOD VOLUME

Using the Evans blue (T1824) dye method upon 50 animals in order, initially, to determine the plasma volume, and using the haematocrit to calculate the

336

blood volume, the following values were obtained by Walker and Dziemian (1950):

Blood volume range: 87·8–93·5 ml/kg with a mean
                     value of 90·2 ml/kg
Mean red cell volume: 27·3 ml/kg
Mean plasma volume: 62·9 ml/kg

8b.2 THE ERYTHROCYTE

8b.2.1 DIAMETER

These extremely small cells have a diameter between 1·5 and 5 μm, with a mean of 3·2 μm (Holman & Dew 1963). MCV varies from 15 to 39 fl with a mean of 20–22 fl depending upon the literature source. The degree of aniso-cytosis is variable. It may be very marked but, more commonly, one encounters a blood film in which almost all the red cells appear similar in size while 2 or 3 in any microscope field are 50 per cent larger in diameter than the majority of their fellows. Anisocytosis is more obvious in kids under one month old. It is not uncommon to see a film in which the cells vary in shape, so that many appear roughly triangular. The cell has a biconcavity which is obvious on focusing.

8b.2.2 NUMBER

The numbers of red cells vary considerably, from 7 to $21 \times 10^{12}/l$, a value for the mean lying between 13 and $15 \times 10^{12}/l$ in the adult goat, again depending upon the source. Figures for Indian goats e.g. mixed Gujarat breed (Vaidya *et al* 1970) lie below this level, and the haemoglobin values for these goats are also low by western standards.

8b.2.3 PACKED CELL VOLUME

Again there are considerable variations. In adult animals the range is from 0·19–0·40 l/l with a mean of 0·29 l/l. To obtain acceptable values with such small cells the centrifugal force must be of the order of that exerted in the microhaematocrit centrifuge. A duration of 10 minutes in such a machine ensures minimal plasma trapping. Schalm *et al* (1975) regard goats with a PCV below 0·22 l/l as anaemic, for such a low PCV usually accompanies a low haemoglobin value.

8b.2.4   FRAGILITY

Perk *et al* (1964) showed that the erythrocytes of young kids were more osmotically resistant and formed a more heterogeneous population in this respect than adult cells. However, there was a progressive change to the homogeneity of cells from the adult by about the 6th week of life. Haemolysis of adult cells began in 0·66 per cent saline and was complete by 0·44 per cent saline. These values compare well with those observed by Holman and Dew (1965a) where extreme values for adults are quoted as 0·60–0·40 per cent saline. The increased resistance of kid cells is also apparent in their results, where, however, the width of the range remains similar despite the changing age of the animal.

8b.2.5   HAEMOGLOBIN

Red cells of adult goats contain A, B, or AB haemoglobins. Fetal haemoglobin (F) is found in kids during the first eight weeks of life. Haemoglobin C is produced in response to heavy bleeding by HbA and HbAB animals and Blunt *et al* (1969) showed, in a limited number of animals, that the goat appeared to produce haemoglobin C more readily than the sheep subjected to similar bleeding over a similar period. HbC was present in the blood of goats at higher concentrations and for longer periods than in the blood of sheep following the same procedures.

The haemoglobin content of goat blood is 8–16 g/dl with a mean of 11 g/dl. It must, however, be pointed out that there are many mean values in the literature from tropical areas which lie well below this figure. Vaidya *et al* (1970) found that the mean adult haemoglobin value of mixed Gujarat-bred goats was 7·7 g/dl. In native Philippine goats Gonzaga and De Guzman (1964) recorded a mean value of 9·7 g/dl, their highest value being 11·03 g/dl. Mukherjee and Bhattacharya (1952) had an upper limit of 7·4 g/dl to their range. These are very low values for healthy animals in more temperate regions, but one must have due regard for the frequency with which such values have been recorded elsewhere.

The following are typical corpuscular values:

MCH   5·3–8·4 pg with a mean of 6·9 pg
MCHC   32–40 g/dl with a mean of 37 g/dl

8b.2.6   SEDIMENTATION

Rouleau formation is rare and sedimentation negligible. Similar comments can be made for the goat as for the sheep where this subject is dealt with more fully. As a clinical aid the ESR is of little value.

8b.2.7 RED CELL CHANGES WITH GROWTH

Holman and Dew (1964, 1965a) and DeShaw *et al* (1969) have measured changes occurring in young goats. In the former series an erythrocyte count of $8\cdot14 \times 10^{12}/l$ at birth fell, by the seventh day to $7\cdot3 \times 10^{12}/l$, only to rise to $20 \times 10^{12}/l$ at 3 months. Adult levels were reached in the 3rd year. DeShaw *et al* (1969), using Spanish goat kids, show in a graph a mean erythrocyte count of $17\cdot6 \times 10^{12}/l$ for the third month of life.

The PCV is high at birth, Holman and Dew (1964) showing that from $0\cdot37$ l/l at birth it fell to $0\cdot24$ l/l at 1 month, rose to $0\cdot34$ l/l at 3 months, and achieved an adult value of $0\cdot28$ l/l in the 3rd year. This was associated with a change in MCV, from large cells at birth (45 fl) to smaller cells by the 3rd month (17 fl), with a succeeding rise to adult values between 2 and 3 years (24 fl). DeShaw *et al* show graphically that the PCV at 1 month is $0\cdot185$ l/l, rising to $0\cdot26$ l/l at 3 months. At 12 months it was $0\cdot284$ l/l. The MCV at 1 month was 20 fl, and at 3 months was $14\cdot8$ fl. At 12 months it was $14\cdot9$ fl.

Holman and Dew (1964) showed that the mean corpuscular diameter of 5 μm at birth falls to 3 μm between the 1st and 2nd month and remains at this value.

Anisocytosis was most apparent in the 1st month, and misshapen cells, seen between the 1st and 3rd month, gave the appearance of sickling, an impression which could be removed by lowering the pH to $6\cdot0$. Immature red cells were rare and some cells displaying punctate basophilia were seen in half the kids studied, but all such cells had vanished by the 7th week.

Haemoglobin fell from $12\cdot25$ g/dl at birth to $8\cdot5$ g/dl at 1 month, and then rose to $12\cdot6$ g/dl at 3 months. An adult level of $10\cdot8$ g/dl was reached at 24 months (Holman & Dew 1965a). MCHC, which was 30 g/dl at birth, rose progressively to 39 g/dl, before falling slowly to an adult level of 36 g/dl at 24–30 months. At birth the erythrocytes were less fragile than cells from adult animals, but there was a progressive change to adult fragility. Perk *et al* (1964), who also observed this greater osmotic resistance of goat erythrocytes at birth, were able to demonstrate a heterogeneous population in respect to fragility, and not two clear-cut populations.

The observations of Wilkins and Hodges (1962) on 6 male kids aged $4\frac{1}{2}$ months show general agreement with the results quoted above.

Holman and Dew (1966b) showed that the fall in haemoglobin levels soon after birth could be prevented by injecting iron dextran, suggesting that there is a relative iron deficiency as the red cell numbers increase.

Reticulocytes are not normally seen in adult goat blood, but they may be seen in the blood of young kids, and in anaemic animals showing a remission.

8b.3 LEUCOCYTES

The total leucocyte count for adult goats has a range of $4 \times 10^9/l$ to $15 \times 10^9/l$, with a mean of $8 \times 10^9/l$. The lymphocytes and neutrophils make a similar percentage contribution, lymphocytes comprising between 45 and 60 per cent and neutrophils between 40 and 50 per cent. These are rough figures, for the ranges for both cell types are considerable Holman and Dew (1965b) found similar percentages for both types in 3-year-old goats (48 per cent). Eosinophil granulocytes compose between 2 and 10 per cent, while the monocytes make up 2 to 6 per cent. Basophils are uncommon cells and do not normally exceed 1 per cent.

8b.3.1 LYMPHOCYTES

These cells are 10 μm in diameter, while a few of 12–14 μm diameter are to be found. The cytoplasm appears less scanty than in some other species, stains blue, and sometimes contains several azurophilic granules. The nucleus contains dark-staining, well-defined and thickly skeined chromatin. The regularly shaped nucleus of the larger cells may appear to contain small rings of chromatin and, occasionally, vacuoles. Binucleate lymphocytes are seen in very small numbers.

8b.3.2 NEUTROPHIL GRANULOCYTES

These have cytoplasm which stains faint pink with Wright–Giemsa stains. Dust-like granules stain very poorly, but can be clearly seen under high-power phase-contrast microscopy. The lobes of the nucleus are connected by thick bands rather than the thread-like nuclear material of other species, which often makes lobe counting difficult. However, 5 nuclear lobes can frequently be distinguished. The diameter of these cells is 10–11 μm.

8b.3.3 EOSINOPHIL GRANULOCYTES

These resemble those of the sheep in the number and small size of their granules. There is an impression, perhaps illusory, that the granules are slightly fewer in number and larger in size than those of the sheep, and while counting them does not tempt as an exercise, measuring them would not be unreasonable. The cytoplasm stains poorly, and the nucleus has 2 or 3 lobes. A not uncommon nuclear form is that in which 2 lobes are joined by a thick band from which arises a slender thread leading to the 3rd lobe. The cell diameter is 12 μm.

8b.3.4 BASOPHIL GRANULOCYTES

These have numerous purple staining granules and a bi- or tri-lobed angular nucleus.

8b.3.5 MONOCYTES

These have granular blue cytoplasm, often containing fine red granules. The diameter is 14–16 μm. There is more diversity in the shape of the nucleus than in most species and this irregularity is one of the most characteristic features of the cell. Dense aggregations of chromatin, which look like nucleoli can be seen, as can circular transparent patches which suggest vacuoles.

8b.3.6 LEUCOCYTE CHANGES WITH GROWTH

The total leucocyte count rises from the birth level to a peak about the 3rd or 4th month, from which it sinks to an adult level similar to that at birth. The early increase appears to be due to a rise in the absolute number of lymphocytes. DeShaw *et al* (1969) showed that the total leucocyte count of the Spanish goat during the 1st month was $7 \cdot 3 \times 10^9/l$ from which it rose to a peak of $16 \cdot 5 \times 10^9/l$ at 4 months. Thereafter the count fell to a fluctuating level of between 12 and $15 \times 10^9/l$. Holman and Dew (1965b) recorded a total leucocyte count of $7 \cdot 5 \times 10^9/l$ during the first 14 days. By 3 months this had risen to $18 \times 10^9/l$, followed by a decrease to $8 \times 10^9/l$ at 2 years. Lymphocyte percentages changed from 41 per cent at birth to 73 per cent at 3 months, and 42 per cent at 2 years. These lymphocyte values are lower than those found by DeShaw *et al* (1969) where a lymphocyte percentage of around 92 per cent at 1 month subsided to 76 per cent at 3 months and continued to decline, with lowest values about 58 per cent at 11 months. (The figures are inexact because they are taken from graphs.)

The $4\frac{1}{2}$-month-old kids of Wilkins and Hodges (1962) had higher total leucocyte counts than adults and a lymphocyte percentage of 68 per cent. All these results show a comparable lymphocyte percentage at the age of 3 or 4 months.

Neutrophils, according to Holman and Dew (1965b), had an initially high level of 55 per cent during the first 14 days, which fell to 23 per cent at 3 months, and rose to 49 per cent at 2 years. The absolute numbers of neutrophils remained remarkably constant. Wilkins and Hodges' (1962) kids had neutrophil levels of 30 per cent but when the absolute numbers of neutrophils of the kids are compared with those of the adult goats, albeit a different group of animals, there is similarity.

Holman and Dew's kids had lymphocyte numbers at 3 months which were 4 times those in the first 14 days, and those at 2 years. The kids of Wilkins and

Hodges had lymphocyte counts almost double those of adults, despite the lymphocyte percentage being raised only 14 per cent. The results of DeShaw *et al* (1969) show the lymphocyte numbers almost doubling by 4 months.

Holman and Dew (1965b) comment upon the steadiness of the percentages of eosinophils, monocytes and basophils in their 3 year study but the adult group of Wilkins and Hodges (1962) showed a trebling of the eosinophil percentage (and a doubling of absolute numbers) over the values in kids.

The patterns described above are not apparent in the Bangladesh goat studies of Ahmed and Rahman (1973), where a consistent absence of change in the 5 age groups studied is the most notable feature.

8b.4 MARROW STUDIES

The bone marrow of goats has been investigated by Winqvist (1954) who carried out sternal marrow punctures upon 10 adults. The cell content resembled that of bovine marrow, as did the cytochemistry. However, the neutrophils had much lower alkaline phosphatase activity. The mean myeloid/erythroid ratio was 0·69:1, eosinophils playing a less prominent part in the marrow population of the goat than in that of the sheep. 4·3 per cent of the nucleated cells belonged to the eosinophil series, only half the lowest percentage quoted for the sheep.

8b.5 PLATELETS AND COAGULATION

These resemble platelets from other species and number $400–500 \times 10^9/l$.

Blood coagulation time in the adult goat has a mean value of 4·5 minutes (Holman & Dew 1965b), while the normal prothrombin time for the goat has a mean of 11·1 seconds (Dorner & Bass 1974).

8b.6 SPECIFIC GRAVITY OF WHOLE BLOOD

For adult goats this lies between 1·040 and 1·060, with a mean of 1·050.

8b.7 PLASMA PROTEINS

The mean value for the *serum* proteins of 40 normal female adult goats was 72·3 g/l (Verma & Tyagi 1974). Plasma values determined by Millson *et al* (1960) gave a range for total protein of 67·0–78·5 g/l, for albumin 32·5–49·0 g/l and for globulin 23·0–46·0 g/l. Changes in the different components of the serum proteins of female goats during the oestrus cycle, gestation and post parturition have been studied by Georgiev *et al* (1973).

8b.8 DISEASES

The goat is susceptible to many of the haematological problems which beset the sheep. However, deficiency anaemias are uncommon and blood disorders associated with toxicity appear to be less of a problem, perhaps because of the animal's browsing habit. While this might at first be thought to offer to the goat a whole new range of poisonous materials, the practice of nibbling no doubt prevents the ingestion of large quantities of poisonous shrubs provided an adequate quantity and variety of food material is available in other forms.

Parasitic anaemias, such as those of *Haemonchus contortus* and fascioliasis occur but, because of browsing and the usually limited number of animals upon the foraging area, goats present fewer serious infestations and less of an overall management problem. Of course, if they are pastured upon land where sheep have been, the incidence of parasitic infestation will rise.

A blood affection not dealt with under the heading of sheep is that caused by ingesting the green leaves of *Ipomoea carnea*, a tropical plant of the family *Convolvulacae*. This plant has caused the death of goats and other domestic animals in the Sudan and its effects upon the blood picture have been studied by Tartour *et al* (1974). Nubian goats were fed the fresh leaves of the plant. Quite rapidly after beginning feeding, the red cell numbers, PCV, haemoglobin and leucocyte count began to fall. Platelets were not counted. The animals differed considerably in the rate at which the haematological changes occurred, but the pattern of the changes did not differ greatly. The MCV was usually within normal limits, if somewhat low, and the authors describe the anaemia as normocytic, and generally normochromic, with lapses to hypochromia if the illness became protracted. When there was a sharp fall in erythrocyte numbers of macrocytic phase appeared, sometimes terminally. As internal haemorrhages have been observed post mortem it is possible that the bouts of red cell depression resulted from bleeding. If there was recovery from this loss the anaemia resumed its normocytic character, but was now hypochromic.

The animals showed nervous system signs in the hind limbs and death was a common outcome.

The toxic factor in *Ipomoea carnea* is not known and the mechanism of its haematological effects, initially suggestive of marrow depression, requires further study.

The goat, like the sheep, suffers from lymphoma, or lymphosarcoma, but the incidence is extremely low in a species far fewer in numbers than the sheep. The condition has usually been diagnosed post mortem by the presence of tumours in lymphatic tissue. Information about the blood picture is limited. Schalm *et al* (1975) describe a case in a 3-year-old female Saanen–Nubian cross. The PCV was 0·185 l/l, and the haemoglobin 6·8 g/dl. The leucocyte count was 15×10^9/l, of which 2 per cent were band neutrophils, 31 per cent mature neutrophils, 6 per cent monocytes, and 61 per cent lymphocytes. Thirteen per cent of the lymphocytes were large and atypical, and some were binucleate. All the lymph nodes were found to be enlarged at post mortem examination.

A lymphatic tumour arising in the mediastinum should provoke suspicion of its being a thymoma, a tumour which, though uncommon, occurs more frequently in the goat than one might expect.

Table 8b.1 Goat: normal values

	Mean	*Range*
Erythrocytes	14×10^{12}/l	$7–21 \times 10^{12}$/l
PCV	0·29 l/l	0·19–0·40 l/l
Diameter	3·2 μm	1·5–5 μm
Volume (MCV)	21 fl	15–39 fl
Hb	11 g/dl	8–16 g/dl
MCH	6·9 pg	5·3–8·4 pg
MCHC	37 g/dl	32–40 g/dl
Leucocytes	8×10^9/l	$4–15 \times 10^9$/l
Lymphocytes %	49	45–60
Neutrophils %	42	40–50
Eosinophils %	6	2–10
Basophils %	<0·5	0–1
Monocytes %	3	2–6
Platelets	450×10^9/l	$400–500 \times 10^9$/l

Table 8b.2 Goat: absolute leucocyte numbers

	Mean absolute numbers
Total	$8·00 \times 10^9$/l
Lymphocytes	$3·90 \times 10^9$/l
Neutrophils	$3·40 \times 10^9$/l
Eosinophils	$0·43 \times 10^9$/l
Basophils	$0·03 \times 10^9$/l
Monocytes	$0·24 \times 10^9$/l

9

HAEMATOLOGY OF THE DEER

D. I. CHAPMAN

9.1 INTRODUCTION

Although deer (Cervidae) are regarded usually as wild animals, some species have been domesticated. The use of reindeer (*Rangifer tarandus*) as draught animals by the Lapps is traditional. In 1949, an experimental moose (*Alces alces*) farm was set up in northern Russia with the aim of raising a domestic animal specialized for the taiga, as the reindeer is for the tundra. These moose have been used to produce milk and meat and as draught animals (Yazan & Knorre 1964). The farming of red deer (*Cervus elaphus*) is currently being studied experimentally in Scotland (Blaxter *et al* 1974). Both fallow deer (*Dama dama*) and red deer are farmed commercially in Australia and New Zealand. These examples show that some species can be domesticated and attempts to farm deer, particularly for meat, are likely to increase. Consequently, a knowledge of their haematology becomes increasingly important.

The taxonomy of deer is confusing. The nomenclature used here is that given by Morris (1965), who lists 41 species of deer in 17 genera. Reindeer (*Rangifer tarandus*) occur in both the Old World and the New World but in the latter they are usually called caribou. Moose (*Alces alces*) also occur in both the Old and New Worlds but in the former they are referred to as elk. This practice leads to confusion because wapiti (*Cervus canadensis*) are referred to in America as elk. In this chapter, the terms reindeer, moose and wapiti are used.

The haematology of only 7 species of deer has been investigated in detail, although limited information is available for a further 18. The haematology of reindeer has been reviewed by Gorodetskii (1962).

The major difficulty in studying the haematology of deer is to decide what are normal values. Even domesticated deer are not always amenable to stand without restraint and allow blood to be removed by venepuncture. What effect does the stress of either capture or restraint of deer have on their haematology? What are the effects of sedation? Can blood taken from deer within a few minutes of death be regarded as normal? Does the blood picture of a wild deer reflect accurately that of a domesticated deer? These are some of the problems that have to be considered when reviewing the haematology of deer.

There are no clear answers to the above questions. Because 'normal' resting blood values are almost impossible to obtain, the effect of the various practices cannot be evaluated. From a practical point of view, however, this is not so serious as at first appears. If deer always have to be sedated before blood is collected, then a knowledge of the 'normal' value of sedated deer is required, not the resting value of unsedated animals.

The blood of deer varies according to whether they are physically restrained or sedated. Significantly lower erythrocyte counts (RBC), haemoglobin concentration (Hb), packed cell volume (PCV) and total serum protein concentration (TSP) were obtained when 3 male white-tailed deer (*Odocoileus virginianus*) were restrained and sedated than when they were only restrained. There were no changes in either mean corpuscular volume (MCV) or mean corpuscular haemoglobin concentration (MCHC). Four female white-tailed deer were restrained, released, restrained again 24 hours later and subsequently sedated. There was a decrease in RBC, Hb concentration, PCV and TSP; a spectacular 3–200-fold increase in creatine kinase (CPK), lactate dehydrogenase (LDH) and aspartate aminotransferase (AAT) but no changes were detected in MCV, MCHC, leucocyte count (WBC), blood urea nitrogen, calcium, cholesterol, glucose, total bilirubin and uric acid at the time of the second restraint compared with the first (Seal *et al* 1972a). The haematological values for sedated deer were closer to those obtained by Seal and Erickson (1969) for deer that had been shot than were the values for the physically restrained animals. The mean RBC,

Hb and PCV also showed small decreases when roe (*Capreolus capreolus*) and red deer were sedated compared with non-sedated animals. No changes were detected in MCV, MCHC, mean corpuscular haemoglobin (MCH) and WBC (Drescher-Kaden & Hoppe 1972, 1973). It appears that initial physical restraint of deer leads to haemoconcentration with a rise in RBC count, Hb and PCV but that subsequent restraint leads to less marked changes. Sedation does not lead to such marked haemoconcentration and the values obtained appear to be similar to those found when undisturbed deer are shot.

Many haematological values for deer are based on blood collected from dead animals. Therefore the behaviour of the animal immediately before death may be important. The blood of deer shot whilst resting may be different from that of animals that have been excited. Mule deer (*Odocoileus hemionus*) that were wounded on shooting and ran several hundred metres before being killed had lower RBC, Hb and PCV than did deer that were killed instantaneously (Rosen & Bischoff 1952). However, Anderson *et al* (1970) concluded that the behaviour of mule deer before being shot did not affect the cellular components of their blood. The high concentration of plasma potassium in white-tailed deer shot through the neck was attributed by Wilber and Robinson (1958) to shock.

Because of the many differences in the physiological states of the deer, the methods used to collect blood and the lack of interlaboratory standardization in analysis, it is impossible to draw many meaningful conclusions about interspecific variations in their haematology. In fact, many of the analytical results leave much to be desired.

9.2 CELLS AND PLATELETS—NORMAL VALUES

9.2.1 HAEMOGLOBIN

Little is known about haematopoiesis in deer. A single embryonic haemoglobin, Hb-P, is present in month-old reindeer embryos. This haemoglobin is replaced at about 6 weeks by a slower moving fetal haemoglobin, Hb-F. In new-born reindeer, the haemoglobin consists of 60 per cent Hb-F and 40 per cent Hb-A, the latter being the typical adult form. The formation of Hb-F apparently does not cease during the first week of life but the amount of Hb-A doubles and so becomes predominant (Irzhak 1973, Irzhak *et al* 1973). Haemoglobins of different electrophoretic mobilities occur in fetal, new-born and adult moose (Irzhak & Kahmarik 1971). Two electrophoretically distinct haemoglobins are present also in 50–170-day-old white-tailed deer fetuses. These fetal haemoglobins comprise 2 different α polypeptide chains, which are electrophoretically similar to the α chains of adult haemoglobin, and 2 γ-like polypeptide chains which were electrophoretically distinct from adult β polypeptide chains (Kitchen *et al* 1964, 1967, Seal & Erickson 1969).

Adult animals of 10 of the 13 species of deer which have been studied appear to have only one type of haemoglobin, although in some cases few specimens have been examined. The electrophoretic mobilities on starch gel of the single haemoglobin from barasingha *Cervus duvauceli* (n = 1), Père David's *Elaphurus davidianus* (n = 1), sika (*Cervus nippon*) (n = 44) and red deer (n = 32) are identical. Fallow deer (n = 62) haemoglobin moves faster than that of roe deer (n = 80) which lies between that of fallow and of the other species (Maughan & Williams 1967). A single haemoglobin component is found also in adult Indian muntjac (*Muntiacus muntjak*) (n = 1, Naik *et al* 1964), moose (Irzhak & Kahmarik 1971), reindeer (n = 64, Gahne & Rendel 1961) and wapiti (n = 2, Miller *et al* 1965).

Multiple haemoglobins occur in Reeves' muntjac (*Muntiacus reevesi*), Chinese water deer (*Hydropotes inermis*) and in white-tailed deer (Maughan & Williams 1967, Miller *et al* 1965, Weisberger 1964). Whether axis deer (*Axis axis*) have multiple haemoglobins is uncertain: Maughan and Williams (1967) examined one animal and found a single haemoglobin whereas Naik *et al* (1964) found 2 haemoglobins in 3 out of 4 animals examined, but the electrophoretogram is not particularly convincing.

White-tailed deer are unusual in that 11 structurally different adult haemoglobins have been identified (Huisman *et al* 1968). These haemoglobins result from the combination of one of 4 types of α polypeptide chain with one of at least 5 types of β polypeptide chain. Individual deer may have either one, 2 or 4 haemoglobin variants. All deer have a major haemoglobin and they may also have one or more minor components. The major haemoglobins are termed II, III, IVa, IVb, V and VII whereas the minor ones are called I-2, I-3, I-4a, I-4b, I-5 and I-7. Major haemoglobins are present in amounts usually exceeding 60 per cent and contain one of the 3 types of α polypeptide chain, all termed $^I\alpha$ (or α), with one of the six types of β polypeptide chain which are termed β^{II}, β^{III}, β^{IVa}, β^{IVb}, β^V and β^{VII}. Minor haemoglobins are present in amounts of 0, 15, 33 or 42 per cent and comprise one type of α chain, termed $^{II}\alpha$ (or α′), and one of the same 6 types of β chain found in the major components (Kitchen *et al* 1966, 1967, 1968).

The α chains differ from each other by one, 2 or 3 amino acids at positions 5, 20 and 24 (Harris *et al* 1972). For any particular haemoglobin molecule, the two α polypeptide chains are identical, as are the two β polypeptide chains. It has been suggested that the $^I\alpha$ and $^{II}\alpha$ chains are produced by non-allelic genes with the $^{II}\alpha$ structural locus sometimes absent or non-operative (Huisman *et al* 1968, Taylor *et al* 1972).

Not all the theoretically possible haemoglobin variants have been found in white-tailed deer; the most frequent in order of occurrence are III + I-3, III and II + I-2 and III + I-3 (Harris *et al* 1973).

9.2.2 ERYTHROCYTES

Values for Hb concentration, the numbers and sizes of erythrocytes, PCV erythrocyte sedimentation rate (ESR), MCH, MCV and MCHC are summarized in Table 9.1. Where values from different studies are in good agreement, only an overall average value and the range have been quoted, together with the source of the information.

There are no obvious interspecific differences in Hb and PCV of deer blood, particularly when possible variations due to age, season and environment are taken into consideration. The RBC of male moose is much lower than in most of the other species of deer studied (Table 9.1), whereas that of axis and hog deer (*Axis porcinus*) are all higher than most. These differences are reflected in the erythrocyte indices MCH and MCV which in moose are higher and in axis and hog deer lower than usual. The MCHC is similar in all species of deer studied. The values for sika deer published by Bartels *et al* (1963) and by Hawkey (1975) suggest that the blood of this species might be similar to that of axis and hog deer in having a high red cell count, but values published by Ochiai and Enoki (1975) for both male and female sika deer are lower and similar to those of most other species of deer.

Less information is available on the ESR than for the other haematological variables of deer blood and there are wide differences in the values quoted (Table 9.1). For 3 groups of captive mule deer fawns, the mean value was less than 1 mm/h whereas for a fourth group the mean value was 6·4 mm/h (range 0·7–20·0 mm/h) (Cowan & Bandy 1969). High values were also recorded for young mule deer by Kitts *et al* (1956) who believed that this difference reflected changes in PCV rather than nutrition, age or disease.

The Hb, RBC and PCV of mule, roe and white-tailed deer and reindeer all increase substantially during the first few weeks of life, whereas the MCH and MCV decrease. The MCHC of mule, roe and white-tailed deer also increases after birth whereas with reindeer there is a slight decrease with increasing age (Table 9.1). There is a small decrease in PCV and possibly a decline in the concentration of erythrocytes during the first 3 days of life of white-tailed deer but thereafter values increase. The MCV and MCH increase from day 1 to day 7 and then decrease (Youatt *et al* 1965). There is also a decline in Hb and RBC in moose during the first week of life due to an increase in plasma volume (Irzhak 1964). In contrast, White and Cook (1974) found no differences in Hb, RBC, PCV and ESR in white-tailed deer of 1–3, 4–7, and 8–14 days old although the values were lower than those of adult deer. This reported lack of change in the first 2 weeks of life is also inconsistent with the findings of Johnson *et al* (1968) and Tumbleson *et al* (1970).

The composition of the blood of mule, roe and white-tailed deer appears

Table 9.1 Cellular constituents of deer blood—normal values

	Species	Age	No.	Hb g/dl	RBC $10^{12}/l$	MCD μm	PCV l/l	ESR mm/h	MCH pg	MCV fl	MC. g/l
(1)	*Alces alces* Moose	4 m	2 ♂	13·5±0·4*	5·3±0·4	—	0·38±0·03	27±13	25±2	72±7	36
		all ages	341	14·1±4·7	6·2±1·2	6·45	0·41±0·12	—	21·5	59±6	36
(2)	*Axis axis* Axis deer	—	3 ♂ 1 ♀	16·3±0·4	18·2±2·2	—	0·52±0·06	3·3±3·3	9±1	29±4	32
		—	2	13·0	13·4	4·99	0·35	8	10	24	3
(3)	*A. porcinus* Hog deer	—	3	16·8	14·3	4·71	0·50	4·5	13	37	3
(4)	*Capreolus capreolus* Roe deer	2 d	—	8·2	6·3	—	0·30	—	13	47	2
		1–2 m	27–41	19·3±2·8	13·0±1·8	—	0·53±0·04	—	15±2	41	3
		6 m	12 ♂♀	14·2	11·1	—	0·44	—	13	33	3
		9 m	3 ♂ 2 ♀	15·6	12·6	—	—	—	13	—	—
		10–12 m	♂♀	19·2	11·7	—	—	—	16	—	—
		8·5 m	4	17·3±1·9	10·3±2·0	—	—	—	17±2	—	—
		2–4 y	—	16·2	12·0	4·9	0·46	—	14	39	3
(5)	*Cervus canadensis* Wapiti	all ages	171 ♂♀	18·8	11·1	—	0·50	13·2	17	47	3
		all ages	—	16·5	5·8	6·14	0·51	—	29	92	3
		—	2	13·3	9·4	5·46	0·36	3·5	15	39	3
(6)	*C. elaphus* Red deer	1 m–2 y	160	16·2 (12·4–20·6)	11·3 (7·1–16·5)	—	0·45 (0·33–0·55)	—	14	40	3
		all ages	78 ♂♀	15·2±1·4	10·7±1·0	5·2±0·9	0·45	—	14	40	3
		<3 y	16	14·5	9·6	—	0·47	—	15	48	3.
		>3 y	14	—	—	—	—	—	—	—	—
(7)	*C. nippon* Sika deer	—	7	16·8	13·3	5 0	0·45	2	13	34	3
		Adult	5 ♂ 4 ♀	14·6±3·4	10·6±2·6	—	0·40±0·06	—	14±2	39±7	36:
(8)	*C. timorensis* Timor deer	—	1	14·5	10·5	4·82	0·41	—	15	40	3
(9)	*C. unicolor* Sambar	—	♂♀	18·0	8·9	6·2±0·9	—	2	19	—	—
(10)	*Dama dama* Fallow deer	—	1 ♂ 1 ♀	22·2	11·2	5·6	—	0·3	20	—	—
		—	3	14·3	10·0	4·9	0·46	0·5	15	46	3.
(11)	*Elaphurus davidianus* Père David's deer	—	10	17·2	9·5	5·6	0·47	3	18	50	3

*The standard deviation is quoted when available.   d = Day, m = month, y = year.

Table 9.1 *continued*

W $10^9/l$	N %	E %	B %	L %	M %	Plts. $10^9/l$	Conditions	References
5·9±1·1	42	4	—	53	—	—	Captive	Dieterich 1970
4·2±2·5	33	—	—	62	—	—	Shot or sedated	Gulliver 1845, LeResche *et al* 1974
4·8±0·8	63±4·4	2	—	35±3·3	1	—	Captive	Naik *et al* 1964
5·0	30	3	0	65	2	410	Captive	Gulliver 1845, Hawkey 1975
3·3	46	15	1	34	4	273	Captive	Gulliver 1845, Hawkey 1975
—	—	—	—	—	—	—		Marmienė 1972
2·9	40±14	4±3	0·5±0·6	54±13	1±1	—	Restrained	Drescher-Kaden & Hoppe 1972, 1973
6·8	—	—	—	—	—	—	Restrained	Marmienė 1972, Valentinčić 1971
5·8	—	—	—	—	—	—	Restrained	Valentinčić 1971
5·5	—	—	—	—	—	280	Restrained	Drescher-Kaden & Hoppe 1972, 1973, Valentinčić 1971
0·8±0·4	44±11	13±10	1·4±2·4	41±3	0·3±0·3	—	Sedated	Drescher-Kaden & Hoppe 1972, 1973, Gulliver 1875
5·7	—	—	—	—	—	—	—	Marmienė 1972
6·9	50	12	1	41	1	—	Restrained, wild and captive	Follis 1972, Herin 1968, Weber & Giacometti 1972
4·0	42	12	5	32	32	—	Sedated	Gulliver 1845, Vaughn *et al* 1973, Weber & Bliss 1972
4·8	60	3	1	35	3	355	Captive	Hawkey 1975
4·4 (1·7–8·6)	—	—	—	—	—	—	Restrained, deer farm	Blaxter *et al* 1974
5·9	28	5	3	62	3	—	Restrained	Drescher-Kaden & Hoppe 1972, Marmienė & Marma 1972
3·4	31	3	—	63	4	—	Shot or sedated	Upcott & Hebert 1965
2·9	50	9	—	35	7	—	Shot or sedated	Upcott & Hebert 1965
3·6	39	4	0	55	2	353	Captive	Bartels *et al* 1963, Hawkey 1975
—	—	—	—	—	—	—	Captive	Ochiai & Enoki 1975
7·4	40	2	2	52	4	420	Captive	Hawkey 1975
4·5	56	5	0	34	6	—	—	Knoll 1932, Undritz 1946, Urbain *et al* 1936
2·0	31	9	6	52	3	—	Captive	Gulliver 1845, Undritz 1946
2·6	81	1	0	15	3	362	Captive	Hawkey 1975
4·2	44	4	1	48	3	247	Captive	Hawkey 1975

D. I. Chapman

Table 9.1 *continued*

	Species	Age	No.	Hb g/dl	RBC $10^{12}/l$	MCD μm	PCV l/l	ESR mm/h	MCH pg	MCV fl	MC g/
(12)	*Hydropotes inermis* Chinese water deer	—	1	16·2	10·2	—	0·42	2	16	42	3
(13)	*Mazama americana* Red brocket	—	1 ♀	—	—	3·6	—	—	—	—	
(14)	*M. gouazoubira* Brown brocket	—	1 ♂	—	—	3·6	—	—	—	—	
(15)	*Moschus moschiferus* Musk deer	—	—	—	—	3·6	—	—	—	—	
(16)	*Muntiacus reevesi* Reeves' muntjac	—	—	—	—	4·0	—	—	—	—	
(17)	*Odocoileus hemionus* Mule deer	1–21 d	23 ♂ 26 ♀	10·1	5·5	—	0·35	—	18	63	2
		45 d (23–68)	28	13·9	10·3	—	0·36	3	14	35	3
		92 d (65–117)	16	15·7	14·2	—	0·43	0·5	11	30	3
		20–100 d	14	10·7	—	—	0·40	10	—	—	2
		13–16 m	6	14·9	—	—	0·58	6	—	—	2
		Adult	355 ♀	16·4±3·0	10·1±2·0	—	0·45±0·10	—	16	44	3
		1–162 m	174	16·4	9·2	5·7	0·47	—	18	53	3
(18)	*O. virginianus* White-tailed deer	1–14 d	31	10·1	7·0	—	0·29	2·2	15	42	3
		0–6 m	ca. 137	18·7	18·0	—	0·52	—	10	29	3
		7 m–Adult	ca. 330	19·9	14·4	—	0·53	—	14	36	3
		Adult	3 ♂ 8 ♀	15·3±2·7	10·7±1·7	—	0·41	—	14	38	3
		9 m–Adult	32 ♂ 39 ♀	14·7±2·6	11·4±2·0	—	0·42±0·07	—	12	37±4	34
		—	1	11·0	7·0	4·6	0·33	—	16	47	3
		—	4 ♂ 5 ♀	21·4±1·9	—	5·0	0·58±0·04	—	—	—	3
(19)	*Rangifer tarandus* Reindeer	new born	6 ♂♀	14·6	8·7	—	0·33	—	17	37	4
		7 d	5 ♂♀	14·9	9·1	—	0·35	—	16	39	4
		6–18 m	22 ♂♀	18·3	11·8	—	0·45	—	16	40	4
		Adult	83 ♂♀	15·2	8·8	—	0·36	—	18	41	4
		3–52 m	234	17·6	9·9	5·6	0·49	—	18	—	3
		1–3 y	15	15·1	9·2	—	0·45	10	17	50	3
		—	10	17·4	9·8	4·9	0·47	0·5	17	48	3
		all	50	16·2	10·4	—	0·47	—	16	45	3
		—	4 ♂ 1 ♀	14·5	10·8	—	—	—	13	—	–

* The standard deviation is quoted when available.   d = Day, m = month, y = year.

Table **9.1** *continued*

W $10^9/l$	N %	E %	B %	L %	M %	Plts. $10^9/l$	Conditions	References
6·4	74	4	1	19	6	370	Captive	Hawkey 1975
—	—	—	—	—	—	—		Gulliver 1848
—	—	—	—	—	—	—		Gulliver 1875
—	—	—	—	—	—	—		Gulliver 1875
—	—	—	—	—	—	—		Gulliver 1875
5·3	41	2	1	39	16	—	Restrained	Cowan & Bandy 1969
5·2	40	0·1	0·4	54	5	—	Restrained	Cowan & Bandy 1969
5·7	41	0·1	0·4	52	4	—	Restrained	Cowan & Bandy 1969
—	—	—	—	—	—	—	Restrained	Kitts *et al* 1956
—	—	—	—	—	—	—	Restrained	Kitts *et al* 1956
—	—	—	—	—	—	—	Shot, jugular	Rosen & Bischoff 1952
3·0	42	8	0·4	43	6	—	Shot, heart	Anderson *et al* 1970, Browman & Sears 1955
3·6	—	—	—	—	—	—	Wild, restrained	White & Cook 1974
3·9	—	—	—	—	—	—	Restrained	Foreyt & Trainer 1970, Johnson *et al* 1968, Tumbleson *et al* 1970
2·5	—	—	—	—	—	—	Restrained	Johnson *et al* 1968, Mathews 1968, Seal *et al* 1972a
1·7	—	—	—	—	—	—	Sedated	Seal *et al* 1972a
—	—	—	—	—	—	—	Shot	Seal & Erickson 1969
3·5	56	7	2	32	3	460	Captive	Hawkey 1975
2·7±1·4	17±12	2±3	0·1	80±13	1±1	512	Restrained	Debbie *et al* 1965, Gulliver 1845, Mathews 1968
—	—	—	—	—	—	—		Gorodetskii 1959a
—	—	—	—	—	—	—		Gorodetskii 1959a
—	—	—	—	—	—	—		Gorodetskii 1959a
—	—	—	—	—	—	—		Gorodetskii 1959a
4·4	52	12	4	29	4	—	Restrained	Drescher-Kaden & Hoppe 1972, 1973, McEwan & Whitehead 1969
7·9	42	11	1	45	0·1	—	Captive, restrained	Dieterich 1970
4·7	57	3	1	38	3	276	Captive	Hawkey 1975
4·6	49	8	1	42	1	—	Sedated	McEwan 1968
4·2	59	2	1	40	2	—	Shot	Gibbs 1960

to reach adult values by about 6 months. With reindeer, the Hb concentration, RBC and PCV increase until about 18 months of age and then decline so that adult values are similar to those of the new-born. The haematological indices of adult reindeer are greater in the autumn than in the spring and Gorodetskii (1959a) believes the changes in blood from birth to 18 months are due to season, not age.

The mean values for Hb, RBC and PCV for female reindeer, mule and white-tailed deer are slightly higher than those for males (Table 9.1) although only one example, the PCV of adult white-tailed deer, shows a statistically significant difference. The MCV of 1-year-old female white-tailed deer was statistically greater than that of males of similar age (Dommert *et al* 1968). The values given for Hb of wapiti by Follis (1972) appear to be unreliable in view of the high standard deviations (males $18·9 \pm 16·8$ g/dl and females $20·4 \pm 18·2$ g/dl). Although most of the differences between the blood of male and female deer are not statistically significant, it is interesting that the mean values for females were consistently higher than those for males. The mean Hb, RBC and PCV of adult female moose were slightly higher than those of adult males in December but the position was reversed in October (LeResche *et al* 1974). Significant differences in the blood of male and female deer may not become apparent until carefully matched samples are examined at the same time of year.

Attempts to investigate seasonal changes in the blood of deer are complicated by physiological and environmental factors. For example, most adult female deer are pregnant and/or lactating throughout the year. Hb and RBC, but not the PCV, of mule deer declined from December to February when a severe winter forced them close to starvation (Rosen & Bischoff 1952). These variables are found to be greater for reindeer in the summer and autumn than in winter and spring whereas the reverse is true for the MCH. These changes affect both sexes and are attributed mainly to shortage of food and more severe climatic conditions in winter and spring. The MCV and MCHC remain constant (Gorodetskii 1959a, Kvitkin 1957). The Hb and PCV of captive, adult male and female reindeer have been measured weekly throughout the year but there were no well-defined seasonal changes. Pregnancy may result in haemoconcentration as both values apparently increase from 5 months pregnant to parturition. It is also claimed that haemoconcentration occurs when reindeer start to rut but similar changes in Hb and PCV also occur at other times of the year (McEwan & Whitehead 1969). A decline in Hb, RBC and PCV of adult male moose from October to December is probably a result of the cessation of rutting as no changes are found in the blood of female moose (LeResche *et al* 1974).

The Hb of pregnant wapiti was significantly greater than in non-pregnant animals (Follis 1972) but no changes were detected in mule and white-tailed deer (Anderson *et al* 1970, Seal & Erickson 1969).

Antler growth does not appear to affect the cellular components of the blood.

The length of life, in days, of the red cells are: mule deer, ca. 145; sika deer, 159; white-tailed deer, 100–155, and wapiti, 149 (Cornelius *et al* 1959, Noyes *et al* 1966).

9.2.3 LEUCOCYTES

One of the most characteristic features of the blood of each species of deer studied is the low concentration of leucocytes. Leucocyte counts of $13.5 \times 10^9/l$ have been reported for an apparently healthy captive reindeer calf (McEwan & Whitehead 1969) but such high values are extremely unusual whereas values of $2\cdot3 \times 10^9/l$ are common. In reindeer, the maximum concentration of leucocytes is reported to occur in the summer and autumn (Kvitkin 1957).

The leucocytes comprise mainly neutrophils, mostly segmented, and lymphocytes. There are no marked species, sex or age differences in the concentration of leucocytes. In red deer, the ratio of neutrophils to lymphocytes increases with increasing age: up to 3 years the ratio is 0·5, whereas in older animals the ratio is 1·4 (Upcott & Hebert 1965). The ratio increases also in wapiti from 0·5 for calves to 0·7 for yearlings and 1·1 for adults (Follis 1972) and in female white-tailed deer the ratios for one, 2 and 3 year olds are 0·5, 0·6 and 0·8 respectively (Dommert *et al* 1968). However, the ratio for four races of mule deer fawns up to 117 days of age ranged from 0·6 to 1·1 (Cowan & Bandy 1969).

9.3 SERUM CONSTITUENTS—NORMAL VALUES

The concentrations of proteins, blood urea nitrogen (BUN), electrolytes, glucose, total bilirubin, cholesterol, creatinine and enzymes in the serum (or plasma) of 13 species of deer are given in Table 9.2. Where several studies have given similar results, a composite value is stated. For several species, either the blood of very few animals has been examined or only a few constituents have been investigated. Consequently, the information for any particular species is frequently an amalgamation from several sources. With few exceptions the concentrations of the various constituents are surprisingly similar for the different species of deer.

9.3.1 PROTEINS

Paper or cellulose acetate membrane electrophoresis of deer serum gives five fractions, namely albumin, α_1, α_2, β and γ globulins. The concentration of

TSP of white-tailed deer and reindeer increase during the first 2 months after birth, whereas that of mule deer fawns decrease. A change in food and environment when the mule deer were caught, however, may have meant that the original values are unrepresentative: they are much higher than those reported for other species of deer of similar age. The serum albumin concentration of mule and white-tailed deer increases rapidly after birth; the globulin concentration falls, mainly because γ globulin levels decline rapidly before increasing to adult values. Changes in the α and β globulins are far less marked (Bandy *et al* 1957, Johnson *et al* 1968, McEwan & Whitehead 1969, Tumbelson *et al* 1970, Youatt *et al* 1965).

Gamma globulin appears to be absent from the serum of white-tailed deer fetuses. The fetal α_1 globulin is of greater concentration than that of the adult deer (Seal & Erickson 1969) and probably contains a protein homologous with the fetuin described by Engle and Woods (1960) in bovine fetal serum. The serum albumin: globulin ratio of adult wapiti is unusually low (Table 9.2), frequently being less than 1, mainly because of high levels of globulins. The serum albumin:globulin ratio of 0·2 reported by Vaughn *et al* (1973) is surprisingly low as are the low albumin concentrations. The concentrations of ceruloplasmin, a copper protein, and of haptoglobin in the serum of white-tailed deer are given by Seal and Erickson (1969).

Serum transferrins have been shown by starch-gel electrophoresis to be polymeric; 2, 3 or 4 bands being present. Those of white-tailed and red deer, reindeer and wapiti are polymorphic whereas those of fallow and sika deer and moose are monomorphic (Braend 1962, 1964, McDougall & Lowe 1968, Miller *et al* 1965). The serum from most white-tailed deer fetuses contains a single transferrin with the same electrophoretic mobility as the slower of the 2 adult proteins, but in some fetuses a small amount of a transferrin with the same mobility as the faster adult protein is present. The post albumins are polymorphic (Seal & Erickson 1969). The post albumins and α_2 globulins of adult red deer exhibit polymorphism (Kravchenko & Kravchenko 1971).

9.3.2   ELECTROLYTES

The concentrations of serum chloride and potassium are more variable than those of the other electrolytes. In most species of mammal that have been examined, the serum chloride concentration is about 100–120 mmol/l, so the concentration reported for hog, sika and red deer (Table 9.2) by Urbain *et al* (1938b) may be misleading although that for fallow deer is reasonable. The wide variation in the concentration of potassium may reflect the stresses involved in collecting blood (see page 347).

Table 9.2 Serum constituents of deer blood—normal values

	Species	Age	No.	Total protein g/l	Alb. g/l	Glob. g/l	Alb: Glob. ratio	Fibrinogen g/l	Ca mmol/l	Mg mmol/l
(1)	*Alces alces*	all ages	3♂ 10♀	64±9*	45±14	19±4	2.3	—	—	—
	Moose	adult	65♂	69±7	33±4	16±6	2.1	—	2.5±0.3	1.0
		all ages	250♂♀	69±9	39±7	30	1.3	—	2.7±0.3	—
(2)	*Axis axis*	—	4	—	—	—	—	—	2.2	1.0
	Axis deer									
(3)	*A. porcinus*	—	4	—	—	—	—	1.9	2.3	1.2
	Hog deer									
(4)	*Capreolus capreolus*	4 m	2♂ 4♀	—	—	—	—	—	2.6±0.4	1.2±0.2
	Roe deer	6–10 m	—	54	35	19	1.8	—	2.9±0.4	—
		>1 y	—	59	34	25	1.4	—	2.6±0.3	1.1±0.1
(5)	*Cervus canadensis*	all ages	—	72±10	31±9	43	0.7	—	2.4±0.1	—
	Wapiti	9 m	2	61±1	33±10	29±9	1.1	—	—	—
		1–1.5 y	2 / 2	60±6	28±3	32±5	0.9	—	—	—
		1–2 y	14	62±1	11±1	51	0.2	—	2.3±0.04	—
		Adult	1♂ 7♀	74±3	26±8	48±9	0.6	—	—	—
		—	21	74±3	15±2	60	0.2	—	2.4±0.05	—
(6)	*C. elaphus*	all ages	♂♀	61	—	—	—	5.1	2.6±0.3	0.9±0.1
	Red deer									
(7)	*C. nippon*	all ages	9	54–88	18–42	28–48	—	7.1	2.4	1.0
	Sika deer									
(8)	*C. unicolor*	—	9	—	—	—	—	—	3.0	—
	Sambar									
(9)	*Dama dama*	all ages	♂ ♀	69	48	25	2.0	4.7	2.6	1.6
	Fallow deer									
(10)	*Elaphurus davidianus*	—	2	—	—	—	—	—	2.7	0.9
	Père David's deer									
(11)	*Odocoileus hemionus*	20 d	—	71	26	47	0.6	4.0	—	—
	Mule deer	1–3 m	—	56	36	17	2.1	4.2	—	—
		13–16 m	6	65	44	18	2.4	3.5	—	—
		all ages	103♂ 165♀	61	—	—	—	—	3.2	1.6
(12)	*O. virginianus*	1–3 d	11	54	22	32	0.7	—	2.8	—
	White-tailed deer	21 d	12	55	30	25	1.2	—	—	—
		5–12 m	18♂ 18♀	76±4	32	44	0.7	—	2.9±0.1	1.5
		1 y	—	62	37	27	1.4	—	2.3±0.3	1.2±0.2
		all ages	—	51±6	33±5	19±2	1.8±0.4	—	—	—
(13)	*Rangifer tarandus*	1–2 m	8	54	33	22	1.4	—	—	—
	Reindeer	3–12 m	—	67	38	28	1.4	—	3.0	1.0
		Adult	—	69	39	36	1.1	1.9–2.5	4.7	0.9

* The standard deviation is quoted when available.
** Because of the wide variety of units employed to express enzyme activity, the reader is advised to consult the original publication.
d = Day, m = month, y = year.

(Table continued on p. 356)

Table 9.2 *continued*

	P mmol/l	K mmol/l	Na mmol/l	Cl mmol/l	AP **	CPK **	LDH **	AAT **	BUN mmol/l	Cholesterol mmol/l	Creatinine μmol/l
(1)	—	—	—	—	—	—	—	—	4·6±1·1	—	—
	2·1±0·4	—	—	—	—	—	—	—	3·0±1·1	1·4±0·3	—
	1·8±0·6	—	—	—	—	—	—	—	4·6±4·3	2·3±0·6	—
(2)	—	10·5	—	—	—	—	—	—	—	—	—
(3)	—	8·5	—	83	—	—	—	—	—	—	—
(4)	2·1±0·3	—	—	—	**	—	—	—	—	—	—
	1·9±0·2	—	—	—	**	—	—	—	—	—	—
	1·7±0·1	—	—	—	**	—	—	—	—	—	—
(5)	0·8±0·4	5·5±0·7	148±9	—	**	—	**	**	10·0±4·9	2·0±0·2	253±35
	—	—	—	—	**	—	**	**	7·1±0·4	2·2±0·2	150±9
	—	—	—	—	**	—	**	**	5·9±0·6	1·8±0·3	202±176
	1·4±0·06	—	—	—	**	—	**	**	11·5±1·1	1·3±0·2	—
	—	—	—	—	**	—	**	**	10·6±2·8	2·5±0·7	228±201
	1·4±0·04	—	—	—	**	—	**	**	13·8±1·0	1·8±0·2	—
(6)	1·7±0·2	7·8	—	79	**	—	—	—	—	1·9	—
(7)	1·5	2·1	172	83	**	—	—	**	5·7–15·4	1·6–3·9	97–211
(8)	—	—	—	—	—	—	—	—	—	1·9	—
(9)	1·5	7·6	—	101	—	—	—	—	—	1·8	—
(10)	1·2	3·8	142	111	—	—	—	—	—	—	—
(11)	—	—	—	—	—	—	—	—	—	—	—
	1·1	—	—	—	—	—	—	—	—	—	—
	1·0	—	—	—	—	—	—	—	—	—	—
	1·5	9·0	149	—	—	—	—	—	—	—	—
(12)	3·6	5·4	156	110	**	—	**	**	7·1	2·1	211
	—	—	—	—	**	—	**	**	—	1·6±0·3	229±44
	2·2±0·2	6·4±0·7	159±4	111±3	**	—	**	**	10·7±1·8	2·1±0·8	220±26
	1·6±0·4	4·8±0·8	150±6	115±6	**	**	**	**	6·4±1·4	1·9±0·5	—
	1·8	10·4	174	101	—	**	—	—	5·0±2·9	1·1±0·3	167±26
(13)	—	—	—	—	—	**	—	**	—	—	—
	1·4	—	—	—	**	**	—	**	—	—	—
	1·4	4·9–9·5	144	—	**	**	**	**	8·7	2·6	—

Table 9.2 *continued*

	Glucose mmol/l	Total bilirubin mmol/l	Conditions	References
(1)	$3 \cdot 5 \pm 0 \cdot 3$	$1 \cdot 8 \pm 0 \cdot 6$	Sedated	Houston 1969
	$4 \cdot 4 \pm 0 \cdot 5$	$8 \cdot 6 \pm 1 \cdot 7$	Shot	LeResche *et al* 1974
	$6 \cdot 7 \pm 3 \cdot 0$	$6 \cdot 8 \pm 3 \cdot 4$	Shot or sedated	LeResche *et al* 1974
(2)	—	$5 \cdot 1$	Captive	Naik *et al* 1964, Pasquier 1947, Urbain & Pasquier 1941a, 1948
(3)	—	—	Captive	Hawkey 1975, Pasquier 1947, Urbain & Pasquier 1941b, 1948, Urbain *et al* 1938b
(4)	—	—	Sedated	Drescher-Kaden 1974, Marmiené 1972
	—	—	Sedated	Drescher-Kaden 1974, Marmiené 1972
	—	—	Sedated	Drescher-Kaden 1974, Marmiené 1972
(5)	$9 \cdot 7 \pm 2 \cdot 7$	$11 \cdot 5 \pm 3 \cdot 4$	Restrained	Follis 1972, Herin 1968
	$9 \cdot 4 \pm 1 \cdot 0$	$22 \cdot 2 \pm 6 \cdot 8$	Sedated	Weber & Bliss 1972
	$12 \cdot 5 \pm 4 \cdot 8$	$17 \cdot 1 \pm 10 \cdot 3$	Sedated	Weber & Bliss 1972
	$7 \cdot 8 \pm 1 \cdot 1$	$8 \cdot 9 \pm 0 \cdot 9$	Sedated	Vaughn *et al* 1973
	$11 \cdot 4 \pm 3 \cdot 8$	—	Sedated	Weber & Bliss 1972
	$8 \cdot 9 \pm 1 \cdot 2$	$8 \cdot 6 \pm 1 \cdot 0$	Sedated	Vaughn *et al* 1973
(6)	$5 \cdot 7$	—	Restrained, shot or sedated	Drescher-Kaden 1974, Hawkey 1975, McDougall & Lowe 1968, Pasquier 1947, Urbain *et al* 1938a b, Urbain & Pasquier 1941a b, 1948
(7)	$4 \cdot 5 \pm 13 \cdot 9$	$3 \cdot 4 \pm 15 \cdot 4$	Restrained or shot	Bartels *et al* 1963, Hawkey 1975, McCandless & Dye 1950, McDougall & Lowe 1968, Parshall *et al* 1975, Pasquier 1947, Urbain *et al* 1938a b Urbain & Pasquier 1941a b, 1948
(8)	—	—	Restrained	Pasquier 1947, Urbain *et al* 1938a
(9)	$5 \cdot 8$	—	Sedated or shot	Drescher-Kaden 1974, Graham *et al* 1962, Hawkey 1975, McDougall & Lowe 1968, Pasquier 1947, Urbain *et al* 1938a b, Urbain & Pasquier 1941a b
(10)	—	—	Captive	Altmann & Dittmer 1974
(11)	$5 \cdot 0$	—	Restrained	Bandy *et al* 1957
	$3 \cdot 5$	—	Restrained	Bandy *et al* 1957
	$2 \cdot 1$	—	Restrained	Bandy *et al* 1957
	—	—	Shot, heart blood	Anderson *et al* 1972a b, Hunter *et al* 1972, Taber *et al* 1959
(12)	$5 \cdot 6$	$15 \cdot 4$	Restrained	Tumbleson *et al* 1970, Youatt *et al* 1965
	$6 \cdot 9$	—	Restrained	Tumbleson *et al* 1970, Youatt *et al* 1965
	$7 \cdot 2 \pm 0 \cdot 7$	$6 \cdot 8 \pm 1 \cdot 7$	Restrained	Sikes *et al* 1972, Tumbleson *et al* 1970, Ullrey *et al* 1973
	$8 \cdot 2 \pm 3 \cdot 4$	$8 \cdot 6 \pm 1 \cdot 7$	Restrained	Mathews 1968, Seal *et al* 1972a b, Sikes *et al* 1969, Tumbleson *et al* 1968a b
	$13 \cdot 9 \pm 8 \cdot 4$	—	Restrained	Seal & Erickson 1969, Wilber & Robinson 1958
(13)	$5 \cdot 9$	—	Restrained	Hyvärinen *et al* 1975, 1976, McEwan & Whitehead 1969
	$5 \cdot 9$	—	Restrained	Drescher-Kaden 1974, Hyvärinen *et al* 1975, 1976, McEwan & Whitehead 1969
	$4 \cdot 5$	$5 \cdot 3$	Restrained or sedated	Drescher-Kaden 1974, Dieterich & Luick 1971, Hawkey 1975, Hyvärinen *et al* 1975, 1976, Hyvärinen & Helle 1974, McEwan 1968, McEwan & Whitehead 1969

9.3.3 ENZYMES AND OTHER CONSTITUENTS

Unfortunately, the serum enzyme levels of the various species have been measured in several different ways and expressed in different units, so can be neither compared nor converted to a standard form. The concentration of AAT in white-tailed deer fawns rises rapidly after birth, reaching a maximum at about 10 weeks, before declining to the original level. Lactate dehydrogenase concentrations follow a similar but less well-defined pattern. Serum alkaline phosphatase (AP) concentrations decrease with increasing age in young fallow and white-tailed deer and wapiti (Graham *et al* 1962, Tumbleson *et al* 1970, Weber & Bliss 1972).

Glucose concentrations vary widely, but this is to be expected when different diets and times of collection of blood are taken into consideration.

The concentrations of corticosteroid-binding globulin, thyroxine-binding globulin, thyroxine, total iodide, protein-bound iodide, iron, protein-bound carbohydrates, fucose, hexose, hexosamine and sialic acid in white-tailed deer serum have been measured (Seal & Erickson 1969, Seal *et al* 1972a b). The thyroxine content of moose serum also has been measured (LeResche *et al* 1974).

Very few differences between the composition of the sera of male and female deer have been reported. In white-tailed deer, the concentration of uric acid is lower in males than in females, both juvenile and adult. The concentration of glucose is lower in adult males than in adult females whereas the reverse is true for cholesterol and creatinine concentrations (Seal & Erickson 1969).

Seasonal differences in the composition of serum may reflect pregnancy in females and antler growth or rutting in males, as well as changes in food and environment. The most marked seasonal change demonstrated in the serum of deer occurs in the concentration of AP during antler growth. The concentration of this enzyme in male fallow, white-tailed and red deer reaches a peak at the time of rapid antler growth in the summer and declines precipitously when the antler velvet is shed in early autumn (Drescher-Kaden 1974, Graham *et al* 1962). No significant seasonal changes are detected in the concentration of this enzyme in female deer. Seasonal changes are observed in the concentrations of blood urea nitrogen, cholesterol, glucose, AAT, LDH and TSP in wapiti (LeResche *et al* 1974). There are no significant seasonal changes in the serum proteins of reindeer (Afanas'ev 1963).

9.4 BLOOD VOLUME

Total blood, red cell and plasma volumes for roe and red deer and reindeer are given in Table 9.3. The discrepancies in the values for reindeer are probably a result of differences in method. Whereas Gorodetskii (1959a) used a

Table 9.3 Blood volume of deer

Species and age	No. and sex	Volume, % of body weight			References
		Blood	Plasma	Cells	
Capreolus capreolus Roe deer					
1 y	4♂ 2♀	7·1 ± 1·0*	—	—	Valentinčić 1971
Cervus elaphus Red deer					
Adult	2♂ 7♀	10·5 ± 0·3	5·7 ± 0·1	4·8 ± 0·2	Marmienė & Marma 1972
Rangifer tarandus Reindeer					
New-born	6 ♂♀	12·4	8·6	3·8	Gorodetskii 1959a
7d	5 ♂♀	14·1	9·4	4·7	Gorodetskii 1959a
6m	16 ♂♀	12·0	6·4	5·6	Gorodetskii 1959a
Adult	85 ♂♀	11·8 ± 1·2	7·5 ± 0·6	4·2 ± 0·5	Gorodetskii 1959a
1·5–4 y	7♀	7·2 ± 1·8	4·0 ± 0·9	2·9 ± 0·9	Cameron & Luick 1972
Adult	castrate ♂♂	10·9	—	—	Gorodetskii 1959b

* Standard deviation.
d = Day, m = month, y = year.

dye to measure plasma volume and calculated the other results, Cameron and Luick (1972) measured the blood volume using erythrocytes labelled with chromium-51.

9.5 COAGULATION AND FIBRINOLYSIS

The concentrations of the various clotting factors and other variables such as prothrombin time, partial thromboplastin time and euglobulin lysis time have been reported by Hawkey (1975), but insufficient animals have been studied to enable normal values to be defined. The plasma concentrations of fibrinogen (factor I) are given in Table 9.2.

The mean clotting time of 58 white-tailed deer was 7·3 minutes (s.e. 0·25) when determined by the capillary tube method (Johnson *et al* 1968) and 8·3 minutes (range 6–10) when determined on glass by the Lee-White method (Debbie *et al* 1965). With 34 wapiti, the mean clotting time by the capillary tube method was 14·2 minutes (range 12·7–15·7) (Herin 1968).

The concentration of platelets in the blood of deer is about $300 \times 10^9/l$ (Hawkey 1975). The mean and standard deviation of the concentration of platelets of 16 male red deer, 2·3 years of age or older, which were shot in August and September, were $270 \pm 75 \times 10^9/l$ (range $138–436 \times 10^9/l$). The mean and standard deviation of the volume of the platelets were $4\cdot34\ \mu m^3 \pm$ $0\cdot55$ (range $3\cdot55$–$5\cdot59$) (Williamson & Chapman, personal communication, 1975).

The amino acid composition of fibrinopeptides has changed rapidly during vertebrate evolution and structural studies are used as taxonomic tools. The amino acid sequence of the A and B peptides of the fibrinogen of moose, muntjac, mule deer, red deer, reindeer, sika deer and wapiti have been given by LeResche *et al* 1974. Red deer and wapiti are often regarded as conspecific and they have identical A and B fibrinopeptides. Also the closely related sika deer differs by only one amino acid in the A peptide (Mross & Doolittle 1967).

9.6 ERYTHROCYTE SICKLING

The erythrocytes of many species of deer exhibit sickling, forming a variety of bizarre shapes (Figs. 9.1 and 9.2). Sickling was first noticed in the blood

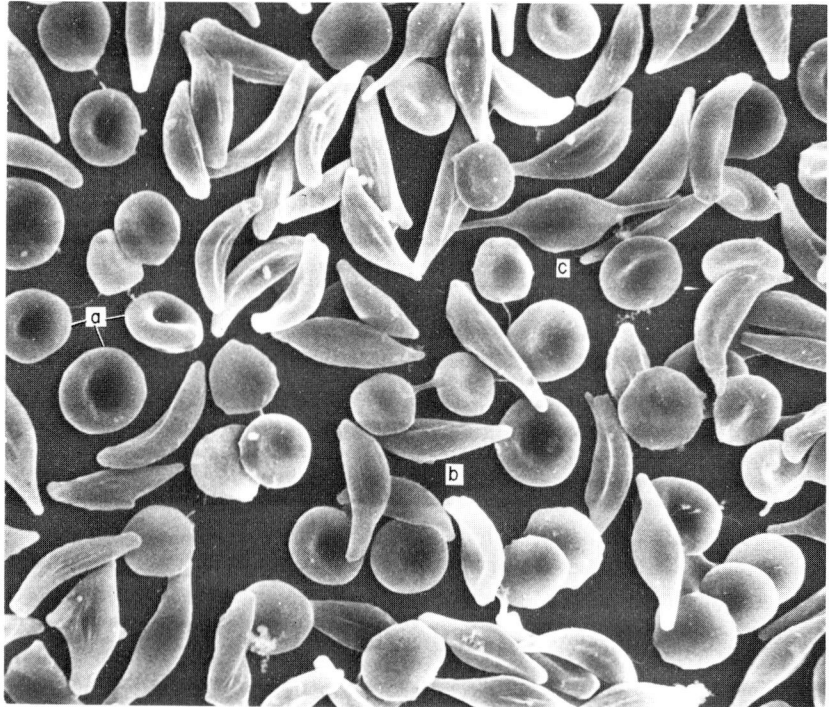

Fig. 9.1 Stereoscan electron micrograph of erythrocytes of an adult barasingha (*Cervus duvauceli*) showing (a) normal cells, (b) classical sickled cells and (c) spindle-shaped or matchstick-type cells. × 1950.

of Reeves' muntjac, hog deer and white-tailed deer by Gulliver (1840) and since then it has been observed in axis deer, barasingha, fallow deer, Indian muntjac, mule deer, Père David's deer, red deer, roe deer, sambar, sika deer and wapiti. The only species of deer examined in which sickling has not been observed are Chinese water deer (Maughan & Williams 1967), moose and reindeer (Undritz *et al* 1960). The sickling of deer erythrocytes is a hereditary, physiological characteristic of the blood but, unlike that of man, it does not result in either haemolytic anaemia or vascular occlusion.

Sickling of white-tailed deer blood is not caused by the presence of a single abnormal haemoglobin, as is the case in man with Hb-S. Haemoglobins II, III and IV are associated with sickling whereas V and VII and Hb-F

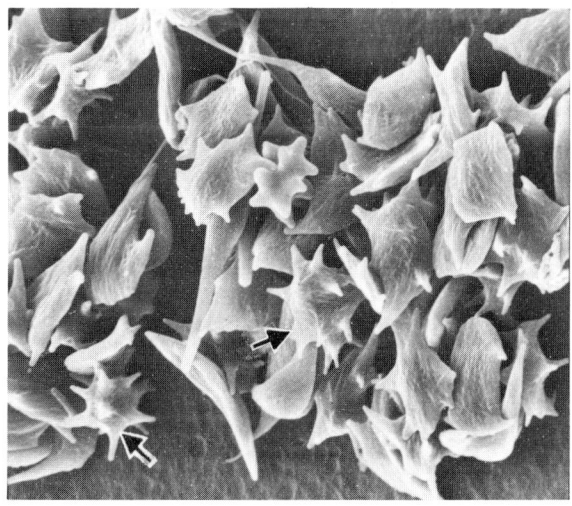

Fig. 9.2 Stereoscan electron micrograph of erythrocytes of a Reeves' muntjac deer (*Muntiacus reevesi*) showing burr-shaped sickle cells. × 1900.

apparently preclude sickling (Kitchen *et al* 1964). In many of the other species of deer whose blood sickles, only a single haemoglobin is found. It should perhaps be referred to therefore as pseudosickling. The sickling of deer erythrocytes can be produced *in vitro* by oxygenation, increasing the pH from 7·0 to 7·5 or lowering the temperature to 4°C. The pH can be raised by bubbling oxygen, nitrogen or carbon monoxide through the blood and causing a 'respiratory alkalosis'. The effect can be reversed by bubbling carbon dioxide through the blood or by the addition of acidic reducing agents (Undritz 1946, Undritz *et al* 1960). The conditions required for the *in vitro* sickling of human Hb-S are the reverse of those required for deer haemoglobin, namely deoxygenation and a reduction in pH to less than 7. Sickled human erythrocytes are more rigid and fragile than non-sickled cells and this is believed to lead to reduced cell life and consequent anaemia. With white-tailed deer, however, sickled red cells are as pliable as and no more fragile than non-sickled cells. These differences in the formation and properties of sickled erythrocytes between deer and man probably explain the absence of clinical sickle cell disease in the former. The viscosity of sickled white-tailed deer blood is 35 to 68 per cent greater than when not sickled. An increase in viscosity of human blood occurs also when sickling takes place (Whitten 1967).

Electron microscopy of sickled, deer erythrocytes shows the haemoglobin to be polymerized and in a highly organized state within the cells whereas in non-sickled cells the haemoglobin appears to be in a fluid state with no apparent orientation (Pritchard *et al* 1963). In typical sickle cells (Fig. 9.1) and in those appearing in the holly leaf shape, the polymerized haemoglobin forms linear aggregates, producing a loose array of multisided tubules with a diameter of $170–190 \times 10^{-1}$ nm. The structure of these 2 types of sickled, deer erythrocyte is similar to that of human sickle cells (Simpson & Taylor 1974). The matchstick type of sickled deer erythrocyte (Fig. 9.1) has a well-ordered intracellular structure, in which the polymerized haemoglobin is arranged in long filaments with a diameter of $75–80 \times 10^{-1}$ nm. These filaments form aggregates which are aligned with the long axis of the cell (Taylor & Simpson 1974).

The different shapes of sickled erythrocytes in white-tailed deer are related to the different types of haemoglobin. The presence of Hb III alone or with Hb I-3 produces classical sickling and the holly leaf shape whereas Hb II and Hb IVa result in the formation of matchstick (Fig. 9.1) and burr (Fig. 9.2) forms respectively (Kitchen *et al* 1964, 1966, 1967). The only difference in chemical composition of human Hb-S from Hb-A is that the negatively charged glutamic acid at position 6 in each of the two β polypeptides is replaced by neutral valine. This small change has far-reaching effects in that it allows intramolecular hydrophobic bonds to form and so change the conformation and solubility of the molecule (Ingram 1957, Murayama 1966). The various haemoglobins of white-tailed deer have even greater differences in composition than do the human ones. It is likely that these differences also result in different molecular conformation and solubility of the haemo-globin molecules, thus accounting for the different shapes of the sickled deer erythrocytes. Changes in pH and pO_2 also affect molecular configuration. The intracellular polymerization of haemoglobin distends the cell membrane, so giving the sickled erythrocyte its characteristic appearance.

9.7 CLINICAL HAEMATOLOGY

Clinical signs related to haematology of deer are almost unknown, it being customary to kill the sick animal rather than treat it. This practice may now change as the farming of deer increases and if the problems often associated with intensive husbandry appear.

9.7.1 EPIZOOTIC HAEMORRHAGIC DISEASE

Epizootic haemorrhagic disease was first identified in white-tailed deer by Shope *et al* in New Jersey in 1955. Outbreaks arise from August to December. It is usually a fatal disease with mortality in experimental infections exceeding 90 per cent. Mule deer are also susceptible but less so than white-tailed deer. The signs are general weakness, inability to stand, fever and haemorrhages throughout the body, particularly in the internal organs. The disease, caused by a virus probably of the picornavirus group, results in multiple haemorrhages probably consequent upon thrombocytopenia. There is a marked thrombocytopenia, the platelet count falling from an average of $512 \times 10^9/l$ (range $380-655 \times 10^9/l$) in healthy animals to $100 \times 10^9/l$ on the 5th day after inoculation, and to about $30 \times 10^9/l$ just before death. The whole-blood clotting time on silicone increases from 16 minutes (9–22) to 35–58 minutes at 1–3 days before death, but the whole-blood clotting time on glass may remain within the normal range of 6–10 minutes. The one-stage prothrombin time may increase from 21 seconds (18–22) to 40 seconds or more but may remain unchanged. Russell's viper venom clotting time increases from 30 seconds (25–39) to 40–50 seconds as the platelet count decreases. In 2 white-tailed deer infected experimentally, the mean RBC declined from $10.5 \times 10^{12}/l$ to $8.4 \times 10^{12}/l$ before increasing to $12.1 \times 10^{12}/l$ on the day of death. There were also marked changes in the neutrophil:lymphocyte ratio (Debbie *et al* 1965, Karstad *et al* 1961).

9.7.2 ARTHRITIS

It has been claimed that arthritis due to infection with *Erysipelothrix insidiosa* leads to changes in the proportions of the various serum proteins (Sikes *et al* 1972) but because only 6 animals were used, 2 of which were controls, the differences could be ascribed to chance.

9.7.3 PARASITISM

Anaplasmosis in mule deer due to a parasite, *Anaplasma marginale*, infecting the red cells, results in a marked anaemia with PCV as low as 0·09 (Osebold *et al* 1959).

Infection of young white-tailed deer fawns with adult lone-star tick, *Amblyomma americanum*, leads to a marked reduction in Hb from 12 to 4 g/dl and in PCV from 0·3 to 0·1 l/l. This type of anaemia probably occurs rather than a microcytic hypochromic one because, in deer of this age, the Hb and PCV usually increase with increasing age. Death may occur if the incidence of infection reaches about 100 ticks per fawn and, in these deer, the PCV may be less than 0·1 l/l. A species of *Theileria* was observed in the red cells and may have contributed to the anaemia (Barker *et al* 1973).

Certain gastrointestinal parasites, such as *Haemonchus contortus*, cause severe anaemia in roe deer and white-tailed deer, with a reduction in Hb, PCV and TSP (Foreyt & Trainer 1970, Valentinčić 1971). Experimental infection of roe deer fawns with liver fluke, *Fasciola hepatica*, resulted in a 6-fold increase in the eosinophil concentration after 12 weeks, the concentration falling to normal values by 26–32 weeks. A second infection at this time caused only a 2-fold increase in the concentration of eosinophils after 12 weeks. The concentrations of the other cellular components were not affected (Berth & Schaich 1973).

9.7.4 MALNUTRITION

Deer may die of starvation in severe winters. The haematology of deer on different planes of nutrition has been studied experimentally but few well-defined differences have been observed. Seasonal changes and the stress of handling may have obscured changes. In white-tailed deer and reindeer, the TSP have been lower in animals on a poorer diet compared with those of better-fed deer (Hyvärinen & Helle 1974, Hyvärinen *et al* 1975; Ullrey *et al* 1964, 1967). The concentrations of blood urea nitrogen in white-tailed deer and plasma urea in reindeer were both reduced in animals on a low protein diet compared with animals receiving a high protein diet (Hove & Jacobsen 1975, Seal *et al* 1972b).

ACKNOWLEDGMENTS

I am most grateful to my wife Norma, Dr J. B. Dixon and J. K. Fawcett for commenting upon the text and to R. McCready for help with translations. I thank P. D. Butcher of the Nuffield Institute of Comparative Medicine for preparing the sickled erythrocytes and P. M. Rowles of the Middlesex Hospital Medical School for taking the stereoscan electron micrographs.

10

THE HAEMATOLOGY OF THE DOG

N. W. SPURLING

10.1   INTRODUCTION

The popularity of the dog as a pet and as an experimental subject for bio-medical research has resulted in the development of a wide knowledge of its haematology in both health and in disease.

10.2   HAEMOPOIESIS

Haemopoiesis during embryonic and fetal development has been studied in Beagles by Andersen and Goldman (1970) and Andersen and Schalm (1970). First evidence of intraembryonic erythropoiesis was observed in the liver on day 25 post coitum. Prior to this the mesoblastic phase of erythropoiesis occurred in extra-embryonic blood-forming tissue and the circulating cells were predominantly primitive nucleated erythrocytes. By day 27 post coitum, hepatic erythropoiesis was taking place in sparse foci and by day 40 was very active. First evidence of the myeloid (bone marrow) phase of haemopoiesis was seen in a 32-day embryo when erythropoiesis was observed both in the marrow and in the liver together with occasional foci in the thymus, mesonephros and gonads.

During the second half of the 60–65-day gestation period there was a gradual progression towards the blood picture observed at birth. There was a decrease in the proportion of circulating nucleated erythrocytes. Leuco-cytes made a gradual appearance, myelopoiesis (granulocyte production) was first observed in the bone marrow on day 35 post coitum. The lymphocytes were the last leucocytes to appear. In the femoral marrow of a 48-day fetus, myelopoiesis was observed but the sinusoids were poorly developed. By day 58 the sinusoids were well developed and organized haemopoietic tissue was present. The leucocyte count was approximately $1 \times 10^9/l$ in the blood of a 50-day fetus. Precisely when splenic erythropoiesis commenced was not clear from these studies by Andersen and Goldman (1970) and Andersen and

Schalm (1970). It was certainly absent as late as day 40 post coitum although on day 45 slight evidence of differentiation of red and white pulp was seen.

During puppyhood there is a progressive reduction in haemopoietic activity. Andersen and Goldman (1970) found that erythropoiesis was still occurring in the liver on day 7 but was absent on day 45. Splenic erythropoiesis was active on day 14 and, although the level of activity was diminished by 45 days it was still detectable until approximately 175 days. Femoral marrow at birth contained little fat and was highly cellular whereas the amount of fat present was increasing by 64 days. Andersen and Schalm (1970) found that early in life haemopoiesis is active in the marrow of all bones of Beagle pups. This declines with maturity in the long bones but it increases in the ribs, vertebrae, pelvis and other flat bones. In my laboratory active marrow has been removed at necropsy from the proximal epiphysis of the femurs of approximately 450 Beagles aged between 5 and 13 months of age as well as from over 100 dogs of mixed breeds. It was not uncommon to encounter difficulty in obtaining a good sample of red marrow, free of obvious fat, from this site in the older dogs in this series despite the fact that the marrow cavity was first exposed by splitting the bone.

Bone marrow biopsy from puppies is practicable using the method of Spranger and Hime (1961). Entry to the femoral medullary cavity is achieved by penetration of the bone in the floor of the trochanteric fossa, as for the insertion of an intramedullary orthopaedic pin. The method has been used for day-old puppies and for adult Beagles. In adult dogs the iliac crest or the ribs and sternum are other sites for withdrawing marrow during life. Although Schermer (1967) warns of the greater care that is necessary when carrying out sternal punctures on dogs, compared with the same procedure on man, Melveger *et al* (1969) and Saar (1973a) have successfully used this site. Brown and Hardy (personal communication, 1975) have also carried out a large number of sternal punctures on young Beagles. Penny (1974) found the external angle of the ilium to be the most satisfactory site. When large amounts of canine marrow are required, without sacrifice of the donor, the surgical resection of ribs (Liegeois & Monaco 1973) may have an application. However, when interpreting results, it should be remembered that the ribs are particularly rich in active marrow (Greenberg *et al* 1966) and that the removal of several ribs would presumably result in compensatory increases in active marrow at other sites.

There have been many publications describing the cellular composition of canine bone marrow (Calhoun 1954, Altman & Dittmer 1961 and Schalm *et al* 1975). Penny and Carlisle (1970) in a comparative study of bone marrow biopsy material obtained from the iliac crest, rib and sternum suggested that there was a statistically significant difference in cellular composition between the sexes based on a study using 10 male and 10 female dogs. Penny (1974),

N. W. Spurling

however, appears to question this earlier finding, stating that the sample number was small and that further work was necessary. The distribution of bone marrow throughout the canine skeleton has been studied by Greenberg *et al* (1966) and by Calvo *et al* (1975). Maximum cellularity occurs in the

Table 10.1 A typical canine myelogram. Derived from the published data of several authors (see text) and embracing 186 individual myelograms. The ranges encompass the smallest and the largest values which occurred among the data collated or in a few instances the author's mean values ± the standard deviation.

Cell type	%	Range %
Myeloblasts	1·24	0– 5·1
Promyelocytes	1·37	0– 5·8
Neutrophilic myelocyte	5·78	0–15·0
Neutrophilic metamyelocyte	5·60	0–24·4
Neutrophilic band cells	25·98	6·8–62·9
Segmented neutrophils	8·15	0–44·2
Eosinophilic myelocyte	1·19	0– 4·2
Eosinophilic metamyelocyte	1·47	0·4– 3·7
Eosinophilic band cells	1·31	0·9– 2·4
Segmented eosinophils	2·35	0– 6·8
Basophils	0·11	0– 1·3
Total myeloid cells	54·55	
Proerythroblasts	1·24	0– 3·4
Early (basophilic) normoblasts	5·79	0·4–11·6
Intermediate (polychromatic) normoblasts	20·13	3·5–27·0
Late (oxyphilic) normoblasts	11·32	0–25·8
Total erythroid cells	38·48	
Reticulum cells	0·39	0– 2·1
Lymphocytes including prolymphocytes	2·80	0–15·1
Monocytes (mature and immature)	0·18	0– 0·4
Plasma cells	1·12	0– 4·3
Damaged and other unidentified cells	2·29	0–15·7
Megakaryocytes	0·20	0– 1·4
Mitotic index	0·62	0– 1·14
M/E ratio	1·42	< 5·64

bones of the trunk with gradual diminution along the limbs, but the differential count was similar in all sites examined.

The data of Stasney and Higgins (1937), Mulligan (1941), Van Loon and Clark (1943), Rekers and Coulter (1948), Schalm (1965) and Penny and

Carlisle (1970) have been collated in Table 10.1 to give a representative canine myelogram based on the data from 186 samples from adult dogs.

Reference has already been made to a series of femoral marrow samples obtained in my laboratory during necropsies on Beagles. I have determined myeloid/erythroid ratios from 93 apparently normal healthy Beagles, aged 5–13 months. Smears were prepared by the rapid method of Berenbaum (1956) in which a fragment of marrow is mixed with a drop of a 10% solution of bovine albumin (Armour) on a slide until the cells are evenly dispersed. The resultant cell suspension is spread in the same manner as a blood film. Homologous serum containing EDTA has also been advocated as a suspending agent for use in preparing films of canine marrow (Fluharty & Uhler 1975). Myeloid/erythroid ratios averaged 1·17 (s.d. 0·40) for male and 1·22 (s.d. 0·59) for female Beagles from our colony. A series of 19 male and 18 female dogs of mixed breeds and unknown age were also examined using the same technique. The myeloid/erythroid ratios of these dogs averaged 1·36 (s.d. 0·81) for male and 1·22 (s.d. 0·49) for female dogs. Giemsa-stained sections prepared from bone marrow were examined to assess architecture and cellularity. Westen (1974) found that cylindrical biopsies, 4 mm in diameter and suitable for sectioning, could be obtained from the iliac crest of Beagles.

It has recently been shown, however, that examination of a stained section may be an insensitive method of assessing marrow cellularity (Morley & Blake 1975). Ideally both a total nucleated cell count and an examination of a film and a stained section should be performed. Few authors cite marrow total nucleated cell counts but Rekers and Coulter (1948) presented mean counts which ranged from 788 to 1795 (mean 1205) $\times 10^9$/l for marrow derived from the ribs and 576 to 2256 (mean 1122) $\times 10^9$/l for marrow derived from the epiphysis of the femur. Meyer and Bloom (1943) reported total white cell counts, which were in fact total nucleated cell counts, averaging 145×10^9/l in ilial marrow of dogs. Brown and Hardy (personal communication 1975) report that on a large number of young Beagles the total nucleated cell count of marrow obtained by sternal puncture averaged 160×10^9/l (range 80–259 $\times 10^9$/l) for male animals and 185×10^9/l (range 75–296 $\times 10^9$/l) for female animals.

Deubelbeiss *et al* (1975a), using a method in which the cellularity of marrow sections was correlated with that of total skeletal marrow by a radio-iron dilution method, found the total number of nucleated red cells in the marrow of 6 mongrels averaged $5·48 \times 10^9$/kg body weight and the total number of cells of the neutrophil series in the marrow averaged $6·6 \times 10^9$/kg. The neutrophil/erythroid ratios of marrow obtained from rib, vertebra and pelvis (average 1·2) did not vary significantly. Daily erythron iron turnover averaged 0·90 mg Fe/dl of whole blood. These data are at variance with those of several earlier workers who used a variety of methods. Deubelbeiss *et al* discussed some of these earlier attempts to quantify haematopoietic tissue in the dog. It has been claimed that approximately 20 per cent of canine erythroid cells die between extrusion of the nucleus and the appearance of the erythrocytes in the blood (Lala *et al* 1966). A similar loss occurs during granulopoiesis (Maloney *et al* 1963). Deubelbeiss *et al* (1975b) in a study of neutrophil kinetics in 6 mongrels, and utilizing [^{3}H] thymidine-labelling of cells, found that the mean transit time of post mitotic neutrophils in the marrow was 82·1 hours. It was estimated that the daily marrow turnover of neutrophils averaged $1·65 \times 10^9$ cells/kg body weight. This corresponded closely with their estimated daily turnover of neutrophils in the blood which was $1·66 \times 10^9$ cells/kg, thus demonstrating that virtually all neutrophils which leave the marrow enter the blood. The peripheral blood of the dog, like that of man, has been shown to contain significant numbers of cells with haemopoietic colony forming potential (Debelak-Fehir *et al* 1975).

Colour photomicrographs of the major cell types which may be found in canine marrow have been published by Lorthioir (1968), Saar (1973b, 1974 1975), and by Schalm *et al* (1975) and descriptions of the cells have been given by Stasney and Higgins (1937), Bloom and Meyer (1944), Rekers and Coulter (1948) and Penny (1974). The canine cells are similar to those present in human marrow and atlases of human haematology such as Heilmeyer and Begemann (1955), McDonald *et al* (1968) or Undritz (1973) are quite satisfactory for use in identifying the canine cells.

The hormone, erythropoietin, which regulates erythropoiesis, is now known to be generated in the plasma by the action of renal erythropoietic factor (REF) on an inactive precursor globulin, erythropoietinogen, which is synthesized in the liver. In dogs REF occurs, as in man, in approximately equal quantities in the renal cortex and in the medulla (Zanjani *et al* 1967). Incubation of kidney fractions containing REF in vitro, with serum containing erythropoietinogen results in the generation of erythropoietin. This reaction does not appear to be species specific among mammalian species (Zanjani *et al* 1969). The erythropoietic response produced in mice or rats by the injection of canine plasma may be used to assay the level of REF or erythropoietin (Abbrecht and Malvin 1966). Mujovic and Fisher (1974) suggested that prostaglandins may be involved in the first stage of a sequence leading to kidney production of REF in dogs.

Naets and Heuse (1964) found that almost total erythroid aplasia occurred in dogs as early as 3 days after bilateral nephrectomy and Mirand *et al* (1968) demonstrated that the increase in the plasma erythropoietin levels, which normally results from hypoxia due to blood loss, did not occur in dogs from which both kidneys had been removed. These findings suggest a difference between the control of erythropoiesis in the dog and that which operates in man and several other species where there is apparently also an extra-renal source of erythropoietic factor.

10.3 THE BLOOD PICTURE OF THE HEALTHY DOG, INCLUDING PHYSIOLOGICAL VARIATION

10.3.1 THE ERYTHROCYTES

10.3.1.1 Blood volume and erythrocyte life-span

Measurements of the blood volume of dogs have been carried out by determining the erythrocyte volume utilizing isotopically labelled erythrocytes or by the less accurate method of determining plasma volume by the Evans' blue (T-1824) dilution or isotopically labelled albumin methods. A more accurate combined method is also used based on both erythrocyte and plasma volume determinations. The literature has been collated by Altman and Dittmer (1961) and by Schalm *et al* (1975). The average value for blood volume was 91·6 ml/kg body weight although figures as low as 55·5 and as high as 134·8 ml/kg have been reported. Direct determinations of erythrocyte volume averaged 38·1 ml/kg but a range of values from 20·4 to 64·8 ml/kg have been recorded. Similarly, direct measurements of plasma volume have averaged 51·8 ml/kg but range from 31·7 to 83·9 ml/kg. Sabourin *et al* (1975), using [131]iodine-labelled albumin, found that the mean values for blood volume, erythrocyte volume and plasma volume in 39 dogs were 92·08 (s.d. 8·85), 39·35 (s.d. 5·79) and 52·14 (s.d. 6·58) ml/kg respectively. Reihart and Reihart (1968) consider the normal blood volume of the dog to be only 80–85 ml/kg. Herczeg *et al* (1974) recently compared the plasma volume of the dog when determined by the Evans' blue (T-1824) method with that determined by the ^{131}I-albumin dilution method. The values obtained, 48·9 ml/kg and 48·6 ml/kg, corresponded very closely. Andersen and Schalm (1970) state that between 50 and 75 per cent of the blood volume of the dog may be collected by exsanguination.

The majority of reports using isotopic methods suggest a life-span of canine erythrocytes of approximately 115 days. Berlin *et al* (1959) quote the average life span as 90–135 days. The half-life, using Cr^{51} labelling, was 21 to 30 days.

10.3.1.2 Reticulocytes

In my laboratory the average reticulocyte count of healthy Beagles, using the method of Dacie and Lewis (1975), was found to be approximately 1·0–1·5 per cent of the circulating erythrocytes. This is in general agreement with the range of values published in the literature (Van Loon & Clark 1943, Brunk 1969, Bushby 1970, Schalm *et al* 1975). Morley and Stohlman (1969) demonstrated that the reticulocyte counts of a proportion of dogs reveal oscillations with a periodicity of approximately 14 days. Canine reticulocytes usually contain definite aggregates of reticulum, rather than the punctate granules which occur in species such as the cat (Laber *et al* 1974). Under normal circumstances the average maturation time of reticulocytes in canine blood (i.e. the time required for them to lose their visible reticulum) is 31 hours (Nizet & Robscheit-Robbins 1950), but in anaemia and dietary deficiency maturation may be grossly abnormal. In these circumstances the reticulocyte count, expressed simply as a percentage of the circulating erythrocytes, will present a distorted impression of erythropoietic activity and the count should be corrected in the manner described by Hillman and Finch (1969). Reticulocytes appear as polychromatophilic erythrocytes when stained in conventional blood films by Romanowsky methods (Dacie & Lewis 1975). Laber *et al* (1974) compared counts of polychromatophilic erythrocytes in Romanowsky stained films with direct counts of reticulocytes as a means of assessing erythrocyte production in the dog. They found no significant difference between the values obtained by these 2 methods.

10.3.1.3 Erythrocyte metabolism

Erythrocyte metabolism in the dog and other mammalian species has been reviewed by Kaneko (1974). Kaneko collated from the literature the levels of the majority of enzymes present in erythrocytes. Values for erythrocyte glucose utilization in the dog range from 1·33 to 2·99 μ mols/h/ml. This rate is intermediate between species which have low overall rates of erythrocyte glucose metabolism (the cow and the sheep) and those with high rates (man, rabbit and rat). The pentose–phosphate pathway is important although it utilizes only some 5 per cent of the glucose-6-phosphate generated in the canine erythrocyte. This pathway protects the erythrocyte membrane, enzymes and haemoglobin against oxidative damage. Heinz bodies, which occur when oxidative damage to haemoglobin has occurred, are not present in the blood of normal healthy dogs (Meyer 1962). Harvey and Kaneko (1974) found that canine and human erythrocytes were less susceptible to methylene blue-induced Heinz body formation in vitro than were those of the cat, but canine and feline erythrocytes were less able than human erythrocytes to concentrate methylene blue intracellularly. In the presence of methylene blue, canine and feline erythrocytes were also unable to maintain normal levels of reduced glutathione. Kaneko (1974) indicated that the level of glucose-6-phosphate dehydrogenase is basically similar in canine and human erythrocytes and a hereditary deficiency of this enzyme in dogs does not appear to have been reported. However, Buonaccorsi *et al* (1973) claimed that a deficiency of glucose-6-phosphate dehydrogenase and 2,3 diphosphoglyceric acid occurred in the erythrocytes of 75 per cent of anaemic dogs with a variety of disorders.

Smith and Kiefer (1973) demonstrated differences between breeds in erythrocytic glyceraldehyde-3-phosphate dehydrogenase and enolase activity and the erythrocytes of Great Pyrenees and Labrador retrievers reduced oxidized glutathione at a faster rate than did erythrocytes of other breeds studied. A variant of erythrocytic soluble aspartate aminotransferase (AAT) was found to occur with high frequency among Basenjis and occasional variants of indophenol oxidase and acid phosphatase occurred in other breeds (Weiden *et al* 1974). Like the erythrocyte of the cat, but unlike that of man, the canine erythrocyte has a virtually inactive sodium pump. Consequently the ion concentrations present in the canine erythrocyte show marked differences from those present in human erythrocytes. Kaneko (1974) showed that the sodium and potassium concentrations within the canine erythrocyte, 121 mmol/l and 9·5 mmol/l respectively, approximate those in serum, 146 and 5 mmol/l respectively. Bost and Magat (1975) claimed that only 73 per cent of canine blood glucose was in solution in the plasma, a considerably lower proportion than was present in the plasma of several other species studied.

10.3.1.4 Haemoglobin

In the dog, as in most species studied (Kitchen & Brett 1974) a distinct embryonic haemoglobin has been found to be associated with the presence of primitive nucleated erythrocytes in the early embryo. Thereafter there is apparently a direct transition to the adult type of haemoglobin (Le Crone 1970). It is possible that, although the haemoglobin present in the fetal erythrocytes is the same as that present in the erythrocytes of the adult dog, its oxygen affinity during fetal life and for a time after birth is increased by decrease of the concentration of 2,3-diphosphoglycerate (2,3-DPG) within the erythrocyte (Dhindsa *et al* 1972, Kaneko 1974, Kitchen & Brett 1974). Kitchen (1974) postulated that, although only one form of the β chain is present in the canine adult haemoglobin molecule, polymorphism of the α chain may occur. Dresler *et al* (1974) defined 2 forms of the canine α chain differing only at a single position. One form had a threonyl residue whereas the other had an alanyl residue in this position. Breeding studies suggested the presence of multiple structural gene loci for the α chain of canine haemoglobin. Haemoglobinopathies, such as occur in man due to the presence of abnormal haemoglobin types, have not been demonstrated in dogs.

During the routine examination of blood films crystals which are presumed to be haemoglobin are occasionally encountered. Lund (1974) observed large numbers of these crystals situated both intra- and extra-erythrocytically in the blood of 11 young dogs and proposed that their presence be due to the immaturity of the reticulo-endothelial system. I have occasionally observed rectangular crystals situated extra-erythrocytically, in films of the peripheral blood of young Beagles.

10.3.1.5 Normal values of red cells

Numerous workers have presented their 'normal' ranges for the erythrocyte count (RBC) haemoglobin (Hb) level and packed cell volume (PCV) of dogs, but the range of such 'normal' values encountered in the clinical diagnostic laboratory will almost certainly be different to that encountered in research laboratories since the latter study only healthy dogs of a single breed in a limited age range (Pick & Eubanks 1965).

It has been reported that the number of erythrocytes present in a sample can be estimated from the PCV since in dogs these values are closely correlated (Uglialoro & Alder 1957). For example a PCV of 0·45 l/l was considered to be equivalent to an erythrocyte count of $7·29 \times 10^{12}$/l. It should be remembered, however, that this method is valid only when the mean cell volume (MCV) is normal.

Typical erythrocyte data presented by Van Loon and Clark (1943), Usacheva (1957), Altman and Dittmer (1961), Doxey (1966a) and Schalm *et al* (1975) have been used to produce the following 'normal' ranges for dogs of mixed breeds and mixed ages.

	Mean value	*Range of values*
Erythrocyte count (RBC)	$6·5 \times 10^{12}$/l	$4·25–8·5 \times 10^{12}$/l
Haemoglobin (Hb)	15·5 g/dl	10·5–21 g/dl
Packed cell volume (PCV)	0·46 l/l	0·34–0·58 l/l

Irfan (1961) and Doxey (1966a) reported that the various breeds of dog, with the exception of the Greyhound, have a similar erythrocyte picture. In the Greyhound the RBC, Hb and PCV are higher than in other dogs of a comparable age. Similar differences between the values for Greyhounds and for mongrels were reported by Porter and Canaday (1971). Haematological values for normal Basenjis were presented by Ewing, Schalm and Smith (1972).

Many studies of the normal haematological picture of the Beagle have been reported according to sex and age but few have analysed their data for sex and age-related differences. Significant differences between the sexes in their Hb level, PCV and RBC may develop as Beagles reach maturity (Andersen & Gee 1958). These values tend to be greater in mature male Beagles than in mature female Beagles. Other authors have reported minor differences between the sexes (Robinson & Ziegler 1968, Michaelson *et al* 1966, Weisse *et al* 1971).

There are considerable differences between the values for young pups and those for mature animals. Haemoglobin levels, PCV and RBC counts are high, close to adult levels, during the first 3 days following birth after which they fall dramatically until days 14–17. From this age RBC begin to increase whereas Hb levels and PCV continue to fall slightly, thus indicating a change in cell volume. These changes during the first weeks of life are also reflected in the total body erythrocyte volume (Deavers *et al* 1971). The precise point at which these 2 values are reported to start increasing varies between 28 and 30 days (Andersen & Gee 1958) and 47 to 52 days (Earl *et al* 1973, Shifrine *et al* 1973) and may well be a result of the pups beginning to consume food provided for the dam (Andersen & Gee 1958). Hb level, PCV and RBC increase in parallel from this age onwards. Andersen and Gee (1958) found that maximum levels were reached at approximately 10 months of age, but Weiner and Bradley (1972) report PCVs which continue to increase until 18 months of age. Bulgin *et al* (1970) show values which remain essentially constant between approximately 10 months and $4\frac{1}{2}$ years of age, with the exception of a very slight fall in PCV. Abel and Schneider's (1973) data indicate that peak levels are reached between 13 months and 2 years of age. Dougherty and Rosenblatt (1965) noticed a steady decline from 2 years onwards which continues at least until the dogs are 9 years of age.

Feeding and excitement may result in an increase in the PCV of dogs (Reece & Wahlstrom 1970). The change which results from feeding is probably due to transient haemoconcentration. No increase in PCV occurred after feeding in splenectomized dogs but their PCV was already higher than that of intact dogs (Reece & Snodgrass 1972). Hamilton and Horvath (1954), however, found no significant difference in the RBC of samples from normal and from splenectomized dogs. A high RBC may result from splenic contraction due to excitement or fear arising from the collection of a blood sample. Schalm *et al* (1975) encountered high counts, which they attributed to this factor, in samples from a number of breeds. Soave and Boyle (1965) found significantly lower Hb levels and PCVs in apparently healthy, newly purchased, pound dogs compared with dogs which had been housed in laboratory kennels for more than 4 months. This difference may have been due, in part, to the improved nutritional status of the laboratory-housed dogs. I found that the Hb levels of a group of dogs increased by more than 1 g/dl after their diet was changed from canned pet food, supplemented with biscuit meal, to a complete dry dog diet with *ad libitum* water. Andersen and Gee (1958) commented on the likelihood of dietary differences being responsible for some of the variation of erythrocyte values reported in the literature.

Andersen and Schalm (1970) reported that the PCV of Beagle puppies varied by approximately 0·05 l/l during each day. The PCV was at its highest in the early morning, declining during the morning but increasing in the evening. This diurnal pattern was less marked in adult Beagles. A seasonal variation of approximately 0·03 l/l in the PCV of Beagles kept in outdoor kennels was reported by Andersen and Schalm (1970). The values were at their lowest point during May, peak values occurring during December. Potkay and Zinn (1969) observed that PCV and Hb values of laboratory-reared Foxhounds were significantly higher in winter than in summer and Thomas

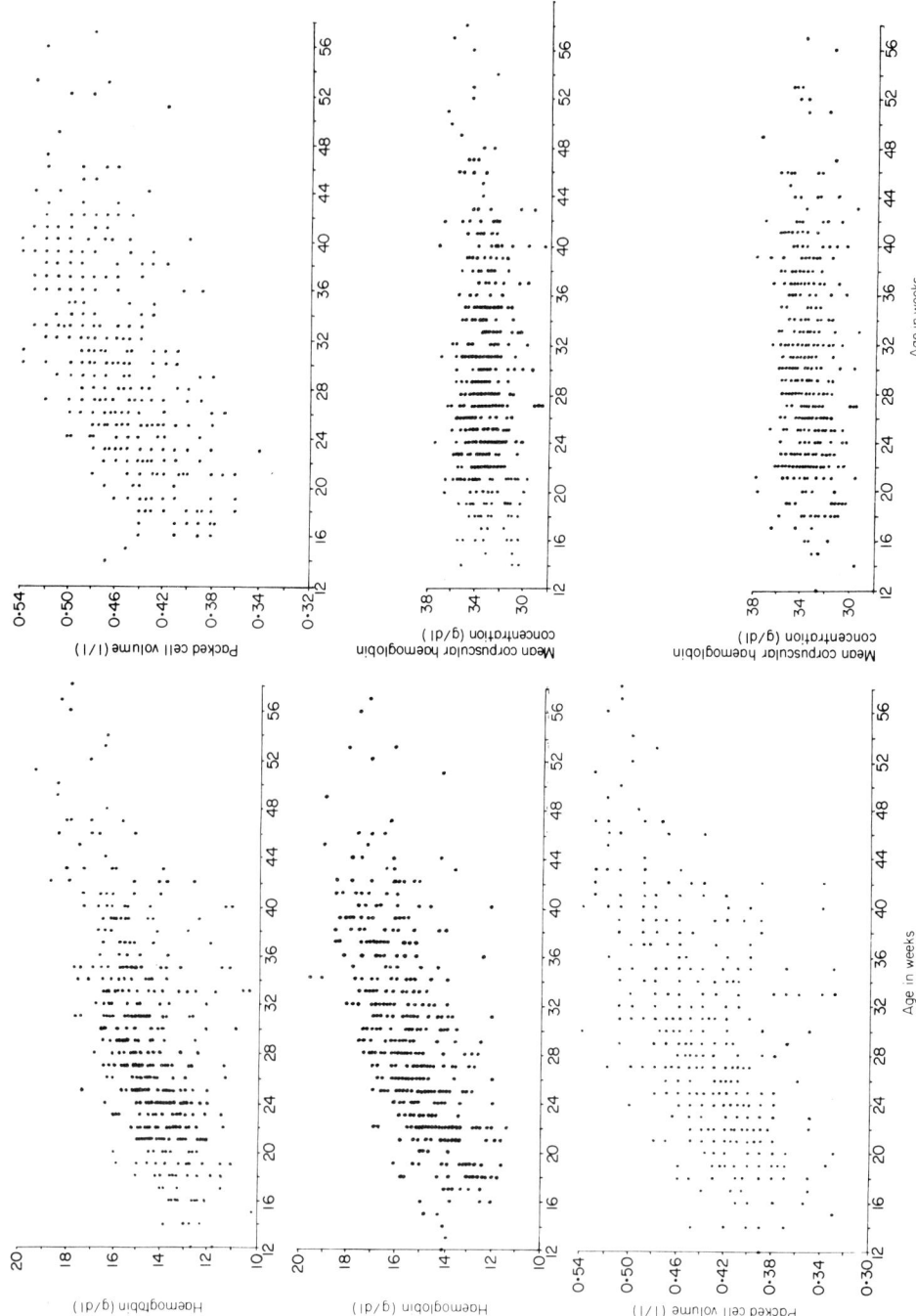

and Kittrell (1966) recorded similar seasonal changes in the erythrocyte parameters of German Shepherd dogs (Alsatians). Considerable daily variation occurs, even when the same dogs are examined at the same time on successive days (Afonsky 1955).

Gibson *et al* (1946) found that 17 per cent of the blood volume of the dog was present in the microvasculature, the greatest amount being present in the liver and skeletal muscle. Overall, the PCV of blood in the arteries and veins was greater than that of blood in the remainder of the circulation. Hamilton and Horvath (1954) found that there was no significant difference between the RBC of samples from the arterial and the venous sides of the circulation. The trapped plasma correction factor for the PCV of the dog was found to be 0.95 ± 0.023 (s.d.) for the macro method and 0.97 ± 0.020 for the micro method (Chien *et al* 1965). Thus the influence of trapped plasma is small when the micro method is employed due to the greater acceleration achieved in the microhaematocrit centrifuge (usually 12,000 *g*). The susceptibility of canine erythrocytes to rouleau formation also assists in reducing the volume of trapped plasma.

Doxey (1966b) and Andersen and Schalm (1970) studied the changes which occur in the blood of bitches during gestation and lactation. The erythrocyte count gradually decreased during gestation, the lowest values occurring at or soon after parturition. El-Hindawy (1948) observed a fall in the RBC of bitches which continued during lactation but this finding may reflect a difference in the nutritional status of his dogs. Both Doxey (1966) and Andersen and Schalm (1970) found that the erythrocyte values had usually returned to normal by approximately the 9th week after parturition.

The Hb level, PCV and mean corpuscular haemoglobin concentration (MCHC) data of Beagles which composed the control group from various long term experiments have been assembled in Figs. 10.1–10.6. The dogs were fed a commercially available complete dry diet, with *ad libitum* water. Erythrocyte counts are not shown since they were not performed on all dogs. A number of the points represent more than one observation. This occurred most often among the PCVs since they were recorded only in steps

---

Fig. **10.1** (top left)   Male Beagles, haemoglobin levels. Relationship with age.
Fig. **10.2** (middle left)   Female Beagles, haemoglobin levels. Relationship with age.
Fig. **10.3** (bottom left)   Male Beagles, packed cell volume (microhaematocrit). Relationship with age.
Fig. **10.4** (top right)   Female Beagles, packed cell volume (microhaematocrit). Relationship with age.
Fig. **10.5** (middle right)   Male Beagles. Mean corpuscular haemoglobin concentration. Relationship with age.
Fig. **10.6** (bottom right)   Female Beagles. Mean corpuscular haemoglobin concentration. Relationship with age.

of 0·01 1/l. These data are in general agreement with published data derived from Beagles or from the general canine population.

Haden (1934) found the mean diameter of canine erythrocytes to be 7·2 μm and Altman and Dittmer (1961) give the mean diameter as 7·1 μm. The thickness of canine erythrocytes was found to be 1·7 μm by Haden (1934). Shifrine *et al* (1973) found that the mean corpuscular haemoglobin (MCH) decreased from 32·7 pg shortly after birth to approximately 22 pg by 2 months of age. Similarly the MCV decreased from 94 fl soon after birth to 64 fl at 2 months of age. The proportionate change in the MCH and the MCV was almost identical thus confirming the findings of Niepage (1974) who showed that in dogs a very close correlation exists between these values. The changes which occur during the first weeks of life are also reflected in the Hb level and in the total bodily erythrocyte volume (Deavers *et al* 1971). According to Shifrine *et al* the MCHC varied only slightly with age, the average value being 34·6 g/dl shortly after birth but decreasing only marginally to approximately 33 g/dl at 2 months of age. Niepage (1974) found that the MCHC remained constant, averaging approximately 32 g/dl, irrespective of changes in the MCV. Schalm *et al* (1975) gave the normal values for the canine erythrocyte as MCH 19·5–24·5 pg (average 22·8 pg); MCV 60–77 fl (average 70 fl) and MCHC 32–36 g/dl (average 34 g/dl). I find no appreciable change of MCHC between 15 and 42 weeks of age, averaging approximately 33·5 g/dl (Figs 10.5 and 10.6). Niepage (1975) claims that the MCV of a dog may fluctuate by as much as 10 fl as a result of physiological variations. It is likely, however, that technical factors contributed to this fluctuation.

10.3.1.6 Red cell fragility

During handling of blood samples in the laboratory, canine erythrocytes appear to be more liable to undergo lysis than do human erythrocytes. Cruz and Baumgarten (1957) found marked variability between dogs in the susceptibility of their erythrocytes to lysis. By replacement of the plasma with buffered saline they showed that canine erythrocytes were far more susceptible to haemolysis due to changes in pH than were human or sheep erythrocytes. Haemolysis begins between pH 8·0 and 8·3 and is complete at pH 10·0. Iampietro *et al* (1967) also demonstrated pH-dependent lysis of canine erythrocytes.

Coldman *et al* (1969) compared the osmotic fragility of the erythrocytes of 8 mammalian species and found that canine erythrocytes were the least susceptible to osmotic lysis. Perk *et al* (1964) gave the concentration of buffered saline in which lysis of cells with 'minimal' and 'maximum' resistance occurred as 5·0 and 2·9 g/l respectively. These workers, however, used the 'gradual haemolysis' method which is known to produce results which cannot be compared with those obtained by conventional methods. I find that maximum haemolysis of normal Beagle erythrocytes occurs at a saline concentration of 3·3 g/l and zero (i.e. minimal) haemolysis at 6·0 g/l respectively (Poynter *et al* 1965). Hall and Follett (1972) reported that the range of saline concentrations causing maximum (100 per cent) and minimum lysis of canine erythrocytes were 1·0–3·5 g/l and 5·5–7·0 g/l respectively and Jain (1972) quoted 2·5–3·5 g/l and 4·8–6·0 g/l.

Two groups of workers have reported a difference between the susceptibility of newly formed canine and human erythrocytes to lysis (Cruz *et al* 1941, Stewart *et al* 1950). Using radioactive iron as a label, these workers found that, in anaemic dogs, the erythrocytes which have recently entered the circulation seem to show increased susceptibility to osmotic lysis compared with older cells. This difference disappeared after the cells had been in the circulation for a few days. Stewart *et al* (1950) also observed that their susceptibility to mechanical lysis was decreased. Towards the end of their life in the circulation their susceptibility to mechanical lysis increased and their susceptibility to osmotic lysis was either unchanged (Stewart *et al* 1950) or decreased (Cruz *et al* 1941).

Jasper and Jain (1965a) reported that whereas the mechanical fragility of canine erythrocytes increased during lipaemia, resulting from a fat-rich diet, osmotic fragility remained normal. Soliman and Amrousi (1966) found that the osmotic fragility of the erythrocytes of various species including the dog was related to cell size, the larger a species' erythrocytes, the greater their resistance to lysis.

10.3.1.7 ESR and plasma viscosity

Determination of the erythrocyte sedimentation rate (ESR) can provide a useful indication of progress during many diseases in the dog, particularly infections, malignancies and diverse inflammatory conditions. The non-specificity of this test is illustrated by the fact that Morgan (1966) listed 13 factors which may increase and 14 which may decrease the ESR.

Pillai and Nair (1974) compared the ESR of 8 species, including the dog, using the Wintrobe and Westergren methods and also the Washburn and Meyers (1957) method. In this latter method, Wintrobe tubes were supported at an angle of 45° from the vertical. One-hour rates for mongrel dogs were 6·5 ± 3·1 mm by the Westergren method, 14·5 ± 5·3 mm by the Wintrobe method and 26·5 ± 8·5 mm by the Washburn and Meyers method. Jain and Kono (1975) found that 1-hour rates with the Wintrobe method were generally greater than those with a capillary tube method when the PCV of canine blood was in the 0·36 to 0·60 l/l range. With lower PCVs this relationship was reversed. A very slight decrease in the ESR resulted if the blood sample was held at 4°C for 2 to 6 hours prior to testing. If held at room temperature the resultant decrease was greater. Osbaldiston (1971), using the Wintrobe method, reported that the canine ESR averages 18 mm in 1 hour, the normal range being 7·5–26 mm. Bild (1965) stated that a young, healthy Beagle should have a zero ESR by the capillary tube method. Morgan (1966) cited normal ranges from the literature of 5–25 mm, 1–4 mm and less than 10 mm in 1 hour. Technical variation may be responsible for a proportion of the variation found but some variation is probably attributable to differences in the health status of the dogs studied.

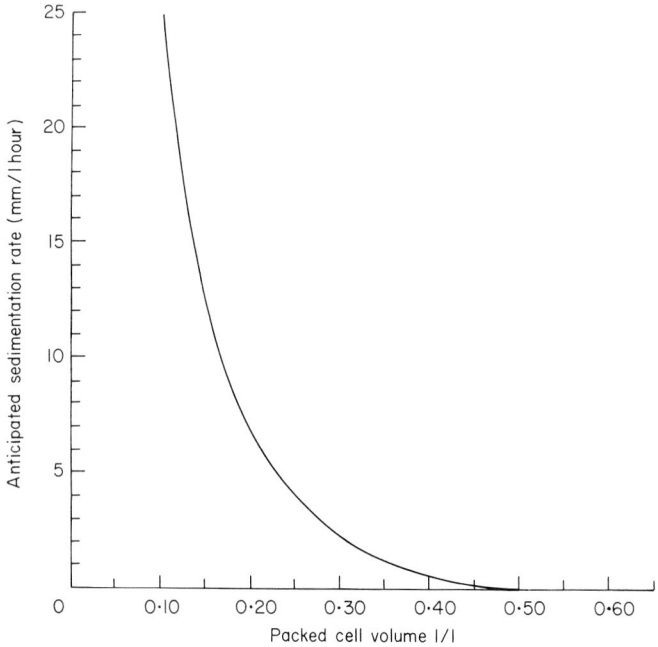

Fig. 10.7 Anticipated ESR for sample with PCV between 0·10 and 0·60 1/1 Westergren (Accu-Tech) method.

I use the Westergren ESR method with disposable Westergren tubes and specimen containers which completely eliminates any handling of the sample after collection (Accu-Tech Ltd, Littleborough, Lancashire, England). By this method the ESR values of healthy 6–13 month old Beagles from our colony normally lie between 0·5 and 1·5 mm in 1 hour. Despite this low normal range for the ESR, an increase in the rate to between 40 and 100 mm in 1 hour is not uncommon following surgery or during infection and, despite a satisfactory rate of clinical recovery, the ESR may sometimes take many weeks to return to normal. A table of anticipated canine ESR values for use with the Wintrobe method when the PCV is abnormal has been published (Schalm *et al* 1975).

The curve shown in Fig. 10.7 gives anticipated Westergren ESR values using the Accu-Tech system and was prepared from mixtures of the separated cells and plasma of normal healthy Beagles.

The determination of plasma viscosity (PV) offers several advantages over the ESR (Harkness 1971). Little information is available on the viscosity of canine plasma although Allen and Archer (personal communication, 1976) examined 7 samples and obtained values ranging between 1·44 and 1·89 (mean 1·69) centipoises.

10.3.1.8 Red cell destruction

According to Cornelius (1970) the interpretation of the van den Bergh test in the dog more closely approximates that of man than that of the other domestic animals. Although most bilirubin is formed and conjugated in the liver, extrahepatic sources of bilirubin formation and conjugation in dogs probably include the spleen, intestine and kidney (Royer *et al* 1974). The amount of bilirubin formed from 1 g of canine haemoglobin has been given as 35 mg (Hawkins & Johnson 1939). Increased levels of mainly unconjugated bilirubin in dogs are usually found in haemolytic disorders. Increased levels of mainly conjugated bilirubin are suggestive of hepatocellular or obstructive disease (Cornelius 1970). Barbier *et al* (1973) investigated the haptoglobin type present in canine blood. Although polyacrylamide or starch gel electrophoresis suggests the presence of 2 forms of haptoglobin, these authors found that these bands represented a single type of haptoglobin complexed with different amounts of haemoglobin. Shifrine and Stormont (1973) also found only one type of haptoglobin in dog plasma. As in man, the canine haptoglobin–haemoglobin complex is too large a molecule to be eliminated by the kidneys and is removed from the circulation by the reticulo-endothial system. Shifrine and Stormont (1973), using starch gel electrophoresis, found that all samples of canine plasma showed identical transferrins.

Coburn and Kane (1968) determined the maximal rate of erythrocyte destruction and haemoglobin catabolism in dogs. They found that the dog was capable of catabolizing a maximum of 70 mg of Hb/kg/h. A 10 kg dog can therefore catabolize as much as 17 g of Hb during a day. Thus the system would theoretically be capable of catabolizing more than 10 per cent of the animal's total circulating Hb in one day. Healthy Beagles from our colony usually have serum bilirubin levels of less than 0·5 mg/dl which is in agreement with published data. Most hepatocellular diseases in dogs result in serum bilirubin levels of less than 4 mg/dl although levels as high as 20 mg/dl do sometimes occur in disorders such as cirrhosis, prolonged extrahepatic obstruction or intrahepatic cholestasis. These rather low levels result from a low renal threshold for bilirubin in the dog (Cornelius 1970). Thus the determination of bilirubin (conjugated) in canine urine is a particularly sensitive method of detecting early hepatocellular disease or bile duct obstruction. Unconjugated bilirubin is not usually filtered by the canine kidney. Haemolysis, unless extensive, does not usually result in bilirubinuria (Stock & Schepper 1968). Allison and Rees (1957) considered that the renal threshold for haemoglobin in dogs was 0·8 to 1·5 g/l of plasma. Thus haemoglobinuria did not occur at plasma concentrations below this level. The kidney clearance mechanism for Hb was apparently operating at its maximum rate when the plasma concentration reached 2·5 g/l (Monke & Yuile 1940).

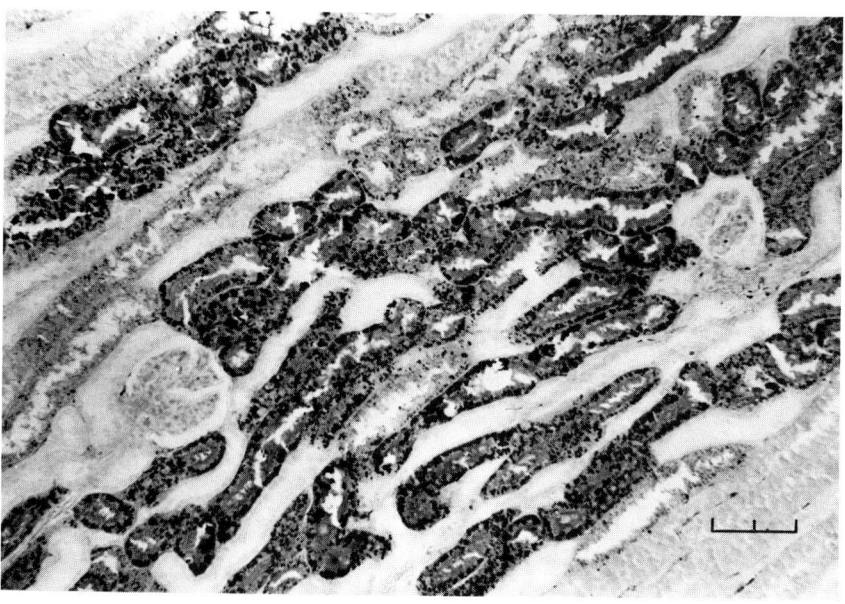

Fig. 10.8 Section of a canine kidney showing haemosiderin in the epithelial cells of the proximal convoluted tubules. The dog had received repeated doses of a haemolytic agent (Perls' Prussian Blue reaction). Scale = 100 μm.

Figure 10.8 shows a section of the renal cortex of a kidney of a Beagle which had suffered chronic intravascular haemolysis resulting from the daily oral administration of a haemolytic agent over a period of 16 weeks immediately prior to it being killed. This substance, *in vitro*, appeared to act directly on the erythrocyte membrane and did not produce Heinz bodies (Poynter *et al* 1965). The section shown in Fig. 10.8 was stained by the Perls' Prussian Blue method and the cells lining the proximal convoluted tubules can be seen to be densely packed with haemosiderin. This deposit remained unstained in similar sections treated by the benzidine reaction. The cells of the proximal convoluted tubules of other dogs killed 7 weeks after the last dose of the haemolytic agent still contained significant quantities of haemosiderin.

10.3.2 THE LEUCOCYTES

The leucocytes present in films of peripheral blood from healthy dogs closely resemble those in human blood. Colour illustrations of the leucocytes have been presented by Lorthioir (1968), Rich (1974) and Schalm *et al* (1975).

Canine neutrophils, lymphocytes and monocytes, when studied under the electron microscope (EM), were found to be basically similar in structure to those present in other mammalian species (Shively *et al* 1969). The granules of canine eosinophils were found to lack a crystalloid internum such as has been described in the eosinophil granules of man and other species (Shively *et al* 1969, Hudson 1970). Jones and Paris (1963) reported that in the eosinophils of the Greyhound there were many vacuoles, slate coloured and about 2 µm in diameter, more frequent in eosinophils from adults. Some showed no granules at all. Some workers have reported that the granules of canine eosinophils do not stain satisfactorily by Romanowsky methods (Irfan 1961, Dawes 1967). In my laboratory May-Grunwald-Giemsa (Pappenheim's) stain has been found to produce the most satisfactory staining of the canine leucocytes. Significant amounts of alkaline phosphatase (AP) activity cannot be demonstrated in normal canine neutrophils and amounts are not increased during leukaemoid reactions whereas the level of this enzyme is markedy, increased in human neutrophils during this disorder (Willson & Brown 1961,5 Atival & McFarland 1967, Jain 1967). However, in some cases of myeloid leukaemia the cells of the neutrophil series do contain demonstrable alkaline phosphatase activity (Schalm *et al* 1975) and this technique does thus have a limited application in canine haematology. The nitroblue tetrazolium (NBT) reduction test is a useful indicator of the presence of bacterial infection or endotoxaemia in dogs (Hallet & Wilson 1973, Banas 1974). Hallet and Wilson (1973) detected increased NBT reduction in the neutrophils in transfused blood and care should be taken in interpreting this test following transfusion. NBT reduction has been reported to be increased in *Dirofilaria immitis* infections, possibly due to a direct action of a component of the parasite on the neutrophils (Farnes *et al* 1972). These authors found the concentration of heparin to be a critical factor in the successful performance of the NBT reduction test on canine cells. Other enzyme histochemical techniques have also been applied to canine leucocytes (Bell 1964, Schalm *et al* 1975).

Many workers have published total and differential leucocyte data derived from clinically normal dogs. The data of Van Loon and Clark (1943), Usacheva (1957), Altman and Dittmer (1961), Doxey (1966a) and Schalm *et al* (1975) have been combined to produce the following 'normal ranges' for dogs of mixed breeds and mixed ages.

	Mean value	*Range of values*
Total leucocyte count $\times 10^9/l$	11·54	5·0–18·0
Neutrophils (band and segmented $\times 10^9/l$	7·80	2·50–12·50
Percentage	67	40–80
Lymphocytes $\times 10^9/l$	2·49	0·50–4·80
Percentage	22	10–34
Monocytes $\times 10^9/l$	0·60	0–1·60
Percentage	5	0–13
Eosinophils $\times 10^9/l$	0·64	0–3·00
Percentage	6	0–20
Basophils $\times 10^9/l$	<0·05	0–0·30
Percentage	<0·5	0–2

Usacheva (1957) and Schalm *et al* (1975) distinguished between immature (band) and mature (segmented) neutrophils in their data. Usacheva found an average of $0·42 \times 10^9/l$ immature forms ($0–1·05 \times 10^9/l$) whereas Schalm *et al* (1975) found an average of $0·07 \times 10^9/l$ ($0–0·30 \times 10^9/l$). This discrepancy is probably due to a difference in these workers' criteria for differentiating the 2 stages.

Some of the variation among published leucocyte data possibly reflects the existence in the dogs of subclinical disease. Evidence suggestive of previous localized minor subclinical infections is a common finding during necropsy of apparently healthy dogs (Hottendorf & Hirth 1974). Soave and Boyle (1965) observed a greater variation in the leucocyte counts (WBC) of newly purchased pound dogs compared with counts of dogs which had been housed in laboratory kennels for at least 4 months. Separate data for mongrels and for Beagles, obtained in the same laboratory, were given by Bushby (1970). This author's range of values for total leucocyte counts and all leucocyte types except eosinophils were narrower by an average 20 per cent in Beagles. The mean value for the WBC and for all cell types except lymphocytes were only slightly lower (approximately 10 per cent) in Beagles and the mean values for both groups of dogs corresponded reasonably well with the compilation of normal data given above. Pick and Eubanks (1965) also demonstrated lower WBC values in colony-bred Beagles than in mongrels.

Andersen and Gee (1958) found that sex-related differences among the leucocyte data were not discernible in their Beagles during the first year of life. Other workers (Weisse *et al* 1971; Michaelson *et al* 1966) have reported certain minor differences between the sexes but no consistent pattern emerges among these findings. Age-related changes are most conspicuous during the first 4 to 6 months after birth. Shifrine *et al* (1973) studied pups of up to 60 days of age and found that the WBC were high, $16·80 \times 10^9/l$, immediately after birth, falling during the first 3 weeks to $12·30 \times 10^9/l$ and then rising to $15·70 \times 10^9/l$ in the 9th week. Neutrophils, $9·20 \times 10^9/l$ at birth, followed the same general pattern. Lymphocytes, however were $3.70 \times 10^9/l$ at birth, rising to $5.10 \times 10^9/l$ on day 7 and increasing gradually to $6.10 \times 10^9/l$ after approximately 6 weeks but declining to $4.00 \times 10^9/l$ on day 60. Earl *et al* (1973) observed generally similar changes although their actual counts differed from those of Shifrine *et al* (1973). Andersen and Gee (1958) found that values during the first 3 months were broadly similar but that the lymphocyte values were shown to rise to an average $6.00 \times 10^9/l$ in the second month and decline only to approximately $4.00 \times 10^9/l$ by the end of the first year of life. From the data of Andersen and Gee (1958), Dougherty and Rosenblatt (1965), Bulgin *et al* (1970) and Weisse *et al* (1971) it is apparent that the WBC, together with the number of neutrophils and lymphocytes, declines between 6 months and 4 years of age. Between 4 years and 7 years of age the differential count remains essentially constant but after this the number of neutrophils, and thus the total count, increases (Dougherty & Rosenblatt 1965). There was no clear age-related pattern among eosinophil or monocyte data.

A comparison of published leucocyte data for Beagles with that for the general canine population shows that WBC and the numbers of neutrophils, monocytes, eosinophils and basophils are in reasonable agreement. The numbers of lymphocytes, however, are sometimes considerably higher in Beagles. Only a few authors present their data in a form which gives the range of values obtained but the following actual ranges, or mean values with standard deviations, are representative of the diversity of the 'normal' lymphocyte data given in the literature. Lymphocyte counts of 1.00 to $5.50 \times 10^9/l$ between 6 months and 54 months of age were reported by Bulgin *et al* (1970). The following mean lymphocyte counts ($\pm$s.d.) were reported: 2.49 (± 0.57)–$5.47(\pm 1.60) \times 10^9/l$ between 6 months and 24 months of age (Weisse *et al* 1971), $4.48(\pm 1.04) \times 10^9/l$ between 6 months and 3 years of age (Michaelson *et al* 1966), $4.97(\pm 2.27) \times 10^9/l$ between 6 months and 12 months of age (Robinson & Ziegler 1968). Irfan (1961) found that the lymphocyte counts of apparently healthy Beagles, under 2 years of age, ranged between 3.8 and 10.5 (mean 6.1) $\times 10^9/l$. These counts were markedly higher than those of other breeds of comparable age. In Beagles over 2 years of age the range was 1.4–5.1 (mean 2.8) $\times 10^9/l$ but these counts were still higher than those of other breeds. Older Beagles also tended to have considerably higher neutrophil counts than the other breeds. These differences were reflected in higher WBC counts for Beagles compared with dogs of other breeds.

I have found that WBCs of healthy Beagles (Figs 10.9 and 10.10) are on average approximately $15.75 \times 10^9/l$ at around 6 months of age, declining to around $13.25 \times 10^9/l$ at around 10 months of age although a considerable number of counts exceeded the upper 'normal' limit of $18 \times 10^9/l$. The average neutrophil count (Figs 10.11 and 10.12) is approximately $9.15 \times 10^9/l$ at around 6 months of age, declining to approximately $7.48 \times 10^9/l$ at around 10 months of age.

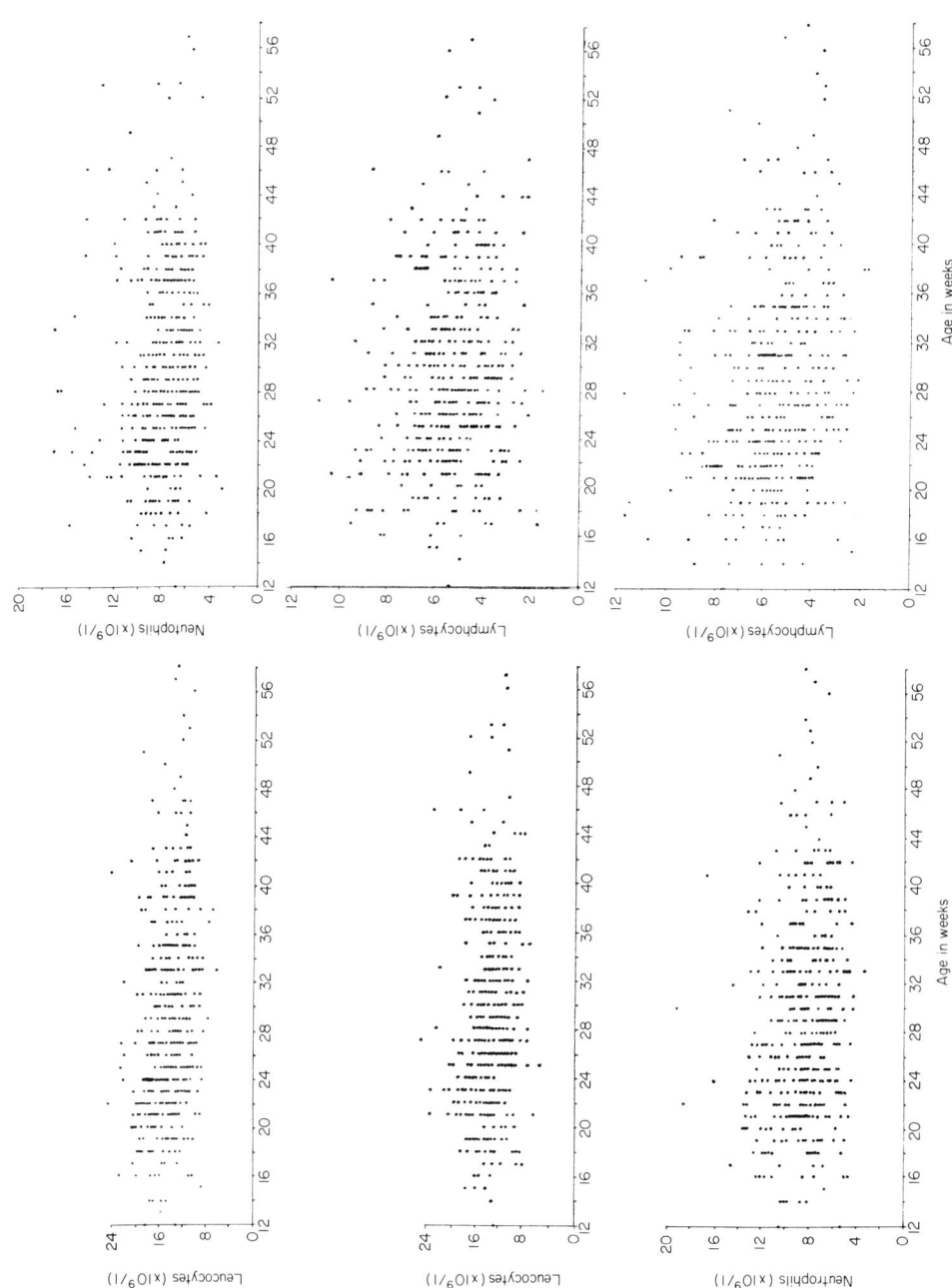

Monocyte and eosinophil counts generally fall in the lower region of the 'normal' range although a high proportion are zero. Much of the rather high total leucocyte count in our Beagles results from the number of lymphocytes present. Highly variable, but averaging approximately $6.0 \times 10^9/l$ in animals of around 6 months of age, they remain appreciably above published 'normal' values for dogs, falling to approximately $5.25 \times 10^9/l$ at around 10 months of age. More than 50 per cent of counts exceed the upper limit of the 'normal' range of $4.81 \times 10^9/l$ (Figs 10.13 and 10.14). This is confirmed by findings in 2 other laboratories. In one, the average lymphocyte count of 2 groups of 24 of our Beagles was 5.6 (3.5–7.7) $\times 10^9/l$ and 3.63 (1.26–5.99) $\times 10^9/l$ (Street 1975, personal communication). In the second laboratory, which has studied substantial numbers of these Beagles, 4-weekly average counts determined separately for each sex remained with only 2 exceptions between 4.0 and $5.0 \times 10^9/l$ throughout the period they were being studied (i.e. until approximately 10 months of age (Mifsud 1976, personal communication)).

Several reports concerning Beagles differentiate immature (band, stab) from mature (segmented) neutrophils. Average counts of $0.5 \times 10^9/l$ (Earl *et al* 1973) or $0.6 \times 10^9/l$ (Shifrine *et al* 1973) occur in Beagle pups during the first week of life. Reported values in older Beagles vary between less than $0.1 \times 10^9/l$ (Andersen & Gee 1958) and $0.44 \times 10^9/l$ (Abel & Schneider 1973).

An investigation of diurnal variation in haematological values (Andersen & Schalm 1970) showed that the WBC counts of young Beagle pups were low at 06.00 h, increasing during the day, with a small peak at 14.00 h, but reaching highest levels at 02.00 h. Much of the variation in counts was attributed to changes in the activity of the pups. A consistent diurnal pattern did not emerge amongst adult Beagles. Seasonal variations in WBC counts were reported by Andersen and Schalm (1970), counts being highest in early summer and lowest during autumn and winter, the average change being approximately $2.5 \times 10^9/l$. This was a general effect on the leucocytes—probably attributable to fluid shift—since the differential count was unchanged. During pregnancy the WBC count increases, reaching almost $20 \times 10^9/l$ at term (Andersen & Gee 1958, Doxey 1966b). Doxey (1966b) found that most of this change was due to an increase in the number of neutrophils. During

Fig. 10.9 (top left)   Male Beagles. Total leucocyte count. Relationship with age.
Fig. 10.10 (middle left)   Female Beagles. Total leucocyte count. Relationship with age.
Fig. 10.11 (bottom left)   Male Beagles. Numbers of neutrophils. Relationship with age.
Fig. 10.12 (top right)   Female Beagles. Numbers of neutrophils. Relationship with age.
Fig. 10.13 (middle right)   Male Beagles. Numbers of lymphocytes. Relationship with age.
Fig. 10.14 (bottom right)   Female Beagles. Numbers of lymphocytes. Relationship with age.

lactation there was a downward trend, although considerable variation occurred, and a complete return to normality was not reached until the pups were weaned. Doxey (1966a) reported that environment may affect the blood picture of dogs. He found higher WBCs among dogs from a large kennel, such as a hunt kennel, than occurred amongst dogs from a small (<50) kennel. The WBC count of pet dogs, particularly those from rural areas, was lower than that of kennel-maintained dogs. Exercise or emotional stress is known to give rise to a marked redistribution of leucocytes in the circulation; the number present in venous and arterial blood increases whereas the number sequestered in the capillaries decreases (Schalm *et al* 1975). Hamilton and Horvath (1954) found that WBCs were the same in arterial and in venous blood samples from dogs. No change in leucocyte distribution resulted from splenectomy.

Schalm *et al* (1975) showed the effect of age on the haematological values of Basenji dogs. The mean WBC was at its highest ($15 \cdot 03 \times 10^9$/l) between 9 and 12 weeks of age, falling to $12 \cdot 16 \times 10^9$/l at ages greater than 2 years. The mean number of lymphocytes reached $5 \cdot 06 \times 10^9$/l between 9 and 12 weeks of age, falling to $2 \cdot 81 \times 10^9$/l at ages greater than 2 years.

10.3.2.1 Neutrophils

Deubelbeiss *et al* (1975b) found that, in dogs, the half-life of neutrophils in the blood averaged $6 \cdot 7$ hours. These authors estimated that of $0 \cdot 75 \times 10^9$ neutrophils/kg in the total blood granulocyte pool, two-thirds are in the circulating pool and one-third are marginated in the microvasculature. The neutrophil storage pool was found to be about $7\frac{1}{2}$ times the blood compartment, representing 3–4 days' supply of neutrophils. Raab *et al* (1964) found that the daily granulocyte turnover rate was $3 \cdot 05 \times 10^9$ cells/kg. Following a sudden depletion of the number of circulating granulocytes, release of cells from the marrow reserve could be detected within 15 minutes (Thomas *et al* 1965). Cells sequestered in the microvasculature are rapidly washed into the main circulation during an increase in bloodflow such as is produced by exercise or emotional stress (Schalm *et al* 1975). A neutrophilia-inducing factor has been detected in the blood of dogs recovering from neutropenia (Boggs *et al* 1966).

In female dogs the nuclei of between 1 and 7 per cent of neutrophils bear drumstick appendages such as occur in the female human neutrophil (Porter 1957, Irfan 1961). If this characteristic is used to determine the sex of a dog, care must be taken to distinguish true 'drumsticks' from other appendages.

10.3.2.2 Lymphocytes

Canine peripheral blood lymphocytes can be differentiated into thymus-dependent cells (T cells) and bone-marrow derived cells (B cells) by their surface characteristics. Braganza *et al* (1975) showed that a proportion of the lymphocytes of many species are capable of forming non-immune rosettes with erythrocytes of certain other species. The highest level of rosette-formation by canine lymphocytes (51·4 per cent) occurred with human erythrocytes. Beall *et al* (1974) concluded that canine non-immune rosette-forming cells are T lymphocytes since they did not stain for surface immunoglobulin. The total proportion of cells bearing immunoglobulin or forming rosettes suggest that it is unlikely that all canine lymphocytes are accounted for by these 2 properties. Repeated assays of samples from 12 normal dogs showed that $21·7 \pm 2·0$ per cent of mononuclear cells in the peripheral blood formed rosettes with human erythrocytes. There was, however, considerable variation between serial examinations of the same dog and also between dogs. Rosette-forming cells (RFC) appeared to be exclusively lymphocytes. An examination of lymphoid tissues of adult dogs showed that RFC were present in the thymus, spleen, lymph node and also bone marrow. Bowles *et al* (1975) reported that between 21 and 55 per cent of canine lymphocytes formed non-immune rosettes with human erythrocytes and 23–43 per cent formed non-immune rosettes with guinea pig erythrocytes. Separate receptors on the same lymphocyte membrane were apparently required for the 2 types of erythrocyte to form rosettes. Canine bone-marrow derived lymphocytes were characterized by the presence of immunoglobulin on the cell membrane and the formation of erythrocyte–antibody-complement (EAC) rosettes (immune rosettes). Between 35 and 63 per cent of the peripheral blood lymphocytes formed EAC rosettes. Zander *et al* (1975) found that 38 per cent of canine peripheral blood lymphocytes formed non-immune rosettes with human erythrocytes whereas 17 per cent formed rosettes with guinea pig erythrocytes. It appeared that not all thymus-derived lymphocytes may have formed rosettes since 68 per cent of lymphocytes were stained by fluorescently labelled antithymocyte globulin. However, since no attempt was made to absorb the antiserum with B cells it is possible that cross reaction with some B cells accounted for the unexpectedly high proportion of stained cells. Zander *et al* found that 22 per cent of peripheral blood lymphocytes formed EAC rosettes and were thus probably a subpopulation of the bone marrow-derived lymphocytes.

Gerber and Brown (1974) found that the T lymphocytes of Beagle pups of up to 4 weeks of age showed less responsiveness to phytohaemagglutinin (PHA) than did T lymphocytes of the same dogs when older. Peak levels of responsiveness occurred when the dogs were between 6 weeks and 6 months of age. This work, however, assumes that PHA responsiveness is similar in dogs and man.

10.4 PATHOLOGICAL CHANGES IN THE HAEMATOLOGICAL PICTURE

10.4.1 THE ERYTHROCYTES

10.4.1.1 Nutritional requirements for normal erythropoiesis

This has been well defined in dogs by Morris (1968) and Corbin *et al* (1972). Corbin *et al* concluded that 1·3 mg of dietary iron/kg body weight each day, equivalent to a minimum of approximately 0·66 mg/kg of absorbable iron, would be sufficient for normal haemoglobin production. It should be remembered when prescribing iron preparations that some iron salts, particularly ferrous sulphate, are quite toxic to dogs (D'Arcy & Howard 1962). The daily requirement of copper, necessary for the incorporation of inorganic iron into haemoglobin, is given by Corbin *et al* as 0·17 mg/kg although more may be required by young puppies. The vitamin B_{12} (cobalamin) molecule contains cobalt and probably provides the total requirement for this element, which is also necessary for the incorporation of iron into haemoglobin. Excess cobalt may hinder haemoglobin synthesis. Iron deficiency in the dog results in microcytic, hypochromic anaemia, sometimes with poikilocytosis. A deficiency of copper or cobalt usually results in normocytic, normochromic anaemia (Morris 1968). The dog is thought to require between 22 and 55 μg/kg body weight of vitamin B_6 (pyridoxine) daily. A deficiency results in microcytic, hypochromic anaemia and a high serum iron level. Folic acid (pteroylglutamic acid) requirements are easily met from any normal diet. Afonsky (1954) observed a case of anaemia possibly due to folic acid deficiency in a dog which was receiving an artificial diet. Morris gives the daily requirement of vitamin B_{12} as 0·7–1 μg/kg. It has been claimed that infection with *Diphyllobothrium latum*, the fish tapeworm, may result in vitamin B_{12} deficiency in the dog (Morgan 1967). Vitamin B_{12} deficiency causes hypochromic, macrocytic anaemia. According to Morris (1968) deficiencies of riboflavin (daily requirement 40–80 μg/kg body weight), niacin or nicotinic acid (220–400 μg) and choline (55 mg) may lead to anaemia.

10.4.1.2 Anaemia

Liver disorders, including hepatic insufficiency, may also result in defective erythropoiesis (Ewing *et al* 1974, Prouty 1975). Normocytic, normochromic anaemia may result from chronic progressive hepatic fibrosis (Cornelius 1970) and intestinal malabsorption may result in the appearance of nutritional anaemia (Kelly & Hill 1975) although removal of the stomach, duodenum and part of the jejunum does not apparently result in vitamin B_{12} deficiency (Bentinck-Smith 1969). Anaemic dogs absorb increased quantities of iron from the gastro-intestinal tract (Stewart *et al* 1953) and during recovery from anaemia it is important to increase the protein content of the diet (Morris 1968). There are no reports of true pernicious anaemia in dogs. Other haematological disorders following dietary changes include slight regenerative anaemia attributed to hypervitaminosis A in dogs (Cho *et al* 1975) and an increase in erythrocyte fragility resulting from a change in erythrocyte lipid composition in dogs which were fed an atherogenic diet (Butkus *et al* 1974).

Schalm *et al* (1975) describe a bone marrow disorder which was seen occasionally in Poodles, particularly Miniature Poodles. Apparently genetically based, it did not seem to effect the health of the dogs. Haematologically the disorder resembled vitamin B_{12} or folic acid deficiency. Macrocytosis resulted in a high PCV in relation to the RBC. Howell–Jolly bodies or other nuclear remnants were present in some erythrocytes. A number of large polychromatophilic erythrocytes and a few hypersegmented neutrophils were also observed. Bone marrow examination revealed abnormal erythropoiesis characterized by incomplete separation of daughter cells after mitosis, large oxyphilic (late) normoblasts with fragmented nuclei and occasional abnormal neutrophils.

A chronic normochromic, normocytic anaemia, which may become severe, develops in many cases of chronic interstitial nephritis. Schalm *et al* (1975) mention one case in which the PCV fell as low as 0·10 l/l. Others showed a severe lymphocytopenia and a raised ESR. Target cells or leptocytes may be seen in such cases (Rich 1974). Hyperfibrinogenaemia, a common finding in inflammatory conditions, also occurs. Biochemical abnormalities include a reduction in urinary specific gravity and a very high blood urea nitrogen value.

Anaemia may also occur as a result of uraemia in cases of leptospirosis although dehydration may mask the low erythrocyte values (Packer & Smith 1968). In common with other species, dogs suffering from infections or related conditions frequently develop a mild or moderate anaemia, the severity of which may be dependent on the duration of the disease. The anaemia is usually of the non-regenerative normochromic, normocytic type. Doxey (1966b) reports its occurrence in chronic (Dow type IV) pyometra and a dog suffering from peritonitis was found by Rich (1974) to have PCV of 0·28 l/l and a reticulocyte count of only 2 per cent. I sometimes observe this type of anaemia in Beagles recovering from surgery. An infective agent is not a prerequisite for this type of anaemia. Robscheit-Robbins and Whipple (1936) found that haemoglobin production was suppressed by the development of a turpentine abscess in the dog. Several explanations have been offered for the development of this type of anaemia. Leucocytosis may cause crowding of the marrow, termed 'myelophthisic' anaemia; toxins may suppress marrow activity and nutritional deficiencies may develop (Loeb 1969). Relative to the latter hypothesis, low plasma iron concentrations have been observed during the anaemia of infections in dogs (Cartwright *et al* 1946). Depressed erythropoiesis, resulting usually in normocytic, normochromic anaemia, may also occur in association with lymphosarcoma and other malignancies, hypothyroidism (Schalm *et al* 1975), Addison's disease (Schalm *et al* 1975) and myocarditis.

In dogs the withdrawal of 10 ml/kg of blood was shown to result firstly in the release of small erythrocytes held in the marrow, causing a fall in MCV and a rise in MCHC (Niepage 1974). Later, as regeneration occurred, the MCV, MCH and reticulocyte count increased and the MCHC fell, the maximum changes being observed between 3 and 7 days. All values had returned to normal when the dogs were examined 20 days after bleeding. The initial fall in the MCV did not occur after severe blood loss since the presence in the blood of an increased proportion of the larger young erythrocytes results in higher MCV and increased erythrocytic enzyme activity (Smith & Agar 1975). Serum alanine aminotransferase (ALAT) and aspartate aminotransferase (AAT) levels increase within 15 minutes of sudden loss of a large volume of blood and remain increased during the period of regeneration (Jayasooriyan & Nair 1971). Chronic haemorrhage, secondary to malignant tumours, may give rise to anaemia accompanied by thrombocytopenia in dogs (Prasse *et al* 1972, Giles *et al* 1974). A case of regenerative anaemia, due to bleeding from a duodenal carcinoma, was reported by Jones and Darke (1975). The bone marrow response may be particularly intense when blood is lost from the circulation but is retained within the body, as occurs in internal haemorrhage or haemangiosarcoma. This is presumably due to rapid re-utilization of the iron and amino acids present in the shed blood. Rich (1974) and Kammermann-Lüscher (1974a) described dogs with haemangiosarcoma and regenerative anaemia with large numbers of normoblasts present in the blood. Acanthocytes were also observed in the blood of Rich's case, a characteristic finding in liver, spleen or kidney disease. Serious blood loss may occur in many of the disorders of haemostasis which are mentioned later in this chapter. Warfarin poisoning is a significant cause of blood loss in dogs, haemorrhages frequently occurring into the gastro-intestinal tract, which is susceptible to irritation by a variety of agents. Aspirin is well known to cause gastric bleeding in dogs (Taylor & Crawford 1968, Bokelman *et al* 1972). I have seen severe gastro-intestinal bleeding produced by a number of non-steroidal anti-inflammatory agents, including indomethacin. Bleeding due to gastritis may also be associated with uraemia in dogs.

A variety of blood-sucking parasites may cause anaemia. Flynn (1973) lists 3 species of *Ancylostoma*, the blood-sucking hookworm, which occur in dogs. Of these, *A. caninum*, which is almost worldwide in its distribution, is the most pathogenic, causing severe iron-deficiency anaemia and even death in heavily infected young dogs. The severity of the anaemia is dependent on the worm burden and the degree of host resistance (Bailey *et al* 1968). In pre-natal infections the anaemia may develop before ova are present in the faeces. McKenna *et al* (1975) reported a fatal case of ancylostomiasis in a Greyhound pup in which the Hb was 1·1 g/dl, PCV was 0·07 l/l, MCHC was 15·7 g/dl and plasma total protein 3 g/dl. Erythropoietic activity was intense. *A. braziliense*, which occurs in the southern United States, central and South America, Asia and southern Africa causes a chronic microcytic hypochromic anaemia (Morgan 1967). Areekul and Tipayamontri (1974), however, found that an experimental infection of *A. braziliense* in dogs did not result in a significant reduction in Hb concentration in the blood. Flynn (1973) states that the pathogenicity to dogs of *A. ceylanicum*, which occurs in South America and Asia, is unknown. *Physaloptera rara* occurs in dogs in the USA. Its presence in the stomach and duodenum causes ulceration and melaena (Flynn 1973). Many other intestinal parasites, including both protozoa and helminths, may cause haemorrhagic diarrhoea and other intestinal disturbances which, if severe, may result in disturbance of the blood picture.

A number of species of blood-sucking ectoparasites are known to feed on dogs. Leeches may occasionally be responsible for blood loss and heavy infestations with *Amblyomma americanum*, the Lone Star Tick, which occurs in parts of the United States, Mexico, central and South America can re-portedly result in exsanguination (Flynn 1973). Rich (1974) reported a case in which a regenerative microcytic hypochromic anaemia was attributed to chronic blood loss and iron deficiency resulting from a heavy infestation with lice.

Many reports have described autoimmune haemolytic anaemia in dogs (Lewis *et al* 1965a, Bull *et al* 1971, Avolt *et al* 1973 and Schalm *et al* 1975). In a typical case described by Kelly and Farrow (1970), the anaemia was macrocytic and hypochromic with reticulocytosis, numerous spherocytes and erythrocytic inclusions. Osmotic fragility was increased and Coombs' test was positive. Normal erythrocytes transfused into the patient were rapidly destroyed. Liver damage, with raised serum enzyme levels, was attributed to the profound anaemia. This particular case did not benefit from steroid therapy although most cases do improve considerably with such treatment. An increase in osmotic fragility may be detected in autoimmune haemolytic anaemia (Jain 1973). Chronic haemolytic disease in which haemosiderinosis or liver damage occurs is often accompanied by bilirubinaemia due to hepatic regurgitation of conjugated bilirubin (Cornelius 1970). The thrombocyto-penia which accompanies this condition is discussed later.

Rich (1974) presented a case history of autoimmune haemolytic anaemia (AHA) in a St Bernard. Spherocytes were present, autoagglutination was marked and Coombs' test was positive. A high level of erythroid regeneration was evident. The presence of increased numbers of monocytes was attributed to their role in removing cellular debris. Erythrophagocytosis was sometimes observed close to the edge of blood films and corticosteroid therapy was successful. Rich (1974) drew attention to the similarity of those cases of AHA in which Coombs' test is positive and apparently similar cases in which Coombs' test is negative. Neutrophilia, with immature cells present, is a common feature of regenerative anaemia (Kammermann-Lüscher 1974b). Mackenzie (1969) presented details of 4 cases of haemolytic anaemia, 3 of which had positive Coombs' tests. Cold haemagglutinins were said to have been present in one of these cases and all were acutely ill. Transfusion produced an initial improvement but this was rapidly reversed due to destruction of the transfused cells. Steroid therapy was successful in all 4 cases. Jones and Darke (1975), due to unfavourable experience with Coombs' test, employed papain-treated erythrocytes for the detection of incomplete erythrocyte auto-antibodies in their investigation of 9 dogs with regenerative anaemia. Six of the 9 dogs gave a positive reaction whereas negative results were obtained for 5/5 normal dogs. Five of the papain test-positive dogs responded to corticosteroid treatment. Canine histoplasmosis may be accompanied by a Coombs' positive anaemia (Shadduck & Weikert 1963).

A number of the early reports of AHA in dogs may in fact have been systemic lupus erythematosus (SLE). An autoimmune disease which is similar to SLE in man occurs in dogs. Lewis *et al* (1965b) observed this disease in 7 dogs of various breeds. The disease in these dogs was mainly characterized by AHA, thrombocytopenic purpura and glomerulonephritis. PCV values as low as 0·115 l/l occurred, together with increased reticulocyte and normoblast counts, erythroid hyperplasia in the marrow and urobilinuria. Facial lesions, polyarthritis and lymphadenopathy sometimes occurred. The haematological changes responded to steroid therapy although the renal lesions were not affected. The direct Coombs' test was always positive in addition to which rheumatoid factor, antithyroid antibody and lupus erythematosus (LE) factor were also demonstrable among these cases. Lewis (1965) performed the test for the LE phenomenon on 100 dogs with a variety of diseases and also on 25 clinically normal dogs. Details of the method of making the LE preparations are given in the paper. Of 17 dogs with a diagnosis of SLE, 16 gave a positive LE cell preparation. Other diseases in which positive results were obtained included polyarthritis, lymphosarcoma including lymphoblastic leukaemia, and dicoumarol poisoning. The LE test was negative in the normal dogs. Jain (1973) also described a case of polyarthritis from which blood samples gave a positive Coombs' test, LE cell preparation and antinuclear antibody test. A proportion of the erythrocytes in this case showed increased fragility. Wilkins *et al* (1973) demonstrated antiplatelet activity in the serum of dogs with AHA and with SLE. Lewis and Schwartz (1971) were unable to find any definite evidence of genetic transmission of canine SLE but the presence of multiple serological abnormalities in the progeny suggested vertical transmission of an infective agent to genetically susceptible individuals.

Haemolytic anaemia in a 7-year-old female toy Pinscher was shown to be due to a cold haemagglutinin. Even at high dilutions of serum, complement was fixed to the erythrocytes of the patient and also to those of normal dogs. The optimum temperature for agglutination of these cells was found to be 0°C. Exposure of the patient to a cold environment resulted in cyanosis followed by gangrene of the ears, nose and feet. Clear evidence of defibrination syndrome was also observed (Slappendel *et al* 1975). I examined a male Beagle which, at 18½ months of age, suddenly developed general malaise without icterus, pyrexia or other specific clinical signs. A blood sample

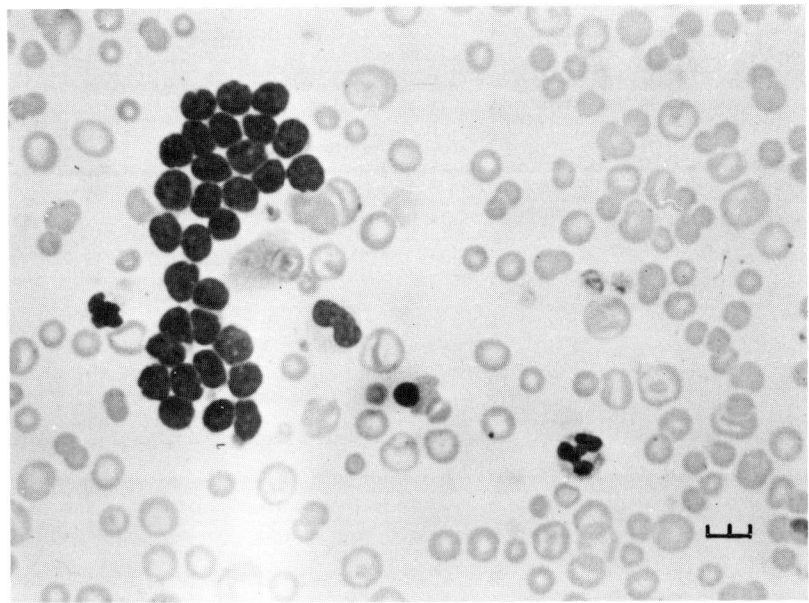

Fig. 10.15 Clusters of lymphocytes in a blood film from the dog which suffered a simultaneous haemolytic episode and leukaemoid reaction. Also shown are 3 immature neutrophils, a late normoblast (damaged) and the marked anisocytosis (Leishman's stain). Scale = 10 μm.

showed an Hb of 3·1 g/dl and a PCV of 0·13 l/l. The WBC was $72·3 \times 10^9$/l. The erythrocytes showed marked macrocytosis, polychromasia, hypochromia, anisocytosis and slight agglutination. Many normoblasts and occasional Howell–Jolly bodies were present. Platelet numbers were assessed to be normal or increased. All stages of neutrophil maturation from promyelocytes to hypersegmented neutrophils were present. Normal mature neutrophils were the predominant type present. A highly conspicuous feature was that more than 90 per cent of the lymphocytes were in clusters averaging approximately 10 cells each on the stained film (Fig. 10.15). In view of the large size of some of these clusters and the fact that they were always arranged in 2-dimensional groups, without any apparent tendency to overlap, it was thought that they probably formed in vitro during preparation of the films. Reagents for performing Coombs' and other immunological tests were not available at that time. No urine samples were examined. Although there was no obvious evidence of an infection, a 2-day course of antibiotics was administered. Re-examinations over the next 2 weeks showed a gradual rise in the erythrocyte values and a fall in the WBC with progressively fewer immature cells present. Clinically, the disorder lasted only 4 or 5 days and haematological normality was restored within 4 weeks. The dog remained in good health for 7 months after recovery at which time it was utilized for experimental surgery. The sudden onset of regenerative macrocytic anaemia, in the absence of obvious blood loss, was thought to be indicative of a haemolytic crisis. The occurrence of lymphocyte clusters and slight haemagglutination suggested to us that an immunological abnormality had occurred. It has since become known that, in man, a cold IgM antibody, cytotoxic for a subpopulation of normal lymphocytes, probably T cells, sometimes develops during cold haemagglutinin disease, SLE, infectious mononucleosis or macroglobulinaemia (Thomas 1973). The possible occurrence of a cold haemagglutinin cannot be ignored in this case. The transient nature of the illness was certainly compatible with cold haemagglutinin disease (Slappendel *et al* 1975) and the illness did occur during winter. Events known to trigger cold haemagglutinin disease, such as infections, are also known to be capable of triggering a leukaemoid reaction, such as occurred in this dog. However, the haemolytic crisis may itself have provided the trigger for the leucocyte response. Neutrophilia often occurs after severe haemorrhage or intravascular haemolysis.

Haemolysis also occurs during canine leptospirosis but this may well be masked by dehydration due to kidney damage. Both *Clostridium welchii* and haemolytic *Streptococci* spp produce a toxin which is a powerful haemolytic agent.

The occurrence of hereditary haemolytic anaemia among Basenji dogs in the USA was first reported by Tasker *et al* (1969) and Ewing (1969). Searcy *et al* (1971) identified the underlying defect of erythrocytic pyruvate kinase activity. A breeding colony of these dogs has now been established (Brown & Teng 1975). Anaemia developed rapidly in puppies, the PCV being 0·20–0·22 l/l at 8 weeks of age and 0·16–0·20 l/l at 6 months of age. Reticulocyte counts were 18–30 per cent at 8 weeks of age and 30–60 per cent at 6 months of age. Erythrocyte half-life was considerably decreased. In affected adult Basenjis the half-life was only 2 or 3 days and splenomegaly was marked. The presence in affected dogs of spherical erythrocytes with uniform spicules on their surface was demonstrated by Chandler *et al* (1975). Heterozygotes could be detected by assaying the level of pyruvate kinase activity (Standerfer *et al* 1974). Brown and Teng (1975) proposed that 4 multiple alleles control the level of pyruvate kinase activity. The haemolytic anaemia appeared to show autosomal recessive inheritance whereas the enzyme defect showed autosomal codominant inheritance. Differences between the defective enzyme and that present in normal dogs were investigated by Standerfer *et al* (1975). Chronic haemolytic anaemia in a 15 month old Beagle was also identified as being due to erythrocyte pyruvate kinase deficiency. Studies of related dogs showed that they were probably heterozygotes for the defect although they were clinically normal (Prasse *et al* 1975).

Hereditary short-limbed dwarfism (chondrodysplasia) and haemolytic anaemia occur as pleiotropic effects of a single gene among Alaskan Malamutes in the United States and Canada. The literature concerning this disorder was recently reviewed by Fletch *et al* (1975). The disorder is characterized by a mild, macrocytic, regenerative anaemia, stomatocytosis, decreased MCHC, decreased erythrocyte survival, splenomegaly and negative Coombs' test. Mechanical and osmotic fragility and autohaemolysis are increased. A membrane defect results in disordered erythrocyte cation transport. Haemosiderin was sometimes present in the urine of affected dogs. The haematological disorder was already present in 2 week old pups, the haemoglobin level, PCV and erythrocyte count all being low. In affected dogs over 6 months of age the Hb level and RBC remained low but the PCV was actually slightly greater than that of normal dogs due to a marked increase in the MCV to an average 96 fl. The reticulocyte count was elevated but the platelet and leucocyte data were normal, with the exception of mild neutrophilia. Stomatocytes averaged 3·7 per cent of cells in blood films of affected dogs but the erythrocyte morphology of heterozygous dogs was indistinguishable from that of normal dogs. Heterozygotes can be detected by their erythrocyte values, a factor which should prove of use in eliminating chondrodysplasia and anaemia from the breed. Necropsy of affected dogs revealed marked deposition of iron in the kidney, liver and spleen and erythroid hyperplasia in the bone marrow. The defect does not present serious problems of management; affected dogs are known to remain healthy until at least 5 years of age (Fletch *et al* 1975).

It is well known that erythropoiesis in dogs is reduced during a period of oestrogen administration (Tyslowitz & Dingemanse 1941) and Chiu (1974) concluded that inhibition of the pluripotential stem cell occurred. The leucocytes and platelets were similarly affected. Haematological changes involving both erythrocytes and leucocytes, similar to those which occur in pregnancy, also occur during the administration of progestagens to dogs (Capel-Edwards *et al* 1973, Weikel *et al* 1975).

The haematological changes which may result from medication are broadly similar to those which occur in man. Repeated administration of chloramphenicol to dogs results in a reversible suppression of bone marrow mitochondrial ferrochelatase activity and also other changes consistent with a block in the final stage of haem synthesis (Manyan *et al* 1972). There was no significant change in the leucocyte and platelet values. Penny *et al* (1973) observed that large doses of chloramphenicol may produce evidence suggestive of reversible bone marrow suppression in dogs. Phenylbutazone has been shown to be capable of causing aplastic anaemia in dogs (Miller & Kind 1962). The administration of certain tranquillizers, barbiturates and other narcotics causes short duration changes in the blood picture (Collette & Meriwether 1965, Soliman *et al* 1965) and blood samples for diagnostic purposes should not be withdrawn shortly after the administration of these agents. Amphotericin B, the antifungal antibiotic used in the treatment of systemic infections in dogs, may also cause anaemia (Ditchfield 1968).

The haematological changes which follow exposure to radiation were described by Brewer (1968). The symptoms of lead poisoning in young dogs may suggest other disorders (Schalm & Holliday 1975) but the presence of nucleated or polychromatic erythrocytes without an unusually low PCV, together with significant numbers of erythrocytes and normoblasts exhibiting basophilic stippling, is suggestive of lead poisoning. Microcytic, hypochromic anaemia may result from chronic lead poisoning. Blood films to be examined for evidence of lead poisoning should be prepared from fresh blood since some anticoagulants, including EDTA, cause a reduction in the number of cells exhibiting stippling (Zook *et al* 1970). Maxfield *et al* (1972) found that erythrocyte regeneration in anaemic dogs was not diminished by the daily administration of large doses of lead acetate per os for 46 weeks. Ingestion of onions is known to give rise to haemolytic anaemia in dogs (Farkas & Farkas 1974). An agent expressed from the parotid glands of *Bufo marinus* and certain other toads is toxic to dogs (Palumbo *et al* 1975). The toxaemia is accompanied by a moderate increase in the erythrocyte parameters and the ESR and neutropenia. Simply mouthing the toad is sufficient for the dog to obtain a toxic dose of this agent. *B. marinus* probably occurs only in tropical regions. A number of other poisons produce haematological changes (Buck *et al* 1968). Arsenic poisoning results in anaemia due to blood loss. Glycols may cause haematuria and leucocytosis. Phenol, in non-corrosive doses, causes anaemia. Castor bean seed (Ricin) causes severe haemolysis and white phosphorus causes icterus.

Marrow aplasia of unknown aetiology affecting only erythroid cells in a 3-year-old dog was described by Lund and Avolt (1972). The dog had been anaemic for one month but normoblasts were absent from marrow smears and iron utilization was disturbed. Leucocyte and platelet data were normal. A similar disorder of a 6 year old dog was described by Watson *et al* (1975). This case was also characterized by severe non-regenerative anaemia with depletion of erythroid cells in the marrow.

Erythroblastic neoplasia has been reported in a dog. Liu and Carb (1968) presented the case history of a Dachshund with severe anaemia which did not respond to therapy. Normoblasts and both hypochromasia and anisocytosis were present in the peripheral blood but there was no reticulocytosis.

Examination of the marrow revealed extensive proliferation of erythroblastic cells and arrested maturation. The spleen was enlarged and was infiltrated with immature erythroid cells and megakaryocytes.

10.4.1.3 Polycythaemia

Several canine cases of polycythaemia rubra (primary polycythaemia) have been reported. McGrath (1974) reviewed 5 cases previously reported in the literature and reported 3 further cases. Haemoglobin levels varied between 21·6 and 28·3 g/dl, PCV between 0·65 and 0·82 l/l and RBCs between 10·1 and $15·4 \times 10^{12}$/l. Total blood volume was also increased. Leucocytosis and thrombocytopenia occurred in some cases. The aetiology of this disorder is unknown. Treatment has usually consisted of the removal of large quantities of blood but some workers have administered myelosuppressive therapy. The development of microcytic cells due to depletion of iron can be beneficial in maintaining the reduction in the PCV.

Schalm *et al* (1975) describe a case of secondary polycythaemia in a dog due to tetralogy of Fallot. A lowered arterial oxygen saturation, 65–69 per cent of normal, occurred as a result of the blood partially bypassing the lungs. Thus tissue hypoxia resulted in abnormal erythropoietic activity causing secondary polycythaemia of equal severity to the cases of polycythaemia rubra mentioned above. The less dramatic effects of slight tissue hypoxia on erythrocyte parameters are occasionally observed. I encountered abnormal erythrocyte values in a 6 month old female Beagle pup which, it was assumed, illustrated this point. This pup's pulse rate, determined from the femoral artery, was found to vary between 56 and 80 beats/minute despite the pup being unaccustomed to this procedure. Other pups of comparable age and temperament, examined at the same time and under the same conditions of restraint, had pulse rates between 96 and 172 beats/minute (mean 136 beats/min). The erythrocyte values obtained from this pup were as follows: Hb, 18 g/dl; PCV 0·51 l/l and RBC $7·3 \times 10^{12}$/l. Comparison with values shown in Figs 10.2 and 10.4 show that the Hb and PCV were above or at the upper limit of our normal range for animals of this age. The RBC was also abnormal giving a normal MCV (70 fl) but a slightly elevated MCH (24·7 pg). There was no biochemical evidence of haemoconcentration. The interpretation placed on these findings was that erythropoiesis was increased in this dog in order to compensate for a reduction in the transportation of blood to the tissues due to reduced cardiac performance. Boccadoro *et al* (1957) described a number of dogs with compensatory increases in the erythrocyte values as a result of cardiac defects and respiratory diseases.

10.4.1.4 Other abnormalities

Intraerythrocytic inclusions have been observed in canine distemper and may be confused with Howell–Jolly bodies although the inclusions are usually larger. Schalm and Gribble (1974) describe an unusual case of canine distemper in which both erythrocytic and leucocytic inclusions were present. Watson and Wright (1974a) reported that EM studies of erythrocytic inclusions in canine distemper showed them to consist of viral nucleocapsid tubules and they were thus identical to the inclusions which occur in the leucocytes.

Erythrocyte sedimentation rate in dogs can be markedly increased in a variety of conditions such as pregnancy (Simms 1940), bacterial and viral infections, other inflammatory conditions and malignancies. Ramakrishnan *et al* (1972) observed a raised ESR in cases of canine eczema, demodectic mange and sarcoptic mange. The ESR may also be increased as a result of the skin changes which occur in hypothroidism and Cushing's syndrome (Schalm *et al* 1975), in myocardial disease (Detweiler *et al* 1968) and in chronic interstitial nephritis (Schalm *et al* 1975). Simms (1940) reported that the ESR is increased in cases of 'Salmon' poisoning.

10.4.2 THE LEUCOCYTES

10.4.2.1 Leucocytosis

Infections with pyogenic organisms such as occur in pyelonephritis, peritonitis, large abscesses, pneumonia, osteomyelitis, meningitis, etc, may produce a marked neutrophilia. Values in the region of $30–40 \times 10^9$ neutrophils/l, with immature (band) cells present are commonly encountered during infections (Kammermann-Lüscher 1974b). Viral and fungal infections may also cause neutrophilia, for example, pneumonia due to *Pneumocystis carinii* (Copland 1974). Severe infection with pyogenic microorganisms may sometimes overwhelm the haemopoietic capacity of the bone marrow and result in a preponderance of immature cells in the blood or leucopenia.

Doxey (1966b) summarized the leucocyte responses seen in the different types of canine pyometra (Dow 1957). In Dow type II the haematological values were within normal limits. In Dow type III (acute) pyometra, WBCs varied between approximately 11 and 72×10^9/l in closed cases and between 7 and 38×10^9/l in open cases. In Dow type IV (chronic pyometra) the counts were between 30 and 116×10^9/l in closed cases and between 6 and 77×10^9/l in open cases. In Dow types III and IV, immature neutrophils, metamyelocytes and myelocytes are often present in the blood but even in these types the blood picture may be normal in early cases. Anaemia is not a constant finding but occurs most often in type IV cases. Monocytosis and eosinopenia are other changes seen in cases of pyometra.

I find that a type of meningitis of unknown aetiology in Beagles may cause neutrophil counts as high as 56×10^9/l, associated with normochromic, normocytic anaemia and a raised ESR. Samples of cerebrospinal fluid contain between 0·2 and 10×10^9 cells/l. In less severe infections, such as minor infected wounds, otitis, upper respiratory tract infections, small abscesses and most urinary tract infections, the leucocyte response is often small. Slight or moderate neutrophilia may occur in many other conditions, for example intestinal lymphangiectasia (Mattheeuws *et al* 1974) and cholangiohepatitis (La Croix & Pulley 1974). Neutrophilia may also occur in both acute and chronic pancreatitis. This disease is particularly common in the dog but the aetiology is in doubt (Medway 1969). In myocarditis, leucocytosis may persist after the primary disease has subsided (Detweiler *et al* 1968). Neutrophilia often occurs in certain types of neoplasm (Kammermann-Lüscher 1974b), particularly when a tumour becomes necrotic. Rich (1974) considered persistent leucocytosis and neutrophilia in a small animal to be suggestive of neoplasia. Moderate to severe neutrophilia occurs during uncomplicated recovery from surgical procedures.

Occasionally leukaemoid reactions, with counts in the region of 100×10^9/l, occur in which blast cells and other immature forms may be present in the blood. This response may affect neutrophils, eosinophils or lymphocytes. Neutrophil leukaemoid reactions may be triggered by a variety of conditions such as infections and malignancies. A typical leukaemoid reaction was described by Willson and Brown (1965) and occurred in a dog which was suffering from widespread neoplasia. The WBC reached $111·6 \times 10^9$/l, 98·6 per cent of the cells being of the neutrophil series, embracing all stages of development.

Haematological investigation may be helpful in distinguishing between the 3 major infectious diseases of dogs although immunological and bacteriological, or virological, tests are required to confirm a diagnosis. In leptospirosis, particularly infections due to *L. icterohaemorrhagiae*, the WBC may reach 50×10^9/l due to neutrophilia with immature forms present (Packer & Smith 1968). The ESR is usually increased. Later, if uraemia develops, the leucocyte count declines to normal or subnormal. Leptospirae may occasionally be seen in blood films. According to Doxey (1966a), haematological investigation in *L. canicola* infections is of less value since the WBC may be normal or only moderately increased, perhaps reaching 30×10^9/l. The erythrocyte values are variable due to dehydration.

10.4.2.2 Leucopenia

In distemper a general leucopenia develops early in the disease, but often by the time the dog is noticeably ill secondary infection has occurred (Gillespie & Carmichael 1968) and neutrophilia and occasionally monocytosis may be present. Schalm and Gribble (1974) found marked lymphopenia to be the most consistent abnormality in the blood of 64 cases with canine distemper.

Anaemia may be seen in some affected dogs. The ESR may be increased, but haemoconcentration due to dehydration is also common. Schalm and Gribble (1974) found that the haematological picture was normal in more than half of their cases. Viral inclusion bodies may sometimes be present in the neutrophils, lymphocytes or monocytes (Schalm & Gribble 1974, Watson & Wright 1974a b). A typical distemper inclusion body in a canine neutrophil is shown in Fig. 10.16. Watson and Wright (1974) showed that these intracellular inclusions consist of viral nucleocapsid tubules.

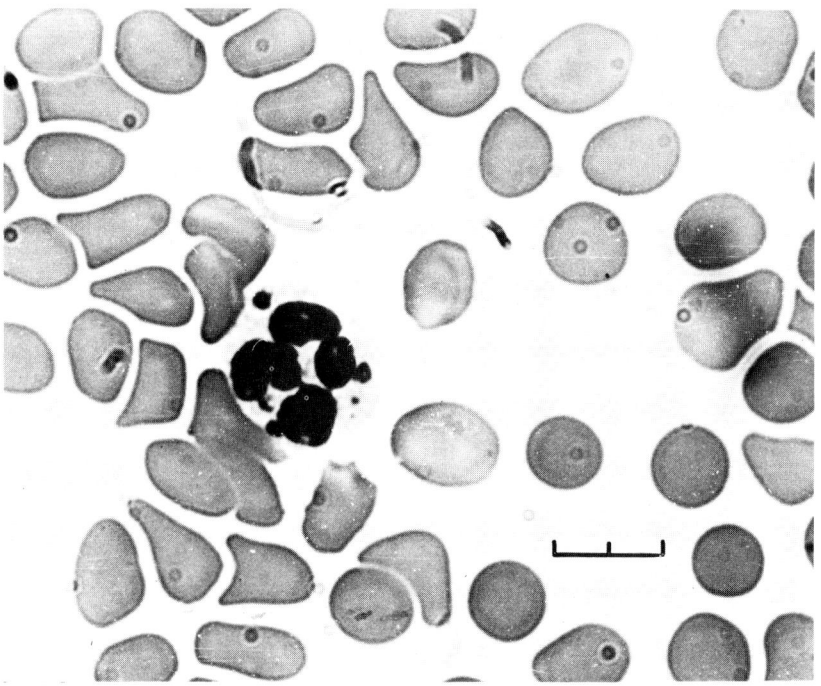

Fig. 10.16 Canine distemper. Neutrophil containing typical inclusions in the cytoplasm. Reproduced by kind permission of Dr D. L. Doxey. Scale = 10 μm.

In canine viral hepatitis (CVH) leucopenia usually persists throughout the febrile period (Lindblad & Bäckgren 1964, Gillespie & Carmichael 1968). In a series of 11 cases studied by Schalm *et al* (1975) the leucopenia was shown to be mainly due to a decrease in the number of lymphocytes present although neutrophils were also affected. Leucocytosis occurs during the recovery phase. Icterus was not observed in any of the cases studied by Schalm *et al.* The ESR was sometimes increased. A number of other changes occur in the plasma, including a disturbance of the albumin/globulin ratio. The levels of serum enzymes are also increased, AAT reaching a peak 2 days earlier than

ALAT (Beckett *et al* 1964). Defective coagulation and thrombocytopenia are also characteristic findings in affected puppies. Schalm *et al* (1975) state that in blood samples from cases of CVH the lymphocytes and monocytes stain more darkly than usual making their differentiation difficult.

The WBC falls during defibrination syndrome or disseminated intra-vascular coagulation (DIC). This is due to the entrapment of leucocytes in the fibrin deposits in the vasculature. Leucopenia, in association with thrombo-cytopenia, reduced levels of coagulation factors and hypotensive shock may be indicative of defibrination (Hardaway 1966).

A single injection of adrenocorticotrophic hormone (ACTH) or cortisone into dogs results in lymphopenia and eosinopenia and a marked neutrophilia and monocytosis (Reinhardt *et al* 1944, Jasper & Jain 1965b). Prednisolone produced a similar effect only after repeated administration. Eosinopenia and lymphopenia occurring in conjunction with elevated serum levels of AP, ALAT and cholesterol, mild hyperglycaemia and reduced urinary relative density are typical laboratory findings in canine Cushing's syndrome (Mulnix & Smith 1975, Kelly & Darke 1976). These findings may sometimes be suffi-cient to establish a provisional diagnosis in a case showing typical symptoms and pot-bellied appearance. Assay of plasma corticosteroid or urinary 17-hydroxycorticosteroids is necessary to confirm the diagnosis. Martin *et al* (1954) found that the injection of between 5 and 50 iu of ACTH into dogs in which no adrenal cortical deficiency was known to exist, resulted in a 75 to 99 per cent decrease in the number of circulating eosinophils within 7 hours. However, Doxey (1971) found that the change in the eosinophil count fol-lowing the administration of ACTH was not always particularly marked in dogs. In hyperadrenocorticism (Cushing's syndrome) the administration of ACTH gives a much bigger increase in plasma cortisol levels than occurs in normal dogs (Kelly & Darke 1976).

It is well known that the effects of oestrogens on the canine marrow are not confined to erythropoiesis. Capel-Edwards *et al* (1971) administered ethynyl-oestradiol to female dogs in sufficient doses to produce persistent signs of oestrus. This treatment resulted in leucocytosis as a result of myeloid hyper-plasia in the bone marrow. Thrombocytopenia gave rise to a haemorrhagic diathesis. Tyslowitz and Dingemanse (1941) administered large doses of oestrogens to dogs and found that the initial period of leucocytosis was followed by aplastic anaemia and agranulocytosis with the development of necrotic lesions in the throat and vagina.

Hereditary cyclic haemopoiesis, due to a stem cell defect, has occurred among English Collies in the United States and is associated with grey or silver hair colour. Ocular lesions are common and pups usually die during the first few days of life. The cause of these deaths is unknown, but although some may survive they usually succumb to infection within a few weeks. The literature concerning this disorder has recently been reviewed by Cheville

(1975) and by Jones *et al* (1975a). Although cyclical changes occur also in platelet and reticulocyte counts, cyclical neutropenia is the major health hazard and first appears not earlier than 7 days after birth and thereafter recurs at intervals of approximately 10–12 days. The Hb and PCV of affected pups is usually lower than that of normal pups and their body weight is also usually less than normal. From 6 to 8 weeks of age infections, particularly ulcers, diarrhoea and respiratory infections, become progressively more serious, resulting in the neutrophil counts between cycles of neutropenia becoming progressively greater. Antibacterial therapy may result in some affected dogs surviving to 2 years of age when they develop anaemia, due to the underlying stem cell defect. There may also be lymphopenia and mono-cytosis, with plasmacytosis of the blood. At this age arthritis, glomeruloneph-ritis and amyloidosis may occur. Whole body irradiation, followed by bone marrow transplantation, has been used experimentally in this disorder (Jones *et al* 1975b). Breeding studies have produced results compatible with simple autosomal recessive inheritance. The neutrophils of Collies with cyclic haemo-poiesis have been found to have metabolic and functional abnormalities including an intracellular bactericidal defect, although phagocytosis was apparently normal (Chusid *et al* 1975). Cyclic neutropenia, but not reticulo-cyte cycling, can be prevented by the daily administration of endotoxin (Maloney *et al* 1974).

Renshaw *et al* (1975) presented the case history of an Irish Setter which suffered recurrent infections due to a dysfunction of the neutrophils. This defect was found to be a failure of intracellular bactericidal activity although phagocytosis was normal. Haematologically, the defect was characterized by persistent leucocytosis with neutrophilia and lymphocytosis. On one occasion the number of neutrophils present in the blood reached $188 \cdot 0 \times 10^9/l$. Nuclear hypersegmentation was prominent. Lymph node biopsy revealed suppurative lymphadenitis with reticuloendothelial hyperplasia. Recurrent, widespread infections occurred but were eventually controlled by antibiotic therapy. It has not been established whether or not this is a genetic defect although 3 littermates of the affected dog died soon after birth.

The Pelger–Huet anomaly of neutrophils and eosinophils has been described in dogs by Carper and Hoffmann (1966) and Kiss and Kómár (1967) but the trait was not associated with any health problems.

10.4.2.3 Infectious mononucleosis

In infectious mononucleosis in the dog, the number of monocytes is often between 20 and 40 per cent of the total leucocyte count and counts between 50 and 65 per cent are not uncommon (Groulade 1972). Plasma cells may also be present. Monocytosis has also been reported to occur in cases of sarcoptic mange in dogs (Ramakrishnan *et al* 1972). Numbers of circulating monocytes are often increased when granulomatous lesions, or lesions containing cellular debris, are present. Acute muscle or liver necrosis may result in neutrophilia and monocytosis.

10.4.2.4 Eosinophilia and basophilia

Helminth infections at almost any site in the body are well known to result in eosinophilia. Morgan (1967) lists *Strongyloides stercoralis* (intestines), *Paragonimus kellicotti* (bronchi), *Filaroides osleri* (trachea and bronchi), *Diphyllobothrium latum* (small intestine) and *Metorchis conjunctus* (bile and pancreatic ducts) as causing eosinophilia in association with a general leucocytosis in dogs. Eikmeier and Manz (1966) found that 38 per cent of dogs with eosinophilia had digestive disturbances. Eosinophilia was present in more than 25 per cent of dogs with diseases of the gastrointestinal tract. Mild or moderate eosinophilia, with leucocytosis, may occur in dogs suffering from eosinophilic myositis and atrophy of the head muscles (Whitney 1957, Irfan 1971). Eosinophilia has been observed in various forms of eczema in dogs (Groulade & Laurian 1957) and also in demodectic mange (Ramakrishnan *et al* 1972). In experimentally induced canine toxocariasis, Hayden and van Kruiningen (1975) observed marked eosinophilia associated with eosinophilic infiltration of the organs.

Basophilia has been produced experimentally in dogs by administering heparin i.v. or i.p. (Begović *et al* 1972). These same workers found that basophilia occurred as a result of injecting 2 strains of *Candida* intraperitoneally. Basophilia is sometimes seen in association with heartworm infection and allergic respiratory disorders in dogs (Rich 1974).

10.4.2.5 The leukaemias, lymphosarcoma and other tumours

In this discussion lymphocytic leukaemia is assumed to represent a phase of lymphosarcoma. Multicentric, thymic and alimentary forms of lymphosarcoma all occur in the dog (Meier 1957, Jarrett & Mackey 1974) and the cell types which may be present include lymphocytes, prolymphocytes, lymphoblasts and also histiocytic cells. In more than half of animals affected with lymphosarcoma the blood picture is normal (Rich 1974). Neutrophilia and non-regenerative anaemia develop in a proportion of affected dogs as a result of necrosis of the affected tissues and leucopenia may occasionally be observed. When leukaemia occurs the cells present in the blood may be classified, as proposed by Jarrett and Mackey, into poorly differentiated, lymphoblastic and lymphocytic and prolymphocytic types. The bone marrow may be extensively infiltrated by invading cells and blood samples may reveal the presence of as many as 600×10^9 lymphocytes or lymphoblasts/l (Owen 1973). The lymphocytic cells present in the blood or bone marrow may be bizarre types. Atypical cells may be present in the blood even when the WBC is not obviously increased. Anaemia and thrombocytopenia commonly occur due to displacement of normal bone marrow by the invading cells. According to Loeb (1969) the incidence of lymphocytic leukaemia is higher in Boxers, Scottish Terriers and Cocker Spaniels than in other breeds.

Lymphosarcoma is one of the most commonly encountered tumours in dogs, but Cohen *et al* (1974) estimated from the literature that leukaemia occurs in less than 10 per cent of cases. This estimated incidence of leukaemia may, however, be misleading because leukaemia is not a constant occurrence in any one case and is not progressive (Jarrett *et al* 1966). Thus leukaemia may be present at one and absent at the next examination. Jarrett *et al* found evidence of leukaemia in 16 among a total of 56 blood samples collected from 13 canine cases of lymphosarcoma, all of which were leukaemic at some stage of the disease. Furthermore, among 6 dogs from which 3 or more samples were examined, only 2 were found to be leukaemic during the terminal stages of the disease. Jarrett *et al* concluded that blood examinations were of little value in the diagnosis of canine lymphosarcoma.

Owen *et al* (1975) found that cases of canine lymphosarcoma seen in their department were usually multicentric. The alimentary form, although also common in dogs, was frequently an acute disease and affected dogs were only occasionally seen by them. Lymph node biopsies were obtained from a number of their cases (Onions 1975) and were used as a source of cells for B and T cell typing. Both B cell and mixed B and T cell multicentric lymphosarcomas were found. The cells obtained from a case of thymic lymphosarcoma proved to be predominantly T cells. Successful transplantation of both the non-leukaemic and leukaemic forms of lymphosarcoma have been achieved in dogs by cellular transmission (Owen 1973). Successful transmission can be achieved by inoculation of cells obtained from the buffy coat of leukaemic cases (Cohen *et al* 1974). Whitaker (1974) reported finding viral particles in the lymph nodes, bone marrow and spleen in canine lymphosarcoma but an attempt at the cell-free transmission of the disease was unsuccessful (Owen 1973). Between 42 and 65 per cent of serum samples from dogs with lymphosarcoma were found to contain precipitating antibodies against various soluble antigens prepared from lymphosarcomatous tissues (Winters & Snow 1974). Serum samples from normal dogs and dogs with adenocarcinoma were consistently negative. Squire *et al* (1973) investigated the relative efficacy of various chemotherapeutic schedules in producing remissions among canine cases of lymphosarcoma. The most effective was a combination of vincristine, cyclophosphamide and prednisone.

Myeloma is occasionally seen in dogs (Schalm 1974, Osborne *et al* 1968). The proliferation of plasma cells within the bone marrow results in normocytic, normochromic anaemia, and thrombocytopenia. Plasma cells and abnormal lymphocytes may occasionally be seen in the blood. Later, as the disease progresses, other tissues and organs become involved. The clone of plasma cells which is present synthesizes a specific protein and electrophoresis of serum will reveal a monoclonal gammopathy. Bence-Jones (light-chain) protein may also be present in the serum and urine. Osteolytic lesions, detectable radiographically, are commonly present in the flat bones and may lead to lameness. The presence of the abnormal protein leads to increased viscosity of the plasma which is thought to interfere with coagulation.

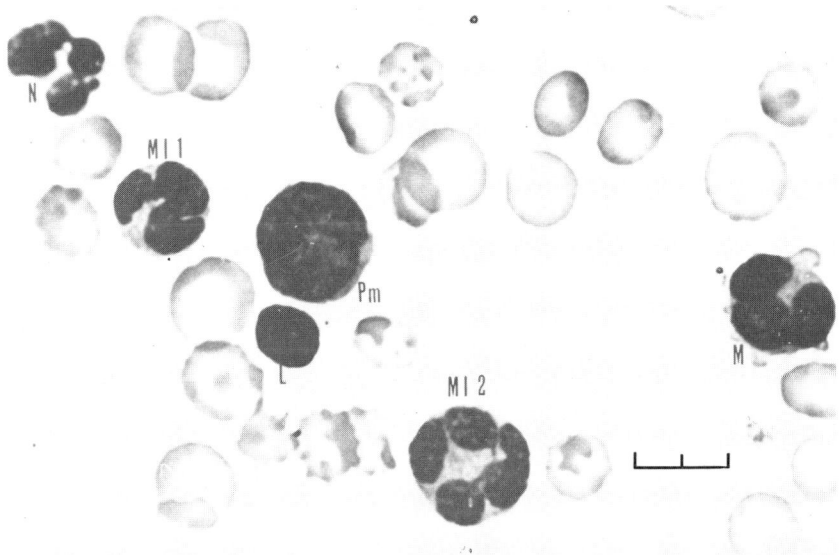

Fig. 10.17 Myelomonocytic leukaemia. Peripheral blood film of a dog showing myelomonocytic intermediates (M11 and M12), a mature monocyte (M), a pro-monocyte (Pm) and a mature neutrophil (N) and lymphocyte (L) (Wright's stain). Scale = 10 μm. From C. H. Barthel: Acute Myelomonocytic Leukemia in a Dog. *Vet. Path.* **11**, 79–86 (Karger, Basel 1974). Reproduced by kind permission of the author and publisher.

Although thrombocytopenia also occurs, the bleeding disorder commonly seen in dogs with myeloma may be due to a platelet function defect (Shepherd *et al* 1972).

The granulocytic or myeloid leukaemias are found occasionally in dogs (Meier 1957, Cooper & Watson 1975). Total leucocyte counts in excess of $400 \times 10^9/l$ occur, but the count may at times be normal despite the presence in the blood of immature cells. Schalm *et al* (1975) found that the typical blood picture of this type of leukaemia in dogs was neutrophilia with all developmental stages present and considerable variation in size and shape of the cells. Hypersegmented and other bizarre nuclear forms were also seen.

Peroxidase staining may prove useful in identifying atypical cells. Bone marrow involvement is variable, some cases showing relatively little alteration of the myeloid/erythroid ratio and others showing extensive replacement of erythroid cells by the neutrophil series (Cooper & Watson 1975). When bone marrow involvement is extensive, a severe non-regenerative anaemia and thrombocytopenia may develop. Extramedullary haemopoiesis in the liver,

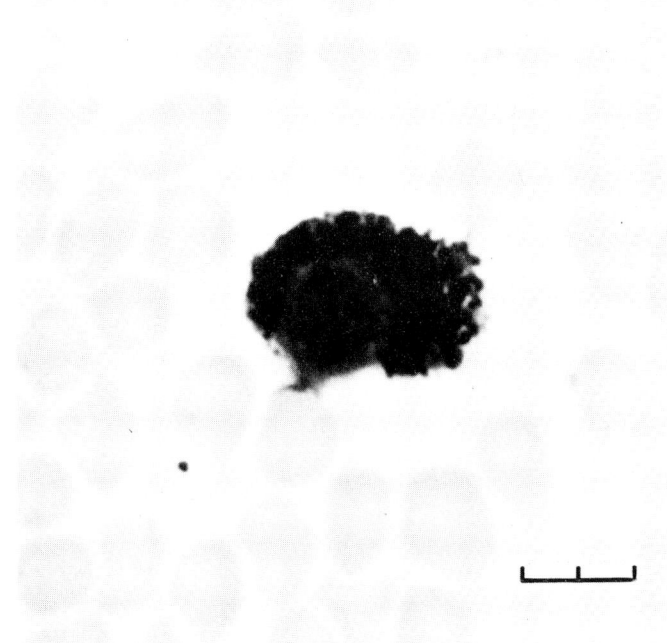

Fig. 10.18 Mastocytaemia. A disrupted mast cell in a peripheral blood film from the case described by Allan *et al* (1974). The nucleus is clearly visible. From a blood film kindly provided by Mr A. D. J. Watson, Department of Veterinary Medicine, University of Sydney, New South Wales, Australia. Scale = 10 μm.

spleen and lymph nodes is a common finding (Schalm *et al* 1975). The haemorrhagic diathesis which develops in some cases is probably a result of the thrombocytopenia. Myeloid leukaemia has been produced experimentally in dogs by exposing them to radiation (Fritz *et al* 1973). Care must be exercised in differentiating true myeloid leukaemia from a leukaemoid reaction, the most common form of which involves the neutrophils (Schalm 1975).

A few cases of basophilic leukaemia have been reported (MacEwen *et al* 1975). Leucocytosis is common and the preponderance of cells present in the blood are the blood basophils. Rich (1974) described a case in which the

WBC was normal ($11.0 \times 10^9/l$), but a differential count showed 85 per cent basophils, including myelocytes, metamyelocytes and mature cells. The majority of cells present in the bone marrow were basophil myelocytes.

Barthel (1974) described an interesting case of leukaemia in a Collie suggestive of concurrent granulocytic and monocytic leukaemia. Furthermore, in the peripheral blood myelomonocytic intermediates were present which possessed characteristics of both granulocytes and monocytes (Fig. 10.17).

A small number of canine cases of monocytic leukaemia have been described (Mackey *et al* 1975c). In 3 cases the WBC varied between 16·8 and $800 \times 10^9/l$ and cells of the monocyte series varied between 6·05 and $744 \times 10^9/l$. Anaemia was slight since there was considerable extramedullary haemopoiesis. Clinically, all 4 cases showed lymph node enlargement and splenomegaly. At necropsy, widespread infiltration by monocytes and monoblasts was found in the spleen, lymph nodes, bone marrow, liver and kidney.

Malignant mastocytoma is a common type of skin neoplasm in dogs. Metastases occur widely, but an accompanying mastocytaemia has been reported only occasionally (Fowler *et al* 1966, Allan *et al* 1974, Schalm *et al* 1975). Fig. 10.18 illustrates a mast cell in a blood film from such a case.

A canine case of megakaryocytic neoplasia was described by Rudolph and Hübner (1972). The dog was anaemic and extramedullary haemopoiesis was present in the spleen. Massive infiltration by megakaryoblasts and megakaryocytes had occurred in the lymph nodes, tonsils, bone marrow and liver. Infarcts were present in the spleen and kidneys.

10.4.3 THE OCCURRENCE OF PARASITES IN THE BLOOD

It is important to recognize the various parasites which may be present in canine blood. When encountered in conventional blood films they stain adequately by standard Romanowsky methods but better differentiation of protozoal cytoplasm and chromatin may be obtained if the buffered water which is used has a pH of 7·2 instead of the usual 6·8. However, for diagnostic purposes the preparation of thick films or wet preparations will often be necessary.

10.4.3.1 *Babesia*

Three species of *Babesia* have been identified in the blood of dogs (Flynn 1973). Probably the most common is *B. canis* which occurs widely in subtropical and tropical areas of all continents but is uncommon in temperate regions. *B. vogeli* and *B. gibsoni* both occur in dogs in parts of Asia and in northern Africa. Spread by ticks, the parasite is found inside the erythrocytes. *B. canis* in the peripheral blood of a dog is shown in Fig. 10.19. Pairs of pyriform trophozoites often almost fill an erythrocyte. *B. vogeli* is indistinguishable from *B. canis* and may not actually be a separate species (Malherbe 1969) but *B. gibsoni* is rather smaller than *B. canis*. Osmotic fragility of erythrocytes is unchanged during *B. canis* infections but mechanical fragility is increased (Maegraith *et al* 1957). Leucocyte inclusion bodies may also occur during *B. canis* infection (Ewing 1963) but their significance is unknown. Extensive phagocytosis of both parasitized and non-parasitized

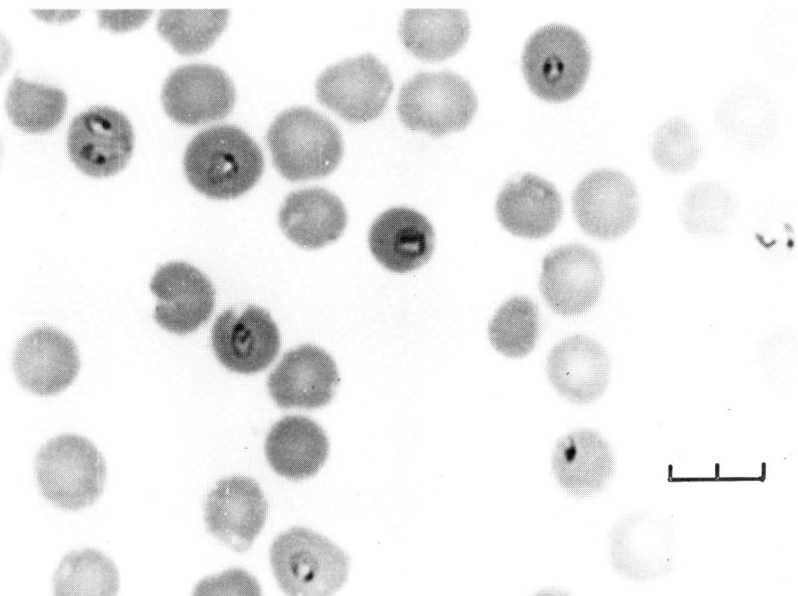

Fig. 10.19 Babesiasis. *Babesia canis* in a peripheral blood film of a dog. From a film kindly provided by the Parasitology Division, The Royal Veterinary College, London. Scale = 10 μm.

erythrocytes by the Küppfer cells may occur, leading to anaemia, haemoglobinuria, splenomegaly and sometimes death. Bilirubinaemia, bilirubinuria and urobilinuria together with a change in the plasma albumin/globulin ratio may occur as a result of liver damage (Gilles *et al* 1953). Haemosiderosis of hepatic cells is a characteristic histopathological finding. The characteristics of *B. gibsoni* infection in dogs, which are essentially similar to those of *B. canis* infection, are described by Botros *et al* (1975).

10.4.3.2 *Haemobartonella canis*

Haemobartonella canis is a rickettsial organism which infects the erythrocytes of dogs. It is probably worldwide in distribution but does not usually cause disease in otherwise healthy dogs. Severe anaemia may occur in splenectomized dogs and the concurrent presence of bacterial or parasitic infections in the blood, may, because of overloading of the reticulo-endothelial system, similarly give rise to overt haemobartonellosis. Malherbe (1969) describes the organism as being a pleomorphic, usually coccoid body occurring singly or in chains which extend across the erythrocyte. Rods, rings and other shapes may also occur. Pryor and Bradbury (1975) reported finding this infection in dogs at 2 widely separated institutes in the United States. The only evidence indicative of infection was intermittent fever, eosinophilia and occasional slight anaemia. Diagnosis was made by injection of blood from affected animals into healthy, splenectomized, animals.

10.4.3.3 *Ehrlichia canis*

Other parasites occur within the leucocytes of dogs. Infections by *E. canis* (*Rickettsia canis*), a tickborne organism which causes tropical canine pancytopenia, have been recorded in the Caribbean (Aruba), Africa, India, Pakistan and countries bordering the Mediterranean (Farrell 1968), south-east Asia (Nims *et al* 1971), the Persian Gulf (Seamer & Snape 1970) and the United States (Schalm & Strombeck 1974, Stephenson *et al* 1975). The infection is often highly persistent and is characterized by severe chronic pancytopenia

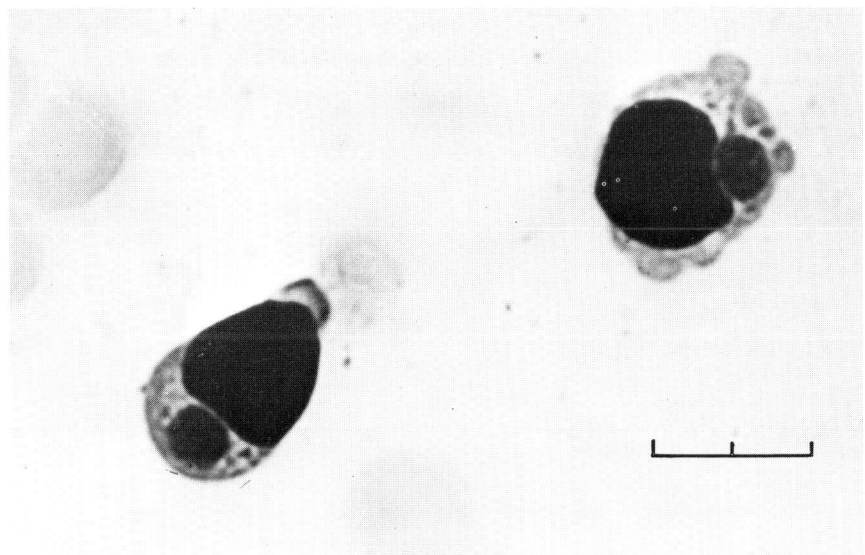

Fig. 10.20 Tropical canine pancytopenia. Peripheral blood film of a dog showing two monocytes each containing a morula of *Ehrlichia canis*. By courtesy of Dr John Seamer, Crown Copyright Reserved. Scale = 10 μm.

with developing anaemia, generalized perivascular plasmocytosis, secondary bacterial infection, hypergammaglobulinaemia and a high antibody titre, although less severe forms of the disease occur in which increased numbers of leucocytes and immature erythrocytes may be present in the blood. Haemorrhagic symptoms have occurred in German Shepherd dogs (Alsatians) but experimentally infected Beagles (Huxsoll *et al* 1970) or mongrels (Seamer & Snape 1970) did not develop haemorrhagic symptoms. Schalm and Strombeck (1974) described a natural *E. canis* infection in a terrier-type dog in which there were no haemorrhagic symptoms. The disease can be diagnosed by the occurrence of large inclusions (morulae) in the cytoplasm of a small proportion of the blood leucocytes, usually the monocytes. The morulae stain a deep lilac shade with Romanowsky stains. Typical morulae within monocytes of an infected dog are shown in Fig. 10.20. At post mortem examination morulae can be found in impression smears of lung, spleen, liver and kidneys. Simpson (1974) observed cell-free morulae in the lumen of the arterioles in the lungs. Diagnosis can also be made by an immunofluorescence method (Carter *et al* 1971). Buhles *et al* (1974) found that the total leucocyte counts of severely ill experimentally infected German Shepherd dogs were between 1 and 4 $\times 10^9$/l, with severe thrombocytopenia. Buhles *et al* (1975) found that during the transient, acute form of the disease the bone marrow was actually producing increased numbers of leucocytes and platelets, suggesting that the leucopenia and thrombocytopenia may result from increased destruction, possibly due to defibrination. During the severe, chronic form of the disease the development of generalized marrow hypoplasia, affecting myeloid and erythroid series and megakaryocytes, was suggestive of aplastic anaemia.

10.4.3.4 *Hepatozoon canis*

H. canis does not usually cause any clinical signs in dogs but may occasionally give rise to fever, anaemia and splenomegaly (Flynn 1973). Distributed in southern Europe, Asia and Africa, the parasite is transmitted as a result of a dog swallowing an infected tick. Schizonts occur mainly in the spleen and bone marrow but the gamonts are found within the neutrophils. Flynn describes them as being elongate and rectangular with rounded ends, 8–12 μm by 3–6 μm.

10.4.3.5 *Leishmania donovani*

The protozoan parasite *L. donovani*, which occurs in tropical and subtropical regions, may infect the bone marrow and also the spleen, lymph nodes and other tissues of dogs (Flynn 1973).

10.4.3.6 *Trypanosoma* spp.

There is little difficulty in recognizing the parasites which occur extracellularly in canine blood. The trypanosomes are highly distinctive organisms and 6 species are known to occur in the blood of dogs. Anaemia is a common feature (Flynn 1973). *T. cruzi*, the cause of Chagas' disease, is known to infect dogs in the southern United States and Mexico but since this parasite also occurs in other species in central and South America and possibly also Asia (Flynn 1973) its distribution in dogs is probably more widespread. Chagas' disease is usually transmitted to dogs by ingestion of infected reduviid bugs, bug faeces or rodents although the parasite can gain access via the skin. Myocarditis, oedema, anaemia, splenomegaly, hepatomegaly and lymphadenitis are among the symptoms. *T. evansi* may occur in the blood and cerebrospinal fluid of dogs in central and South America, northern Africa and Asia (Flynn 1973). Transmitted by the bite of the Tabanid fly, symptoms include fever, anaemia, oedema, emaciation, incoordination or paralysis, blindness and death. *T. brucei*, *T. congolense* and *T. dimorphon* may occur in the blood and the cerebrospinal fluid of dogs in Africa and are transmitted by the bite of the Tsetse fly (Flynn 1973). The clinical symptoms are identical to those of *T. evansi* infection. *T. rangeli* also occurs in the blood of dogs in central and South America but is apparently non-pathogenic. The vectors are the reduviid bugs.

10.4.3.7 Microfilariae (*Dirofilaria immitis*)

Microfilariae, the larval stage of the filarial (Onchocercid) nematodes, may occur in the blood of dogs. Nelson (1966) and Flynn (1973) collectively list 9 species, the microfilariae of which have been recorded in canine blood in various regions of the world. *D. immitis* is the only one of these parasites which is known to produce serious clinical symptoms in the dog (Nelson 1966). It is worldwide in its distribution being especially prevalent in the tropics and subtropics (Flynn 1973). The major pathological effects are produced as a result of the restriction by the microfilariae of the blood-flow to the lungs and liver although the adult worms seriously interfere with cardiac function. The adult *D. immitis* is situated in the right ventricle, pulmonary artery or vena cava. The adults of the other species which infect dogs occur in the lymphatics, skin or peritoneal cavity. *D. immitis* and most of the other species which infect the dog are transmitted by mosquitoes. A microfilaria of *D. immitis* in a thick (haemolysed) blood film from a dog is shown in Fig. 10.21. Although microfilariae may be encountered during routine examination of blood films this is not the best method of diagnosing these infections. Diagnostic and other aspects of canine dirofilariasis have been discussed by Garlick (1975). The 2 species present in North America are quite easily distinguished. The microfilariae of *D. reconditum* has a blunt head whereas that of *D. immitis* has a tapered, almost conical, head.

10.4.3.8   *Histoplasma capsulatum*

The fungus *H. capsulatum*, which causes systemic disease throughout America and in Europe, Africa, Asia, Australia and the Philippines, may be found within the monocytes in buffy-coat preparations of the blood of infected dogs. Bone marrow infections also occur and anaemia is a common feature of this disease (Ditchfield 1968).

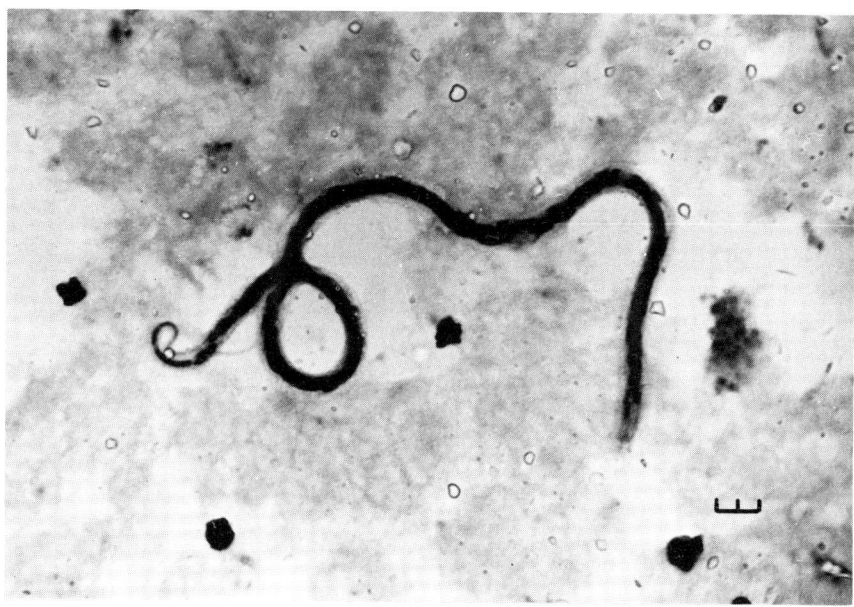

Fig. 10.21 Dirofilariasis. Thick (haemolysed) blood film of a dog showing a microfilaria of *Dirofilaria immitis* (Giemsa's stain). From a blood film kindly provided by Professor G. S. Nelson, The London School of Hygiene and Tropical Medicine. Scale = 10 μm.

10.5   CANINE BLOOD GROUPS, TRANSFUSION AND HAEMOLYTIC DISEASE OF THE NEW-BORN

The literature concerning canine blood groups has been reviewed by Swisher and Young (1961), Swisher *et al* (1962) and Swisher *et al* (1973). The usual system of nomenclature of the canine blood groups uses letters A, B etc for each group but there is no relationship with the human ABO groups. The canine Tr antigen, however, is serologically related to the human A blood group. A new system of nomenclature has been introduced for the canine erythrocyte antigens. This is given in Table 10.2 which was compiled from Swisher *et al* (1973) and Vriesendorp *et al* (1974). Bowdler *et al* (1973) demonstrated the presence of canine blood group substance H activity in saliva but this substance could not be detected on canine erythrocytes. Other canine erythrocyte antigens are known but are poorly defined. Canine anti-A serum may be produced by immunizing an animal of A-negative phenotype

Table 10.2 The canine blood groups

Blood group	Alleles	Antigen (new nomenclature)
A	A_1	* CEA1
	A_2	CEA2
	a	(A-negative or O)
B	B	CEA3
	b	(B-negative)
C	C	CEA4
	c	(C-negative)
D	D	CEA5
	d	(D-negative)
F	F	CEA6
	f	(F-negative)
Tr	—	—
He	—	—

* CEA = Canine erythrocyte antigen.

with group A_1 cells. The A_1 antigen (CEA1) is strongly reactive and a specific antiserum may be produced by immunizing an animal of A_2 phenotype with A_1 cells. The A_2 antigen appears to embrace a series of more weakly reactive grades. The E and G antigens are mentioned in earlier publications but specific antisera are no longer available (Swisher & Young 1961, Swisher *et al* 1973).

Immunization of animals with the B, C, D, F, Tr and He antigens gives rise to antisera which contain saline-active agglutinins (Swisher *et al* 1973). The agglutination reaction with anti-F serum is enhanced by the addition of fresh normal serum, the remainder of these are unaffected by fresh serum (Swisher & Young 1961). Canine anti-A serum will cause gross haemolysis and strong agglutination of A_1 cells suspended in fresh autologous serum as a source of complement. A_2 cells usually show weak agglutination without haemolysis. The agglutination may be visible only under a microscope. The very weak A_2 antigens can only be detected by means of the antiglobulin test. Technical details of this differentiation of the A antigens was given by Dudot de Wit *et al* (1967). The optimum temperature for the reaction with anti-A or anti-A_1 sera is 37°C. If both anti-A and anti-A_1 sera are produced, canine A_1 cells will react with both anti-A and anti-A_1 sera, whereas A_2 cells will react only with anti-A serum.

Swisher *et al* (1973) reported that random screening of dogs in the United States showed that the A_1 antigen was present in approximately 40 per cent, the A_2 antigen in 20 per cent and 40 per cent were a (A-negative). Thus a total of approximately 60 per cent are A-positive. Approximately 98 per cent of dogs in the USA possess the F and C antigens so problems of incompatibility involving these antigens will be extremely rare (Swisher *et al* 1973). Mears *et al* (1969) screened 150 mongrels in Australia and found 64 (42·7 per cent) to be A-positive. These workers did not attempt to differentiate between A_1 and A_2 antigens although 24 were detected by complete haemolysis and were presumably A_1. The remainder were detected by direct agglutination or by a positive indirect Coombs' test. Chappuis and Terré (1970) found that of 115 dogs in a large kennel in France, 63 per cent were A-positive and 37 per cent a (A-negative). Inheritance of the canine A, B, C and D antigens appears to be autosomal and dominant (Swisher & Young 1961).

Swisher and Young (1961) compared the in vivo manifestations resulting from the administration of incompatible cells to previously sensitized dogs. Only the A_1 cells evoke a major clinical reaction with rapid destruction of the transfused erythrocytes and haemoglobinuria. The reaction to A_2 cells is variable, usually slight, although destruction of the transfused erythrocytes occurs moderately rapidly. The remaining antigens usually give rise to very much less severe clinical reactions although in most cases the transfused erythrocytes are eventually destroyed. Naturally occurring isoantibodies to canine erythrocyte antigens occur in the blood of less than 10 per cent of dogs (Swisher *et al* 1962). Swisher and Young (1961) mention 3 dogs with naturally occurring anti-B activity, 14 dogs with anti-D activity and 5 dogs with antibodies to unidentified antigens. Naturally occurring anti-A activity was not encountered. Thus a dog can be transfused with the blood of any canine donor on a single occasion with relatively little risk. It should be realized, however, that if the cells are incompatible and sensitization occurs, these cells will be destroyed as the antibody appears approximately 10 days after transfusion. Swisher *et al* (1962) estimated that 22 per cent of dogs would become sensitized to the A antigen as a result of random transfusions. The clinical reaction following the transfusion of A_1 cells to previously sensitized donors, although rarely fatal, occurs within minutes of commencing transfusion and is characterized by tremors, respiratory distress, vomiting, incontinence of urine and faeces, haemoglobinuria, transient prostration and fever (Swisher & Young 1961). Defibrination, probably initiated by the presence of erythrocyte stroma in the circulation, may give rise to a haemor-rhagic diathesis (Friesen *et al* 1952). This subject is discussed later in this chapter. The infusion of plasma containing anti-A activity into a dog posses-sing the A erythrocyte antigen will evoke a dramatic response since in this case the recipient's own cells will be destroyed (Young *et al* 1949).

Suitable techniques for producing antisera, including Coombs' serum, and for cell-typing and cross-matching have been described by Swisher and Young (1961), Wright (1962), Dudok de Wit *et al* (1967), Mears *et al* (1969), Rasmusen (1969), Hall (1970b) and Suzuki *et al* (1975). Jackson *et al* (1971) described a highly sensitive haemolysis test for detecting the A_1 canine ery-throcyte antigen and for measuring isoantibody activity. An adaptation of an automated method using Polybrene, a positively charged polymer which aggregates erythrocytes, was developed for canine blood typing by Huang *et al* (1974).

Swisher *et al* (1962), Foster (1967) and Coulon (1973) recommended the routine use of A-negative blood for transfusion since this would eliminate any risk of severe incompatibility reactions. Crossmatching is advisable, however, particularly if a dog is likely to receive further transfusions. Using ^{51}Cr-labelled cells, Owen and Holmes (1972) found that the *in vivo* survival time of autologously transfused canine erythrocytes was not reduced following storage in acid–citrate dextrose solution at 4°C for periods of up to 6 weeks. Coulon (1973), however, recommended storage for no more than 15 days. Eisenbrandt and Smith (1974) and Ou *et al* (1975) studied the preservation of canine blood in a variety of solutions and found that citrate–phosphate–dextrose was superior to the customary acid–citrate dextrose solution. Foster (1967) recommends as an approximate guide the administration of 11–17·5 ml of blood/kg body weight according to the amount of blood which has been lost.

Haemolytic disease of the new-born only occurs when an A-negative bitch has been previously sensitized by the transfusion of group A cells so that anti-A activity has developed (Young *et al* 1951, Swisher & Young 1961, Hime 1963). If the bitch is subsequently fertilized by a dog which possesses the A erythrocyte antigen, a high level of anti-A activity will accumulate in the colostrum prior to parturition. Any A_1 pup which suckles the dam during the first day of life may receive sufficient anti-A to evoke a serious, possibly fatal, haemolytic anaemia. The reaction in group A_2 dogs is usually more mild and may only be detectable by the antiglobulin reaction. There was no evidence of transplacental isoimmunization or of transfer of antibody across the placenta from mother to pup. Consequently haemolytic disease is easily avoidable by fostering pups to a non-immunized bitch or by artificial feeding during the first few days of life.

10.6 THE HAEMOSTATIC MECHANISM

10.6.1 HAEMOSTASIS IN THE HEALTHY DOG

The haemostatic mechanism in the dog is essentially similar to that of man. The 3 principal components of the mechanism, the response of the injured vessels, the platelet response and the coagulation of blood, all play their role in arresting bleeding and a defect of any one of these must be considered when investigating disordered haemostasis in a dog.

The constriction of vessels and the diversion of blood flow by anastomatic dilatation of other vessels has been fully described in man (Macfarlane 1972). In most animal species which have been studied, the walls of the arteries and veins contain a thromboplastic ingredient. In the dog, however, Astrup and Buluk (1963) found that the vessel walls contained negligible quantities of thromboplastic activity but no relationship has been established between this finding and the incidence of cardiovascular disease in the dog. Hovig *et al* (1967) found that in normal dogs the initial arrest of bleeding occurred about 3 minutes after transection of a vessel and secondary bleeding was infrequent. Each plug was composed of a mass of platelets attached to perivascular connective tissue. Fibrin was present around the periphery of the plug and in the contact zone between the platelet mass and the perivascular connective tissue. Hovig *et al* found that a defective intrinsic pathway of coagulation, such as is present in haemophilia, resulted in the production of a plug which was insufficiently strong to withstand intravascular pressure and thus recanalization and secondary bleeding occurred. In vitro studies indicated that there was no abnormality of platelet aggregation associated with these disorders although spontaneous aggregation, dependent on the generation of thrombin, is known to be delayed in canine factor VIII and factor IX deficiency (Rowsell 1969).

10.6.1.1 Platelets

Canine platelets can be counted by conventional methods and their preservation is satisfactory in blood samples in EDTA (Weed *et al* 1965). Jain (1975) found that after storage of EDTA blood samples for 1 hour, platelet morphology as revealed by scanning electron microscopy was markedly affected. I use ammonium oxalate solution as diluent and counting is performed, as described by Brecher and Cronkite (1964), with phase contrast microscopy. Typical platelet counts of normal, healthy Beagles between 5 and 13 months of age are $311 \times 10^9/l$ (SD $71 \times 10^9/l$) (see also Belleville *et al* 1966, Doxey 1966a, Brunk 1969, Bushby 1970, Hall 1972, Kaše 1972, Cade & Robinson 1975, Schalm *et al* 1975).

Andersen and Gee (1958) found that the platelet counts of Beagles from their colony increased from an average $280 \times 10^9/l$ at 6 months of age to $446 \times 10^9/l$ at 4 years of age. Dougherty and Rosenblatt (1965) found that a small but statistically significant ($p < ·001$) fall occurred in the number of circulating platelets in their Beagles between $1\frac{1}{2}$ years ($400 \times 10^9/l$) and $9\frac{1}{2}$ years of age ($300 \times 10^9/l$). Tocantins (1938) reported that the platelet count may fluctuate by as much as 12 per cent between days. He found that in adult dogs the average platelet count was $468 \times 10^9/l$ in venous blood and $550 \times 10^9/l$ in arterial blood. In nursing pups the average count was $269 \times 10^9/l$. Attempts in my laboratory to count canine platelets using a Coulter counter have been disappointing. Although with the majority of samples there was reasonable correlation between manual and machine counts, a small proportion of samples gave widely divergent counts by the 2 methods.

Canine and human platelets show some differences in their response in vitro to aggregating agents. Aggregation after adenosine diphosphate (ADP) has been found to be variable in whether or not disaggregation later occurs (Hall, 1972), which may be due to differences in the levels of ADP inhibitor present. Hovig *et al* (1967) could not regularly induce aggregation in canine plasma with a standard collagen suspension, but aggregation could be induced by winding a fragment of collagen around the stir bar of their turbidimetric instrument. Hall (1972) reported that thrombin induced marked aggregation which was usually irreversible. The response to adrenalin was variable and both noradrenalin and 5-hydroxytryptamine (5-HT, serotonin) were inactive. Hall's findings are essentially similar to those of Mason and Read (1967) although there were considerable differences in the techniques used. Sinakos and Caen (1967) found that, although 5-HT did not directly aggregate the platelets of dogs, ADP-induced aggregation was potentiated by 5-HT. Calkins *et al* (1974) confirmed the activity of ADP and adrenalin in aggregating canine platelets although greater concentrations of both reagents were generally necessary to cause secondary aggregation of canine platelets compared with those of man and other primates. Macmillan and Sim (1970) found that high concentrations of ADP produced secondary aggregation in only 50 per cent of dogs and with high concentrations of adrenalin only 17 per cent showed a secondary response. The secondary response of canine platelets differed from that of the other species studied as it was slower and disaggregation usually occurred. The infusion into dogs of homologous fibrinogen breakdown product caused temporary platelet depletion due to aggregation but these platelets reappeared in the circulation within 1–5 hours (Barnhart *et al* 1967). Calkins *et al* (1974) found that the action of dipyridamole in inhibiting ADP-induced aggregation was similar in dogs and man.

For studies of the adhesiveness of canine platelets Dodds (1974a) recommended a modification of the glass bead column method of Salzman (1963) in which whole blood is pumped under standardized conditions through the column and collected into plastic tubes containing citrate anticoagulant. In samples from normal animals, more than 75 per cent of the platelets are retained on the glass beads. Belleville *et al* (1966), using the glass bead column method of Hellem (1960), found between 45 and 57 per cent (mean 52 per cent) adhesion of canine platelets compared with 36 per cent adhesion of human platelets.

Schulz (1968) found platelet morphology to be broadly similar among a number of species of mammal, including man and the dog. Jain (1975), in a comparative study of the platelets of 6 species, reported that the mean diameter of normal canine platelets was 2·98 μm (range 2·2–3·7 μm). Their thickness was about 0·5 μm. Scanning electron microscopy revealed 2 morphological forms defined here briefly as smooth, discoid and irregular, spheroidal. The vast majority of platelets were of the smooth, discoid form. Since the proportion of irregular, spheroidal platelets varied according to the fixation conditions, their true significance is unknown. Belleville *et al* (1966) had earlier found that, in conventional blood smears, the mean diameter of canine platelets was 2·5 μm for round forms and 3·5 μm for oval forms.

The production of platelets in the bone marrow was studied in dogs by Craddock *et al* (1955). Depletion of the number of circulating platelets resulted in an increase in the megakaryocyte population of the bone marrow. The platelet count was restored to normal after 3–4 days, the authors interpreting this finding as representing the time required for megakaryocyte maturation. Adelson *et al* (1961) found the average functional half-life of canine platelets in vivo to be 2·2 days. Rowsell *et al* (1967) found the half-life to be between 2 and 5 days, but this could be considerably increased by administering moderate doses of heparin. Platelets containing punctate condensations may be present following acute blood loss (Ingram & Coopersmith 1969). Megakaryocytes are often encountered during the microscopic examination of sections of canine lung. These are thought to deliver platelets to the circulation (Kaufman *et al* 1965). These megakaryocytes are probably transported to the lungs in the blood since small numbers can often be found in buffy-coat preparations of canine blood (Roszel *et al* 1965).

10.6.1.2 Specific coagulation factors

The blood coagulation system of the dog is in most respects very similar to that of man. Specific deficiencies of factors XI, IX, VIII, X, VII and I (fibrinogen) have been identified in dogs. Factor XII (Hageman factor) activity was identified in dogs by Didisheim *et al* (1959) and contact activation of the intrinsic pathway of coagulation is simply demonstrated. In my laboratory, using a modification of the glass contact activation test of Margolis (1957), a 1 in 27 mixture of glass-contacted in non-contacted Beagle plasma resulted in a 200-second reduction in the calcium clotting time of the non-contacted plasma (273 s). Factor-V activity in canine blood has been demonstrated by several groups of workers (Quick & Stefanini 1948, Murphy & Seegers 1948, Stormorken 1957a, Didisheim *et al* 1959, Garner & Conning 1970, Hwang & Wosilait 1970). There can be no doubt concerning the presence of factor II (prothrombin), the precursor of thrombin. Both the two-stage prothrombin assay method of Biggs and Douglas (1953) and the specific one-stage assay method of Denson *et al* (1971), which utilizes Taipan (*Oxyuranus scutellatus*) venom, have been successfully used by several workers. A modification of Lorand's (1964) clot-solubility test was evaluated in my laboratory for its suitability for use in assaying factor-XIII activity in canine plasma. Factor-XIII-free fibrinogen was prepared from bovine fibrinogen.

Table 10.3 Evaluation of the method of Mandel and Gerhold (1969) for assaying canine factor XIII activity

Incubation time prior to addition of 0·106 *mol/l* (10·0 *g/l*) *monochloracetic acid*	*Clot solubility* *Time after addition of monochloracetic acid*		
	6 seconds	*5 minutes*	*22 hours*
1 minute	−	−	−
2 minutes	−	−	−
3 minutes	+	−	−
4 minutes	+	−	−
5 minutes	+	−	−
10 minutes	+ + + +	+ + + +	+ + + +
15 minutes et seq.	+ + + +	+ + + +	+ + + +

+ + + + Clot broken into <4 fragments but no obvious reduction in volume. + Flecks only. − Complete dissolution.

Monochloracetic acid was added at intervals to clots, commencing shortly after their formation. The result is shown in Table 10.3. Following incubation periods of between 3 and 5 minutes, evidence of slight and transient resistance to the action of monochloracetic acid was obtained. After 10 minutes' incubation the clots resisted dissolution for periods up to 22 hours providing clear evidence of factor XIII activity.

It is important that a worker investigating the activation of coagulation in dogs should be aware of differences which exist between man and dog in the role of the plasma kallikrein–kinin system. Fletcher factor, the activity of which in human coagulation has been clearly demonstrated (Ratnoff 1974), probably represents plasma prekallikrein, the precursor of kallikrein (Saito & Ratnoff 1974). Saito *et al* (1974) found that the plasma of dogs contained virtually no Fletcher factor activity. Vogt (1966) considered that a glass-activated kinin-forming system, which in human plasma is mediated by kallikrein, is absent from dog plasma. Nakahara (1974), however, reported the presence of potent kininogenase inhibitors in dog plasma and claimed that glass-activation of the kinin-forming system did not otherwise differ qualitatively from that which occurs in human plasma. Furthermore cold-activation of factor VII, which can occur in certain circumstances in human plasma and which is preceded by the generation of kallikrein activity (Laake *et al* 1974), cannot be reproduced in canine plasma (Gjønnaess 1970, personal communication).

Most commercially available tissue thromboplastins are derived from rabbit brain and vary considerably in their suitability for use in determining the one-stage-prothrombin time of canine plasma (Hall 1970a, Poller *et al* 1971). In my laboratory, using one particular brain thromboplastin, the mean prothrombin time of 996 samples of Beagle plasma was 7·96 seconds (s.d. 1·51 s). In 33 cases of factor VII deficiency (Spurling *et al* 1972) the mean prothrombin time was only 12·02 (s.d. 0·94 s). Thus this brand of thromboplastin was not capable of distinguishing reliably between normal and factor-VII deficient dogs. The sensitivity ratio of 1·51 was very close to that reported by Hall (1970a) and by Poller *et al* (1971) for this reagent. Abel and Schneider (1973), using a different brand of thromboplastin, found that the prothrombin time of Beagles purchased from a British colony varied between 6·4 and 12·4 seconds (mean 7·6 s, s.d. 0·6 s). The relationship of the range to the mean prothrombin time suggests that their dogs may well have been composed of 2 different populations. Factor-VII deficiency is now known to have been present in the colony from which the dogs were obtained and, assuming that the second population comprised factor-VII deficient animals, the sensitivity of the thromboplastin used appears to have been very similar to that first mentioned above. Careful selection of a thromboplastin for use with dog plasma is thus of the greatest importance. A number of workers have suggested that thromboplastin should be prepared from tissue of the species under investigation and this, although not always practicable, eliminates any difficulties which might arise due to species specificity of proteins. For this reason, in my laboratory it has been the practice for several years now to prepare either a saline extract of Beagle brain as described by Poller and Thomson (1969) or acetone-dried Beagle brain, as described by Denson (1972). With the latter reagent factor-VII deficient plasma samples regularly give prothrombin times at least twice those given by normal plasma. I have found that when acetone-dried reagent is prepared from the brains of factor-VII deficient Beagles, the sensitivity to a deficiency of factor VII is considerably increased compared with similar reagent prepared from normal brains. This finding suggests that some of the sensitivity of thromboplastin is normally lost during preparation, due to the presence of factor VII in the tissue.

Factor VII, because of its short half-life, is a sensitive indicator of changes in the plasma levels of the vitamin K-dependent coagulation factors. Fortunately, some brands of commercially available rabbit brain thromboplastin are quite adequately sensitive to canine factor VII for them to be safely used for routine purposes (Hall 1970a, Poller *et al* 1971). The thromboplastin which, in my experience, possesses the greatest sensitivity to canine factor VII is that prepared from human brain. A sample of the British Comparative Thromboplastin kindly provided by Dr L. Poller gave a sensitivity ratio of 6·9 or 12·1 according to whether 0·1 or 0·2 ml of plasma was used in conjunction with 0·1 ml of reagent and 0·1 ml of calcium chloride solution. This sensitivity is rather greater than that reported for human brain by Mustard *et al* (1962), Garner and Conning (1970), Hall (1970a) or Poller *et al* (1971) but agrees closely with that found by Hougie (1971, personal communication), working in his department with Beagles from our colony.

The range of whole blood clotting times for normal dogs quoted by various authors varies from 0(*sic*)–3·15 minutes (Brunk 1969) to 12–14 minutes (Wurzel & Lawrence 1961). In a comparative study by Didisheim *et al* (1959) the clotting times of human and canine blood were found to be 7·5 and 8·6 minutes respectively. However, Rowsell and Mustard (1963), Belleville *et al* (1966), Osbaldiston *et al* (1970) and Kaše (1972) all found that the whole blood clotting time of the dog was considerably shorter than that of man. Furthermore the plasma recalcification time of the dog was found to be shorter than that of man by De Nicola *et al* (1957a b), Caillard *et al* (1962), Belleville *et al* (1966) and Kaše (1972). Thromboelastography provides a valuable basis for comparison between species. Human and canine thromboelastograms have been compared by De Nicola *et al* (1957a b), Caillard *et al* (1962), Belleville *et al* (1966), Poller *et al* (1971) and Kaše (1972). Although some workers have used whole blood and others plasma, there is general agreement on the form of the thromboelastogram. Most data indicate that intrinsic coagulation in the dog is much more active than that in man. Further evidence of the higher level of activity of the intrinsic pathway in dogs when compared with man was produced by Ur (1974) who used impedence coagulography and by Hawkey (1974) who assayed the plasma levels of activity of factors XII, XI, IX, VIII, X, V and II (prothrombin), all of which were present in higher concentration in the plasma of the Canidae. Fibrinogen (factor I) levels in dogs are generally similar to those found in man (Hawkey 1975). The high plasma levels of activity of factors X, V and II in the dog have also been documented by a number of earlier workers (Quick & Stefanini 1948, Stormorken 1957a, Didisheim *et al* 1959, Belleville *et al* 1966, Garner & Conning 1970) although Stormorken (1957b) did not find an increased level of factor II in dogs.

A meaningful comparison of extrinsic coagulation between species is more difficult since a tissue-derived activator (thromboplastin) is essential and it is clearly impossible to devise a single test system which would be homologous for each of the species being compared. Nevertheless, a large number of

N. W. Spurling

comparative studies of one-stage prothrombin times utilizing a variety of types of thromboplastin do leave little doubt that extrinsic coagulation in the domestic dog is also faster than that in man (Quick 1941, Rowsell & Mustard 1963, De Nicola *et al* 1957a b, Stormorken 1957c, Didisheim *et al* 1959, Caillard *et al* 1962, Belleville *et al* 1966, Osbaldiston *et al* 1970, Kaše 1972). Assays of plasma factor-VII activity in dogs by De Nicola (1953), Didisheim *et al* (1959) and Belleville *et al* (1966) and in the Carnivora generally by Hawkey (1974) all indicated high levels and, when considered in conjunction with the high levels of factors X, V and II already mentioned, tend to confirm the higher level of activity of extrinsic coagulation suggested by the one-stage prothrombin time. The conversion, by thrombin, of canine fibrinogen to fibrin is also very fast when compared with that of man and other species (Teger-Nilsson & Blombäck 1974). Finally, it is worth noting that both Poller *et al* (1971) and Hawkey (1974) have, in making comparisons with the human system, used the term *hypercoagulable* to describe coagulation in dogs. Thus what is clearly a normal level of activity in dogs would represent a pathological elevation of activity in man.

I have found that 2 modifications to diagnostic tests have proved necessary because of quantitative differences between the human and canine systems. Thrombotest reagent has been used at various times in studies involving dogs, rats and gerbils but it proved necessary to change the blood/reagent ratio in order to attain the level of sensitivity obtained when the test is performed on human blood (Spurling *et al* 1974a). Using the method described by Denson (1972) for the prothrombin consumption index, prothrombin conversion in canine serum is virtually complete 1 hour after clotting has occurred. In my laboratory 8 tubes are set up, coagulation being arrested by the addition of trisodium citrate solution to pairs of tubes at 0, 20, 40 and 60 minutes incubation from withdrawal of the sample, as recommended by Graham *et al* (1964). Following centrifugation the amount of prothrombin remaining in each of the samples is determined as described by Denson (1972). The result of a typical prothrombin consumption test is given in Table 10.4.

10.6.1.3 Fibrinolysis

The fibrinolytic system of the dog has been compared with that of man by several workers (Belleville *et al* 1966, Hawkey 1970, Baillie & Sim 1971, Mason & Read 1971, Hedlin *et al* 1972) and Cade and Robinson (1975) and Irfan (1968) studied fibrinolysis in several species of mammals. The fibrinolytic system of the dog appears to be qualitatively similar to that of man although quantitative differences certainly exist. Proactivator appears to be present in canine blood since streptokinase activates fibrinolysis in the dog both in vitro and in vivo (Irfan 1968). Holemans (1965) suggested that the origin of plasminogen activator was the vascular endothelium, a view which is in agreement with the earlier findings of Astrup and Buluk (1963). Hawkey (1970) found that the level of plasminogen activator was the factor which varied most among the species of mammals studied by her.

Irfan (1968) reported that the dilute (1 in 10) whole blood clot lysis time of canine blood was 14–22 hours (mean 16 h) which is similar to the lysis time of dilute human blood clots (Fearnley 1965). In contrast Irfan (1968) found that the euglobulin clot lysis time of canine blood was only 30 to 55 (mean 45) minutes. Hedlin *et al* (1972) also observed a discrepancy in dogs between the dilute whole blood clot lysis time and the euglobulin clot lysis time, reporting that dilute blood clots of dogs, rats and rabbits failed to undergo spontaneous lysis unless a high concentration of urokinase or streptokinase was provided as an activator. These workers concluded that the blood of these species contained higher levels of inhibitory activity than is present in human blood. Gallimore *et al* (1965) had earlier reported that dog serum contains greater antiplasmin activity than does human serum. Hawkey (1970), however, using a fibrin plate method, found that the level of inhibitory activity present in the blood of the carnivores was similar to that present in human blood. The difference between these findings probably results from differences in the techniques used. Several other workers have reported short euglobulin clot lysis times with canine plasma (Rahn & von Kaulla 1964, Belleville *et al* 1966, Celander & Celander 1968, Baillie & Sim 1971).

Baillie and Sim (1971) emphasized the difficulties inherent in defining a normal euglobulin clot lysis time due particularly to the effect of variations in the concentration of sodium citrate solution used. Mean lysis times for normal dogs were 283 minutes with 19 g/l, 72 minutes with 38 g/l and 43 minutes with 76 g/l sodium citrate solution. After Hawkey (1975), I use a 38 g/l solution of trisodium citrate. The euglobulin clot lysis times of apparently healthy Beagles varies between 30 and 65 minutes (mean 47 min). Belleville *et al* (1966) compared the lysis times of several other workers and found considerable variation (3 to 190 min) which they attributed to differences in the methods used. Rahn and von Kaulla (1964) found that laboratory conditioned dogs showed less variation in their euglobulin clot lysis times than did non-conditioned dogs. It is well known that stress can increase fibrinolytic activity in man and it is thus possibly significant that Hawkey (1970) reported euglobulin clot lysis times within the range 1–8 hours in samples from 26 of the 29 members of the Canidae included in her study since many of her subjects were tranquillized or anaesthetized before the samples were withdrawn. Cade and Robinson (1975) reported a mean euglobulin clot lysis of 93 minutes (SD 33 min) for their dogs, all of which were tranquillized and lightly anaesthetized. Exercise may also increase fibrinolytic activity in dogs (Bedrak 1965).

Hawkey (1970) reported that the range of plasminogen levels found in the plasma of carnivores by the caseinolytic assay method, using urokinase as an activator, varied between 3·1 and 8·4 units/ml (mean 5·8 units/ml) of plasma compared with a range of 1·8–4·6 units/ml (mean 3·4 units/ml) in human plasma. Mason and Read (1971) found that the plasminogen level of canine plasma, assayed by the caseinolytic method using urokinase, was 1·12±0·06 units/ml compared with 0·56±0·08 units/ml in human plasma. Allowing for apparent quantitative differences which are due to the units used, the findings of Hawkey (1970) and of Mason and Read (1971) are in basic agreement, demonstrating that the dog possesses a high level of plasminogen, and therefore a high level of fibrinolytic potential. Both Hawkey, and Mason and Read, found that free plasmin could not be demonstrated in the blood of any of the species of mammal studied by them. Barnhart *et al* (1967) and Owen *et al* (1971) reported much higher levels of fibrinogen split products in the blood of dogs than are normally present in human blood. Cade and Robinson. (1975), however, found low levels, similar to those present in man, in the blood of dogs which were tranquillized and lightly anaesthetized.

Canine plasminogen, like that of several other species, is less susceptible to activation by streptokinase in vitro than is human plasminogen (Hawkey 1970, Mason & Read 1971, Baillie & Sim 1971, Hedlin *et al* 1972). Human urokinase was found to be a highly potent activator of canine plasminogen in vitro when the caseinolytic assay method was used (Mason & Read 1971, Baillie & Sim 1971) but Hedlin *et al* (1972), using the dilute whole blood clot lysis method, found that canine plasminogen was more resistant than human plasminogen to activation by urokinase. Both urokinase and streptokinase are effective in vivo in the dog as activators of fibrinolysis (Tsapogas & Flute 1964). Other substances which enhance fibrinolysis both in dogs and in man are adrenalin, noradrenalin, histamine and a number of other vasoactive drugs (Rahn & von Kaulla 1964, Holemans 1965), and also the antidiabetic agents chlorpropamide (Irfan 1968) and phenformin (Back *et al* 1968).

10.6.2 ABNORMAL HAEMOSTASIS

10.6.2.1 Disorders of the vessels

Although cardiac lesions are not uncommon among older dogs (Detweiler & Patterson 1965) and spontaneous lesions are known to occur in the aorta and coronary arteries (Lindsay *et al* 1952), clinically obvious embolic complications are very rare and usually occur only in those cases in which some precipitating event acts as the trigger for the formation of a thrombus (Luginbühl & Detweiler 1965). Diets rich in cholesterol and saturated fats can give rise to rapidly developing atherosclerotic lesions in dogs (Flaherty *et al* 1972, Nandan *et al* 1975) and hypercholesterolaemia is known to occur among dogs kept as pets (Schiller *et al* 1964). Hypercholesterolaemia also develops in female Beagles between the 3rd and 8th week after oestrus, irrespective of whether or not pregnancy occurs (Tietz *et al* 1967). The injection of adrenalin into dogs gives rise to increased plasma levels of cholesterol, phospholipid and β lipoprotein (Steinberg 1963) and arterial disease may develop in dogs as a result of the repeated administration of adrenalin (Davies & Reinert 1965). A discrepancy between Normotest and Thrombotest values occurs during active thrombosis in dogs (Rø & Flatmark 1972) and this could occasionally have an application in the diagnosis of some thrombotic disorders.

Purpuric bleeding is usually due to thrombocytopenia but Medway and Rapp (1962) reported the occurrence of increased capillary fragility in addition to thrombocytopenia in a Dachsund which was suffering from granulocytic leukaemia. A defect of the capillary wall and thrombocytopenia giving rise to widespread bleeding, develops in dogs as a result of exposure to a high level of radiation (Hall 1972).

A hereditary disease of connective tissue resembling Ehlers–Danlos syndrome in man has been described in Springer Spaniels in Washington, USA by Hegreberg *et al* (1969). The disease is inherited as an autosomal dominant trait. Its chief characteristics are fragility, hyperextensibility and laxity of the skin (Hegreberg *et al* 1970, Hegreberg 1975). Lacerations and abrasions occur frequently. Hardisty and Ingram (1965), investigating this disease in man, considered that the bleeding arose from a defect of the connective tissue in and around the blood vessels.

10.6.2.2 Disorders of the platelets

When the platelet count falls below $60 \times 10^9/l$ it is likely that bleeding will occur (Kammermann-Lüscher 1970). Thrombocytopenia sometimes develops in dogs as an apparently idiopathic condition but it more often occurs during the course of other diseases, particularly those with an autoimmune basis. Lewis *et al* (1963), Brodey (1964), Schalm and Ling (1971) and Wilkins *et al* (1973) intimated an immunological basis for a number of cases of acquired thrombocytopenia in dogs. Wilkins *et al* (1973) were able to demonstrate serum antiplatelet activity in more than half of a group of 26 canine patients which included cases of SLE and Coombs-positive AHA as well as possible cases of amphetamine, digoxin and phenylbutazone-induced thrombocytopenia. More than half of their cases were classified as idiopathic thrombocytopenic purpura. Lewis *et al* (1965a b) described 7 cases of SLE in which thrombocytopenia was a common finding and purpuric bleeding, presumably thrombocytopenic, occurred among the cases of AHA described by Lewis *et al* (1963).

The cytotoxic drugs used in the treatment of leukaemia can lead to reduced platelet production. Only a relatively small number of drugs have been conclusively shown to cause thrombocytopenia in dogs although in man the number is very much larger (Gynn *et al* 1972). Hall (1972) found that mega-karyocytes decline early in treatment with oestrogens and severe thrombo-cytopenic purpura often leads to death. Diseases of dogs during which thrombo-cytopenia is known to occur include tropical canine pancytopenia due to *Ehrlichia canis* infection (Smith *et al* 1975) and canine herpes virus infection (Kakkuk & Conner 1970). Thrombocytopenia may occur in dogs infected with *Haemobartonella* spp. if they are subsequently splenectomized (Brodey & Schalm 1963). It has also been reported that thrombocytopenia may occur during leptospirosis in dogs (Finco & Low 1968). Lindblad and Bäckgren (1964) attributed the haemorrhagic diathesis which occurs in canine hepatitis to vascular damage and thrombocytopenia associated with reduced mega-karyopoiesis. Thrombocytopenia may result from bone marrow invasion in cases of lymphosarcoma, myeloid leukaemia and myeloma (Meier 1957, Medway & Rapp 1962, Rouse *et al* 1967, Squire 1969, Schalm 1974). Cyclical thrombocytopenia occurs in association with cyclical neutropenia in grey English Collies (Cheville 1975, Jones *et al* 1975a).

Thrombocythaemia has been recorded in the dog. Dodds (1974b) cites a platelet count of $1000 \times 10^9/l$ in a dog suffering from a mild bleeding disorder. Jones and Darke (1975) mention a further case. Hall (1972) reported high platelet counts in dogs suffering from pyometra.

In many of the conditions in which a gross change in the platelet count occurs there is also a defect in function (Rowsell 1969). Shepherd *et al* (1972) observed defective platelet adhesiveness and a prolonged partial thrombo-plastin time and bleeding time in a dog suffering from gamma A myeloma. Phenylbutazone, in addition to causing thrombocytopenia, is also known to affect platelet function (Packham *et al* 1967). This could be a contributory factor in the gastro-intestinal bleeding which may sometimes be caused in dogs by high doses of phenylbutazone (Kirsner & Ford 1955). Dodds (1971) states that a therapeutic dose of aspirin may affect platelet function in dogs for 4–5 days. Repeated dosage of aspirin to dogs may cause gastro-intestinal irritation and bleeding (Taylor & Crawford 1968) and the platelet defect may then represent an additional hazard.

Yakely and Streeter (1972) described the occurrence of transient throm-basthenia in a 3-year-old female Vizla. Symptoms included petechiation of the oral mucous membrane, ecchymosis of the flanks and other pressure points, haematuria, melaena and haematomas in the iris together with a diffusion of blood in an eyelid. The onset of symptoms occurred during early metoes-trus and the authors suggested that the condition was related to hormonal change. The bleeding time was markedly prolonged and clot retraction was reduced. The platelet count and laboratory tests for coagulation defects were all normal.

Only 2 investigations, that of Dodds (1966, 1967, 1970a, 1974b) and that of Lotz *et al* (1972), have presented sufficient laboratory and pedigree data satisfactorily to identify hereditary platelet function defects in dogs. Dodds investigated a bleeding disorder which was shown to be hereditary thrombasthenic thrombocytopathy, probably with an autosomal inheritance, in a family of Otterhounds in New York. The laboratory findings included a reduced platelet count, prolonged bleeding time, decreased clot retraction and reduced platelet aggregation and adhesiveness. Although screening tests for a coagulation abnormality were normal, there was a defect in platelet factor 3 release giving rise to impaired prothrombin consumption. Abnormal platelet morphology was observed and there appeared to be 2 populations of platelets present. A disorder similar to that observed in Otterhounds occurred also in a Foxhound (Dodds 1974b). Lotz *et al* (1972) described a disorder of platelet function in a family of Bassett Hounds in Guelph, Canada. Three related animals had a history of recurrent bleeding. Platelet aggregation and adhesiveness was defective and the bleeding time was prolonged. Platelet factor 3 availability and screening tests for disorders of coagulation were all normal.

Other bleeding disorders have been described in dogs which appear to have been due to defects of platelet function, but without evidence of inheritance. Thrombocytopathy was identified in a German Shepherd (Alsatian) in Ottawa by Rowsell (1969). The only laboratory finding reported was an impairment of prothrombin consumption. In Louisiana a Scottish Terrier which suffered recurrent bleeding episodes was investigated by Myers *et al* (1972). All tests of coagulation were reported to be normal, as was the platelet count, but the bleeding time was markedly prolonged. The evidence suggests that a disorder of platelet function, or possibly a vascular defect, was responsible for the bleeding. As stated by Dodds (1974b), there appeared to be no evidence to support the authors' suggestion that the disorder was von Willebrand's disease, nor that it was hereditary. Jones and Hill (1974) reported suspected thrombasthenia in a Shetland Sheepdog in Bristol, England. Two episodes of gingival bleeding had occurred and haematomas had sometimes developed in the mouth. Tests for defective coagulation were normal with the exception of the activated partial thromboplastin time when the patient's own platelets replaced the usual platelet substitute.

10.6.2.3 Disorders of coagulation

According to Corbin *et al* (1972), dogs normally synthesize their total requirement of vitamin K in their intestines. Hall (1972) knew of no authenticated cases of nutritionally induced vitamin K deficiency in dogs. In adult dogs in which a cholecystonephrostomy had been performed, Quick *et al* (1954) demonstrated that only 0.5 μg of vitamin K_1/kg body weight was required to maintain normal prothrombin synthesis, whereas the growing pup requires

10 or more times this amount (Quick *et al* 1962). A deficit of factors II (pro-thrombin), VII, V, X and possibly IX which exists in the new-born dog (Link 1944, Quick 1946, Hathaway *et al* 1964) closely resembles the deficit which is known to exist in the new-born human infant and which is readily corrected by administering vitamin K_1. The only significant difference appears to be that the new-born pup is deficient in factor V whereas the human infant has adult levels of this factor.

A survey has suggested that during the period July 1971 to July 1972 as many as 3500 to 4000 suspected cases of warfarin poisoning in dogs may have been encountered by all the veterinary practices in the United Kingdom (Ashworth 1973). Dogs represented 80 per cent of all cases. Clark and Halli-well (1963) found that administration for 3 days of approximately 2 mg/kg day of warfarin resulted in a marked prolongation of the prothrombin time with haemorrhage in some dogs. The prolongation of the prothrombin time was detectable in samples taken during the morning of the day following the first dose although at this stage the effect was insufficient to represent any hazard to health. Forbes *et al* (1973) also studied haemostasis in dogs experi-mentally poisoned by repeated daily administrations of 10 mg/kg of warfarin administered by feeding tablets in their food. A profound prolongation of the prothrombin time, resulting from a depression of the plasma levels of factors VII, IX, X and II, was observed and haemorrhage occurred in some dogs. Clark and Halliwell (1963) and Anderson and Barnhart (1964) found that a single i.v. dose of 2 mg/kg or 5 mg/kg of vitamin K_1 to warfarin-treated dogs resulted in a fall in the prothrombin time within 4 hours. One of Clark and Halliwell's dogs had developed respiratory distress and haemoptysis but was clinically normal only 2 hours after the i.v. administration of 2 mg/kg of vitamin K_1. Only the i.v. route proved suitable for the emergency treat-ment of warfarin poisoning. The response which resulted from a single dose was not, however, sustained, repeated doses over 4 days being required to effect a permanent correction of the prolonged prothrombin time.

There is now ample evidence to indicate that in the dog, as in man, the liver is the major organ for the synthesis of most of the proteins which are essential for the coagulation system (Hall 1972, Webster *et al* 1975). Both human and canine factor VII have probably the shortest half-life of any of the coagulation factors. Dodds *et al* (1967) found that the half-life in vivo of canine factor VII was between 1 and 4 hours. Earlier, Hellemans *et al* (1963), using synthesis-blocking doses of coumarin derivatives, had found that the half-lives of canine factors VII, IX, X and II (prothrombin) were approxi-mately 6, 14, 17, and 41 hours respectively. Thus any major reduction in the synthesizing capacity of the liver would very soon be reflected in the levels present in the plasma. The canine liver probably has considerable reserve capacity for synthesizing the coagulation factors. Anderson and Barnhart (1964) reported that in normal dogs only 10 per cent of the hepatic parenchymal cells were actively participating in prothrombin synthesis at any one time. These workers found that in normal dogs the rate of synthesis may be increased above the normal by administering vitamin K_1. Thus in severe hepatocellular disease, the administration of vitamin K_1 may have a beneficial effect by increasing the rate of synthesis in remaining healthy parenchymal cells. The considerable reserve capacity of the canine liver means that extensive liver damage must occur before the prothrombin time becomes prolonged. Hoe (1969) stated that determinations of plasma levels of hepatic enzymes are a more sensitive indicator of liver damage in dogs. However, careful selection of the enzymes to be measured is essential (Harvey 1967, Street, 1970, Rico *et al* 1973).

In severe hepatocellular disease in dogs, such as results from poisoning, infections, etc., screening tests for coagulation disorders do detect a defect in the plasma but by this time the disease is usually clinically apparent and there may well be a haemorrhagic disorder. The hepatic poison, aflatoxin, has sometimes been a contaminant of animal foodstuffs and may cause severe liver damage with jaundice and widespread haemorrhages. The experimental administration of aflatoxin to dogs resulted in a marked prolongation of the prothrombin time (Chaffee *et al* 1969, Armbrecht *et al* 1971). There were also increases in plasma levels of isocitric dehydrogenase and alkaline phosphatase. Carbon tetrachloride is capable of causing severe liver damage in dogs with prolongation of the prothrombin time (Drill & Ivy 1944). Canine hepatitis and leptospirosis are frequently accompanied by haemorrhagic symptoms but it is probable that these are usually attributable to a platelet disorder, as already mentioned. However, when the liver is severely damaged it is possible that a disorder of coagulation may develop which will have an exacerbating effect on the haemorrhagic disorder.

Dodds (1974b) stated that defibrination syndrome (DIC, consumption coagulopathy) is probably more common in animals than the infrequent reports suggest. Several groups of workers have produced defibrination syndrome in dogs by infusing thrombin (Rø & Flatmark 1972) or tissue thromboplastin. During infusion of concentrated thromboplastin there is a decrease in the levels of coagulation factors XII, XI, VIII, VII, V, XIII and fibrinogen. Thrombocytopenia occurs and increased levels of fibrin/fibrinogen degradation products (FDP) may be detected. When the infusion is stopped the levels of all coagulation factors increase to normal or above normal levels (Cooper *et al* 1973). A depletion of plasminogen activator occurs in most organs (Sun *et al* 1974) and increased turnover of fibrinogen and platelets has been demonstrated (Owen *et al* 1973). Defibrination and hypotensive shock induced by bacterial toxin was studied by Gilbert (1966) and by Hardaway (1966). The effects have been shown to be far less severe in factor-VII deficient than in normal Beagles (Garner & Evensen 1974). Garner *et al* (1974) reported that prior depletion of complement factor 3 also resulted in a reduction of defibrination and a modified vascular response during the administration of bacterial toxin to Beagles.

Hall (1972) and Dodds (1974b) have reviewed the literature concerning defibrination syndrome in dogs and in other animals. I am unaware of any reports of primary defibrination syndrome occurring naturally in dogs but various workers have reported this disorder occurring secondarily to pre-existing disease. Defibrination in these cases were often sufficiently severe to cause a haemorrhagic diathesis and was usually associated with malignancy, but uraemia, heat-stroke and disorders of various organs (Slappendel et al 1970, Kammerman et al 1971, Slappendel et al 1972, Prasse et al 1972, Slappendel & von Dijk 1973) and heartworm disease (Kociba & Hathaway 1974) have also been involved. Spaulding et al (1975) attributed defibrination in a case of heartworm disease to hepatic damage caused by the medication administered. Dodds (1974b) mentioned a case of thoracic granulomatous disease in which defibrination occurred. A foreign body was found to be present in the mediastinum. In the majority of these cases thrombocytopenia and a typical depression of the levels of various coagulation factors was reported. Fibrinogen levels varied between being undetectable and greater than normal and fibrin degradation products (FDPs) were often increased. Canine FDPs are known to affect platelets (Kowalski et al 1964, Barnhart et al 1967), thus possibly exacerbating a haemorrhagic diathesis. The immunological assay of fibrinogen in one of the above cases was facilitated by the fact that rabbit anti-human fibrinogen serum, which is commercially available, also reacts with canine fibrinogen (Slappendel et al 1970). The methods of assay of fibrinogen in canine plasma were investigated by von Schaewen (1974) although, in acute defibrination, observation of the blood clot in vitro is normally sufficient (Dacie & Lewis 1975). It should be remembered that a fibrinogen level derived from the thrombin clotting time may be inaccurate when FDPs are present in the sample.

The presence of fibrin in the microvasculature may give rise to erythrocyte fragmentation. Dodds (1974b) studied a case of suspected thrombotic microangiopathic anaemia in a puppy which had developed thrombosis of the extremities. The cause was thought to be hyperosmolarity induced by feeding concentrated evaporated milk. The injection of autologous haemolysates into dogs has been shown to result in defibrination (Dosne et al 1968). The reaction in dogs to incompatible blood transfusion, during which erythrocyte debris is often formed in the bloodstream, may include a bleeding disorder (Friesen et al 1952) and laboratory investigations have shown that thrombocytopenia, hypofibrinogenaemia and other evidence of hypocoagulability may be present (McKay et al 1955). Hardaway (1966) proposed that the defibrination syndrome which develops in untreated acute haemorrhagic shock in dogs may also be related to the presence of erythrocyte stroma which possess potent thromboplastic activity in dogs (Rabiner & Friedman 1968).

There is also a risk of defibrination due to the formation of stroma following trauma such as fractures (Bergentz & Nilsson 1961) or surgery. In obstetrical disorders it is possible that thromboplastic material may enter the blood-stream with serious consequences (Ratnoff & Conley 1951). Many snake venoms are potent coagulants and a few reports have described defibrination-like syndromes in dogs poisoned either by bites or experimentally by injection (Hall 1972, Isard 1974). Ancrod, a purified fraction of the venom of the Malayan Pit Viper, *Agkistrodon rhodostoma*, is available for the therapeutic induction of anticoagulation by controlled defibrination and has been used in dogs (Slade *et al* 1973). The venom of the scorpion *Buthus tanulus* has also produced defibrination in dogs (Devi *et al* 1970).

The treatment of defibrination syndrome must be aimed at arresting the transformation of fibrinogen to fibrin. Paradoxically therefore, an anti-coagulant such as heparin must often be administered despite the haemor-rhagic diathesis. Until veterinary surgeons become familiar with the nature and diagnostic features of this disorder, cases are unlikely to receive the cor-rect treatment since administration of heparin to a bleeding animal necessi-tates considerable confidence in the correctness of the diagnosis.

The laboratory and genetic features of inherited disorders of coagulation in dogs are virtually identical to those of the corresponding defects in man.

Of 5 early reports of canine 'haemophilia', concerning a Fox Terrier in France (Taskin 1935), Aberdeen Terriers in Huddersfield (McKinna 1936), Greyhounds in Indonesia (Merkens 1938), Scotch Terriers in Copenhagen (Andreassen 1943) and a St Bernard in Berkshire (Lewis & Holman 1951), only two, those of McKinna and of Merkens, include evidence sufficient to suggest that the dogs were suffering from an X chromosome (sex-) linked defect such as factor-VIII or factor-IX deficiency.

Factor-VIII deficiency or haemophilia, although a rare disorder, is un-doubtedly the most commonly described of the hereditary defects of coagula-tion in dogs, having been the subject of almost 30 reports. As in man, this de-fect is inherited as an X-chromosome-(sex-)linked recessive trait. Dodds (1975) reported that the level of factor-VIII related antigen is increased in haemophilic dogs whereas it is decreased in dogs with von Willebrand's disease. Hovig *et al* (1967) found that platelet plug formation was defective in haemophilic dogs. When the plasma factor VIII level is low, bleeding is often severe. Treatment includes fresh-frozen dog plasma, cryoprecipitate or other special concentrates (Dodds 1968).

Haemophilia has been reported in Irish Terriers (Field *et al* 1946, Hutt *et al* 1948, Graham *et al* 1949, Parkes *et al* 1964), a Shetland Sheepdog (Wurzel & Lawrence, 1961), Beagles (Brock *et al* 1963, Rowsell 1963, Hampton *et al* 1973, Dodds 1974), Collies (Rowsell 1963, Rowsell & Mustard 1963), a Chihuahua/Pomeranian cross (Didisheim & Bunting 1964), a Samoyed (Stormorken *et al* 1965), a Chihuahua and Weimaraners (Kaneko *et al*

1967), Vizlas (Buckner *et al* 1967), German Shepherds (Alsatians) (Greenlee & Carper 1968, Rowsell 1963, Rowsell & Mustard 1966, Rowsell 1969, Aufderheide *et al* 1975), English Setters (Rowsell 1963, Sherwood *et al* 1966), Labradors (Archer & Bowden 1959, Howell & Lambert 1964); Greyhounds (Sharp & Dike 1964); Huskies (Bellars 1969) and several other breeds (Dodds, 1974).

Factor IX deficiency (haemophilia B, Christmas Disease) in dogs, like factor VIII deficiency, is an X-chromosome-(sex-)linked recessive trait. Platelet plug formation in factor-IX deficient dogs is defective (Hovig *et al* 1967) and in each of the reports cited below the factor IX level has been less than 1 per cent of normal and the severity of the bleeding was clearly related to the size of the breed. As treatment, Dodds (1968, 1974b) recommends fresh-frozen dog plasma, supernatant from cryoprecipitates, or special factor IX concentrates. Rowsell *et al* (1960), Mustard *et al* (1960), Brinkhous *et al* (1973) and Dodds (1974b) have studied this defect in Cairn Terriers from Toronto, Canada. It has also been described in Black and Tan Coonhounds in Albany, New York (Dodds 1968, Rowsell 1969, Brinkhouse *et al* 1973) and in a St Bernard in New Haven, Connecticut (Dodds & Kaneko 1971, Dodds 1974b). Bleeding in the St Bernard was extremely severe, making maintenance difficult.

The only full report of canine hypofibrinogenaemia concerned a family of Dürrbacks in Zurich, Switzerland (Kammerman *et al* 1971). Fatal, severe bleeding occurred in the propositus whose fibrinogen level, determined immunologically, was less than 6 mg/dl. The mode of transmission in dogs is not known, but in man it is probably autosomal recessive. Fresh-frozen dog plasma, cryoprecipitate or fibrinogen concentrate is recommended as treatment (Dodds 1968).

Factor X deficiency was identified in American Cocker Spaniels by Dodds (1973, 1974b) in Albany, New York State, USA. The defect appears to be inherited as an autosomal dominant trait. The bleeding symptoms are moderately severe, new-born pups being particularly at risk. There is evidence to suggest that the animals studied by Dodds, all buff-coloured, were heterozygotes for the defect and that the homozygous condition may be lethal. Dodds (1974b) suggests that the only way to maintain new-born affected puppies is by transfusion of special concentrates via the umbilical vein, a procedure unlikely to be widely used. Many dogs of this breed have now been examined but the defect has so far been confined to dogs related to the buff line. However, the involvement of buff coloured animals in the pedigrees of many good black, black and tan and parti-coloured lines is considerable. Contact I have had with breeders of American Cocker Spaniels in Britain indicates concern over the close relationship of some of their animals to those described in Dodds' original paper and veterinary surgeons in Britain should be vigilant for the possible emergence of this defect.

Canine factor XI deficiency was identified by Dodds and Kull (1971) in a family of Springer Sapniels in New Haven, Connecticut, USA. Inheritance of this defect is autosomal and bleeding symptoms are usually moderate, but serious, possibly life-threatening, haemorrhage may result from surgery or other trauma. Moderate symptoms were also observed among heterozygotes

Table 10.4 Results of laboratory investigations* on the factor-VII deficient propositus (Peter/19) from the Smith, Kline and French Laboratories colony.

Test (*units*)	Peter/19	Normal Beagles†
Whole blood clotting time in glass (s)	275	157–305
Platelet count ($\times 10^9$/l)	376	215–360
Celite partial thromboplastin (cephalin) time(s)	22·2	22·8–30·4
One-stage prothrombin time (s)	23·8	10·0–11·8
Additions to one-stage prothrombin time test:		
10% of aluminium hydroxide-treated plasma(s)	27·6	—
10% of incubated normal Beagle serum (s)	9·9	—
1:1 mixture with plasma of VII-deficient		
homozygote from Allen and Hanburys' colony	22·1	10·1
Russell's viper venom (+cephalin) time(s)	10·8	11·0–11·7
Thromboplastin generation test (see Fig. 10.22)	Normal	—
Prothrombin consumption test (index) after 20 min	30·4	—
after 40 min	6·6	—
after 60 min	<1	—
Factor II assay (Taipan) (% normal Beagle)	92	—
Factor VII assay (% normal Beagle)	1	—
Factor IX assay (% normal Beagle)	110	—
Factor X assay (% normal Beagle)	101	—
Plasma total protein (g/dl)	6·4	4·5–7·0
Plasma alkaline phosphatase (iu)	105	50–120
Plasma alanine aminotransferase (iu)	16	5–20

* Most techniques were as described by Spurling *et al* (1972). Human substrate plasma (Dade) was used for factor IX assays. Filtered bovine plasma (Diagen) was used as a substrate for factor X assays.
† Healthy Beagles examined at the same time as the propositus. The number examined differed between tests.

for this trait. Although no specific therapy is recommended, Dodds (1974) states that transfused canine factor XI has a relatively long half-life.

Dodds (1970, 1975) fully investigated a family of German Shepherds (Alsatians) in Detroit, USA in which von Willebrand's disease occurred. The pedigree suggested that the disease was transmitted as an autosomal dominant trait with variable expressivity although Dodds (1975) proposed the possibility of polygenic inheritance. The severity of symptoms has been variable but severe, sometimes fatal, bleeding has occurred although it tended to become less severe with increasing age or with repeated pregnancies. Recommended treatment is fresh-frozen dog plasma or the supernatant from cryoprecipitates (Dodds 1968). Many of the laboratory features which, in man, have recently facilitated the differentiation of von Willebrand's disease from haemophilia, have been observed during investigation of affected dogs. Thus

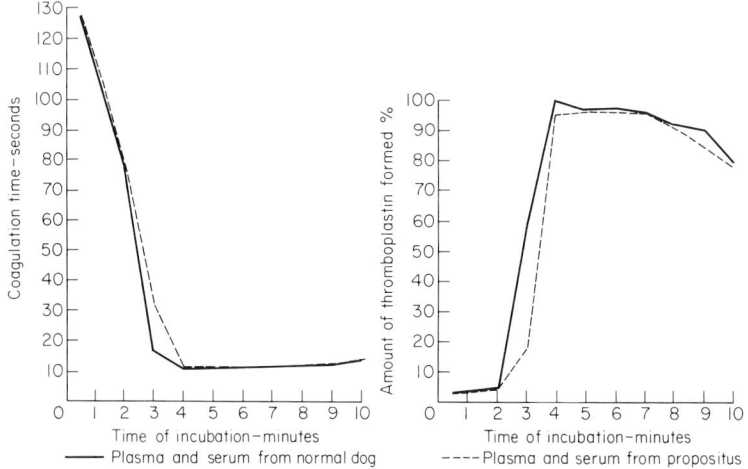

Fig. 10.22   Thromboplastin generation test on the factor-VII deficient propositus in the Smith, Kline and French Laboratories' colony.

the bleeding time was prolonged, factor-VIII activity and the level of factor-VIII related antigen were reduced. Both prothrombin consumption and platelet adhesiveness induced by Ristocetin were abnormal and plasma factor VIII levels over-responded to the transfusion of normal or haemophilic plasma.

Factor VII deficiency presents interesting differences from other hereditary defects of coagulation in dogs in that it is not usually associated with bleeding symptoms and does not normally necessitate treatment. As mentioned earlier this defect even appears to convey a measure of protection during bacterial toxin-induced defibrination. The defect is transmitted autosomally, and is phenotypically recessive although genotypically codominant (Spurling *et al* 1972). Platelet plug formation in factor VII deficient dogs is indistinguishable from that in normal dogs (Hovig *et al* 1967).

Of 8 definite reports of this defect in dogs, 7 concern Beagles. Mustard *et al* (1962) in Canada discovered this defect fortuitously. The pedigree suggested that 2 dogs, one from Fort Worth and the other from Toronto, introduced the trait. Only later was a very mild haemorrhagic diathesis recognized. Dodds (1974b) also mentions its presence among Beagles in a large colony in North Rose, New York. Factor VII deficiency has been found on 6 occasions in Beagles in Britain. Garner *et al* (1967), Garner and Conning (1970) and Poller *et al* (1971) reported its presence in a colony in Cheshire and

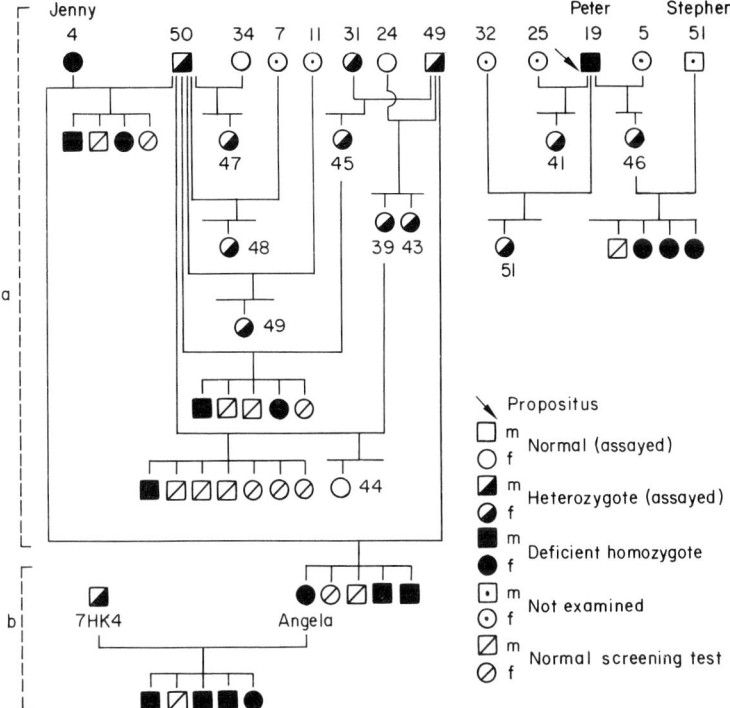

Fig. 10.23 Pedigree of factor-VII deficiency in the Smith, Kline and French (SKF) Laboratories Colony.

a = Breeding in the SKF colony

b = Jenny/4, was moved, whilst pregnant, to another site. Angela was mated with a factor-VII deficient heterozygote (7HK4) from the Allen and Hanburys' colony.

Capel-Edwards and Hall (1968) identified this defect in 2 Beagles purchased from different unidentified British sources. The presence of this defect in the Allen and Hanburys' Beagle colony has been the subject of several reports. Originally identified by Spurling (1971) and Spurling *et al* (1972), pedigree and other genetic studies were reported by Spurling *et al* (1974a) and the defect

N. W. Spurling

was found to be associated with a low level of factor VII antigen (Spurling 1973). Factor VII deficiency is also known to have been present until 1974 in the colony of the largest commercial breeder of Beagles in Britain (Appleton 1976 personal communication) but this breeder no longer provides dogs for research purposes. I have confirmed the deficiency of factor VII in a plasma sample from a dog from this colony. Beagles from this colony were studied by Abel and Schneider (1973) and the inclusion of a small proportion of prolonged prothrombin times among their data suggests that they may have had some factor-VII deficient animals. In 1970 I investigated the prolonged prothrombin times of Beagles from a colony maintained elsewhere in Britain by Smith, Kline and French Laboratories Ltd. This defect also proved to be factor VII deficiency. Laboratory findings on the propositus (Peter/19) are presented in Table 10.4 and Fig. 10.22 and the pedigree is shown in Fig. 10.23.

It is highly probable that factor VII deficiency is widely present not only in colonies maintained for research purposes but also among the general Beagle population in Britain. The defect is only rarely associated with bleeding (Spurling *et al* 1974b) and it does not have any characteristic which would serve as an 'indicator' of the abnormal gene (Spurling 1971). If human brain thromboplastin is available, canine heterozygotes and homozygotes for factor VII deficiency can be separately identified with reasonable confidence by their prothrombin times (Dodds 1974b). An attempt to confirm this observation in my laboratory utilizing British Comparative Thromboplastin has been only partially successful. Alternatively, factor VII assays must be carried out (Spurling *et al* 1974a). Samples of plasma of factor VII deficient Beagles derived from every source mentioned above have been compared in my laboratory. Every plasma was mixed with plasma from each of the other sources but no cross-correction of the coagulation defect occurred. Immunological determination of factor VII antigen revealed low levels in all the samples.

One other report of canine factor VII deficiency concerned a litter of Malamute pups, briefly mentioned by Dodds (1974b) in Albany, New York, USA. One pup developed widespread haematomas and evidence suggestive of haemarthrosis shortly before the onset of symptoms of a severe distemper infection. An isolated factor VII deficiency was identified. Thromboplastin generation, platelet count and platelet function were all normal. It seemed likely that the concomitant distemper infection was responsible for the severity of the symptoms in this animal. Treatment with fresh-frozen plasma resulted in a partial but temporary correction of the plasma defect. The pup was killed, necropsy revealing focal haematomas. The remaining pups in the litter did not contract distemper and, although also factor-VII deficient, were symptomless (Dodds, Hurvitz & Wilkins, 1972, personal communication).

This review of hereditary defects of coagulation has, for reasons of available space, omitted much interesting information. For further information see Rowsell (1969), Guelfi *et al* (1972), Hall (1972) and Dodds (1974b).

10.6.2.4 Disorders of fibrinolysis

Increased fibrinolysis is not often reported although it undoubtedly accompanies the defibrination syndrome and other thrombotic disorders. If prolonged, plasminogen activator levels may become depleted (Sun *et al* 1974). Abnormalities of fibrinolysis occurring in the absence of thrombotic disorders are rare. Engen *et al* (1974) detected increased fibrinolytic activity in a dog suffering from a diaphragmatic hernia. No haemorrhagic diathesis was observed and the authors proposed that the normal platelet count and clotting tests of this dog suggested that defibrination was not responsible for the increased activity and that a primary activation of fibrinolysis had occurred. This was possibly due to a reduction in the levels of fibrinolytic inhibitors, a result of the marked congestion of the liver which had developed due to the hernia. In preparation for surgery, fibrinolytic activity was reduced by administering epsilon-aminocaproic acid. After surgery fibrinolytic activity returned to normal. The administration of a minute dose of the histamine liberator 48/80 to a Boxer with multiple mast-cell tumours resulted in an unexplained dramatic increase in fibrinolytic activity (Ende & Auditore 1964). Bergentz and Nilsson (1961), studying the effect of trauma on coagulation and fibrinolysis in dogs, found that after an initial increase in fibrinolytic activity there followed a period of decreased activity during which the euglobulin lysis time was prolonged and the levels of fibrinogen and urokinase inhibitors in the plasma were increased.

Worowski (1968) reported inhibition of the fibrinolytic system during the hypercoagulable condition which developed during mercury-induced nephrosis in dogs. There was no evidence of defibrination in these dogs.

ACKNOWLEDGMENTS

The following colleagues in Allen and Hanbury's Research Limited are thanked for their collaboration during the preparation of this chapter. Mrs Vanessa Brooks of the Statistics Unit and Miss Susan J. Roberts and Mrs Ann V. Walsham of the Department of Pathology compiled Figures 10.1 to 10.6 and 10.9 to 10.14. Dr A. Mackenzie of the Biochemistry Department gave valuable advice on lymphocyte subtypes. Miss Janet Savory and Mrs Linda K. Burton of the Department of Pathology carried out many of the laboratory investigations mentioned. I thank Miss P. A. Daybell, Librarian, and staff for finding many of the references to the literature and Mrs Doreen Newton for typing the manuscript.

Dr L. Poller of the Withington Hospital, Manchester, generously supplied a quantity of the British Comparative Thromboplastin. Dr W. Jean Dodds of the State of New York Department of Health, the late Mr R. Garner of Imperial Chemical Industries Limited, Mr D. E. Hall of the University of Surrey and Mr A. E. Street of the Huntingdon Research Centre kindly provided samples of plasma from factor VII deficient Beagles. I thank Dr W. A. M. Duncan for permission to mention the findings on the Smith, Kline and French (SKF) Laboratories Beagle colony and Messrs A. Camplin, A. B. Hallam, E. H. Quinn and T. Walker, also of SKF, for their collaboration during this investigation.

I am indebted to Dr D. Poynter and to the Directors of Allen and Hanburys Research Limited for generously consenting to the writing of this chapter.

11

HAEMATOLOGY OF THE CAT

LINDSAY MACKEY

11.1 INTRODUCTION

Diseases of the haemopoietic system constitute a major source of morbidity and mortality in the cat. It has been well known for many years that several forms of anaemia and leukaemia are common in cats. Recently, haematological studies have received added impetus because of widespread interest in feline viral leukaemia. The naturally occurring haemopoietic diseases of the cat are receiving greater attention than previously and the cat is being used extensively in research studies of leukaemia and related diseases. Several disorders of the blood are now known to be associated with feline leukaemia virus (FeLV) infection, including both malignant and non-neoplastic conditions. Haematological and allied examinations therefore have important applications both in clinical medicine and in research.

The earliest published data on normal feline haematological values were fully reviewed by Schalm (1965); in this chapter, emphasis will be placed on relatively recent developments, to give an account of current knowledge of the feline haemopoietic system in health and disease.

11.2 NORMAL HAEMATOLOGICAL FEATURES OF THE CAT

Several studies have been made of the blood and bone marrow of normal cats. The relevant literature has been reviewed by Penny *et al* (1970), who compared the results in relatively recent publications, and by Schalm (1965), who tabulated the data from preceding reports. The published findings show some differences in the mean normal values obtained by the various authors and most have found a considerable range in both erythrocyte and white blood cell values in apparently normal cats. Comparison of data from studies of bone marrow composition is complicated by differences in nomenclature used by individual authors, particularly as applied to cells of the erythroid series.

11.2.1 HAEMATOLOGICAL VALUES FOR FELINE BLOOD

Results from a series of over 100 normal adult cats were published by Penny *et al* (1970) who also correlated their own findings with other relatively recent reports. For details, the reader is referred to their paper and to the

Table 11.1 Recent estimates of haematological values in normal cats

	Schalm (1965)		Penny et al (1970)		Anderson et al (1971)	
	Mean	Range	Mean	s.d.	Mean	s.d.
PCV (l/l)	0·37	0·240–0·450	0·3615	0·0494	0·366	0·036
RBC ($\times 10^{12}$/l)	7·5	5·0–10·0	6·45	0·87	7·7	0·8
Hb (gd/l)	12·0	8·0–15·0	12·48	1·72	13·3	1·8
MCV	45·0	39·0–55·0	56·16	6·22	4·7	3·9
MCHC	33·2	30·0–36·0	34·53	3·26	36	3·1
WBC ($\times 10^9$/l)	12·5	5·5–19·5	13·86	5·18	24·0	12·5
Neutrophils %	59·5	35–75	61·14	15·38	70	14·4
Lymphocytes %	32	20–55	28·4	12·24	27	12
Monocytes %	3	1–4	1·87	1·78	—	—
Eosinophils %	5·5	2–12	8·92	2·41	—	—
Basophils %	0	Rare	0·03	0·11	—	—

literature cited in it. Earlier studies are reviewed by Schalm (1965). Because of marked disparity between certain of the results obtained by individual authors, it is not possible to give a definitive statement as to the true limits of the normal values in cats. For this reason, recent studies are summarized separately in Table 11.1. The particular discrepancies to be noted are in the PCV, RBC and Hb values, where the lower estimate of the normal limit by Schalm would be considered anaemic according to the results of Penny *et al* and Anderson *et al* (1971). The MCV value of Penny *et al* is substantially higher than that in either of the other studies and also shows a much wider range than in the latter. The WBC is considerably higher in the series of Anderson *et al* than the other 2 results and shows a very wide range; this may reflect the fact that the cats studied by Anderson *et al* were from a cat colony, in which minor subclinical infections could have been present in the group. These cats were kept under constant veterinary supervision and it is therefore interesting to note that high WBC levels may occur in the absence of any overt clinical abnormality. In the author's experience, the eosinophil counts towards the upper end of the ranges given by Schalm and Penny *et al* are seen typically in cats with parasitic infestations or chronic skin conditions,

Table 11.2   Erythrocyte values in kittens and adult cats

	Kitten	*Adult*
PCV (l/l)	0·262 ± 0·051	0·366 ± 0·036
RBC (× 10^{12}/l)	4·8 ± 0·53	7·7 ± 0·8
Hb (gd/l)	7·5 ± 0·5	13·3 ± 1·8
MCV	54 ± 10·7	47 ± 3·9
MCHC	30 ± 5·7	36 ± 3·1

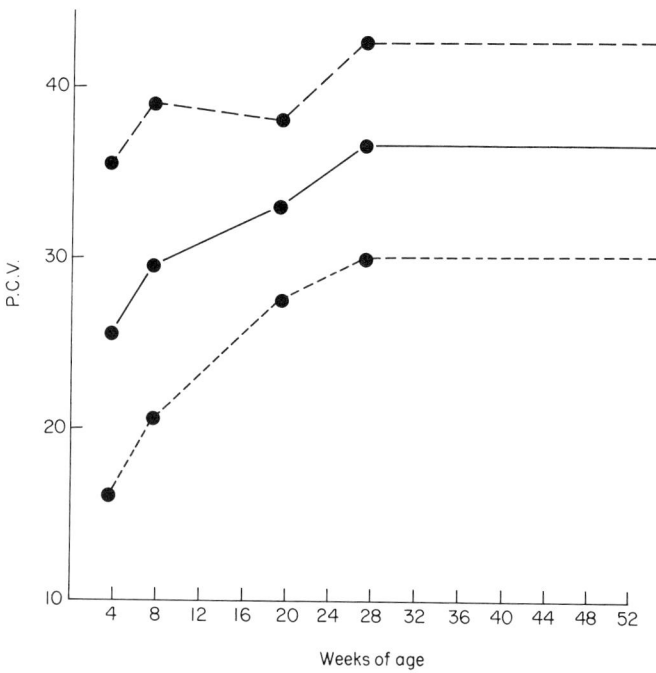

Fig. 11.1   Normal haematocrit values in relation to age in cats from 4 weeks to 1 year of age. Mean values are joined by a solid line, with 2 s.d. values above and below the mean joined by broken lines.

and otherwise eosinophil proportions of 0·5–1·0 per cent would be more usual. Substantial helminth infestations may of course be present in clinically normal cats.

As pointed out by Schalm (1965) there has been general agreement that the PCV, RBC and Hb values are lower in young kittens than in adult cats, but that the MCV is higher in kittens than in adults. This is illustrated by the findings of Anderson *et al* (1971), who examined normal cats from 4 weeks to 1 year of age. They found a statistically significant difference between the erythrocyte values at 4 and 8 weeks of age and in cats aged 12 weeks and over. The results from 4 week old kittens and 1 year old cats from that study are shown in Table 11.2. Based on the data from the same study, Fig. 11.1 shows the normal mean PCV value in relation to age; the solid line shows the mean, with 2 SDs on either side shown by broken lines. A graph of this type provides an easy means of assessing whether individual PCV measurements fall within the normal range, particularly in kittens. Anderson *et al* also found significant changes in the neutrophil leucocyte and lymphocyte populations

Table 11.3 Leucocyte values in kittens and adult cats

	Kitten	Adult
WBC ($\times 10^9$/l)	$11 \cdot 7 \pm 2 \cdot 5$	$24 \pm 12 \cdot 5$
Neutrophil %	$39 \pm 8 \cdot 8$	$70 \pm 14 \cdot 4$
Lymphocyte %	$60 \pm 7 \cdot 1$	$27 \pm 15 \cdot 2$

with age. In young kittens, lymphocytes formed a majority of the WBC while in older cats, neutrophil leucocytes predominated. The results from 4 week old kittens and 1 year cats are shown in Table 11.3.

In most studies, reticulocyte counts in normal cats have been well below 1·0 per cent. Schalm (1965) found a mean count of 0·2 per cent and a range of 0·1–1·0 per cent, while in the series of Penny *et al* the count was $0·05 \pm 0·9$ per cent. However, Kramer and Lewis (1972) considered that 2 types of reticulocyte could be identified in the cat. In one type, the reticulum occurred as dense aggregates and in the other as fine punctate foci. If both types were counted, they found a normal mean of 4·6 per cent and a range of 1·4–10·8 per cent, but only 0–0·4 per cent were of the coarsely reticulated variety. Those with fine punctate reticulum were considered to be maturing cells. From studies on cats with artificially induced anaemia, they concluded that the feline reticulocyte has an unusually prolonged maturation time. When 30 ml blood/kg body weight were removed (i.e. approximately half of the total blood volume) a mean reticulocyte response of 50 per cent was reached by 11 days; this was sustained for a further 9 days, followed by gradual reversion to normal in the subsequent 5–9 days. The proportion of heavily reticulated cells was greatest in the early phase of the erythropoietic response. The same authors cite Krafka (1931) as claiming that all erythrocytes of new-born kittens are reticulocytes. In the author's experience, at 2–3 months of age, approximately 50 per cent of feline erythrocytes are reticulocytes.

OSMOTIC FRAGILITY
In a study by Jain (1972), the mean corpuscular fragility of normal feline erythrocytes (i.e. the concentration of saline required to produce 50 per cent haemolysis) was found to be 0·54 (range 0·46–0·64).

ERYTHROCYTE LIFE SPAN
In the cat, this has been estimated as 68–77 days (Schalm 1965).

ERYTHROCYTE SEDIMENTATION RATE
There are no published data on the ESR of cats.

11.2.2   MYELOGRAM

There have been several estimates of the cellular composition of normal adult feline bone marrow (as reviewed by Schalm 1965). Comparison of data is complicated by the lack of uniformity in terminology in these reports. The largest study, and also the most recent, was that of Penny *et al* (1970) who prepared myelograms from 60 normal cats and compared their data with those in earlier studies. They concluded that their results did not differ significantly from others previously published, except that their estimate of the myeloid/erythroid (M/E) ratio as $2·47\pm0·91$ was somewhat higher than the figure of 1·6 (range 0·1–3·9) found by Gilmore *et al* (1964), who had examined 15 cats. The results of Penny *et al* (1970) are reproduced in Table 11.4, which shows the normal myelogram based on differential counts of 1000 cells.

11.2.3   CYTOLOGY OF HAEMOPOIETIC CELLS

The cytology of feline haemopoietic cells has been described by Gilmore *et al* (1964) and Schalm (1972) who used different nomenclature for cells of the erythroid series than is used in this chapter. Here the main distinguishing features of cells in each series at different stages of maturation are described. The divisions between categories are of course rather arbitrary, since the precursors of the mature, end stage, cell progress through a spectrum of morphological changes during maturation.

ERYTHROCYTE SERIES
Cells in the erythroid series are the proerythroblast, early, intermediate and late normoblast, reticulocyte and the mature erythrocyte. Normally, only erythrocytes and very small numbers of reticulocytes appear in the blood.

The proerythroblast, derived from a pluripotential stem cell, is the earliest recognizable member of the series. It is 10–14 μ in diameter, has a large central round or slightly ovoid nucleus which almost fills the cell, and strongly basophilic cytoplasm. The nuclear chromatin has an interwoven, somewhat granular appearance; nucleoli are present. The proerythroblast gives rise by cell division to normoblasts. As the series progresses, these cells become

Table 11.4 Myelogram of normal cats (Penny *et al* 1970)

Cell type	Mean	Range or s.d.
Myeloblast	1·74	0·6–4·6
Pro-myelocyte	0·88	0·0–2·2
Neutrophil myelocyte	9·76	4·2–15·6
Neutrophil metamyelocyte juvenile	7·32	3·0–14·6
Neutrophil metamyelocyte band	25·8	18·6–40·0
Neutrophil polymorph	9·24	2·0–22·3
Eosinophil myelocyte	1·47	0·3–5·7
Eosinophil metamyelocyte	1·52	0·2–4·0
Eosinophil	0·81	0·0–2·8
Basophil	0·002	0·0–0·1
Total myeloid	58·53	±6·95
Pro-erythroblast	1·71	0·2–3·6
Early normoblast	3·83	1·5–7·4
Intermediate normoblast	8·67	3·9–16·0
Late normoblast	11·68	6·4–19·0
Total erythroid	25·88	±6·51
Plasma cell	1·61	0·2–4·6
Reticulum cell	0·13	0·0–0·6
Lymphocyte	7·63	±3·7
Others	1·62	0·2–5·9
Damaged or undifferentiated	4·60	±2·43
M/E ratio	2·47	±0·91
i/m ratio	0·32	±0·11
Mitosis	0·61	±0·16
Vacuolated myeloid	0·21	±0·29

Except for the ratios, the values are expressed as percentages.

smaller in size and have increasingly densely staining nuclei without nucleoli; the nuclear/cytoplasmic ratio is reduced and the cytoplasm gradually loses its basophilia as it becomes haemoglobinized. The reticulocyte is an immature erythrocyte, slightly larger than the latter, and it may be faintly basophilic; the reticulum content is shown by supravital staining with new methylene blue or brilliant cresyl blue. The erythrocyte is 5·5–5·6 μ in diameter and stains orthochromatically. In the mid-portion of the blood film, the erythrocytes show a central pale zone, which reflects the biconcave of the shape of the cell. A small proportion of feline erythrocytes contain Howell–Jolly bodies. These nuclear remnants are seen as purple dots of approximately $0.5\,\mu$ diameter. They may be seen in up to 1.0 per cent of erythrocytes in normal cats (Schalm 1965) and their frequency rises when erythrocyte production is increased in response to certain anaemias.

Macronormoblasts are abnormally large normoblasts and may be seen in response to haemolytic anaemia and in myeloproliferative diseases. Megaloblasts are also larger than normoblasts and have more open nuclei; they often show a marked degree of cytoplasmic haemoglobinization which is out of the normal phase for the maturity of the nucleus. They are seen in malignancies involving erythroid cells, in which other bizarre cytological appearances are also found. Macrocytes are larger than normal erythrocytes; they are often slightly basophilic and usually prove to be reticulocytes. They are seen in the haemolytic and haemorrhagic anaemias.

GRANULOCYTE SERIES

Cells in this series are the myeloblast, promyelocyte, myelocyte, meta-myelocyte, immature (band) polymorph and the mature polymorphonuclear leucocyte. Normally, only mature polymorphs and a few band cells are seen in the blood.

The myeloblast is a large cell of 15–$20\,\mu$ diameter, round or slightly ovoid in shape, containing a large ovoid reticulated nucleus with nucleoli. The cytoplasm is more abundant than in proerythroblasts and less deeply staining. Granules are not usually visible with Romanowsky stains. Pro-myelocytes and myelocytes show progressive reduction in size, absence of nucleoli and reduction of nuclear/cytoplasmic ratio. The cytoplasm gradually acquires more specific granules. In the metamyelocyte, the nucleus is indented or kidney-shaped and cytoplasmic granulation is more conspicuous. The band cell is the same size as the mature polymorph. The nucleus is much reduced in size and assumes an elongated, U shape or twisted shape; it stains much more densely than nuclei of earlier cells. Specific granules are obvious. The mature polymorph is 6–$9\,\mu$ in diameter and contains a fully lobulated nucleus. In the cat, it is notable that the granules of the neutrophil polymorph stain only poorly with Romanowsky methods (Fig. 11.2). Eosinophil granules in the cat have a slender rod shape and stain a dull orange colour (Fig. 11.2). Basophil polymorphs are rare and are identified by dense basophilic granules filling the cytoplasm and overlaying the nucleus; they are slightly smaller than other granulocytes.

MONOCYTIC SERIES

Mature monocytes are readily identified in normal blood films by their large size, being 15–$22\,\mu$ in diameter (Fig. 11.3). The nucleus is pale-staining and may appear indented, twisted or clover leaf in shape. The cytoplasm is

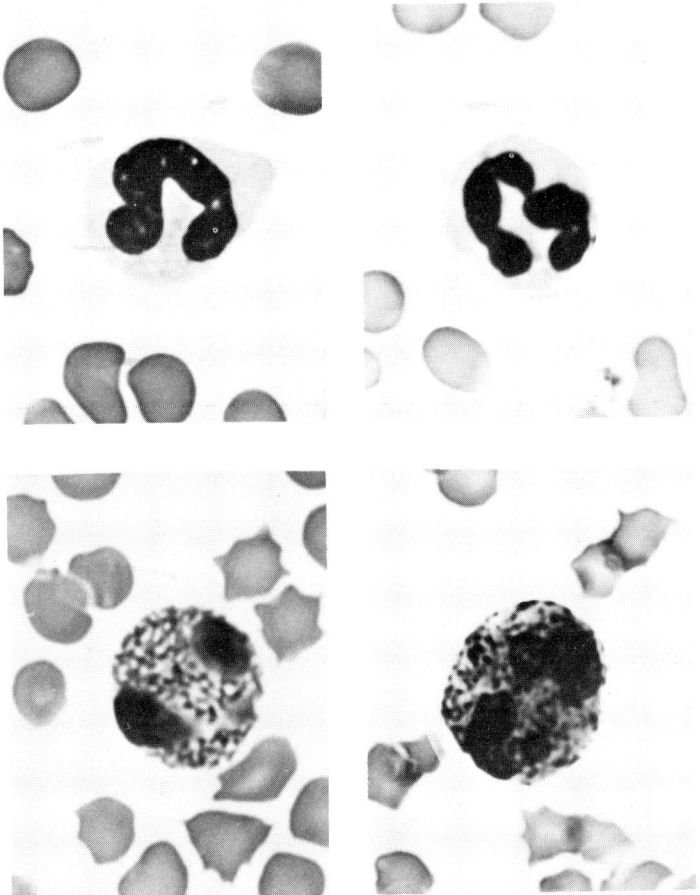

Fig. 11.2 (a) Immature neutrophil polymorphonuclear leucocyte with band nucleus.
(b) Mature neutrophil polymorphonuclear leucocyte with fully lobulated nucleus.
(c) Eosinophil polymorphonuclear leucocyte, showing rod-shaped granules.
(d) Basophil polymorphonuclear leucocyte with round azurophil granules obscuring the nucleus.
Leishman × 1000.

abundant and only faintly basophilic, with a ground glass appearance. A few tiny azurophilic granules may be present, usually localized to one area of the cytoplasm. Small vacuoles are not uncommon. The monocyte precursors, the monoblast and promonocyte, are not normally found in blood. They may be difficult to distinguish from granulocyte precursors in the marrow, and in the blood in certain leukaemias. They are smaller than mature monocytes and the nuclei contain nucleoli. Cytochemical methods are often necessary to identify these cells.

MEGAKARYOCYTES

These cells are normally confined to the bone marrow, and are easily recognized by their extremely large size and multiple or partially lobulated nuclei. Megakaryoblasts are much smaller and resemble other myeloid precursors.

LYMPHOID CELLS

Lymphocytes are found in the blood and bone marrow. Small numbers of lymphoblasts occur in the marrow and are occasionally seen in normal feline blood.

Lymphocytes are the smallest nucleated cells in normal blood, being 7–9 μ in diameter. The nucleus almost completely fills the cell; it is round in shape and densely basophilic with a coarsely granular appearance. A narrow rim of basophilic cytoplasm is usually visible at one edge of the cell (Fig. 11.3). Lymphoblasts are larger, 12–15 μ in diameter, and have more abundant cytoplasm, although the nuclear/cytoplasmic ratio is high in all lymphoid cells. The nucleus is round or slightly ovoid with a smooth, well defined outline. The chromatin is coarsely clumped and a single nucleolus is present. Cleavage of the nucleus is seldom obvious in feline lymphoblasts. The cytoplasm is basophilic and can be seen around the circumference of the nuclei. Occasionally, a few fine azurophilic granules are present. Malignant lymphoblasts may have slightly indented nuclei and sometimes contain cytoplasmic vacuoles. Lymphoblasts are no longer considered to be precursor cells, or poorly differentiated forms, since following stimulation by antigen or mitogen, small lymphocytes transform to become lymphoblasts.

PLASMA CELLS

These occur in small numbers in the bone marrow and not in the blood. They are oval cells, maximum diameter 12 μ, with basophilic cytoplasm and eccentric nuclei. The nuclei are round, strongly staining and contain coarsely clumped chromatin. In the cytoplasm close to the nucleus, a paler-staining zone can often be seen (the Golgi region). In the malignant state (myeloma), numerous cytological irregularities may be found. There is often considerable variation in cell size and binucleated or multinucleated cells occur.

11.2.4 CYTOCHEMISTRY OF HAEMOPOIETIC CELLS

The use of cytochemical methods is extremely valuable for the identification of early members of the various haemopoietic cell series. This is particularly so in the case of certain haemopoietic malignancies, where the cells may be

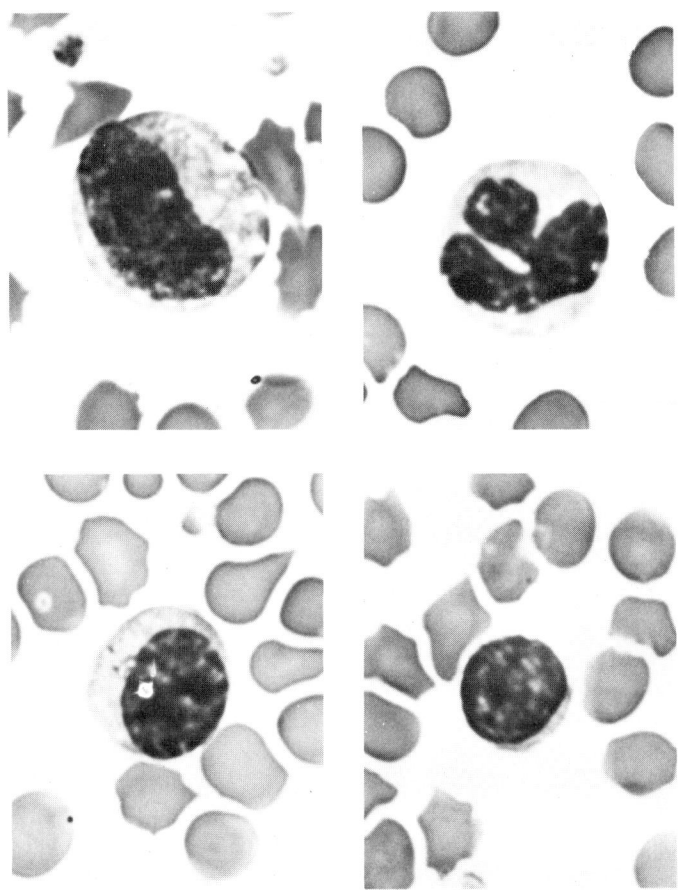

Fig. 11.3 (a) Monocyte with oval, slightly indented nucleus and small cytoplasmic vacuoles.
(b) Monocyte with clover-leaf shaped nucleus.
(c) Large lymphocyte with small azurophilic cytoplasmic granules.
(d) Small lymphocyte.
Leishman × 1000.

very poorly differentiated and not readily classifiable in Romanowsky stained films. The use of special techniques will usually show cytoplasmic features which identify the cell series to which the primitive, poorly differentiated, or blast cells belong. Particularly useful methods are (i) the peroxidase technique, (ii) Sudan black B for lipids, (iii) periodic acid–Schiff (PAS) for glycogen and (iv) Prussian blue for free iron. The technical details are given in the section on techniques (para. 14.8.4). In practice, the main diagnostic difficulties involve the differentiation of monocytes, myeloid and erythroid precursors, particularly in the malignant state. Certain types of malignant lymphoid cell may also be difficult to classify with Romanowsky stains. The cytochemical characteristics of cells in these groups are described below. As a general rule, malignant cells tend to show similar reactions to the normal precursor cells of the same series, although the degree or intensity of the reaction may vary from normal.

MONOCYTES

The cytoplasm of monocytes and their precursors is peroxidase and Prussian blue negative. With Sudan black, fine punctate staining occurs. The positive granules are discrete and not densely clumped as in cells of the granulocyte series. Monoblasts in monocytoid leukaemia may show reduced or negative staining. The PAS reaction in monocytes and their precursors may be faintly positive or negative.

NEUTROPHIL PRECURSORS

These are well shown by the peroxidase technique. Mature neutrophils show heavy granular cytoplasmic staining. Positive granules occur in cells of the whole series from the myeloblast onwards, with the intensity of staining increasing as the cells mature. In cases of myeloid leukaemia, the degree of positivity may be less than in normal cells. The Sudan black method is also useful. Mature neutrophils show densely positive, coarsely granular cytoplasmic staining. Positivity is seen in all members of the series, varying from small numbers of fine granules in the promyeloblast, through increasingly numerous and enlarging granules in the metamyelocyte stages to reach the intense reaction of the mature cell. PAS staining also shows increasing positivity through the neutrophil maturation series. Myeloblasts and promyelocytes show negative reactions or the cytoplasm may be faintly diffusely positive. In mature neutrophils there is diffuse staining of moderate intensity. Prussian blue staining is negative in cells of this series.

ERYTHROCYTE PRECURSORS

These are negative with the peroxidase and Sudan black methods. Prussian blue staining is negative in normal mature erythrocytes and normal late stage normoblasts. However, earlier members show positive cytoplasmic staining and in malignant erythroid cells, there may be some staining in normoblasts also. Normal erythroblasts are PAS negative, but glycogen may be demonstrable in malignant erythroblasts.

LYMPHOID CELLS

Lymphocytes and lymphoblasts are completely negative in the peroxidase reaction and with Sudan black and Prussian blue staining. Normal and malignant lymphoblasts may contain a small number of PAS positive fine cytoplasmic granules.

11.3 FELINE HAEMOGLOBINS

Two types of haemoglobin, termed HbA and HbB, occur in normal blood of domestic cats (Lessard & Taketa 1969). They occur in ratios in individual cats varying from 1:1 to 1:9. The 2 proteins have identical alpha but different beta chains. The cat is unusual in showing such a wide variation in the relative amounts of the haemoglobins. In most species where multiple haemoglobins occur, the relative proportions tend to be fairly constant between individuals. Haemoglobins of the adult type and ratios are present in fetal cats from 26–30 days' gestation. No haemoglobin analogous to HbF found in late human and some other mammalian fetuses has been identified electrophoretically in cats.

Compared to many species, feline Hb has a low oxygen affinity and the cat is unusually susceptible to anoxic conditions. Reeves *et al* (1963) found that cats invariably died within 2 months of being moved to an altitude of 14,000 ft (4600 m). Considerable variation has been found in the oxygen carrying capacity of the different Hb components in cats (Taketa 1974). In addition to HbA and HbB, 3 minor components termed HbB_1, HbB_2 and HbB_3 have been identified, and all of these have much higher oxygen affinities than either HbA or HbB. Taketa (1974) found that in response to anaemia, the proportion of HbB_1 was increased. In a further study, Mauk *et al* (1974) examined cats with phenylhydrazine-induced anaemia and found that both HbB_1 and HbB_2 are increased while HbB is decreased and that the amount of HbA remained unchanged. On recovery from anaemia, the ratio reverted to pre-existing values. These authors concluded that the feline response to anaemia is somewhat paradoxical in this respect, in view of the general assumption that the efficiency of tissue oxygenation is improved by reduction in Hb oxygen affinity. The feline response effectively raises the oxygen loading potential of the blood. Mauk *et al* (1974) suggested that this may be important in conditions of oxygen deprivation since normal cat blood, with its low oxygen affinity, would be difficult to oxygenate under these circumstances.

11.4 FELINE BLOOD GROUPS

No information has been published on the blood group systems of the cat.

11.5 THE ANAEMIAS

It is widely recognized that anaemia is common in cats and is an important cause of mortality. The types of anaemia seen most commonly in the cat are haemolytic of infectious or immunological origin, myelophthisic resulting from malignancies of the haemopoietic system, and aplastic which may be associated with FeLV infection, though the etiology is often unknown. Anaemias due to mineral or vitamin deficiencies do not appear to be important in cats. Pernicious anaemia has not been found in cats and in a study of intrinsic factor activity in stomach preparations from several species, Hippe and Schwartz (1971) were unable to demonstrate any activity in the cat. It is not known whether vitamin B_{12} absorption requires intrinsic factor in cats and deficiency of this vitamin is not recognized in the cat.

In several reports, the term 'non-regenerative' has been applied to anaemias in cats; the haematological data in some of these cases suggested an aplastic basis for the disease but in others, the information did not allow categorization. Since 'non-regenerative' is non-specific and describes a secondary feature which may supervene in several types of anaemia, this is not an appropriate diagnostic term.

In haemolytic or haemorrhagic anaemias where a compensatory erythro-poietic response is usual, the feline haemopoietic system appears to be particularly labile in its reaction to a need for increased erythrocyte production. Reticulocyte counts often exceed 50 per cent in clinically anaemic cats and may reach almost 100 per cent. Extramedullary haemopoiesis is readily established in anaemic cats and is seen in marked degree in the spleen but may also develop in the liver and lymph nodes. When extramedullary haemopoiesis occurs, it leads to the escape of many normoblasts and even erythroblasts into the circulation and on occasion, nucleated red blood cells may compose as much as 50 per cent of all nucleated cells in the blood. Care must be taken to distinguish normal erythroid cells in such cases from leukaemic blast cells.

The main forms of anaemia currently recognized in the cat are as follows.

11.5.1 FELINE INFECTIOUS ANAEMIA

This condition was first described in South Africa by Clark (1942) and is now recognized in many parts of the world. It is an important disease of the cat, although its prevalence is not known precisely. The causal organism is a parasite of erythrocytes, now most commonly termed *Haemobartonella felis* (*H. felis*) but also known as *Eperythrozoon felis*. The taxonomy and classification of the group of organisms to which this belongs has presented some difficulty, with certain authorities favouring their inclusion in the rickettsial group and others considering them more akin to the protozoa.

Furthermore, there has been doubt as to whether *Haemobartonella* and *Eperythrozoon* represent 2 distinct genera. For practical purposes, in the cat, the organisms recognized in this category in different countries are morphologically alike and induce the same type of disease in infected cats. In stained blood films, the organisms appear attached to the erythrocyte membrane; they are highly pleomorphic, often appearing as single or multiple

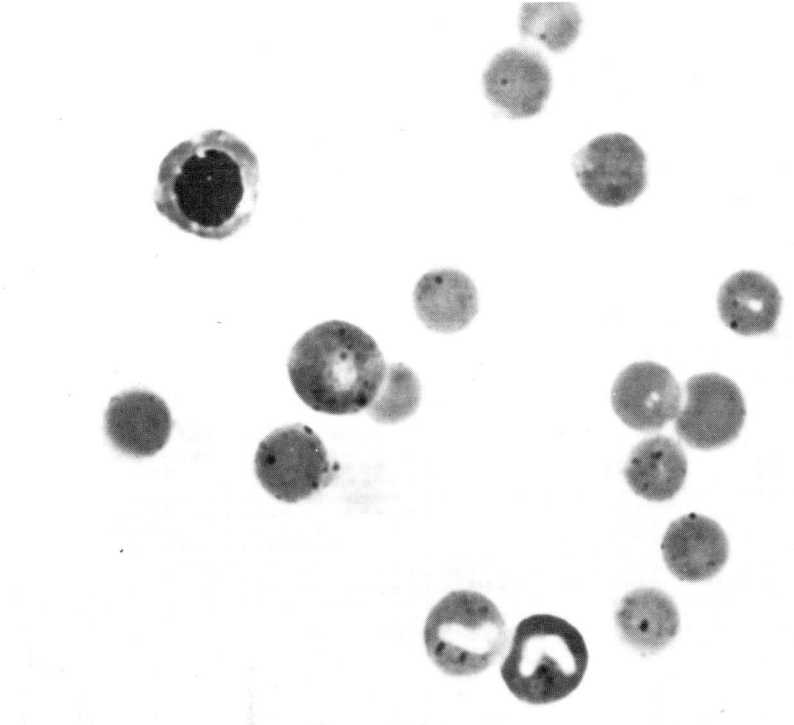

Fig. 11.4 Feline infectious anaemia. Blood film showing large numbers of Haemobartonella organisms on the erythrocytes. Macrocytic erythrocytes and a normoblast are present. Giemsa × 1000.

coccoid bodies of 0·8–1 μ diameter, but also as tiny dots or as rods up to 1·5 μ in length (Fig. 11.4). They are well shown by Romanowsky stains, and in Giemsa stained preparations they are purple in colour. To avoid confusion with artifacts produced by stain deposit or dust, it is essential to use only well filtered stains and absolutely clean, grease-free slides.

Electron microscopic studies have confirmed the eperythrocytic localization of the parasites, where they cause shallow indentation in the erythrocyte membrane (Small & Ristic 1967). Both mature and immature erythrocytes may be parasitized and, in a heavy infection, up to 100 per cent of the erythrocytes may contain organisms. Acridine orange staining indicates the presence of both DNA and RNA in the organisms, which are however non-nucleated. A fluorescent antibody technique can also be used to diagnose the infection. Using directly labelled serum obtained from cats 2–4 weeks after experimental infection, Small and Ristic (1967) were able to demonstrate the organisms and considered the method much more sensitive than routine staining techniques. They found a high degree of correlation between the results obtained with the fluorescent antibody technique and with acridine orange staining and therefore concluded that the methods were equally accurate for diagnostic purposes, although the latter is, of course, non-specific.

The method of replication of *H. felis* is unknown; both binary fission and a budding process have been suggested, but since the parasite has not yet been propagated in vitro much remains to be learned about its life cycle. The means of transmission is also unknown. Experimental infections are readily established by inoculation of small samples of infected blood. Under natural conditions, transmission by bites and scratches, by arthropod vectors or congenital infection are possibilities, but unproved. The infection may induce an acute illness with fatal haemolytic anaemia. In other cases, the disease takes a more chronic form, with relapses and remissions extending over a period of months, even when therapy is maintained. It has not been shown that true cure, with total elimination of all parasites, can in fact be achieved. Cats may also become chronic carriers of infection in the absence of clinical abnormality. It has been suggested that inter-current stress factors may precipitate overt disease in chronically infected cats.

It is well recognized that parasitaemia is not always readily demonstrable in the infected animal. Even in cats with clinical illness, parasites may not always be visible. Typically, the infection undulates, with parasites present in a high proportion of the erythrocytes for several days, but with intervening intervals when they may apparently disappear. In a suspected case therefore, a single negative result does not prove freedom from infection. Under these circumstances, it is essential to examine further blood films on subsequent days, or after a few days' interval, before reaching any conclusion as to the presence of *H. felis*.

In a severe acute case the cat shows fever, apathy, anorexia, severe anaemia and splenomegaly. In occasional cases only, jaundice and haemoglobinuria are seen. The haematological features are those typical of haemolytic anaemia. The RBC may fall below $1 \times 10^{12}/l$. The anaemia is macrocytic (MCV values may exceed 90) normochromic with anisocytosis and poikilocytosis. Numerous Howell–Jolly bodies are seen in the erythrocytes, many of which show polychromasia. There is a marked degree of reticulocytosis, with the reticulocyte count often approaching 100 per cent. There is always an accompanying extramedullary haemopoiesis, with numerous normoblasts and occasional erythroblasts present in the blood. Initially, there may be a neutrophilia, but this is usually followed by neutropenia. In the author's experience, once a cat becomes severely ill, neutropenia is a typical finding. Care must be taken to avoid confusion of the erythrocyte precursors in the blood with malignant blast cells, since the clinical features of haemobartonellosis and the leukaemias are alike. In the most severe cases, blood transfusions and tetracycline therapy provides only transient relief and death from profound anaemia ensues within days or a week or 2 at most. In less severe cases, treatment is beneficial but relapses often occur in subsequent weeks and months; as already noted, there is some doubt as to the completeness of cure in such cats.

Necropsy examination of cats which die of haemobartonellosis shows pallor of the mucous membranes and the parenchymal organs. There is splenomegaly resulting from expansion of the red pulp and extension of erythropoietic marrow in the long bones. The lymph nodes are usually slightly enlarged and may reach twice normal size. Jaundice is appreciable only in occasional cases. Histologically, the spleen shows a marked degree of haemopoiesis, haemosiderosis and erythrophagocytosis; there is also an intense plasma cell reaction. The lymph node enlargement is due to the presence of large numbers of plasma cells. In the liver, the parenchyma commonly shows centrilobular degeneration; haemopoiesis may extend to the liver and also to the lymph nodes. The bone marrow shows increased erythropoietic activity. Schalm (1965) noted that in some cases, no compensatory erythropoietic response is seen and it is possible that the response may sometimes become exhausted.

The lysis which follows infection of the red cell by *H. felis* is probably related to the focal damage which can be seen in the cell membrane (Jain & Keeton 1973). It has been found that the osmotic fragility of the cells may be increased in haemobartonellosis (Jain 1973). The normal splenic phagocytic response would be expected to remove such damaged cells from the blood stream.

Nothing is known of protective immune responses in haemobartonellosis. Despite the dramatic plasma cell response which accompanies the disease, and the production of complement fixing antibodies, the cat may remain chronically infected for many months. Since it is not known whether clinically recovered cats completely eliminate the infection, it is also not known whether such animals are resistant to subsequent re-infection.

A relationship has recently been found between haemobartonellosis and feline leukaemia. Priester and Hayes (1973) found a higher than expected frequency of leukaemia in cats with haemobartonellosis. Since the duration of the *H. felis* infection was not known and tests for the presence of FeLV were not made, no conclusion could be drawn as to which condition predisposed to the other. However, it has subsequently been found that cats with haemobartonellosis have a higher frequency of FeLV infection than cats in the same population; Essex *et al* (1974) found FeLV group specific antigen in 10 of 17 cats with haemobartonellosis. Again, no firm conclusion can yet be reached as to the nature of the interaction of *H. felis* and FeLV infection. It is well known that FeLV has an immunosuppressive effect, which may possibly predisopose cats to *H. felis* (Anderson *et al* 1971, Perryman *et al* 1972). At present, for practical purposes, it is advisable to follow apparently recovered or chronic cases of haemobartonellosis for evidence of developing leukaemia. The importance of distinguishing reactive erythropoietic cells in the blood from leukaemic blast cells has already been noted. In addition, it may be considered appropriate to test such cats for evidence of FeLV infection.

11.5.2   ANAEMIA ASSOCIATED WITH FELINE LEUKAEMIA VIRUS

Anaemia is a common consequence of leukaemia virus infection in several species, including FeLV infection in cats. It is now well established that FeLV may induce anaemia as a primary disease, which may prove fatal, or may precede the onset of lymphoid malignancy (Hoover *et al* 1974, Mackey *et al* 1975a). In experimental infections, anaemia occurs with much higher frequency than neoplasia. In some experiments, 100 per cent of infected cats became anaemic (Hoover *et al* 1974, Mackey *et al* 1975a). The importance of FeLV as a cause of anaemia in cat populations under natural conditions is not yet clear, but is the subject of current research. In a study in Boston, evidence of FeLV infection was found in 70 per cent of 76 cats with anaemias of unknown cause (Essex *et al* 1975). The available evidence therefore strongly suggests that anaemia may be a frequent pathogenic effect of naturally acquired FeLV infection. Furthermore, 2 distinctly different forms of anaemia are seen in FeLV infected cats (Hoover *et al* 1974, Mackey *et al* 1975a); the haematological features of one form indicate a haemolytic basis, while the other is an aplastic or erythroblastopenic anaemia. The various circumstances in which FeLV associated anaemias occur are described below.

(a) Anaemia coincident with leukaemia. Anaemia is invariably present in association with any form of leukaemia, as a simple consequence of the destruction and replacement of normal bone marrow by malignant cells. This may be termed myelophthisic anaemia. In such cases, the anaemia is not directly related to FeLV infection, or to the particular form of leukaemia. Severe anaemia is usually the main presenting clinical sign in both lymphoid and myeloid leukaemias and other myeloproliferative neoplasms (see later). The anaemia is macrocytic and normochromic with reticulocytosis. Because of a compensatory extra-medullary haemopoietic response, large numbers of normoblasts and some erythroblasts appear in the peripheral blood. Terminally, the PCV and RBC values usually fall to extremely low levels and thrombocytopenia is also present; the other haematological features of the various leukaemias are described later. Bone marrow aspirates show an over-whelming preponderance of leukaemic cells and a deficiency of normal elements. (b) Anaemia in non-leukaemic lymphosarcoma. Anaemia is commonly

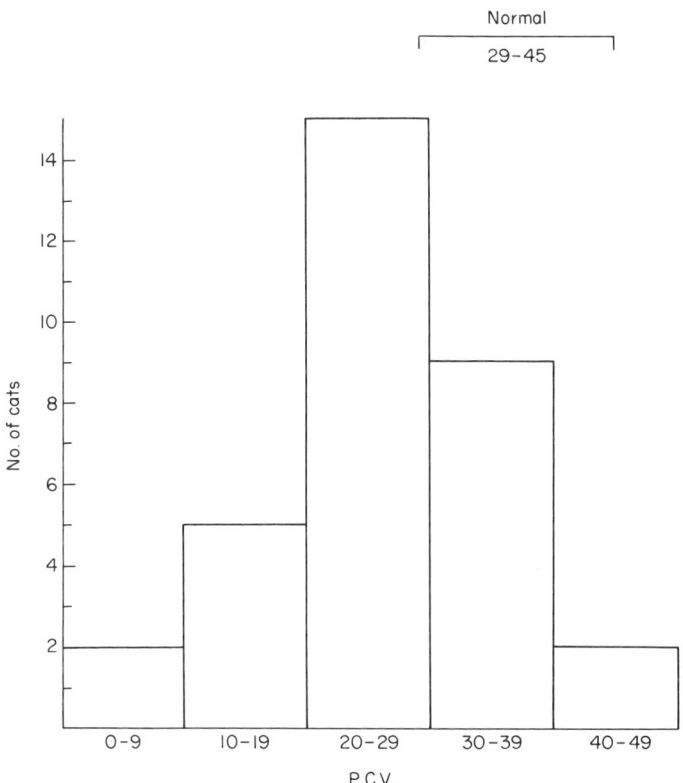

Fig. 11.5 Haematocrit values of cats with non-leukaemic lymphosarcoma, shown in relation to the normal adult range.

found in cats which have lymphoid neoplasms involving lymphoid and other organs, but where there is no infiltration of the bone marrow by malignant cells. In a series of 33 cats with naturally acquired lymphosarcomas in which careful examination of the bone marrow post mortem showed no involvement in the neoplastic disease, 54 per cent had anaemia during their illness (Mackey *et al* 1975a). In one case, the anaemia was severe enough to be the main cause of illness and the lymphosarcoma was only at an early stage when the cat died. In this series, the anaemia was of haemolytic type (i.e. macrocytosis, normochromia, reticulocytosis, extramedullary haemopoiesis and haemosiderosis were usually present). In the majority of cats with non-leukaemic lymphosarcoma, the anaemia is not severe and may not present as a major clinical feature. The PCV values from the 33 cases studied by Mackey *et al* (1975a) are shown in Fig. 11.5. Since anaemia can be expected in at least half of all cats with lymphosarcoma, haematological examination is valuable in suspected cases. The presence of anaemia is a helpful finding and if, in addition, malignant cells can be identified on cytological examination, the diagnosis is certain (see later).

(c) Anaemia without neoplasia. Anaemia commonly occurs in cats with naturally acquired FeLV infection in the absence of lymphoid neoplasia (Gardner 1971, Hardy *et al* 1973, Essex *et al* 1974). The anaemia in such cases has not always been fully characterized haematologically. In some instances the term 'non-regenerative' has been applied to the condition, when the available haematological data suggests an aplastic basis for the anaemia.

From experimental studies, it has been found that FeLV infection may induce both haemolytic and aplastic forms of anaemia. The haemolytic form was often transient and of only moderate severity (Mackey *et al* 1975a). It usually occurred 2–4 months after infection, and sometimes preceded the onset of lymphoid neoplasia. Typical RBC values were approximately $4 \times 10^{12}/l$ and PCV values $0.2–0.25$ l/l. Although ferrokinetic and RBC survival studies were not done in these experiments, haematological features consistent with haemolytic anaemia were present (i.e. macrocytosis, normochromia, reticulocytosis, extramedullary haemopoiesis and haemosiderosis). Cats which developed this type of anaemia had all been inoculated with isolated of FeLV containing either virus of the A sub-group alone, or a combination of A and B. In an experiment in which purified virus of the B sub-group alone was used as the inoculum, no anaemia occurred in any of 39 infected cats (Mackey *et al* 1975).

Aplastic anaemia has also been produced by experimental infection of neonatal cats with FeLV (Hoover *et al* 1974, Mackey *et al* 1975a). In these cases, the virus inoculum consisted either of sub-group C only (Mackey *et al* 1975a) or a combination of A, B and C (Hoover *et al* 1974). Although conclusions cannot yet be reached as to any specific pathogenic effects of the individual sub-groups of FeLV, it is interesting that distinctive anaemia syndromes were associated with particular virus sub-groups in these studies. In both series, the aplastic anaemia was characterized by a short latency and very high incidence in the infected cats. The disease progressed rapidly with death occurring between 1 and 5 months of age. Profound reductions in the erythrocyte values took place; the PCV values in one of these experiments are shown in Fig. 11.6. There was no evidence of any compensatory erythropoietic response. Reticulocytosis was absent and normoblasts did not appear in the blood. On post-mortem examination, the bone marrow was severely depleted of erythroid tissue, while the myeloid components appeared

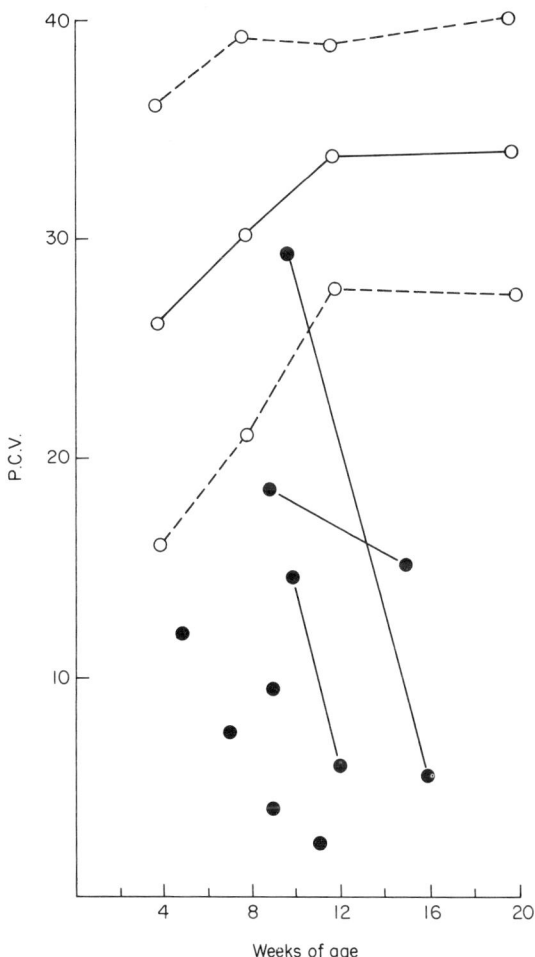

Fig. 11.6 Haematocrit values in kittens with aplastic anaemia resulting from experimental infection with feline leukaemia virus, shown in relation to the normal range in kittens of the same age.

normal. There was no sign of EMH, although erythrophagocytosis was evident. Death was due to congestive cardiac failure as a direct result of anaemia.

At present, it is not known how FeLV induces anaemia. The virus can infect and replicate in cells of the erythroid series (Oshiro *et al* 1972), but it is still not known whether this may damage them directly, or perhaps indirectly by means of an immunological reaction on the cell membrane.

11.5.3 AUTOIMMUNE HAEMOLYTIC ANAEMIA

This disease results from the presence of immunoglobulin (Ig) on the erythrocyte membrane. An immune reaction involving complement may cause lysis of the cells within the blood stream, or the affected cells may be removed from the blood by phagocytosis in the spleen, where they are then destroyed. Severe intravascular lysis produces jaundice and haemoglobinuria; these are generally not seen if the erythrocytes are removed by phagocytosis before destruction. Diagnosis of autoimmune haemolytic anaemia depends on the identification of surface Ig on the erythrocytes, which may be shown by the direct or indirect Coombs tests.

The disease is recognized in cats but few cases have been described in the literature. Based on a study of 7 affected cats, Scott *et al* (1973) found the disease to be characterized by intermittent acute haemolytic crises during which the cats showed fever, anorexia, pallor, depression and splenomegaly. Haematologically, the typical features of haemolytic anaemia were present, most cases being macrocytic and normochromic with reticulocytosis and evidence of extramedullary haemopoiesis. Bone marrow aspirates showed erythroid hyperplasia. Jaundice was seldom evident. Six of the 7 gave positive results in the direct Coombs test and the seventh had a high titre of cold agglutinins. Some cases responded well to corticosteroid therapy and recovered, apparently completely, and converted to Coombs-negative. In other instances there were succeeding relapses regardless of therapy and the disease proved fatal.

More cases will have to be studied in detail before this syndrome in cats can be fully delineated. The series of Scott *et al* 1973 was complicated by the fact that 4 of the 7 cats were found to be infected with FeLV and 2 of them developed lymphosarcoma. Cats with FeLV-associated anaemia are usually negative on Coombs testing, but clearly there is a possibility that the virus played a part in the aetiology of these apparently autoimmune anaemias.

11.5.4 CONGENITAL ERYTHROPOIETIC PORPHYRIA

Porphyrin compounds are precursors of heme and are synthesized by normoblasts. Porphyria is a condition in which abnormal porphyrins, which cannot be utilized in heme production, accumulate and become deposited in the tissues. Porphyria may be of erythropoietic type, in which there is a defect in the biosynthetic pathway, or of hepatic type, when the disease results from disordered porphyrin metabolism. Normal precursors of heme are Type III isomer porphyrins; in erythropoietic porphyria, Type I isomers of uroporphyrin and coproporphyrin are produced in large amounts. In man, both congenital and acquired porphyrias are recognized. In the cat, only congenital erythropoietic porphyria has been described. In a study of the descendants of an affected cat, Glenn *et al* (1968) concluded that the pattern of inheritance was compatible with that of simple mendelian autosomal dominance. Giddens *et al* (1975) studied a family in which the dam and 2 of 3 offspring had porphyria, but the data did not permit any conclusion as to whether the inheritance was of autosomal dominant or recessive type.

The main features of the disease are anaemia and pink or brown discoloration of the teeth, bones and other tissues. The accumulation of abnormal porphyrins in the erythrocytes leads to their removal and destruction by phagocytosis in the spleen. The resulting haemolytic anaemia is macrocytic and hypochromic, the latter feature being due to failure of normal haemoglobin production. The degree of anaemia has varied from moderate to extremely severe in the reported cases. Anisocytosis, poikilocytosis, target cells, normoblasts and an increased frequency of Howell–Jolly bodies may be seen, according to the severity of the anaemia. Splenomegaly results from erythrophagocytosis and extramedullary haemopoiesis. The brown discoloration of the tissues results from porphyrin deposition; the pigment fluoresces a bright pink or red colour in ultra-violet light. The urine may show brown discoloration as a result of porphyrin excretion.

The anaemia may be severe enough to be fatal. At necropsy, the bones show brown discoloration. There is also generalized brownish discoloration of the bone marrow and all other major organs, to varying degrees. In histological section, the pigment appears as aggregates of golden brown material and does not stain with Prussian blue. Autofluorescence in ultraviolet light can be seen in both fresh frozen sections and in unstained formalin-fixed paraffin sections. As well as porphyrin pigment, there may be a marked degree of haemosiderosis. In one of the cases described by Giddens *et al* 1975, extramedullary haemopoiesis was not found. The disease in the families studied by them differed from cases reported by Glenn *et al* (1968) and Tobias (1964) in that severe renal dysfunction occurred and there was some evidence to suggest the presence of photophobia. The renal lesion was a form of glomerulonephritis, characterized by thickening of the basement membranes of Bowman's capsule and convoluted tubules, increased mesangial matrix and some mesangial hypercellularity; immunofluorescent staining for Ig proved negative. Proteinuria and uraemia were found in these cases.

11.5.5 HEINZ BODY HAEMOLYTIC ANAEMIA

Heinz bodies are also known as erythrocyte refractile bodies or Schmauch bodies. They are crystalline erythrocytic inclusions which have a refractile appearance when stained supravitally with new methylene blue. They do not stain with Romanowsky stains, but appear as pale areas within the cell. In healthy cats, they seldom exceed $1 \cdot 0 \, \mu$ diameter. They vary in shape and may appear circular or irregular in outline, and are readily distinguished from Howell–Jolly bodies by the positive Romanowsky staining of the latter. Heinz bodies usually occur singly within the cell and are found near the periphery. They are seen typically in mature erythrocytes and not in reticulocytes. Widely differing estimates of the frequency of Heinz bodies in normal cat blood have been published. Schalm (1965) noted that they are sometimes present and occur in up to 10 per cent of cells in individual cases. On the other hand, Beritić (1965) found the inclusions in all but 1 of 94 cats, with an extremely wide range of frequency within individuals ($0 \cdot 3$–$96 \cdot 1$ per cent).

Heinz body haemolytic anaemia is a disease in which haemolysis is associated with the presence of Heinz bodies in a large proportion of the erythrocytes. The crystals tend to be larger than those occasionally seen in normal cats. The condition has been described as a spontaneous disease of the cat (Altman 1974) and it may occur as a consequence of ingestion of phenylhydrazine or methylene blue (Schechter *et al* 1973). Heinz bodies are considered to consist of denatured haemoglobin, produced by irreversible oxidation. The cat appears to be particularly susceptible in this respect of the action of oxidant drugs.

The naturally occurring disease described by Altman (1974) was found in a family of Siamese cats; the findings in these cases were considered to be closely akin to those in HbC disease of man. In the affected litter, one kitten became severely anaemic at 8 weeks of age and large crystalline inclusions were found in many of the erythrocytes. They were usually rectangular and straight edged and often large enough to stretch and distort the cell membrane. The same type of crystalloid inclusions appeared in the erythrocytes of a litter mate following splenectomy. No difference was found on electrophoresis between the haemoglobin in this kitten and in control normal cat blood.

The cases described by Schechter *et al* (1973) were associated with the use of urinary antiseptic drugs containing methylene blue. Experimental studies showed that the severity of anaemia was related to the dose of methylene blue. However, individual cats given the enteric-coated urinary antiseptic preparation showed a considerable range in the latency and degree of anaemia. Although larger than seen in normal cats, the Heinz bodies observed in these cases were approximately $3 \, \mu$ in diameter and therefore much smaller than the crystalloid bodies described by Altman, who did however equate the crystalloids in his cases with Heinz bodies.

11.5.6 HAEMORRHAGIC ANAEMIA

Anaemia due to loss of whole blood usually occurs when the blood loss is repeated or chronic. This is not a common situation in the cat. The extravasated blood may be lost from the body, as in chronic haemorrhagic enteritis, or in heavy infestations by blood-sucking parasites. Haemorrhage without external blood loss may occur as a result of rupture of fragile visceral tumours, particularly haemangiosarcomas, which sometimes develop in the mesenteric lymph nodes of the cat and tend to metastasize to the liver. The tumour is composed of delicate vascular spaces lined by a single layer of malignant endothelial cells, and is therefore liable to spontaneous rupture and haemorrhage. Haemorrhagic anaemia is macrocytic and is accompanied by a compensatory erythropoietic response leading to reticulocytosis and normoblastosis, as extramedullary haemopoiesis becomes established. Initially the anaemia is normochromic but if iron is continually lost from the body, as in haemorrhagic enteritis, it may become hypochromic.

11.5.7 IRON DEFICIENCY ANAEMIA

A transient anaemia is not uncommon in kittens prior to weaning. It is typically normocytic, normochromic and only mild in degree, with PCV values approximately 0·2–0·25 l/l. In some cases, a slight reduction in MCHC may be seen (Anderson *et al* 1971). All members of a litter may not be affected. This picture suggests that at about 4 weeks of age, the iron intake may be marginal, falling below the anaemia threshold in a proportion of cases. Iron deficiency anaemia of dietary origin is rare in older cats (Holzworth 1956). It may supervene in anaemias due to chronic blood loss.

11.5.8 OTHER ANAEMIAS

Anaemia is a common secondary feature of many diseases in the cat. These include acute infections and chronic debilitating conditions. Severe anaemia may occur in haemolytic coliform infections. In other infections, the cause of anaemia is less obvious, as for example in feline infectious peritonitis, where anaemia of moderate severity is a usual feature. Holzworth (1956) noted that in the small proportion of cases of feline infectious enteritis (panleucopenia) which pursue a relatively chronic course, anaemia may develop apparently as a result of bone marrow inactivity. Anaemia of normocytic normochromic type frequently occurs in association with chronic renal failure, where it is probably due to a combination of reduced erythropoietin production together with toxic depression of the bone marrow. Daily administration of chloramphenicol to cats for 21 days led to vacuolation of both myeloid and erythroid cells and to a reduction in the erythroblast population of the marrow (Penny *et al* 1967). Normocytic normochromic anaemia is seen as part of the cachectic syndrome in several forms of cancer.

11.6 COAGULATION DISORDERS

Coagulation defects have not been reported as naturally occurring diseases of the cat. Soloman *et al* (1974) found that the normal level of vitamin K-dependent clotting factors are higher in cats than in man; in the case of factor V, the level is 6 times the human level. They reported a normal prothrombin time of 9·8 seconds and activated prothrombin time of 24·5 seconds in new-born kittens. Experimentally, they showed reduction of vitamin K dependent clotting factors following administration of phenobarbital.

Warfarin poisoning may occur rarely in cats, resulting in a haemorrhagic disease due to failure of the clotting mechanism.

Disseminated intravascular coagulation has been reported as a histological finding in cats dying of feline infectious enteritis (panleucopenia) (Hoffman 1973).

11.7 DISORDERS OF WHITE BLOOD CELLS

11.7.1 LEUCOCYTOSIS

The increased leucocyte population may comprise any one of the white cell categories.

11.7.2 NEUTROPHILIA

When the number of circulating neutrophil polymorphonuclear leucocytes is increased, immature neutrophil leucocytes are usually present in the peripheral blood. Cells without fully lobulated nuclei—band cells—are common. In addition, during intense neutrophil leucocyte responses in cats, it is not unusual to find metamyelocytes. The neutrophil leucocyte response appears to be very readily mobilized in the cat and absolute counts of $20 \times 10^9/l$ or more are reached in association with relatively minor infections of, for example, the respiratory tract. Counts as high as $60 \times 10^9/l$ may be found in cats with pyometra. Schalm (1969) reported haematological findings in the 2 cats which showed leucopenia and a subsequent resurgence of granulopoiesis leading to the establishment of neutrophilia. One cat had a febrile illness of unknown cause and the other became febrile following hysterectomy. It was found that in the recovery phase, a dramatic rise in WBC values could take place within as short a period as three days, in one case from $1·1–36·1 \times 10^9/l$. Myelocytes and metamyelocytes formed up to 45 per cent of the WBC in the leucopenic phase, falling to approximately 7 per cent as leucocytosis became established.

Pronounced neutrophilia must be differentiated from the developing stages of myeloid leukaemia involving cells of the neutrophil series. Where the count is very high and metamyelocytes common, this can present some difficulty in differential diagnosis at the first examination. Anaemia is a constant feature of myeloid leukaemia but may also be present in infections which give rise to neutrophilia. The presence of very early members of the neutrophil leucocyte series, including primitive blast cells, is indicative of malignancy. The problem can be resolved by examining one or more blood samples from the case after an interval of a few days. Neutrophilia may remain as before or may by then show signs of resolution, whereas the diagnostic features of myeloid leukaemia will have become established and usually readily observable.

11.7.3 EOSINOPHILIA

Increased numbers of circulating eosinophil polymorphonuclear leucocytes are seen most commonly in association with parasite infestations and in chronic skin conditions. The numbers of eosinophils are seldom great enough to cause a significant rise in the WBC, but the proportion of eosinophils may rise to 10 per cent and occasionally as high as 15 per cent. Under such circumstances, many of the eosinophils have incompletely lobulated or band nuclei.

11.7.4 MONOCYTOSIS

An increase in the number of circulating monocytes is most commonly found in association with lymphocytosis and/or neutrophilia. The number of monocytes is not usually sufficient to cause a marked rise in the WBC *per se*, but the proportion of monocytes may reach 5–10 per cent. As a proportion of an increased WBC, this represents a substantial rise in the monocyte population in the blood. The presence of monocytosis may give rise to problems in differential diagnosis, since the augmented monocyte population generally includes a considerable number of monoblasts, with prominent nucleoli. With routine staining techniques it may be difficult to distinguish these cells from early members of the neutrophil series. Thus, in cases of neutrophilia with coexistent monocytosis, where immature neutrophils and monoblasts are present, the cytological features bear some resemblance to those of myeloid leukaemia. In such cases, special staining methods are an extremely valuable aid to diagnosis. The cytochemical reactions of monocytoid and myeloid cells have already been described. As with other situations where the differentiation of reactive cellular proliferation and neoplasia may be difficult on the initial examination, the diagnosis usually becomes obvious if further blood samples are studied after a few days' interval.

11.7.5 BASOPHILIA

This has not been reported in the cat. It is now generally recognized that the disease formerly termed basophil leukaemia of cats is in fact malignant mastocytosis, in which neoplastic mast cells may appear in the peripheral blood as part of a widespread disease involving lymphoid, haemopoietic and other organs (see later).

11.7.6 LYMPHOCYTOSIS

This does not occur commonly in the cat but is seen particularly in association with chronic eczematous skin conditions and occasionally in various chronic infections. The absolute lymphocyte count may reach $10 \times 10^9/l$ and the circulating lymphoid cells in such cases often include a small proportion of large lymphoblasts. It must therefore be emphasized that the presence of occasional lymphoblasts is not pathognomonic of malignancy in the cat. Furthermore, in normal young cats up to 1 year of age, lymphoblasts frequently compose 2–3 per cent of the lymphocyte count. A picture very similar to that of lymphocytosis may be found in cats with non-leukaemic lymphosarcoma. Without supporting clinical information, it may be impossible to make an accurate differential diagnosis solely on haematological features, particularly on a single examination. If subsequent examinations are made, the proportion of lymphoblasts is likely to increase in cases of lymphosarcoma and coexisting anaemia is a helpful feature.

11.7.7 LEUKAEMOID REACTIONS

This term is sometimes used to describe conditions whose haematological features bear some resemblance to the early stages of leukaemias and which are found during certain phases of increased white blood cell production; the cell production is reactive in character and not neoplastic, but precursors of the mature cell type appear in the blood, giving the 'leukaemoid' picture and often causing diagnostic difficulties. The increased cell population may be composed of either neutrophil leucocytes, which are often accompanied by an increase in monocyte numbers, or lymphocytes.

Problems of differential diagnosis in neutrophil responses are encountered in 2 main situations. Firstly, during the most active outpouring of cells in a reactive process, the WBC rises significantly, perhaps to 4 or 5 times normal and, at the same time, immature and precursor cells may be found in the blood. The cytological picture is further complicated when monocytes and monoblasts participate in the reaction. The differentiation of neutrophilia from myeloid leukaemia has been discussed. The second circumstance in which difficulty may arise is in the aftermath of an intense neutrophilia.

Then there is often a transient depletion of neutrophil leucocytes, which in turn is followed after a few days by a recovery phase in which the WBC rises again towards normal and again many precursor cells appear in the peripheral blood. The relatively high proportion of primitive cells in such cases may make differentiation from early myeloid leukaemia virtually impossible on a single examination. The problem is resolved by examining a further sample after a few days, by which time a leukaemoid phase will show reversion towards normal, whereas in a leukaemia, the diagnostic features are likely to have become more evident.

Leukaemoid reactions involving lymphocytes must be distinguished from conditions of lymphoid neoplasia. The presence of substantial numbers of lymphoblasts in the blood when the absolute lymphocyte count is either normal or slightly increased, is consistent with reactive lymphocytosis but also with either non-leukaemic lymphosarcoma or the earliest stage of lymphoid leukaemia. Clinical information is an essential adjunct to haematological examination in assessing such cases. As with myeloid leukaemia, lymphoid leukaemia will quickly become overt and obvious on later examinations.

Finally, it is worth noting that among the domestic animals, leukaemoid reactions probably present diagnostic problems most commonly in the cat. The feline haemopoietic system appears to be particularly labile, so that in any circumstances where there is increased production of granulocytes and monocytes, immature and precursor forms tend to become conspicuous in the peripheral blood.

11.7.8 AGRANULOCYTOSIS

A deficiency of circulating granulocytes occurs in several diseases and is usually accompanied by a reduction in the lymphocyte count. The main circumstances in which agranulocytosis is recognized in cats are the following.

11.7.8.1 Feline panleucopenia (feline infectious enteritis)

This occurs typically as a hyperacute disease with a high mortality rate, in which affected cats may die within hours of onset having shown no specific clinical signs other than fever and prostration. In slightly less acute cases, which may survive for a few days, anorexia, vomiting, diarrhoea and dehydration often occur in addition to fever and severe depression. Haematological examination in this type of case shows a profound reduction in WBC values. Counts are usually below $1 \times 10^9/l$ and often below $0.5 \times 10^9/l$. The reduction is due to loss principally of granulocytes but also of lymphocytes. In the cases detailed by Schalm (1965), granulocytes formed from 0 to 53 per cent of the WBC. Thrombocytopenia may also be found, but anaemia is not a feature and the PCV may be increased as a result of dehydration. While typical of this disease, an extremely low WBC is not pathognomonic and equally low values are seen in certain other infections.

In experimental infections using purified virus in germ-free cats, the disease was only mild and was characterized by transient fever and pan-leucopenia, with subsequent recovery. Enteritis did not occur (Rohovsky & Fowler 1971).

11.7.8.2   Salmonellosis

In acute salmonellosis, particularly in kittens, dramatic reductions in WBC values are commonly found. The levels reached may be below $1 \times 10^9/l$ and therefore in the same range as found in feline panleucopenia. As in the latter disease, the reduction is mainly due to loss of granulocytes, though the lymphocyte population is also depleted.

11.7.8.3   Others

Reduced granulocyte production results from destruction of the bone marrow precursors, which can be caused by cytotoxic drugs, by ionizing irradiation and by replacement of normal bone marrow constituents by malignant cells as in lymphoid leukaemia.

11.7.9   LYMPHOPENIA

Deficiency of circulating lymphocytes contributes to the panleucopenia seen in feline panleucopenia, salmonellosis and other toxaemias.

A specific deficiency of normal lymphocytes is often present in the early stages of lymphoid neoplasia. At the onset of lymphoid leukaemia, before the full clinical and haematological syndrome is established, the WBC often falls due to depletion of lymphocytes. Typical WBC values in such cases are $3–4 \times 10^9/l$. The granulocyte population is normal. Anaemia at this stage is only mild. Cytologically, the picture is interesting and often clearly diag-nostic, since a high percentage of the lymphoid cells present are abnormal large lymphoblasts, while normal small lymphocytes are scarce.

From experimental studies of FeLV infections, it was found that in young kittens, the virus often induced a syndrome characterized by atrophy of the thymus and depletion of thymus-dependent lymphocytes from the blood and peripheral lymphoid organs (Anderson *et al* 1971). The resulting immuno-logical deficiency predisposed these kittens to intercurrent infections which would have been otherwise trivial. When FeLV was inoculated in the neo-natal period, the kittens often died at 3–4 months of age; in individual experiments the mortality rate has reached 50 per cent due to this syndrome. Even when no intercurrent infection was readily demonstrable, affected kittens showed a reduced growth rate and high mortality. The WBC was usually approximately $3 \times 10^9/l$ in these cases, the reduction being mainly due to a depletion of lymphocytes. At present it is not known how important this syndrome might be under natural conditions, though it is known that high mortality rates among kittens occur in a number of breeding establishments where FeLV infection is present in the breeding cats Also it is not known whether FeLV infection may result in a similar lymphocyte depletion in older cats, although it has been shown that FeLV-infected cats have a higher mortality rate from other diseases than FeLV-free cats (Essex *et al* 1975). The role of immunological deficiency in leukaemia virus infections is a subject of much current research interest. In the cat, recently developed techniques allow T and B lymphocytes to be differentiated (Mackey *et al* 1975b d), so permitting detailed studies of the lymphocyte population in health and disease.

11.8 NEOPLASTIC DISEASES OF THE HAEMOPOIETIC SYSTEM

11.8.1 LYMPHOID NEOPLASMS

Comprising approximately 80 per cent of all neoplasms in the lympho-haemopoietic group, lymphoid neoplasms constitute the most frequent form of cancer in cats. Dorn *et al* (1967) found that lymphoid neoplasms form one third of all neoplasms in this species. In the majority of cases, haematological abnormalities can be found. These take several forms, the details of which are discussed later.

In contrast to most forms of cancer, lymphoid malignancies may occur at any age and are recognized in cats from a few months to advanced old age. In a series of 50 cats with naturally acquired disease, FeLV could be isolated from half of the cases (Jarrett 1976); there was no clinical, haematological or pathological difference between cases where virus was demonstrable and those in which it was not. All of the types of neoplasm that are found as naturally occurring conditions have also been reproduced experimentally by inoculation of purified FeLV (Jarrett *et al* 1964, Richard *et al* 1969, Theilen *et al* 1970, Mackey *et al* 1972). In experimental infections the latent period before the onset of malignancy is extremely variable. In the longest experiment carried out, neonatally infected cats were followed for almost 4 years, at which time lymphoid neoplasms were still occurring (Mackey *et al* 1972).

The incidence of lymphoid neoplasia is of course very much lower than the prevalence of infection with FeLV. The best available estimate of the incidence of lymphoid neoplasia, based on a study of tumours in 2 counties in California where the total cat population was known, indicated an annual mortality rate of 0·05 per cent (Dorn *et al* 1968). On the other hand, the frequency of FeLV infection may reach 50 per cent or more among town cats which are allowed to roam fairly freely (Rogerson *et al* 1975, Essex *et al* 1975). Infected cats may develop other diseases as a direct result of the infection, some of which are discussed elsewhere in this chapter. The range of pathogenic effects of FeLV is described more fully by Mackey (1975). Many infected cats mount an immune response, do not develop disease and may eliminate the virus. Thus, evidence of FeLV infection alone does not give any prognostic indication as to whether disease will occur. The immune status of the cat is a critical factor in this situation, as discussed by Jarrett (1975).

From the haematological point of view, lymphoid neoplasms can be usefully subdivided into (a) *lymphoid leukaemia*, a primary disease of the haemopoietic system, and (b) *lymphosarcoma*, a primary disease of the lymphoid system, which may or may not produce haematological abnormalities; lymphosarcoma is further subdivided into 3 main clinicopathological syndromes. The terminology used in describing these conditions is that recommended by the World Health Organization International Committee on Histological Classification of Animal Tumours; the histological and cytological typing of lymphoid and haemopoietic neoplasms of domestic animals was detailed by Jarrett & Mackey (1974).

11.8.1.1 Lymphoid leukaemia

The fully developed case of lymphoid leukaemia is characterized by expansion and replacement of the normal bone marrow by malignant lymphoblasts, which disseminate via the blood stream and appear in large numbers in the peripheral blood (Fig. 11.7). The leading clinical signs relate to the loss of normal marrow constituents, which results in severe anaemia, thrombocytopenia and neutropenia. Profound anaemia and the appearance of petechial haemorrhages in the skin and mucous membranes are typical clinical features. Haematologically, the WBC is increased. A wide range of values is encountered in individual cases, but levels of approximately $70 \times 10^9/l$ are common. The great majority of the circulating white cells are lymphoblasts, which may compose as much as 95 per cent of the WBC, the high percentage being partly due to deficiency of the other normal elements. The malignant cells are readily identified by their large size, being approximately $12\,\mu$ in diameter, round shape, high nuclear/cytoplasmic ratio and basophilia; the nuclei are round or slightly indented and contain prominent nucleoli. The cytoplasm may contain small scattered azurophilic granules and, occasionally, small vacuoles are present.

The anaemia accompanying leukaemia is macrocytic and normochromic. In the late stages of the disease, the RBC may fall as low as $1 \times 10^{12}/l$. The reticulocyte count rises and may reach 20 per cent or more. Extramedullary haemopoiesis becomes established in response to bone marrow destruction, and normoblasts are found in large numbers in the blood. Erythroblasts may also appear in the blood.

Once the disease becomes clinically overt, the course is invariably acute, with death occurring within days or a few weeks at most. Little information is available on the duration of the sub-clinical or prodromal phase but in

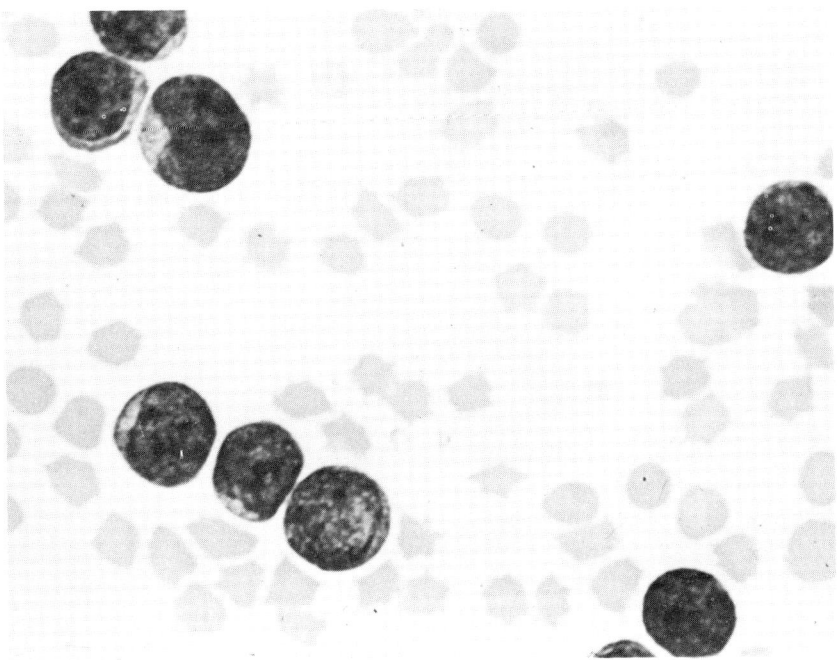

Fig. 11.7 Lymphoid leukaemia. Blood film showing numerous lymphoid cells, including lymphoblasts and large lymphocytes. Leishman × 1000.

experimentally induced cases, the time between first detection of malignant cells in the blood and the onset of clinical disease has been short, and has generally not exceeded a month. As discussed under 'lymphopenia' the prodromal period may be characterized by a transient reduction in the WBC. At this stage, malignant lymphoblasts can be identified in blood films. There is a deficiency of normal small lymphocytes, while other white cells may be normal or somewhat reduced in number. Anaemia of moderate degree is present. If such a case is examined during subsequent days, the picture rapidly changes, with the lymphoblast population increasing to cause a rise in the

WBC and the anaemia quickly becoming more severe. Examination of bone marrow shows a striking degree of hypercellularity and an overwhelming preponderance of lymphoblasts. Cytologically, the great majority of feline lymphoid leukaemias are lymphoblastic in type. There appears to be no counterpart of chronic lymphoid leukaemia in man.

At necropsy, there is diffuse splenomegaly and hepatomegaly and moderate enlargement of the lymph nodes. The spleen and liver are pale in colour and mottled in appearance. The bone marrow is extremely cellular, pale pink or pale grey in colour and fills the medullary cavity of the long bones. Histologically, the malignant cells characteristically infiltrate the splenic red pulp, sparing the white pulp, and permeate the liver sinusoids. In the lymph nodes, the malignant cells localize principally in the medullary cords (Mackey & Jarrett 1972). Involvement of other organs is variable in individual cases.

11.8.1.2 Lymphosarcoma

This disease occurs in cats in three principal forms: multicentric, alimentary and thymic lymphosarcoma. In **multicentric lymphosarcoma,** all of the lymph nodes and the white pulp of the spleen are infiltrated and expanded by malignant lymphoid cells. The clinical syndrome is one of progressive apathy, weight loss, anorexia, anaemia and lymphadenopathy, usually without more specific signs. In **alimentary lymphosarcoma,** the neoplasm arises in lymphoid tissue of the lamina propria of the gastrointestinal tract and also involves the mesenteric lymph nodes. The disease may present as a localized complex involving only the bowel and mesenteric nodes but individual cases show different degrees of further dissemination, particularly to spleen, liver and kidneys. Very occasionally, the mesenteric nodes may be affected without any obvious bowel tumour. Clinically, these cases generally show evidence of gastro-intestinal disturbance. According to the level of the tract involved, vomiting or diarrhoea may be leading signs. The bowel tumour may be palpable and can often be visualized radiographically. In **thymic lymphosarcoma,** the neoplasm develops in the thymus and grows to produce a large anterior mediastinal mass. The thoracic lymph nodes are always infiltrated and usually also the prescapular and axillary nodes; further dissemination to other organs may or may not take place. In this form, the clinical signs are those of respiratory embarrassment produced by the thoracic mass. Cats become depressed, reluctant to take exercise, and show tachypnoea and finally dyspnoea. Fluid often accumulates in the thoracic cavity in considerable volumes. Cytological examination of the fluid is a valuable aid to diagnosis, since it contains large numbers of lymphoblasts.

Histologically, different patterns of infiltration can be seen in the lymph nodes in these forms of lymphosarcoma. In both multicentric and thymic lymphosarcoma, the malignant cells in the early stages of the disease occupy and proliferate in the paracortical, or thymus-dependent area of the nodes. On the other hand, in alimentary lymphosarcoma, tumour cells in the mesenteric node are often localized to the germinal follicles before other parts of the node are affected. These morphological features probably reflect differences in the T or B cell origin of the neoplasm and in the route of migration taken by the malignant cells in different compartments of the immune system. The pathology, cytology and developmental stages of these conditions have been described in detail by Mackey and Jarrett (1972) and Jarrett and Mackey (1974).

From the haematological point of view, several quite different situations may be found in cats with lymphosarcoma. Firstly, in approximately one third of these cases, no haematological abnormality can be detected. Perfectly normal haematological findings therefore do not exclude a diagnosis of lymphosarcoma. In such cases, the bone marrow is not infiltrated by malignant cells, so that there is no interference with normal haemopoietic function, nor do malignant cells escape into the blood stream in appreciable numbers. However, in approximately 20 per cent of cases of lymphosarcoma, a co-existing leukaemia is present. In the author's experience, this is most often in association with the thymic form of lymphosarcoma. Here, the clinical features include those associated with leukaemia and haematological examination is, of course, diagnostic. In a further proportion of cases of lymphosarcoma, leukaemia is not evident but on careful examination of the blood film small numbers of malignant lymphoblasts can be seen. On rare occasions, the bone marrow is found on post-mortem examination to be infiltrated by large numbers of malignant cells in cases where no cytological abnormality was detected in the peripheral blood during life.

An additional and more common complication of lymphosarcoma is anaemia, which is usually of macrocytic normochromic type. In a series of cats with naturally acquired non-leukaemia lymphosarcomas, where careful examination of the bone marrow was carried out post mortem anaemia was present in 54 per cent of cases where no infiltration of the marrow by malignant cells was detectable (Mackey *et al* 1975a). The anaemia was of moderate degree, with RBC values of approximately $3 \times 10^{12}/l$ a common finding; the haematological findings suggested that the anaemia was of haemolytic type. From the diagnostic point of view, in a suspected case of lymphosarcoma, the presence of macrocytic normochromic anaemia is helpful supporting evidence and if, in addition, a substantial number of circulating lymphoblasts can be found, the diagnosis is then virtually certain.

As discussed earlier in the description of anaemias, anaemia may occur in FeLV affected cats in the absence of lymphoid malignancy. In some cases, anaemia has been found as a prodromal feature, preceding the onset of lymphoid malignancy.

11.8.2 MYELOPROLIFERATIVE NEOPLASMS

This term is often applied to a group of malignancies arising from non-lymphoid bone marrow cells. These are sometimes grouped together without more specific sub-division because in the cat, difficulty may arise in the differential diagnosis and categorization of malignancies of myeloid and erythroid cells. In some instances, these neoplasms include cells of more than one series and the predominant cell type may change during the progression of the disease in an individual animal. The features of the main types of neoplasm in this group recognized in cats will be described separately. While these syndromes do occur as malignancies affecting cells of a single series, it must be borne in mind that in some cases the disease is more complex, and apparently involves malignant transformation of more than one type of bone marrow cell, or of a pluripotential stem cell, so that malignant precursors of more than one cell series appear in the peripheral blood. In addition, the haematological features invariably include evidence of a marked extramedullary haemopoietic response, resulting from destruction of normal marrow constituents. Hence, early normoblasts and also erythroblasts are seen in considerable numbers, making the distinction between, for example, myeloid leukaemia with extramedullary haemopoiesis and erythroleukaemia very difficult on haematological examination alone. The general term myeloproliferative disease is, however, inappropriate unless attempts have been made to reach a more specific diagnosis by careful cytological examination, including the use of cytochemical methods where necessary to identify accurately the type of cells involved in the neoplastic process.

The aetiology of myeloid and related leukaemias is less well established than in the case of the lymphoid group. Fewer naturally acquired cases are available for study and myeloid leukaemia has only occasionally been produced experimentally. However, FeLV has been demonstrated in cats with various myeloproliferative disorders (Hertz *et al* 1970) and myeloid leukaemia has resulted from experimental infection with FeLV (Mackey *et al* 1972). The latter case was of particular interest in that a single virus isolate induced a wide range of pathological and cytological types of lymphoid neoplasia, as well as myeloid leukaemia, in the course of the experiment.

The clinical and gross pathological features of the various conditions in this group tend to be alike, since in all cases the syndrome is essentially one of replacement of normal bone marrow cells and haematogeneous dissemination of malignant cells. Destruction of normal marrow leads to progressive anaemia which becomes profound, to thrombocytopenia and to a deficiency of normal granulocytes. Affected cats are often pyrexic and depressed and show extreme pallor and petechial haemorrhages in the skin and mucous membranes. Diffuse splenomegaly and hepatomegaly with varying degrees of lymph node enlargement are seen at necropsy. The bone marrow is grossly hypercellular and fills the medullary cavities of the long bones. Histologically, the pattern of infiltration of the lymphoid and other organs reflects the primarily haematogenous dissemination of these malignancies, as described in lymphoid leukaemia. Thus malignant cells are found mainly in the splenic red pulp, the hepatic sinusoids and the medullary cords of lymph nodes. Precise diagnosis of the diseases in the myeloproliferative group depends on cytological examination of blood and bone marrow films.

11.8.2.1 Myeloid leukaemia

This systemic neoplasm of granulocytic cells usually involves cells of the neutrophil series. Neutrophil precursors multiply within the bone marrow, gradually encroaching upon and replacing normal constituents, and appearing in large numbers in the blood (Fig. 11.8). The degree of maturation varies considerably in individual cases. Usually myelocytes and metamyelocytes are most frequent, but in some instances myeloblasts predominate. Where

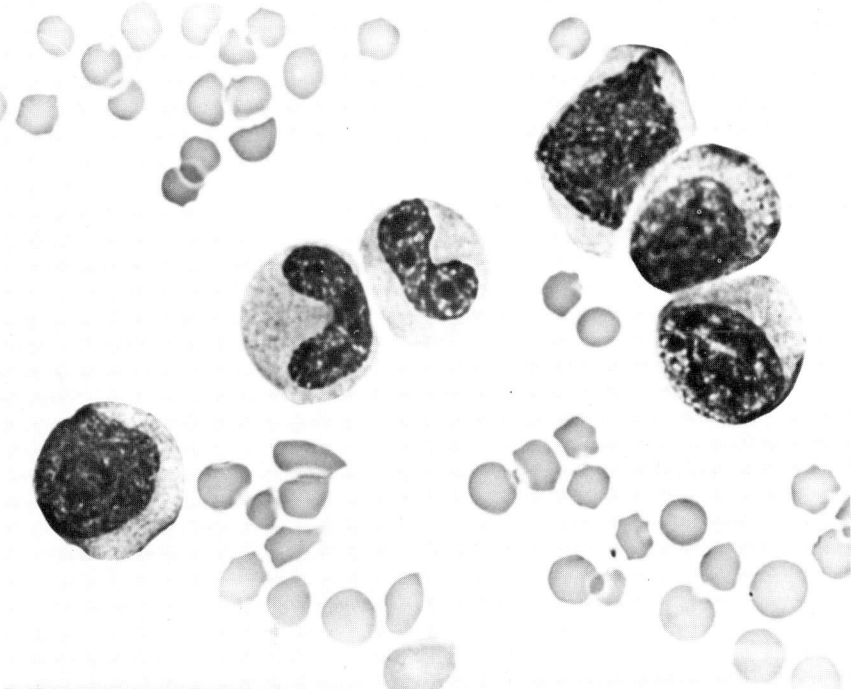

Fig. 11.8 Myeloid leukaemia. Blood film showing neutrophil leucocyte precursors, ranging from myeloblast to metamyelocytes. Leishman × 1000.

the cells are very immature, accurate identification is not possible on routinely stained blood films, and special techniques should be used. The cytochemical reactions of neutrophil precursors have been described. The clinical course of the disease may extend over several weeks or even months, during which time the WBC may fluctuate considerably, with peak levels of approximately $70 \times 10^9/l$, consisting mainly of malignant cells. The sub-terminal phase may therefore extend over a longer period than is usually evident in lymphoid leukaemia.

The anaemia accompanying myeloid leukaemia is macrocytic and normochromic with reticulocytosis. In the final stages of the disease, it becomes extremely severe and is accompanied by thrombocytopenia. The establishment of extramedullary haemopoiesis results in the appearance of many normoblasts and even erythroblasts in the peripheral blood. As already discussed, this may cause difficulty in differentiating the syndrome from erythroleukaemia.

Eosinophilic leukaemia has not been reported in the cat. The disease formerly termed basophilic leukaemia proved to be malignant mastocytosis, in which malignant mast cells may appear in the blood.

11.8.2.2 Erythroleukaemia

Malignant proliferation of cells of both the granulocyte and erythroid series produces a complex haematological picture in this rare disease. The clinical and gross pathological features closely resemble those of myeloid leukaemia. Haematologically, the degree of maturation of the malignant cells is variable. The myeloid component shows differentiation towards neutrophil leucocytes; the confirmatory cytochemical reactions have been described. The erythroid component must be distinguished from reactive erythroblasts and normoblasts which invariably accompany myeloid and other leukaemias. Malignant erythrocyte precursors generally show marked cytological aberration, with many megaloblastic and abnormal forms including multinucleated cells and bizarre mitoses. Also, more primitive precursors may be seen than is usual in an extramedullary haemopoietic response; these can be identified cytochemically as described. At postmortem examination the diagnosis is confirmed by the presence of malignant cells in sites where haemopoiesis does not occur.

11.8.2.3 Acute erythraemia

Also termed erythraemic myelosis or di Guglielmo's syndrome, this malignancy of erythroid cells has been reported in several instances in cats and was first described by Zawidska *et al* (1964). Since the disease involves replacement of the bone marrow by malignant erythroid cells, the syndrome has clinical features in common with myeloid leukaemia. Anaemia results from a deficiency of normal mature erythrocytes. In the blood, large numbers of blast cells, erythroblasts and early normoblasts are present. Aberrant cytological forms are common, with megalocytosis a marked feature. Bone marrow films show a preponderance of early and abnormal erythroid cells with maturation arrest (Fig. 11.9). In man, the diagnosis of acute erythraemia can be made only after failure to respond to folic acid and vitamin B_{12}

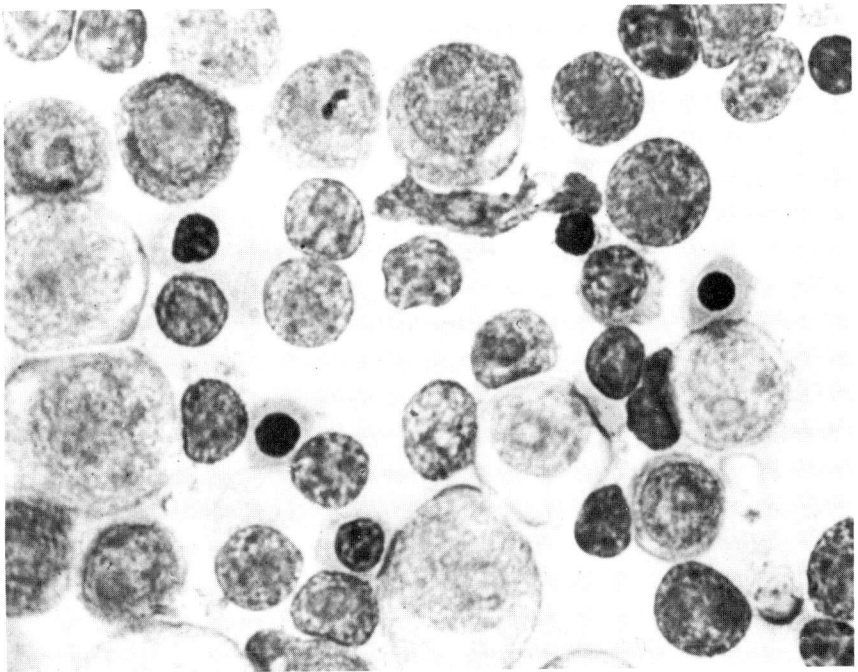

Fig. 11.9 Acute erythraemia. Bone marrow showing preponderance of erythrocyte precursors. Giemsa × 1000.

therapy has been demonstrated. The same criteria should be applied in feline cases, although anaemias due to folic acid or vitamin B_{12} deficiency have not been recognised in the cat. The cytochemical reactions of malignant erythroid cells have been described earlier in this chapter.

11.8.2.4 Polycythaemia vera

This rare condition is characterized by an absolute increase in erythron mass. The expansion of the erythroid population leads to increased production of mature erythrocytes and consequent hypervolemia with a raised packed cell volume. Leucocytosis and thrombocytosis may also occur. This disease may develop into frank malignancy, terminating in erythroleukaemia or myeloid leukaemia.

11.8.2.5 Panmyelosis

In this rare malignancy, cells of the granulocytic, erythroid, monocytic and megakaryocytic series participate in the proliferative process. The megakaryocytic component distinguishes this from erythroleukaemia. The malignant cells grow in and disseminate from the bone marrow as in the other forms of leukaemia already described. This disease may be difficult to distinguish from myeloid leukaemia with advanced extramedullary haemopoiesis. On pathological examination, the diagnosis is confirmed by the presence of proliferating haemopoietic cells in various unusual sites.

11.8.2.6 Monocytoid leukaemia

Neoplasia of monocytes, or histiocytes, in the cat usually takes the form of a solid lymphosarcoma rather than leukaemia. Both multicentric and alimentary lymphosarcoma may occur as predominantly histiocytic neoplasms. In such cases, small numbers of malignant cells may be present in the blood.

Monocytoid leukaemia appears to be rare in cats. Monoblasts and monocytes proliferate in the bone marrow, destroying other constituents and disseminate in the blood stream. The WBC may reach extremely high levels, with associated anaemia. Cytologically, monoblasts are identified by their general similarity to monocytes, except that the nucleus may be less indented and the cytoplasm somewhat less abundant. Prominent nucleoli are always present in the nuclei. The cytochemical techniques described earlier may be necessary to distinguish these cells from other blast cells, as in poorly differentiated myeloid leukaemia.

11.8.3 MYELOMA

Monoclonal gammopathy due to myeloma has been described in the cat by Schultz (1974), who reported that cases of IgG class and a possible IgA producing myeloma had been identified in this species. The proliferation of malignant plasma cells and their precursors in the bone marrow may be focally or diffusely distributed, thereby producing varying degrees of replacement of the normal marrow. Osteoporosis and compression fractures may result from invasion of bone by malignant cells from the medullary cavity. The spleen, lymph nodes and viscera are also involved. There may be renal complications resulting from proteinuria and light chain complexes

(Bence Jones protein) generally appear in the urine. The haematological aspects of this disease depend upon the degree of bone marrow replacement, which in severe cases may lead to anaemia and agranulocytosis. Plasma cells are not usually demonstrable in the peripheral blood and definitive diagnosis depends on examination of the bone marrow.

11.8.4   MALIGNANT MASTOCYTOSIS

Mast cell tumours are relatively uncommon in the cat. In this species they usually present as disseminated malignancies involving the lymphoid and/or haemopoietic systems, together with infiltration of other major organs. The gross pathological findings closely resemble those of either multicentric lymphosarcoma or lymphoid leukaemia, and typically include diffuse splenomegaly, variable degrees of lymph node enlargement and generalized liver involvement. Histologically, in the author's experience, 2 main patterns of organ infiltration are seen. In one, the tumour cells form ill-defined foci which often coalesce and are irregularly distributed in the parenchyma of the liver and spleen and cause varying degrees of lymph node destruction. In the second, the malignant cells appear to behave in a truly leukaemic fashion, with extensive infiltration of the bone marrow and diffuse permeation of the splenic red pulp and hepatic sinusoids; these features indicate haematogenous dissemination. In this second form, malignant mast cells may appear in the peripheral blood. These are mononuclear cells and with Romanowsky stains the cytoplasm is packed with basophilic granules. The diagnosis is confirmed by the use of toluidine blue or astra blue/safranin staining methods. In a case described by Meier and Gourley (1957), mast cells formed 35 per cent of the WBC of $30 \times 10^9/l$ and 6·3 per cent of nucleated cells in the bone marrow. Because of histamine and 5HT production by the tumour cells, cats with malignant mastocytosis may develop peptic ulcers.

11.9   DISORDERS OF THROMBOCYTES

Abnormalities in the number of circulating thrombocytes reflect lesions affecting the megakaryocytes in the bone marrow.

11.9.1   THROMBOCYTOPENIA

11.9.1.1   In haemopoietic malignancies

In lymphoid and myeloid leukaemia and other forms of myeloproliferative malignancy involving cells other than megakaryocytes, destruction and replacement of the bone marrow by malignant cells leads to a deficiency of normal marrow components. Loss of megakaryocytes leads to failure of thrombocyte production and thrombocytopenia. The thrombocyte count may fall below $100 \times 10^9/l$ and may reach $50 \times 10^9/l$. Thus major presenting clinical signs in leukaemias are anaemia and thrombocytopenia. The latter causes petechial haemorrhages which can be seen in the skin and mucous membranes.

11.9.1.2   In feline panleucopenia (feline infectious enteritis)

Megakaryocytes are destroyed along with other white cells in the bone marrow. A very similar picture may be seen in certain other acute systemic infections, particularly salmonellosis. Other forms of severe toxic bone depression may also lead to thrombocytopenia. If the circulating thrombocyte count falls much below $100 \times 10^9/l$ petechial haemorrhages may be seen in the skin and mucous membranes.

11.9.2   THROMBOCYTOSIS

An abnormally high thrombocyte count is an extremely rare situation in the cat. It may be seen in occasional cases of myeloproliferative disease in which abnormal production of megakaryocytes occurs. These diseases are poly-cythaemia vera, megakaryocytoid leukaemia and panmyelosis, which are described elsewhere in this chapter.

12

NORMAL AVIAN (POULTRY) HAEMATOLOGY

R. D. HODGES

12.1 INTRODUCTION

Avian blood is very similar in many ways to that of the mammal but there are certain characteristics by which it differs from mammalian blood. The most important of these differences are as follows:

1. The erythrocytes are nucleated.
2. The cells associated with blood coagulation are not platelets but are nucleated thrombocytes closely resembling erythrocytes in appearance.
3. The initial pathways of blood coagulation differ considerably.
4. The most commonly occurring of the polymorphonuclear granulocytes, the equivalent of the mammalian neutrophil, possesses acid-staining cytoplasmic granules and is called the heterophil.

These and other, minor, differences reflect birds' reptilian ancestry although, like mammals, they are homoiothermic animals. These differences also result in the need for some modifications of certain haematological techniques when examining avian blood (see pages 553, 571 and 577).

The greater part of this chapter is concerned with the normal haematology of the domestic fowl (*Gallus gallus domesticus*), partly because this species is of greatest commercial importance among domesticated species of birds, and partly because a very large proportion of the literature on avian haematology concerns the fowl. However, where possible information on other domesticated species, particularly the duck, the turkey and the quail, has been included.

12.2 GENERAL BLOOD CHARACTERISTICS

12.2.1 BLOOD VOLUME

In much earlier work determinations of blood volume in poultry species were carried out by the dye dilution technique using Evans' Blue (T-1824). This technique was used by Newell and Shaffner (1950), Sturkie and Newman (1951), McCartney (1952), Medway and Kare (1959) and De Shazer and Weiss (1963). More recent investigations have used radioactive tracers to measure blood volume (e.g. I^{131}—Kotula and Helbacka (1966) and Burton *et al* (1967); or Cr^{51}—Cohen (1967c) and Hunsaker (1968)). A comparison of the Evans' Blue and radioiodine methods by Kotula and Helbacka (1968) demonstrated that the radioactive tracer method was more precise than the dye dilution technique. Similarly, Wels *et al* (1967) compared the Cr^{51} and T-1824 methods and found that the tracer method gave lower results. One form of error arising from the dye dilution technique, and resulting in too high values, was an excessive delay in sampling blood after mixing had occurred (Sturkie 1965).

Medway and Kare (1959), using White Leghorn females, demonstrated that blood volume is initially high in young birds and falls progressively during growth and maturation. At one week old blood volume was 12·0 per cent of body weight whilst at 32 weeks of age it had fallen to 6·5 per cent of body weight. Very similar figures for White Leghorn hens were found by De Shazer and Weiss (1963) in 6·5–6·8 per cent, and by Burton *et al* (1967) in 6·3 per cent of body weight. Gilbert (1963) demonstrated a blood volume of 7·8 per cent of body weight in 30 week old Brown Leghorn cocks. Intermediate figures, suggesting that blood volume is inversely related to body weight, were found by Kotula and Helbacka (1968) using 8 to 12 week-old male broilers. Birds weighing 1·0 kg contained about 11·6 per cent of body weight as blood and those weighing 2·0 kg contained about 7·3 per cent. The effects of sex hormones on blood volume have been reported as being somewhat variable. Common *et al* (1948) found that oestrogen administered to chickens greatly increased the blood volume but Sturkie and Newman (1951) considered that neither thyroxine plus oestrogen nor oestrogen alone affected the blood volume. In geese both diethylstilboestrol and testosterone propionate increased total blood volume slightly in males, females and castrates, but in diethylstilboestrol treated males and poulards the increase was significant (Hunsaker 1968). The possible causes of these variations are discussed by Sturkie (1965).

Plasma volume drops progressively though gently from 8·7 per cent of body weight in 1 week old chicks to 4·6 per cent in the 32 week old adult (Medway & Kare 1959). A similar trend in plasma volume occurs in growing ducks (Portman *et al* 1952). Young ducks, 3 weeks old and 150–450 g in weight had a plasma volume of 69·4 ml/kg body weight. At 700–1100 g weight this had fallen to 64·5 ml/kg, and at 1100–2000 g weight, about one year old, plasma volume averaged 55·2 ml/kg body weight.

12.2.2 PACKED CELL VOLUME

Blood packed cell volume (PCV) may be measured using either the macro- or the microhaematocrit methods and employing standard conditions of centrifugation speed and time in order to reduce the error caused by variations in trapped plasma. With the macrohaematocrit method, Hunsaker (1969a) found the optimum conditions to be 3,215 *g* for 30 minutes; giving trapped plasma values of 0·0285 l/l for chickens and 0·0249 l/l for geese. Using the microhaematocrit method Cohen (1967a b) found that 12,800 *g* for 5 minutes gave complete packing of chicken red cells with only 0·0212 l/l trapped plasma. The general trend in PCV with age in poultry is for a low value at hatch to increase during growth and for a significant difference between the sexes to develop only at maturity. However, the initial trend is more marked in geese and quail than in chickens. Medway and Kare (1959) found with White Leghorn female chicks that the PCV increased from 0·275 1/l at one week old to 0·311 1/l at 16 weeks old but that the rise was very irregular. Lucas & Jamroz (1961), again with White Leghorn females, found no differences in PCV at 6 and 12 weeks old and when adult, all values being about 0·3 1/l. In adult chickens a clear and significant difference in PCV is apparent between the sexes. With White Leghorns, Lucas and Jamroz (1961) found values of 0·308 1/l for female and 0·4 1/l for male birds, while Hunsaker (1969b) gave values of 0·255 1/l and 0·408 1/l females and males respectively. In 8-month-old commercial hybrids Abdul-Hameed and Neat (1972) found the PCV to be 0·308 1/l in females and 0·408 1/l in males. Statistically significant changes in PCV are found in laying hens in relation to the laying cycle (Bell *et al* 1965). A rise in haematocrit occurs during the 10 days prior to the final oviposition before a bird stops laying, and a continued rise takes place for the subsequent 20 days or so. A progressive fall commences about 30 days before lay recommences and this drop is pronounced during the on-set of lay. Differences in PCV between laying and non-laying hens have been quoted by Bell (1957) as 0·25 1/l and 0·297 1/l respectively.

With quail (Atwal *et al* 1964) a decrease in PCV occurred during the first 4 days post-hatch in both sexes, followed by a sustained rise until 36 days of age but with no significant sex difference. When mature, at 43 days old, males at 0·45 1/l were significantly higher than females at 0·4 1/l. Hunsaker *et al* (1964) found that young geese of both sexes had similar haematocrits during growth, values rising from about 0·245 1/l at 1 week old to about 0·472 1/l at 20 weeks old. During and after sexual maturation, however, the males continued to increase, reaching a maximum of 0·497 1/l at 43 weeks old, whilst the females fell to 0·395 1/l at 43 weeks. The increased PCV in males at maturation may be due to the increased secretion of androgen (Sturkie 1965) which is known to increase the numbers and volume of red cells in the chicken (Newell & Shaffner 1950, Sturkie & Newman 1951). The lowered PCV in hens at maturity could be caused by higher circulating oestrogen levels (Gilbert 1966). PCV is also affected by environmental temperature. Huston (1965) and Moye *et al* (1969) have shown that PCV in chickens is decreased by raised temperatures and is increased by lowered temperatures.

The leucocytes separate out on top of the haematocrit tube to form a separate layer, the buffy coat. The value for packed leucocyte volume in healthy birds is normally 0·01–0·015 1/l (Lucas & Jamroz 1961, Löliger & Schubert 1967, Freeman 1971).

12.2.3 ERYTHROCYTE SEDIMENTATION RATE (ESR)

The rate of sedimentation of erythrocytes is dependent mainly upon two opposing forces (Sturkie & Textor 1960). These are the force of gravity causing the cells to settle and the frictional resistance of the surrounding plasma which holds the cells in suspension. It has been demonstrated that ESR values obtained by holding the tubes in a vertical position during sedimentation are low (Swenson 1951, Gray *et al* 1954, Burton *et al* 1966) and that a 2 hour sedimentation time is necessary to obtain a good result (Burton *et al* 1966). The preferred method of measuring the ESR in poultry is to incline the tubes at a 45° angle and to read the result after 1 hour (Sturkie & Textor 1958). With tubes held vertically Burton *et al* (1966) described a logarithmic relationship between ESR and PCV but when they are held at 45° the relationship is linear (Gilbert 1968). Gilbert (1969) considered that the method used by Sturkie and Textor (1958) was at least 6 times more sensitive than the method using vertical tubes.

Sturkie and Textor (1958) measured ESR in White Leghorn adult cocks, hens and capons. The hens, with a mean value of 10·58 mm/h, were significantly higher than the cocks at 3·91 mm/h, while the capons (6·90 mm/h) were intermediate. A detailed study of the goose by Hunsaker *et al* (1964) demonstrated a steady fall in ESR between 1 and 20 weeks of age (35·4 mm/h at 1 week old to 10·9 mm/h at 20 weeks old in the case of the male), with no obvious differences between the sexes. However, at maturity the ESR of the females increased considerably (males, 10·0 mm/h and females, 22·3 mm/h at 43 weeks of age) and this difference remained until 59 weeks of age when the males' ESR increased to equal those of the females.

Among the factors which may influence the sedimentation rate of erythrocytes are cell size, shape and number, the difference in specific gravity of plasma and cells, and the level and type of plasma proteins and lipids (Sturkie & Textor 1960). These authors suggested that total corpuscular volume and number of cells influenced the sedimentation rate most and the actual cell size to a much lesser degree. The greatly increased ESR found in mature females is positively correlated with the degree of lipaemia and the latter is related to levels of circulating oestrogen. Gilbert (1962) injected cocks with oestrogen and observed considerable increases in ESR (8·2 mm/h in control birds; 45·6 mm/h in oestrogenized birds). These increases are brought about by the reduction in red cells and by the production of hyperlipaemia, both of which are responses to oestrogens. The change in sedimentation rate is approximately proportional to the degree of lipaemia (Gilbert 1962). An increase in ESR has been reported in turkeys under heat stress by Parker and Boone (1971), the increase following a haemodilution response to the raised temperature. Both Burton *et al* (1966) and Gilbert (1968) consider that ESR measurements are of little clinical value. However, Gilbert (1968) believes that the ESR together with the erythrocyte volume can give some useful information.

12.2.4 SPECIFIC GRAVITY AND VISCOSITY

The specific gravity of whole blood in female chickens ranges from 1·0421 at 1 week old to 1·0459 at 32 weeks old with no obvious pattern of change during this period (Medway & Kare 1959). In geese, however, Hunsaker *et al* (1964) found that whole blood specific gravity increases steadily in both sexes up to 20 weeks old (from 1·034 at 1 week old to 1·062 at 20 weeks old). Thereafter the sexes separate somewhat, the female being lower but by 59 weeks old both sexes again have the same specific gravity (1·055). Plasma specific gravity in the female fowl rises from 1·0150 at 1 week old to 1·0177 at 32 weeks old (Medway & Kare 1959). The values for hens are somewhat lower than those for cocks (Sturkie & Textor 1960), which is unusual since the female plasma contains significantly higher levels of plasma proteins. These lower values may be associated with the hyperlipaemia of hens' blood (Sturkie 1965).

Whole blood relative viscosity is mainly influenced by the number of erythrocytes and by their shape. It is highest in the cock, intermediate in the hen and lowest in the capon, being 3·67, 3·08 and 2·47 cP respectively (Vogel 1961). Fowl plasma relative viscosity is influenced by plasma protein levels and is thus significantly higher in the female (1·51) than in the male (1·42) (Sturkie 1965).

12.3 ERYTHROCYTES AND THROMBOCYTES

12.3.1 ERYTHROCYTES

12.3.1.1 Structure and ultrastructure

The avian erythrocyte differs from its mammalian counterpart in being a nucleated cell and is therefore normally larger in size. When viewed in a stained smear these cells appear as flattened, regularly oval structures with oval nuclei (Fig. 12.1) but when seen in histological sections they are clearly less flattened, irregularly ovoidal cells. The normal, mature erythrocyte possesses palely staining cytoplasm with a clear homogeneous structure and a centrally placed nucleus composed of a uniform network of chromatin clumps. The nuclear appearance varies with the age of the cell, becoming more condensed and darkly staining as the erythrocyte matures and eventually ages. Detailed accounts of the histology of fowl erythrocytes have been given by Lucas and Jamroz (1961) and Hodges (1974).

When examined ultrastructurally the erythrocyte can be seen to have a somewhat irregular lenticular profile in longitudinal section (Fig. 12.2). The nucleus has an indented oval shape with many masses of heavily condensed chromatin lying both peripherally and throughout the nucleoplasm. There is a

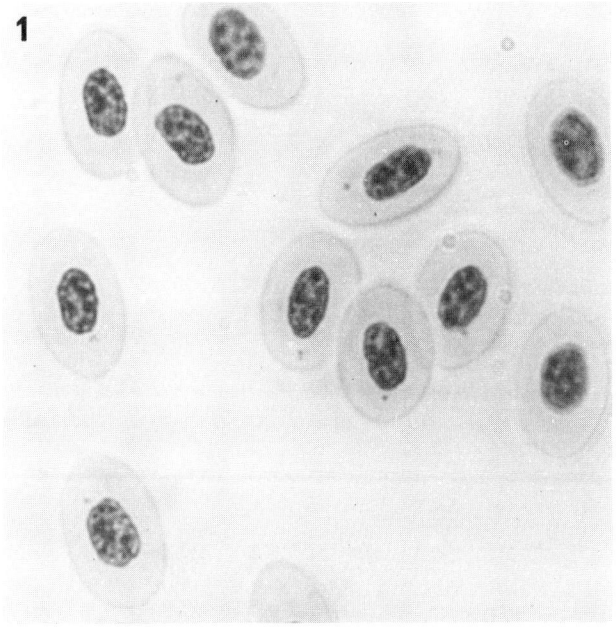

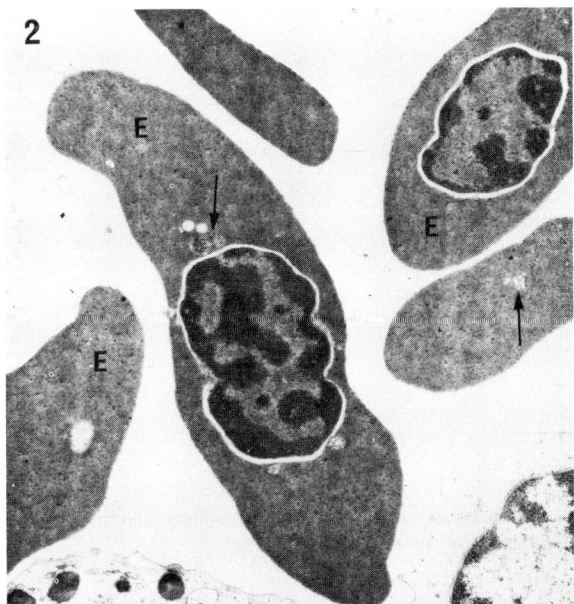

Fig. 12.1 Typical mature chicken erythrocytes. Wright's stain. × 1800.

Fig. 12.2 Electron micrograph of chicken erythrocytes (E). Cytoplasmic detail is obscured by the haemoglobin content although a few organelles (arrows) can be seen. The condensed nucleus is separated from the cytoplasm by a clear gap. × 8000.

well-defined gap between the nucleus and the cytoplasm but the nuclear membranes are obscured by the density of the adjacent chromatin and cyto-plasm (Harris 1971). In the red cell ghost these membranes are clearly visible (Harris & Brown 1971a, b). Within the cytoplasm the haemoglobin content almost entirely obscures structural detail, including the plasma membrane (Fig. 12.2). However, a few organelles are visible in the intact cell and, particularly after extraction of the haemoglobin, some mitochondria and, rarely, a Golgi complex can be seen (Harris 1971). Groups of peripheral microtubules also occur (Behnke 1970).

12.3.1.2 Physical characteristics

Red cell size in the fowl varies considerably not only from breed to breed but also within breeds and between individuals. Figures quoted by Lucas and Jamroz (1961) give the range of erythrocyte length as $9 \cdot 2 - 14 \cdot 2$ μm and that of erythrocyte width as $4 \cdot 6 - 8 \cdot 3$ μm, with mean values of $10 \cdot 6$ μm and $6 \cdot 6$ μm respectively. Further data on cell and nuclear sizes are given in Table 12.1. It has been reported by Kashiwabara (1974) that there is a positive relation-ship between cell size and breed, the dimensions generally being greater in heavier breeds but Keller (1933) concluded that breed size has no influence upon cell size while Mehner (1938) obtained a negative correlation between cell size and body weight. Cell size is related to sex, erythrocytes being significantly larger in the mature male than in the hen (Gilbert 1965, Abdel-Hameed et al 1971). Erythrocyte size is not so well documented in poultry species other than the fowl. Figures for the turkey, duck and quail are given in Table 12.1.

Considerable variation in erythrocyte numbers is found between individual birds even within groups of a fairly uniform character (Biely & Palmer 1935, Lucas & Jamroz 1961). However, when mean values are obtained from a large sample it can be seen that a number of factors, such as age, sex and environment, do affect erythrocyte numbers significantly. Dixon and Torbert (1958) reported day old chicks as having mean red cell numbers of $2 \cdot 48 \times 10^{12}/l$, that this fell to $2 \cdot 17 \times 10^{12}/l$ on the 5th day and that the figure increased again to the 12th day and remained steady thereafter. Biely and Palmer (1935) gave a mean red cell count of $2 \cdot 48 \times 10^{12}/l$ for 1–2 day old chicks and $2 \cdot 78 \times 10^{12}/l$ for mature hens, the difference being significant. Lange (1919) obtained adult red cell counts after about 7 days of age whilst Männel (1967) reported adult erythrocyte levels by 2 days of age. No sex differences in erythrocyte numbers become apparent until sexual maturity when the males develop a higher red cell count (e.g. $3 \cdot 24 - 3 \cdot 8 \times 10^{12}/l$ in adult males as compared to $2 \cdot 72 - 3 \cdot 0 \times 10^{12}/l$ in adult females, Freeman 1971). This sex difference is almost certainly due to the effects of male hormones (Domm & Taber 1946). Significant differences in erythrocyte number between breeds are usually not

Table 12.1 Avian erythrocyte dimensions in poultry species

Species	Cell length μm	Cell width μm	Cell thickness μm	Nuclear length μm	Nuclear width μm	Author	Remarks
Fowl							
3 day old	12·5	7·0	3·8	—	—	Lange (1919)	Breed unknown
25 day old	13·0	7·2	3·5	—	—	Lange (1919)	Breed unknown
70 day old	13·0	6·5	3·5	—	—	Lange (1919)	Breed unknown
Mature male and female	12·8	6·9	3·6	—	—	Lange (1919)	Breed unknown
Mature White Leghorn	10·6	6·6	—	4·2	3·1	Lucas & Jamroz (1961)	Sex not stated
Mature New Hampshires	12·2	6·8	—	5·1	3·3	Lucas & Jamroz (1961)	Sex not stated
Breed unknown	12·0	7·5	—	5·5	3·5	Schermer (1958)	
Brown Leghorn*	12·2	7·4	2·5	—	—	Gilbert (1965)	Wet film
Mature hens	11·0	7·3	—	—	—	Gilbert (1965)	Dry film
Mature cocks	12·8	7·9	2·4	—	—	Gilbert (1965)	Wet film
Mature cocks	11·5	7·5	—	—	—	Gilbert (1965)	Dry film
Commercial hybrid males	10·6	6·2	—	4·6	3·0	Abdel-Hameed et al (1971)	
Commercial hybrid females	9·88	6·1	—	4·8	2·6	Abdel-Hameed et al (1971)	
Turkey							
Male	15·5	7·5	—	—	—	Venzlaff	
Female	15·5	7·0	—	—	—	Venzlaff	
Duck	12·8	6·6	—	—	—	Malasez	Sex not given
Quail	8·8	5·5	—	—	—	Atwal & McFarland (1966)	Up to 14 days old

* The differences in cell length and width between males and females in both wet and dry film groups are significant.

apparent (Männel 1967) but Jaffe (1960) has reported such differences between inbred lines of White Leghorns. Other factors affecting levels of red blood cells are season (Olson 1937), time of day (Domm & Taber 1946), environmental temperature (Moye et al 1969) and state of lay (Bell et al 1965).

In Coturnix quail erythrocyte numbers are significantly higher in the male than in the female at 1 day old ($3 \cdot 0 \times 10^{12}/l$ in the male and $2 \cdot 5 \times 10^{12}/l$ in the female) and remain higher until 10 days old. Between then and sexual maturity there are no significant sex differences but after maturity a difference again appears (male—$5 \cdot 0 \times 10^{12}/l$; female—$4 \cdot 2 \times 10^{12}/l$; Atwal et al 1964). Turkey poults have been reported (Venkataratnam & Clarkson 1962) as possessing an erythrocyte count of $3 \times 10^{12}/l$ at hatch, falling to $2 \cdot 6 \times 10^{12}/l$ after 2 weeks and then remaining steady. Mature males had mean red cells of $2 \cdot 65 \times 10^{12}/l$ and laying females $2 \cdot 48 \times 10^{12}/l$.

Mean corpuscular volume (MCV) values reported for the domestic fowl have shown a wide range, from 137 fl (Wintrobe 1933) down to 92 fl (Abou-Ashour & Edwards 1972). Reported values for mature birds from different breeds suggest that there are considerable breed differences. For example New Hampshire hens—108 fl (Männel 1967); Brown Leghorn hens—120 fl (Gilbert 1965), but light and heavy breeds grown under similar conditions have shown no significant differences between strains within a breed or between breeds, all having values close to 108 fl (Washburn & Guill 1972). Clear cut differences between the sexes have been demonstrated, with the cock being higher than the hen. Such differences have been reported as being significant (Gilbert 1965) or non-significant (Männel 1967). In the quail MCV values are greater in the young bird than in the mature bird, with values decreasing up to maturity (Atwal et al 1964, Nirmalan & Robinson 1971). However, superimposed upon this change are sexual variations occurring during growth and maturation and ending with the mature female having a greater value than the male (Atwal et al 1964). Values for other species are: turkey (male)—$160 \cdot 2$ fl (Ferguson et al 1964) and duck (8–10 months old)—$99 \cdot 7$ fl (Soliman et al 1966).

The osmotic fragility of avian erythrocytes has been discussed by Sturkie (1965) and values for resistance to haemolysis in the fowl have been given by Wirth (1950), Jaffe (1960), March et al (1966) and Abou-Ashour and Edwards (1972). March et al (1966) have demonstrated a greater susceptibility to haemolysis in mature males than in mature females.

12.3.1.3 Haemoglobin values

BLOOD HAEMOGLOBIN VALUES

The fact that birds possess nucleated erythrocytes has presented problems in the measurement of haemoglobin (Hb) levels and resulted in highly variable reports, particularly in the older literature. Much of this variation can be

Species	Age (weeks)	Sex	Hb g/dl	Author	Breed
Chickens	18	M	9·81	Tanaka & Rosenberg (1954)	New Hampshire
	18	F	8·92		
	Mature	M	13·19		
	Mature	F	8·61		
	Non-laying hens	F	8·67		
	1	Both	7·1	Frederickson et al (1957)	White Rock
	4	Both	7·4		
	9	Both	7·4		
	Mature	M	11·8	Olson (1937)	Not stated
	Mature	F	9·1		
	1	Both	9·28	Deaton et al (1969)	Broiler chicks
	4	Both	9·92		
	8	Both	9·75		
Geese	1	M	6·7	Hunsaker et al (1964)	Pilgrim
	1	F	6·6		
	8	M	11·3		
	8	F	11·5		
	16	M	13·7		
	16	F	13·4		
	43	M	15·7		
	43	F	12·7		
Quail	4	M	8·4	Atwal et al (1964)	*Coturnix c. japonica*
	4	F	8·7		
	15	M	10·4		
	15	F	10·8		
	50	M	15·3		
	50	F	12·3		
Turkeys	1	—	7·7	Wolterink et al (1947)	Beltsville Small White
	6	—	10·2	Malewitz & Calhoun (1957)	Beltsville White
	8–12	—	9·3	McGuire & Cavett (1952)	Not stated
	Adult	M	13·9	Rhian et al (1944)	Bronze
	Adult	F	10·5		
Ducks	Adult	—	10·3	Soliman et al (1966)	Not stated
	Adult	—	15·6	Magath & Higgins (1934)	Mallards

attributed to the unsuitable methods of determination used (Sturkie 1965). Values from the early literature have been presented by Olson (1937).

In newly hatched chicks blood Hb levels have been reported as starting at a low level and gradually increasing with age (Tanaka & Rosenberg 1954, Deaton *et al* 1969. See Table 12.2), and similar reports have been given for the turkey (Wolterink *et al* 1947), the goose (Hunsaker *et al* 1964) and the quail (Atwal *et al* 1964). However, Dixon and Torbert (1958) have stated that there is an initially high Hb (13·9 g/dl) in the day-old chick which falls to 10·3 g/dl at day 5 and which recovers again by day 12. Männel (1966) states that adult Hb levels are reached by the chick within 2 days of hatching. Other patterns of change in Hb levels during the first weeks of age have been described by Olson (1937) and Fredrickson *et al* (1957). Despite some variation, no significant differences have been reported in poultry species between the sexes prior to maturation (Wolterink *et al* 1947, Tanaka & Rosenberg 1954, Hunsaker *et al* 1964, Atwal *et al* 1964, Männel 1966). The only exception to this was in the case of day old quail where the male Hb was significantly higher than the female (Atwal *et al* 1964). During and after the period of maturation a difference in Hb values appears between the sexes, with the male having the higher level (Table 12.2). However, considerable fluctuations in Hb values can occur after maturity (Olson 1937, Tanaka & Rosenberg 1954, Hunsaker *et al* 1964).

HAEMOGLOBIN CONTENT OF ERYTHROCYTES

The mean corpuscular haemoglobin (MCH) represents the average amount of Hb contained within each red cell and values are given in picograms (pg). In chickens values of 30·2 pg were reported for 8 week old birds (Soliman *et al* 1966) and 41 and 36 pg for male and female birds respectively (Wintrobe 1933). In the quail Atwal *et al* (1964) noted that hatch values decrease during growth, especially in the male, reaching an adult value of 27–28 pg for both sexes. Rostorfer and Rigdon (1947) noted a similar age change in the duck, with adults averaging 42·6 pg of haemoglobin.

The mean corpuscular haemoglobin concentration (MCHC) expresses the volume of the erythrocyte occupied by the Hb and values are given as grams per decilitre (g/dl). Most poultry (chickens, ducks, turkeys) show values ranging from 30–40 g/dl (Jones & Johansen 1972), although Soliman *et al* (1966) quoted 23·9 g/dl for 8 week old chickens and Abou-Ashour and Edwards (1972) gave a value of 29·5 g/dl for mature hens. Values for mature quail (Atwal *et al* 1964) are male—36·4 g/dl and female—33·2 g/dl. Bell *et al* (1965) have demonstrated that the MCHC may undergo considerable fluctuations in the laying hen, depending particularly upon the state of lay.

HAEMOGLOBIN TYPES

The different types of haemoglobins occurring in the embryonic and adult chicken and the changes which take place during development have been reviewed by Allen (1971) and Bruns & Ingram (1973). In the 2–5 day embryo the haemoglobins consist of a major component P and a minor component E, and these occur in the primitive erythroid cells (Bruns & Ingram 1973). At 6–7 days of incubation, as definitive erythroid cells begin to appear in the blood, the adult components, haemoglobins A and D, become demonstrable. The adult haemoglobins gradually increase until, at 16 days of incubation when definitive erythrocytes have replaced the primitive erythroid cells, no trace of haemoglobins P and E is detectable (Bruns & Ingram 1973). Adult chicken haemoglobin can be resolved into 2 components by starch gel electrophoresis and two components plus a trace component by ion exchange chromatography. Haemoglobin A comprises about 70 per cent, haemoglobin D about 30 per cent and haemoglobin H comprises about 1–9 per cent of the total. Other, minor, haemoglobins that have been detected are probably artifacts of the preparation procedure (Manwell *et al* 1963). A somewhat similar haemoglobin picture has been demonstrated in the White Pekin duck (Borgese & Bertles 1964, 1965).

12.3.1.4 Factors affecting erythrocyte values

The changes in erythrocyte values due to age and sex have already been described. The relationships between male and female red cell values and the hormones responsible for their occurrence have been discussed by Hunsaker *et al* (1964) for geese, Sturkie (1965) for chickens and Nirmalan and Robinson (1971) for quail.

Erythrocyte values are also affected by season and environmental temperature. Olson (1937) reported that red cell numbers in chickens are increased during the winter in comparison with the summer, and Domm and Taber (1946) observed a higher number of red cells during the autumn than during the winter and spring; they also noted a diurnal variation in erythrocytes, with highest values at midnight and lowest values at noon. Olson (1937), however, reported no daily or weekly variations in red cell numbers. Vogel (1961) demonstrated higher red cell volumes for males and females in winter.

Winter (1935) found that during cold weather the Hb content of the blood of hens increased significantly. Under controlled environment conditions Huston (1960, 1965) and Washburn and Huston (1968) found that the haematocrits of chickens at an ambient temperature of 30°C were significantly lower than those of birds grown in cooler environments and that the latter had higher erythrocyte concentrations. Parker and Boone (1971) demonstrated a definite haemodilution effect in turkeys held at 37·8°C, with lowered red cell count, PCV and Hb, but in birds at 10°C the red cell count increased. Analysing these temperature effects Moye *et al* (1969) determined that the increase in PCV with lower temperature is due to increases in both red cell numbers and MCV. The reverse occurs with birds at high environmental temperatures. Similar temperature effects were found with haematocrit and haemoglobin values in broilers by Deaton *et al* (1969).

Other factors affecting erythrocyte values have been described by Sturkie (1965).

12.3.1.5 Erythropoiesis

Central erythropoiesis takes place solely within the lumen of the medullary sinuses of the bone marrow in the post-hatched bird; in the embryo the primary site of erythropoiesis is in the yolk sac and only secondarily within the marrow. Lucas and Jamroz (1961) define the developmental cell line as: erythroblast, early, mid and late polychromatic erythrocytes, reticulocyte and mature erythrocyte. Erythroblasts can be further subdivided into early (proerythroblasts) and late types (Lucas 1959). The early developmental stages lie peripherally along the sinus wall and frequently appear to be attached to it; later stages lie more centrally within the sinus lumen and are not obviously attached to other cells (Campbell 1967). Normally only mature erythrocytes and, to a lesser extent, reticulocytes are released into the general circulation, although occasional early developmental stages may occur in the blood of a healthy fowl (Lucas & Jamroz 1961). The control of avian erythropoiesis has been briefly reviewed by Freeman (1971). As in the mammal the production of red cells is controlled by the humoral substance erythropoietin but erythropoietin in birds is not identical to that in mammals (Rosse & Waldman 1966).

Peripheral erythropoiesis has been reported as occurring to a relatively limited extent in the young chicken (Smith & Engelbert 1969) but much more extensively in certain species of wild birds (Engelbert & Young 1970). In this process new erythrocytes arise directly as nuclear membrane buds from young, mature, circulating erythrocytes. These cells, called clone cells, are released from the mother cell as relatively undifferentiated erythrocytes containing nuclear material contributed by the mother nucleus and then differentiate to form mature erythrocytes. The frequency of such clone cells in the peripheral blood of chick embryos and young hatched chicks averages 5·2 per cent (Smith & Engelbert 1969).

Besides the mature erythrocytes, the penultimate developmental stage, the reticulocyte, is commonly found in the normal circulation. Reticulocyte numbers are highest in the newly hatched chick (up to 35 per cent) and decrease as the bird grows (Coates & March 1966). Although Lucas and Jamroz (1961) considered that reticulocytes only occur rarely in the normal adult, Coates and March (1966) described between 7 and 20 per cent reticulocytes in the total adult red cell count of a number of breeds of fowl. In the adult duck Magath and Higgins (1934) found an average of 20·7 per cent reticulocytes. Reticulocytes resemble the mature erythrocyte in size and shape but possess fine cytoplasmic granules specifically stainable by Brilliant Cresyl Blue and also possess less condensed chromatin in the nucleus.

The life span of the erythrocyte has been studied in the fowl by Hevesy and Ottesen (1945), Ottesen (1948), Shemin (1948), Rodnan *et al* (1957) and Reddy *et al* (1975), in the duck by Brace and Altland (1956) and Rodnan *et al* (1957) and in the quail by Nirmalan and Robinson (1973). Values from these investigations are given in Table 12.3. The process of erythrocyte aging and destruction is little understood (Freeman 1971). As red cells age their nuclei become more condensed and eventually pyknotic and vacuolated

Table 12.3   Values for erythrocyte life span in poultry

Species	Life span in days	Authors
Chicken	28	Hevesy & Ottesen (1945)
	32	Ottesen (1948)
	28	Shemin (1948)
	35 (maximum)	Rodnan *et al* (1957)
(4 strains)	27·5–31·5	Reddy *et al* (1975)
Duck	39	Bruce & Altland (1956)
	42 (maximum)	Rodnan *et al* (1957)
Coturnix quail	35 (male)	Nirmalan & Robinson (1973)
	33 (female)	Nirmalan & Robinson (1973)

but only a few such cells can be seen in normal blood (Lucas & Jamroz 1961). Together with these morphological changes the enzyme levels decrease and fragility increases (Walter *et al* 1965). They are probably finally phagocytosed by macrophages.

12.3.2   THROMBOCYTES

12.3.2.1   Structure and ultrastructure

Thrombocytes are cells which superficially bear a considerable resemblance to erythrocytes. They are essentially oval cells but are smaller and more rounded in appearance than red cells and have a larger more rounded nucleus (Fig. 12.3). Considerable variation in size and shape occurs within the normal range of thrombocytes as they may vary from round through irregular to elongated in shape (Lucas & Jamroz 1961). The cytoplasm is not homogeneous in structure, possessing a reticulated appearance and containing

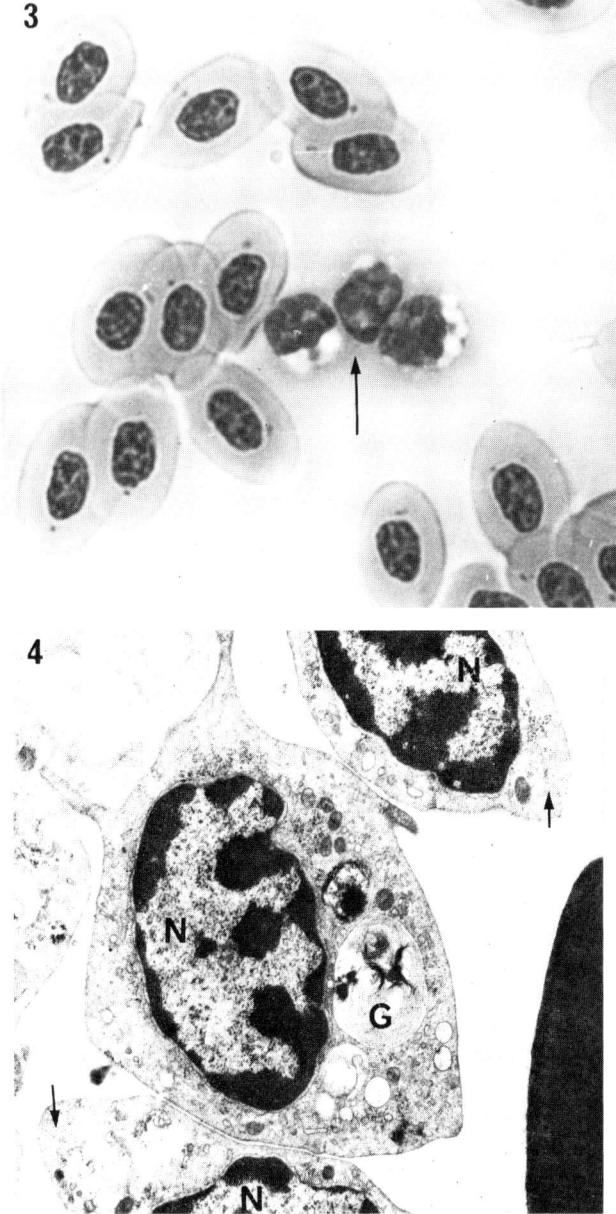

Fig. 12.3 A group of three fowl thrombocytes (arrow) surrounded by erythrocytes. Wright's stain. × 1800.

Fig. 12.4 Electron micrograph of a fowl thrombocyte and parts of two others. G, large partially degenerate specific granule; N, nuclei; arrows, bundles of peripheral microtubules. × 10,000.

one or more specific granules varying in shape from single compact forms to multiple or diffuse forms. The rounded nucleus contains much condensed chromatin giving it a dark, coarsely granular appearance.

When examined with the electron microscope the thrombocyte appears as an irregularly rounded, oval or sometimes elongated cell with a variable number of fine, peripheral cytoplasmic processes or pseudopodia. The round to oval nucleus composes about one third of the total volume of the cell and contains much heavily condensed chromatin (Fig. 12.4). Typical organelles found in the cytoplasm are small numbers of mitochondria, a Golgi complex, much smooth endoplasmic reticulum but little rough endoplasmic reticulum, and many groups of microtubules. However, the largest and most characteristic organelles are the specific granules which may vary from 0·2 to 3 μm in diameter (Sweeny & Carlson 1968, Maxwell 1974). The contents of these membrane-bound granules normally consists of dense osmiophilic granules or tightly-packed arrays of osmiophilic membranes (Simpson 1968, Enbergs & Kriesten 1968a) but once blood has been shed the granules begin to degenerate, breaking down to give vacuolated structures and, finally, empty vacuoles. Other ultrastructural studies on thrombocytes have been published by Carlson *et al* (1968), Enbergs and Kriesten (1968b) Maxwell and Trejo (1970), Kuruma *et al* (1970), Enbergs (1973) and Sterz and Weiss (1973).

12.3.2.2 Physical characteristics

Corresponding to their considerable variation in shape, the dimensions of thrombocytes have also been described as being very variable. Lucas and Jamroz (1961) have reported for the fowl that thrombocyte length varies from 6·1 to 11·5 μm whilst the width varies from 3·0 to 6·1 μm, and that there is some difference in average dimensions between breeds. Blount (1939) described cell length as 10 μm and cell width as 5 μm, whilst Kuruma *et al* (1970), using electron micrographs, gave the range of thrombocyte 'diameters' as 10 to 15 μm.

The number of thrombocytes in the circulating blood of fowls has been found to be slightly higher in adult female chicken (26×10^9 cells/l) than in adult males ($25\cdot4 \times 10^9$/l), with young birds having even higher values ($32\cdot7 \times 10^9$/l; Olson, 1937). Heinson (1930) demonstrated a similar, though greater, sex difference, $30\cdot6 \times 10^9$/l for males and $41\cdot6 \times 10^9$/l for females, and Lucas and Jamroz (1961) confirmed the sex differential in adult White Leghorns but not the increased cell count in young birds. Much higher thrombocyte values than these have been reported by Lucas and Jamroz (1961; $60\cdot3 \times 10^9$/l in Rhode Island Red hens) and from the literature by Schermer (1958).

Nirmalan and Robinson (1971) describe very high thrombocyte levels in

Coturnix quail, $117 \times 10^9/l$ in adult males, $113 \times 10^9/l$ in non-laying females and $132 \times 10^9/l$ for laying females. Although there was a sex difference between males and laying females this was not significant. However, the considerably lower value for 2-week-old quail, $70 \times 10^9/l$, was significant. In the duck, Magath and Higgins (1934) have reported a thrombocyte level of $30 \cdot 7 \times 10^9/l$ of blood.

12.3.2.3 Development

Thrombocytes develop in the bone marrow together with erythrocytes and granulocytes. Although it was originally considered that both erythrocytes and thrombocytes possessed a common developmental line, due to the considerable similarity between the 2 mature cells (Blount 1939), detailed studies by Lucas and Jamroz (1961) have demonstrated that thrombocytes have a developmental line of their own. This originates in the thromboblast, a cell differing from the erythroblast particularly in its more condensed, punctate nuclear chromatin, passes through early, mid and late immature thrombocyte stages, and terminates in the mature, circulating thrombocyte. However, more recent studies by Archer (1971) suggest the possibility that large multinucleate cells within the marrow, resembling mammalian megakaryocytes, may be thrombocyte precursors.

12.3.2.4 Thrombocyte function and blood coagulation

Although the thrombocyte has frequently been described as having the same function as the blood platelet in mammals (Olson 1959, Bradley & Grahame 1960, Lucas & Jamroz 1961) it appears to play little part in the process of initiation of clotting (Archer 1971). Thrombocytes seem to behave physically very similarly to platelets after blood has been shed; the specific granules break down, the thrombocytes clump together, the nucleus becomes pyknotic and eventually the cell degenerates (Lucas & Jamroz 1961). However, the rate of clumping of thrombocytes is not as rapid as that of platelets. The specific granules are apparently identical to the dense osmiophilic granules seen with the electron microscope; the latter degenerate rapidly, leaving large clear vacuoles in the cytoplasm (Schumacher 1965), and the process is most marked in running blood obtained after decapitation (Kuruma *et al* 1970). These granules, however, apparently consist largely of 5-hydroxytryptamine (Kuruma *et al* 1970) and are unlikely to be a source of thromboplastin, which occurs at considerably lower levels in chicken blood than in mammalian blood (Bigland & Triantaphyllopoulos 1960). Quite apart from their uncertain involvement in clotting mechanisms thrombocytes possess a phagocytic function. In vivo they are constantly on the move and protruding pseudopodia

(Kuruma *et al* 1970), and they can phagocytose dyes, bacteria (Carlson *et al* 1968) and viruses (Sterz & Weiss 1973).

The processes of blood coagulation in avian species have been reviewed by Griminger (1965) and Archer (1971). The initial pathways of clot formation in birds are considerably different from those in mammals (Archer 1971, Fig. 12.5). Whereas mammalian shed blood produces relatively large amounts

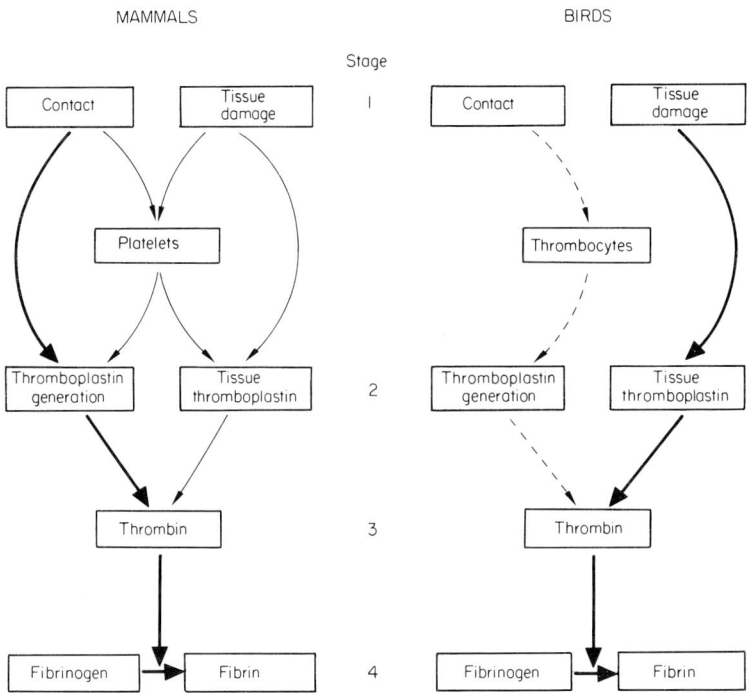

Fig. 12.5 A simplified scheme of blood coagulation in which avian and mammalian systems are contrasted. Stages 1 and 2 are clearly different in the 2 systems. From Archer (1971).

of intrinsic thromboplastin on contact with surfaces other than vascular endothelium, avian shed blood produces only small amounts of intrinsic thromboplastin and consequently is relatively unreactive to foreign surfaces. In birds, extrinsic thromboplastin production, that occurring in tissue juices from damaged tissue cells, is the major source of thromboplastin, and rapid and efficient clotting of avian blood relies on the mixing of tissue juices with the shed blood. Because of this various clotting tests in birds (e.g. prothrombin time) can only be performed successfully by the addition of a thromboplastin extract normally obtained from brain tissue of the same species. Later stages of coagulation, the formation of thrombin and the production of fibrin from fibrinogen, appear to have been little studied in birds (Archer 1971).

12.4 LEUCOCYTES

12.4.1 NON-GRANULAR LEUCOCYTES

12.4.1.1 Lymphocytes

Lymphocytes are the most frequently occurring leucocyte in avian blood. They have a wide range of size, being divided into large, medium and small types but the normal, mature lymphocytes are the medium and small types which have a mean diameter of 7·7 μm (Table 12.4). Large lymphocytes are infrequently found in the blood and are probably immature cells (Lucas & Jamroz 1961). Typical lymphocytes may be round and regular cells or may be somewhat irregular due to peripheral pseudopodia or blebs of cytoplasm. The nucleus is centrally placed and rounded with only rarely a distinct indentation (Fig. 12.6). The amount of cytoplasm varies from a moderately wide band in the medium lymphocyte to only the narrowest rim surrounding the nucleus in the small lymphocyte. In appearance the cytoplasm is normally weakly basophilic and homogeneous although some granular structures may be visible, particularly magenta-staining granules.

Studies on the ultrastructure of avian circulating lymphocytes have been carried out by Schumacher (1965), Simpson (1968), Enbergs and Kriesten (1968b), Kriesten and Enbergs (1970), Maxwell and Trejo (1970) and Maxwell (1974). The medium lymphocyte is a round to oval cell with some peripheral pseudopodia and a large nucleo-cytoplasmic ratio (Maxwell 1974). The rounded nucleus, sometimes indented, possesses a narrow rim of hetero-chromatin surrounding abundant central euchromatin and one or more nucleoli. Within the cytoplasm is a relatively small complement of organelles (Fig. 12.7); some mitochrondria, short strands of rough endoplasmic reticulum, microtubules and numerous ribosomes. The Golgi apparatus, usually moderately well developed, is often located opposite an indentation of the nucleus (Maxwell & Trejo 1970). The small lymphocyte is a rounded cell with only a narrow rim of perinuclear cytoplasm frequently developed into extensive pseudopodia. The round, irregular or indented nucleus consists of roughly equal quantities of heterochromatin and euchromatin, the former arranged more peripherally in clumps. Cytoplasmic organelles are very similar to those of the medium lymphocyte but Maxwell (1974) has reported the presence of structures composed of particles and fibrils and termed 'tyre-tracks' in the small lymphocytes of all domesticated species of birds but the

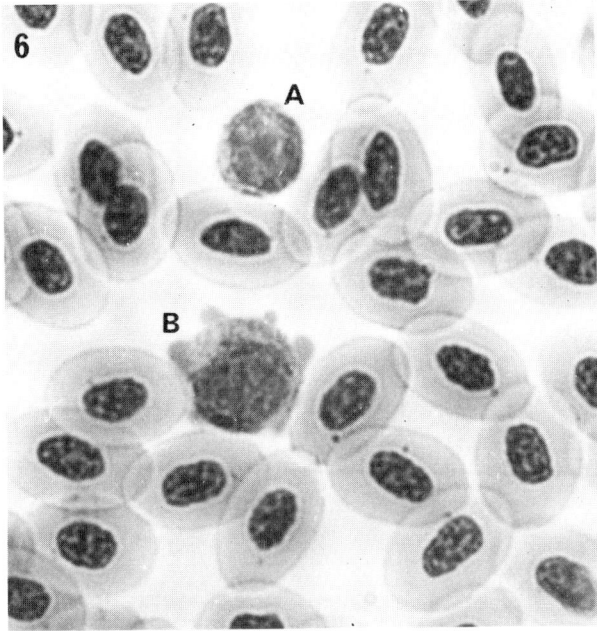

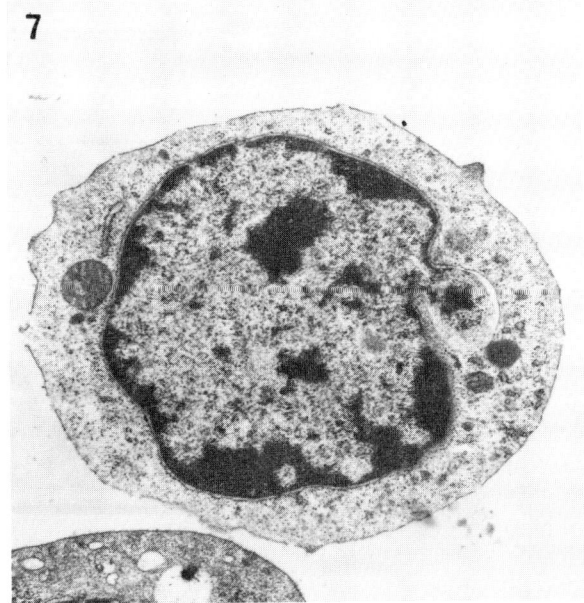

Fig. 12.6 Two chicken lymphocytes. A, typical small lymphocyte with little peripheral cytoplasm; B, medium lymphocyte with pseudopodial cytoplasm. Wright's stain. × 1800.

Fig. 12.7 Electron micrograph of a fowl small lymphocyte. Both cytoplasm and cytoplasmic organelles are sparse. × 13,000.

turkey. Both types of lymphocyte possess dense, membrane-bound cytoplasmic granules of variable morphology up to 1·0 μm in diameter (Kriesten & Enbergs 1970, Maxwell 1974).

Lymphocytes also form the major cellular component of the lymphoid organs of birds, the more important of which are the thymus, the cloacal bursa and the spleen (Payne 1971). The ultrastructural differences between the thymic and bursal lymphocytes have been described by Clawson *et al* (1967).

12.4.1.2 Monocytes

Monocytes are larger in size than lymphocytes and are normally also larger than heterophils, being on average about 12 μm in diameter (Table 12.4). In shape monocytes are normally round, or slightly irregular due to the

Table 12.4 Mean diameters of lymphocytes and monocytes from mature chickens (Lucas & Jamroz 1961)

Breed	Lymphocytes (μm)		Monocytes (μm)	
	Cytosome diameter	Nuclear diameter	Cytosome diameter	Nuclear diameter
Single Comb White Leghorn	8·1	6·8	12·7	8·5
New Hampshire	6·6	5·7	11·4	8·0
Columbian Plymouth Rock	8·1	6·5	11·3	7·9

presence of cytoplasmic blebs (Fig. 12.8). The nucleus is round to elongated with frequently a flattening or indentation on one side, resulting in an overall kidney shape. It is normally eccentrically placed within the cell such that the nuclear indentation faces the greater cytoplasmic width. Adjacent to the indentation is frequently a vacuolated, palely staining area of cytoplasm called the Hof. The general cytoplasm is of an alveolar or reticular structure and may be divided into an outer, hyaline mantle and an inner, more deeply staining core (Lucas & Jamroz 1961). Scattered throughout the cytoplasm are fine, pink-staining dust-like particles.

When examined ultrastructurally the monocyte appears as a round to elongated cell with peripheral pseudopodia and lobopodia (Maxwell 1974). Cytoplasmic organelles are much more prominent in the monocyte than in the lymphocyte (Fig. 12.9). Numbers of mitochondria, short and long strands of rough endoplasmic reticulum, pinocytotic vesicles, ribosomes and dense, membrane-bound granules between 0·1 and 0·5 μm in diameter occur throughout the cytosome. Bundles of fine wavy filaments run longitudinally close

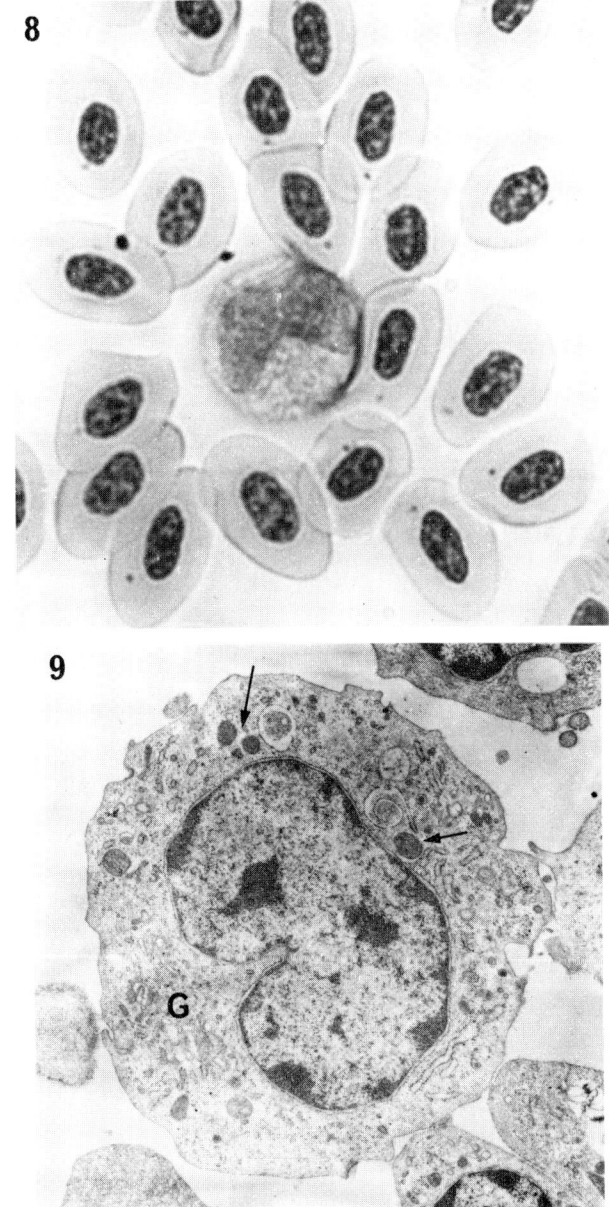

Fig. 12.8 A fowl monocyte containing a clearly indented nucleus. Wright's stain. × 1800.

Fig. 12.9 Electron micrograph of a fowl monocyte. A large Golgi complex (G) lies opposite the indented nucleus and there are a number of cytoplasmic granules (arrows) visible. × 8000.

to the nuclear membrane (Enbergs & Kriesten 1969, Maxwell 1974) and one or more well-developed Golgi complexes lie in the cytoplasm adjacent to the nuclear indentation. This latter region apparently corresponds to the Hof seen with the light microscope and thus the Hof is closely correlated with the Golgi complex of the monocyte. The nucleus is clearly indented and kidney-shaped and contains more euchromatin than heterochromatin, so that in general the nucleus is not so dense as that of the lymphocyte. One or two large nucleoli occur centrally (Maxwell & Trejo 1970).

12.4.1.3 Lymphocytopoiesis

Although some formation of lymphocytes takes place within the bone marrow tissue, it is not the main site of formation of these cells. Jordan (1935, 1936) has described the bone marrow as containing numerous dense lymphoid nodules with germinal centres and Taliaferro and Taliaferro (1955) have seen both nodular and non-nodular lymphatic tissue within the marrow. Campbell (1967), however, did not find any nodules in adult chicken marrow, the non-nodular tissue being composed of numerous small, medium and large lymphocytes densely but indiscriminately arranged throughout the tissue.

Lymphocytes are normally formed within the main lymphoid organs of the body. These are the 'central' lymphoid structures, the cloacal bursa and the thymus, and the 'peripheral' structures, the spleen, caecal tonsils and other intestinal lymphoid tissues (Payne 1971). Lucas and Jamroz (1961) have described the lymphocyte developmental series as consisting of lymphoblasts, immature lymphocytes and mature lymphocytes, both medium and small. Monocytes are formed within the same organs where lymphocytes have their origin; the developmental stages of these cells appear to be monoblast, early and late immature monocytes and mature monocytes (Lucas & Jamroz 1961).

12.4.2 GRANULAR LEUCOCYTES

12.4.2.1 Heterophils

The avian heterophil is equivalent to the mammalian neutrophil although the structure and staining affinity of the heterophil specific granules are different to those of the neutrophil. In fixed and stained preparations for both light and electron microscopes heterophils usually appear as rounded cells with lobed nuclei but Kelly and Dearstyne (1935) have demonstrated by supravital staining that living heterophils are active cells possessing a constantly changing amoeboid shape. Heterophils in the fowl have been reported as being about 8·0–10·0 μm in diameter (Lucas & Jamroz 1961, Table 12.5), with colourless cytoplasm and a multilobed nucleus of 1–5 lobes joined together by narrow bands (Fig. 12.10). The Arneth index for the fowl is 2·44 (Lucas & Jamroz 1961). Lying within the cytoplasm are large numbers of acidophilic granules which, when properly fixed, are frequently rod or spindle-shaped with a central spherical core. Partial breakdown of the granules may occur leaving the spherical cores closely resembling eosinophil granules.

When examined with the electron microscope the heterophil can be seen to possess an irregularly rounded shape with small pseudopodia and an occasional lobopodium projecting from the cellular periphery (Maxwell & Trejo 1970, Maxwell 1973) (Fig. 12.11). The lobed nucleus possesses dense accumulations of heterochromatin and a single nucleolus, whilst cytoplasmic organelles such as mitochondria, endoplasmic reticulum and the Golgi complex are small and relatively poorly developed. Three types of membrane-bound cytoplasmic granules have been described as occurring in the fowl

Table 12.5 Mean diameters of granular leucocytes from mature chickens (Lucas & Jamroz 1961)

Breed	Heterophils µm	Eosinophils µm	Basophils µm
Single Comb White Leghorn	7·9	7·0	7·8
New Hampshire	9·9	7·8	8·1
Columbian Plymouth Rock	8·8	7·9	9·1

heterophil (Dhingra *et al* 1969, Ericsson & Nair 1973). These are: large dense granules, round to fusiform bodies up to 3·5 µm long with a dense granular matrix and, in some cases, an internal electron-dense core; small dense granules, small bodies up to 0·2 µm in diameter with a dense core and a more electron-lucent periphery; and light granules, round to oval structures intermediate in size between the other two types and possessing a pale fibrillar matrix (Ericsson & Nair 1973). Similar types of granules have been described in heterophils from the duck, goose, turkey, quail and guinea fowl by Maxwell (1973). Other ultrastructural studies of fowl heterophils have been reported by Enbergs and Kriesten (1968b), Osculati (1970) and MacRae and Spitznagel (1975), and on the heterophils of other domesticated birds by Enbergs (1973b).

12.4.2.2 Eosinophils

The eosinophil is an essentially rounded cell with some tendency towards irregularity or oval shape (Fig. 12.12). In the fowl it has a mean diameter of 7·3 µm but there is a wide range of variation (4 to 11 µm; Lucas & Jamroz 1961; see Table 12.5). The cytoplasm stains a pale blue colour with Wright's

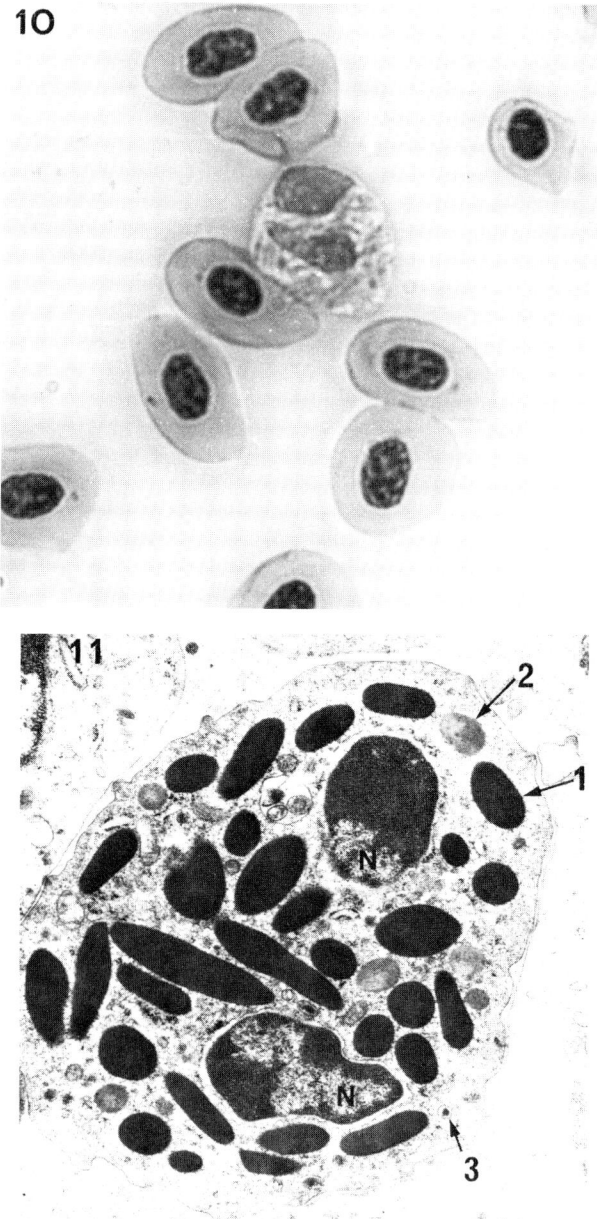

Fig. 12.10 Chicken heterophil. The multilobed nucleus and rod-shaped granules are visible. Wright's stain. × 1800.

Fig. 12.11 Electron micrograph of a chicken heterophil. 1, 2 & 3, the three different types of cytoplasmic granules; N, nuclear lobes. × 13,000.

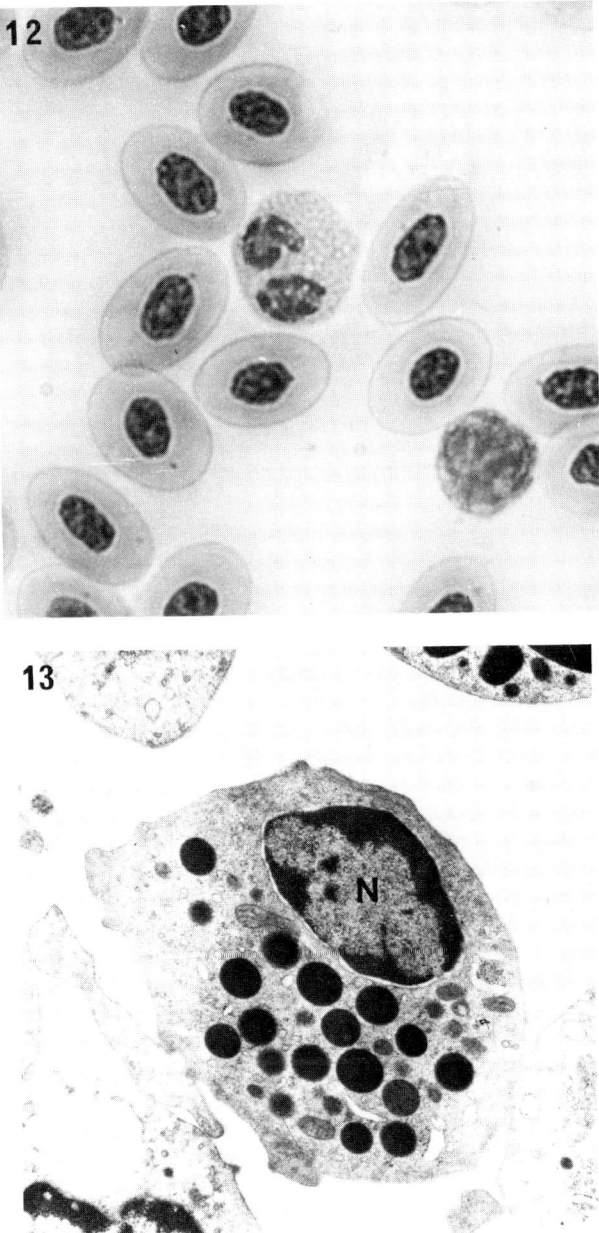

Fig. 12.12   Fowl eosinophil granulocyte. The bilobed nucleus is surrounded by relatively unstained, rounded granules. Wright's stain. × 1800.

Fig. 12.13   Electron micrograph of a chicken eosinophil. The cytoplasmic granules are of one type only and are normally round in profile. N, nuclear lobe. × 10,000.

stain and the nuclear lobes are composed of many dense chromatin clumps. The average Arneth Index is less than that of the heterophil, being slightly below 2·0 (Lucas & Jamroz 1961), so that the typical eosinophil nucleus is bilobed. In stained preparations both the nucleus and cytoplasm are normally obscured by large numbers of spherical cytoplasmic granules which are stained red by blood stains. Although these cells are termed eosinophils their granular staining affinity is not necessarily more eosinophilic than that of the heterophils; it has been considered that eosinophil granules stain a dull red in contrast to the brilliant red of the heterophil (Hodges 1974).

A number of ultrastructural studies have been carried out on eosinophils from several domesticated birds, in particular the fowl (Enbergs & Kriesten 1968b 1970, Kelényi & Németh 1969, Dhingra *et al* 1969, Maxwell & Trejo 1970), the duck (Maxwell & Siller 1972, Enbergs 1973a b), the goose (Enbergs & Beardi 1971, Maxwell & Siller 1972) and the quail, guinea fowl and turkey (Maxwell & Siller 1972). Electron micrographs of eosinophils normally show irregularly rounded cells with variable numbers of short pseudopodia extending from the cytoplasmic periphery, and between 1 and 3 profiles of nuclear lobes with heavy condensation of chromatin (Fig. 12.13). The characteristic cytoplasmic organelles are rounded, oval or elongated, dense osmiophilic granules which frequently show considerable intra- or inter-specific morphological variation (Maxwell & Siller 1972). The main variations in these membrane-bound granules are the homogeneous, dense granular core found in the fowl, guinea fowl, quail and turkey and the crystalline core found in the duck and goose. Other cytoplasmic organelles are mitochondria, abundant rough endoplasmic reticulum, free ribosomes and a well-developed Golgi apparatus.

12.4.2.3 Basophils

Basophils are rounded cells slightly smaller in size than heterophils and slightly larger than eosinophils, being 8 μm in mean diameter (Table 12.5). The clear colourless cytoplasm is normally obscured by large numbers of spherical, basophilic granules up to 0·8 μm in diameter (Fig. 12.14) but the latter are easily broken down by aqueous solutions of stains and may appear in a stained preparation in a state of partial or total dissolution (Hodges 1974). The nucleus in many species is normally eccentrically placed, lying towards one pole of the cell, and consists of a single lobe containing chromatin which is not strongly condensed. Although some nuclei are indented on one side, very few are constricted enough to be termed bilobed. The Arneth Index for fowl basophils is 1·01 (Lucas & Jamroz 1961).

When examined ultrastructurally the basophil appears as a regularly rounded cell with normally only a few small pseudopodia projecting peripherally. The nucleus, frequently laterally placed in the duck, goose, turkey,

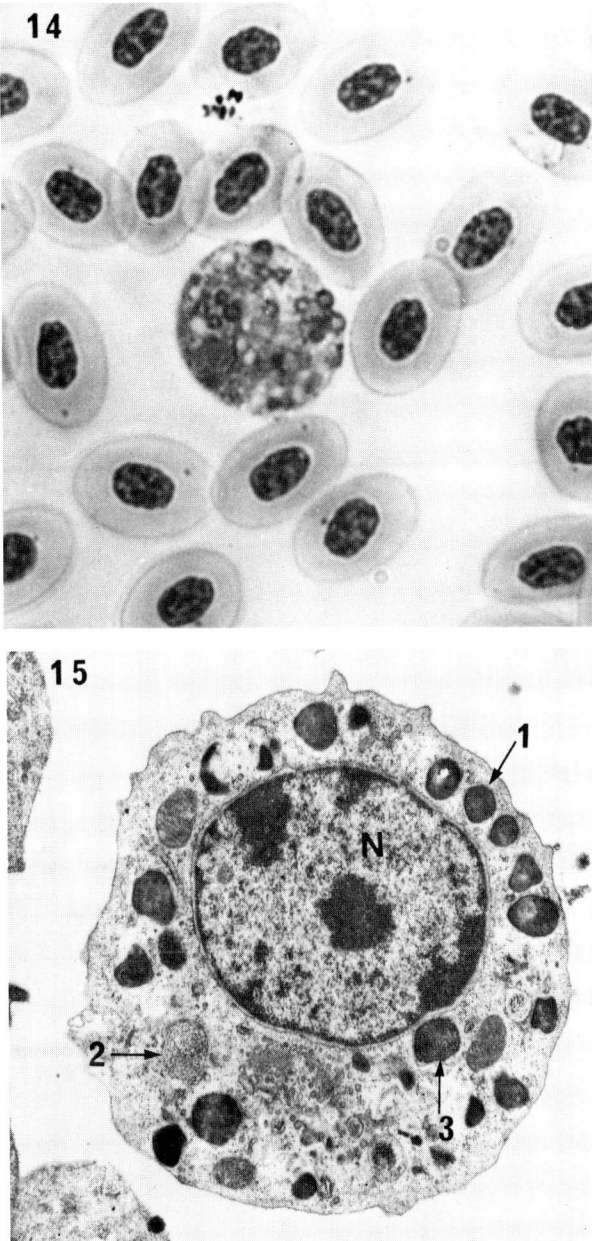

Fig. 12.14 Fowl basophil granulocyte. The large cytoplasmic granules obscure all other structures. Wright's stain. × 1800.

Fig. 12.15 Electron micrograph of a fowl basophil. N, single nuclear lobe; 1, 2 & 3, different types of cytoplasmic granules. × 13,000.

quail and guinea fowl (Maxwell 1973) but more centrally placed in the fowl (Fig. 12.15), is variably indented and contains 1 or 2 irregular nucleoli. Apart from the characteristic cytoplasmic granules, the cell contains a few rounded mitochondria, short strands of rough endoplasmic reticulum, occasional small lipid droplets, glycogen granules and a poorly developed Golgi complex frequently located opposite the nuclear indentation (Maxwell & Trejo 1970). The basophil granules have been described as occurring as 4 distinct types in the fowl (Maxwell & Trejo 1970) but not all of these types have been found in other domesticated species (Maxwell 1973). The granules are rounded or crescent-shaped in cross-section and frequently show signs of dissolution. The first type of granule is very dense with little obvious internal structure; the second is less dense and mottled in appearance; the third type has its substance arranged in a network; and the fourth type has it arranged in myelin-like whorls (Maxwell & Trejo 1970). The types of granule occurring in basophils are, to some extent, correlated with the type of fixation used, and it also has yet to be established whether the variations in basophil granules represent distinct populations or only different stages of development (Maxwell 1973). Other electron microscope studies have been carried out by Enbergs and Kriesten (1968b), Dhingra *et al* (1969), Kriesten and Enbergs (1970) and Enbergs (1973b).

12.4.2.4 Granulocytopoiesis

The processes of granulocyte formation take place within the extravascular spaces of the bone marrow away from the blood sinusoids. The stem cells from which the granulocytes develop have been called haemocytoblasts (Campbell 1967) or, more specifically, granuloblasts (Lucas & Jamroz 1961). Campbell (1967) has shown that the structure of the extravascular haemocytoblasts (granuloblasts) is identical to that of the intrasinusoidal haemocytoblasts (erythroblasts) although Lucas and Jamroz (1961) consider that the two are separable by their appearances in stained smears. The developing granulocyte passes through a number of stages from granuloblast through metagranuloblast, promyelocyte, mesomyelocyte, metamyelocyte to mature granulocyte. The specific granules for the different cell types begin to appear at the mesomyelocyte stage and can be recognized with both light and electron microscopes. By the metamyelocyte stage many of the cells begin to pass through the sinus walls into the circulation and presumably finish their maturation within the sinuses.

12.4.3 LEUCOCYTE FUNCTION

12.4.3.1 Granulocytes

The most commonly occurring of the granular leucocytes, the heterophils, are motile amoeboid cells which act as the body's first line of defence against invading organisms. They actively phagocytose organisms such as *E. coli* (Gross 1961) and *Staphylococcus aureus* (Topp & Carlson 1972b), both within the blood stream and at sites of infection within the tissues (Carlson & Allen 1969). The presence of acid hydrolases, such as acid phosphatase and β glucuronidase, has been demonstrated both histochemically (Topp & Carlson 1972a) and cytochemically (Osculati 1970, Ericsson & Nair 1973) within some of the heterophil granules, suggesting that these structures are lysosomal in nature. The substance of these granules has been demonstrated to take part in the heterophil's attack upon phagocytosed bacteria (MacRae & Spitznagel 1975).

Not a great deal is known about the functions of eosinophil granulocytes in birds. Olson in 1959 stated that their functions were not well understood and since then little further clarification of this position has occurred. It is believed that they act as a detoxifying mechanism and that they increase in tissues where there are parasitic infections and in certain allergic conditions.

Basophil granulocytes have been considered to be the circulating component and the mast cell to be the tissue component of a single cell line in both birds (Michels 1938, Olson 1959) and mammals (Selye 1965). However, although there is considerable ultrastructural similarity between avian basophils (Maxwell & Trejo 1970, Maxwell 1973) and tissue mast cells (Wight 1970), particularly in the structure of the specific granules from both cell types, there are some histological differences between the two (Hunt & Hunt 1959, Wight & Mackenzie 1970, Carlson & Hacking 1972). Basophil function in birds is by no means clear; in mammals the structurally very similar cells participate in anaphylaxis by discharging their granules (histamine) as a response to antigen-antibody reactions (Selye 1965).

12.4.3.2 Non-granular leucocytes

Lymphocytes can be functionally divided into two lines, the B, or bursa-dependent, and the T, or thymus-dependent, lines. Both these lines function as part of the immune system of the bird and each line derives its competency at an early age from the lymphoid organ on which it is dependent. Thus bursectomy of the embryo or young chick will result in a depletion or absence of the bursa-dependent lymphocyte series and eventual agammaglobulinaemia (Cooper *et al* 1967). The bursa-dependent lymphocyte series consists of cells bearing surface immunoglobulins or immunoglobulin receptors (Cooper *et al* 1967, Kincade *et al* 1971) which appear to function as antibody receptors for antigens from bacteria, viruses etc. The thymus-dependent line, the cells of which bear no obvious immunoglobulins on their surfaces, appears to be involved in various mechanisms of cell-mediated immunity such as homograft rejection.

Monocytes in mammals are clearly recognized as being the circulating counterparts of tissue macrophages, and that after a short life in the blood stream the monocytes migrate into the tissues to become macrophages (Nichols *et al* 1971, Nichols & Bainton 1975). Although the evidence for a similar relationship between avian monocytes and macrophages is not so clear cut, it seems fairly certain that avian monocytes are only a transient phase in the formation of macrophages. Monocytes are actively phagocytic cells which can take up other cells, bacteria or particulate material and possess lysosome-like bodies which are presumably associated with the breakdown of phagocytosed material (Maxwell & Trejo 1970, Maxwell 1974).

12.4.3 LEUCOCYTE NUMBERS AND DIFFERENTIAL COUNTS

12.4.4.1 Leucocyte numbers

Total leucocyte numbers in birds tend to show a wide range of variation between individuals; consequently studies concerning leucocyte numbers should be made with large groups of birds in order that significant differences may become apparent (Diesem *et al* 1958, Lucas & Jamroz 1961). Reports generally suggest that the total leucocyte count is relatively low in young birds and that it rises as the birds grow and mature. For example, Fredrickson *et al* (1957) counted $12 \cdot 5 \times 10^9/l$ leucocytes in 1 week old White Rock chickens and this increased, somewhat irregularly, to $33 \cdot 9 \times 10^9/l$ at 10 weeks of age. Similarly, Chubb and Rowell (1959) measured total leucocytes in hatched chicks at about $10 \times 10^9/l$ rising to about $35 \times 10^9/l$ at 7 weeks of age. Biely and Palmer (1935) noted that the mean leucocyte count of 1–2 day old White Leghorn chicks was lower than that of adult birds, the difference being statistically significant. In turkeys (Venkataratnam & Clarkson 1962) total leucocyte numbers rose from $15 \times 10^9/l$ at 3 days of age to $30 \times 10^9/l$ at 2 weeks and to $37 \times 10^9/l$ when adult. In quail this rise during growth was not so pronounced (Nirmalan & Robinson 1971), or there may even have been a slight decrease during the growth period which was regained by the beginning of sexual maturity to give the highest values in adult birds (Atwal *et al* 1964). However, none of the changes in leucocyte count reported by Atwal *et al* 1964) was significant. In contradistinction to the above, Olson (1959) states that total leucocyte numbers are greater in young chickens than in adult birds, and Kaleta and Bernhardt (1968) in geese have shown that the leucocyte count at 5 days old ($25 \times 10^9/l$) rose to $38 \cdot 6 \times 10^9/l$ at 10 days and then fell to achieve a relatively stable level ($16 \times 10^9/l$) by 30 days of age.

Although no significant difference in total leucocyte numbers has been shown to occur between mature male and female birds in a number of reports (Olson 1937, chickens; Atwal *et al* 1964, quail; Venkataratnam & Clarkson 1962, turkeys), others have demonstrated a considerably higher value in the adult female than in the adult male (Lucas & Jamroz 1961, chickens). Other factors affecting leucocyte numbers, such as environment, diet and hormonal influences, have been discussed by Sturkie (1965).

12.4.4.2 Differential leucocyte counts

Considerable changes take place in the differential leucocyte count of chickens immediately after hatch and during the first few weeks of life (Burton & Harrison 1969). At hatch the percentage of heterophils is high (72·4 per cent) and conversely that of lymphocytes is low (15·9 per cent), but over a period of 3 to 4 weeks these positions are completely reversed giving values of about 70 per cent lymphocytes and about 25 per cent heterophils. The basophil population also changes considerably over this period, falling from 8 per cent at hatch to about 3 per cent. Burton and Harrison (1969) consider that the high heterophil and basophil levels immediately post hatching indicate a haematological defence mechanism orientated specifically towards an inflammatory response, the capacity for antibody production developing only as the levels of circulating lymphocytes rise. The chick thus appears to achieve 'haematological maturity' at about 20 days of age (Burton & Harrison 1969). Details of changes in chick differential counts are given in Table 12.6. A fairly similar picture was noted by Chubb and Rowell (1959) in chickens from hatch to 50 days old, except that there was no dramatic fall in basophils during the first week. However, in a study of immature chickens, taken at weekly intervals between the ages of 1 and 10 weeks, Fredrickson *et al* (1957) found relatively stable values for lymphocytes, heterophils and basophils throughout the whole period (approximately 70, 25 and 1 per cent respectively), suggesting that haematological maturation had occurred within the first week. The only clearly determined change was the reduction in the ratio of large to small lymphocytes that occurred throughout the whole period.

Similar changes in differential counts during growth and development have not been reported in other poultry species (Kaleta & Bernhardt 1968, goose; Atwal *et al* 1964 and Nirmalan & Robinson 1971, quail), although in geese there is a small drop in heterophils between 5 and 30 days of age (Kaleta & Bernhardt 1968). In fact in quail (Atwal *et al* 1964) the low levels of heterophils (about 25 per cent) and the high levels of lymphocytes (about 70 per cent) found at 1 day old gradually increase and decrease respectively until at and after sexual maturity the 2 cell types are present in nearly equal numbers. However, in the Bob-white quail (*Colinus virginianus*), although not strictly speaking a domesticated species, Ernst *et al* (1971) have determined post-hatching heterophil and lymphocyte trends very similar to those of the fowl.

Clearly defined trends in eosinophils and monocytes have not been demonstrated in poultry species during the period of growth and maturation.

Differential leucocyte counts have been reported as being very similar

Table 12.6 Total and differential leucocyte counts in the blood of poultry species in relation to age and sex. Total counts expressed as 10^9 cells per litre and differentials expressed as percentages

Species	Sex	Total leuco-cytes	Differential counts					Authors
			Lympho-cytes	Hetero-phils	Eosino-phils	Baso-phils	Mono-cytes	
Chicken								
0 day old	—	—	15.9	72.4	2.5	1.1	8.1	Burton & Harrison (1969)
3 day old	—	—	38.7	52.7	1.6	0.67	6.4	
8 day old	—	—	48.3	50.0	0.25	0	1.5	
20 day old	—	—	68.6	26.7	1.7	0.64	2.3	
1 week old	—	—	75	24	0	0	1	Fredrickson et al (1957)
6 week old	—	—	69	26	0	1	3	
10 week old	—	—	61	33	0	1	1	
Adult	M	19.8	59.1	27.2	1.9	1.7	10.2	Olson (1937)
Adult	F	19.8	64.6	22.8	1.9	1.7	8.9	
Adult	M	16.6	64.0	25.8	1.4	2.4	6.4	Lucas & Jamroz (1961)
Adult	F	29.4	76.1	13.3	2.5	2.4	5.7	
Quail								
1 day old	M	18	72	23	3	2	0	Atwal et al (1964)
1 day old	F	20	66	29	1	3	1	
12 day old	M	17	63	24	1	1	1	
12 day old	F	20	64	33	3	0	0	
43 day old	M	22	51	46	0	1	2	
43 day old	F	23	46	52	2	0	0	
Goose								
5 day old	—	25	37	53	0.4	1.4	8	Kaleta & Bernhardt (1969)
15 day old	—	13.7	38.8	48.2	3.5	2.7	5.2	
30 day old	—	16	55	36	4	3	7	
8 months old	—	16.8	38	44.2	5.1	3.1	10	
Duck								
6 months old	—	20.7	66.2	20.7	4.6	3.7	3.3	Soliman et al (1966)
Adult	—	23.4	61.7	24.3	2.1	1.5	10.8	
Turkey								
0.5 week old	—	15.8	40.4*	51	0.03	6	1.8	Venkataratnam & Clarkson (1962)
4 week old	—	30.7	59.8	32.4	0.3	4.9	2.1	
8 week old	—	30.4	65.1	28.5	0.8	2.6	3.0	
Adult	M	37.2	56.2	37.8	0.3	4.2	1.5	
Adult	F	37.3	56.3	38	0.3	4.4	1.3	

in mature males and females of many poultry species (Olson 1937, chicken; Venkataratnam & Clarkson 1962, turkey; Atwal *et al* 1964, quail; see Table 12.6). However, in the chicken lymphocytes in the male tend to be lower whilst heterophils tend to be higher than in the female (Olson 1937) and these trends are particularly marked in the figures quoted for White Leghorns by Lucas and Jamroz (1961). On the other hand there is a tendency in mature quail for heterophils in the female to be slightly higher and lymphocytes to be slightly lower than in the male (Atwal *et al* 1964). Monocytes are more numerous in the blood of cocks than of hens (Olson 1959).

Various factors can affect the different cellular components of the differential count, and the effects of such factors as environment, hormones, drugs and X-irradiation have been discussed by Sturkie (1965) and Freeman (1971). The most important of these factors, however, is disease, and this subject is not relevant to this chapter.

PATHOLOGY AND PATHOGENESIS OF THE AVIAN LEUCOSIS COMPLEX AND ITS DIAGNOSIS

C. le Q. DARCEL

13.1 INTRODUCTION

This chapter is concerned with diseases of the cellular elements of the blood produced by 2 groups of oncogenic viruses affecting poultry. The first is the leucosis and sarcoma group (L-S viruses) which produce tumours and leukaemias in the chicken. The second group is the herpesvirus group (H viruses), which cause neoplastic and inflammatory lesions of the lymphoid system of chickens—in which the disease is most commonly known as Marek's disease (MD)—and also in turkeys.

The L-S viruses are endogenous viruses which can be experimentally induced in morphologically normal chicken cells by physical and chemical carcinogens (Weiss *et al* 1971). Antigens denoting the presence of the virus genome can be detected in normal as well as infected cells (Vaheri & Ruoslahti 1973, Chen & Hanafusa 1974, Baluda 1972, Allen & Sarma 1972). In nature the L-S viruses are probably released and become pathogenic for the host following other unknown triggering factors.

H viruses are transmitted horizontally; it is possible that L-S viruses, by altering cell susceptibility, may be involved in the pathogenesis of H viruses (Frankel & Groupé 1971, Peters *et al* 1973, Hirumi *et al* 1974).

Avian leucosis is studied to obtain information in viral carcinogenesis, and because the leucoses cause serious losses in the poultry industry. Recent reviews on the L-S viruses and H viruses and the diseases they produce include those by Purchase (1972) and Biggs (1973) in which will be found many references to aspects not fully discussed here.

Ellerman and Bang (Ellerman 1922), in advancing the first classification of avian leucosis, distinguished the following forms: lymphogenous leukaemia (lymphoid leucosis), myelogeneous leukaemia (myeloblastosis), and a form characterized by anaemia with many erythroblasts which would now be termed erythroblastosis. Marek's disease was recognized in 1907 and for some years was grouped as neural lymphomatosis with lymphoid leucosis ('visceral lymphomatosis') but separated again when the H and L-S viruses were differentiated.

The present classification of these diseases has been aided by the application of modern virological tests, for instance, the RIF test (Resistance Inducing Factor) and Complement Fixation Test for Avian Leucosis (COFAL test). Accordingly the 'leucosis complex' in fowls has been classified as follows (Burmester & Witter 1966):

DISEASES CAUSED BY RIF-POSITIVE AGENTS (L-S VIRUSES)
   lymphoid leucosis;
   myeloblastosis;
   myelocytomatosis;
   erythroblastosis, proliferative and anaemic;
   fibrosarcoma, endothelioma, nephroblastoma, and osteopetrosis*

DISEASES CAUSED BY RIF-NEGATIVE AGENTS (H VIRUSES)
   Marek's disease.

* Osteopetrosis is a virus-induced bone disease closely associated with the leucoses.

13.2 L-S VIRUS-INDUCED TUMOURS

Most chickens contain in their cells the genetic information necessary for the endogenous production of the L-S viruses, the multiplication of which may or may not be followed by the development of tumours or leukaemias. In other species it is known that these viruses may induce non-neoplastic diseases such as glomerulonephritis and autoimmune haemolytic anaemia. It is not known whether similar non-neoplastic conditions caused by the L-S viruses exist in the fowl but osteopetrosis and erythroblastosis may fall into this category. The definitely neoplastic conditions caused by the L-S viruses tend to occur in the older bird and, as will be noted later, may be hormone dependent. Where solid tumours develop in an intramuscular or subcutaneous location, they grow quickly to a size where birds carrying them can be recognized without difficulty. The thickening of the leg bones caused by the virus inducing osteopetrosis also makes it possible to detect affected birds before death. With these exceptions, however, most cases of disease caused by these viruses are not detected until they reach the autopsy table.

13.2.1 ROUS SARCOMA

Both neoplastic and non-neoplastic lesions develop within 48–72 hours after the subcutaneous injection of partly purified Rous sarcoma virus (RSV) into chicks. Fibroblasts are altered morphologically into fusiform and round cells. A lymphocytic response develops around the periphery of the lesion consisting of perivascular infiltrations, lymphoid plaques or dense aggregations of lymphocytes. The latter begin to disappear after the 6th day.

Palpable tumours appear 5–6 days after inoculation of large doses of RSV into the breast muscle and rapidly increase in size due to production of mucin. The mucin production is not a host defence mechanism since fast-growing tumours produce more mucopolysaccharide and more virus than slow-growing tumours. There is early metastasis to the lungs, liver and spleen. Virus is present in the induced tumours and in apparently normal tissues such as plasma, buffy coat and bone marrow.

Age (Cotter *et al* 1973) and the route of inoculation influence the pathogenesis of RSV. A haemorrhagic disease may follow when the virus is inoculated intravenously into embryos or young chicks, but when RSV is inoculated intracerebrally the loose connective tissue of the pia arachnoid space at first shows indefinite and transitory hyperplastic changes, which later become neoplastic and metastatic. Bursectomy does not influence the pathogenesis of the disease induced by the virus (McArthur *et al* 1972). Birds with RSV-induced sarcomas show a great increase in plasma lactate dehydrogenase and there are also changes in nucleoside kinase activity.

C. le Q. Darcel

13.2.2 LYMPHOID LEUCOSIS

This condition is now recognized as a lymphoblastoma caused by lymphoid leucosis virus (LLV), originating in the bursa of Fabricius and spreading to other organs with enlargement of the liver (Fig. 13.1) and tumour involvement of other organs. Bursectomy at an early age prevents the disease from developing when LLV is injected into chicks. Changes first occur in the bursa of Fabricius at 5–8 weeks after infection when the lymphoid follicles become engorged with lymphoblasts. When the bird reaches sexual maturity the cells

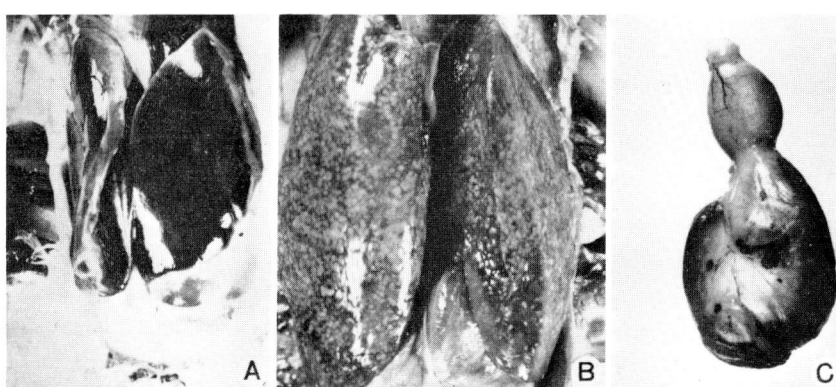

Fig. 13.1 Birds infected with LLV develop a variety of neoplastic conditions, lymphoid leucosis, haemangiomas and osteopetrosis. A—A typical congested appearance of liver in erythroblastosis with a gelatinous transudate covering surface of the liver, often observed in those birds developing an ascites. Also typical of erythroblastosis is a greatly enlarged and congested spleen. B—Involvement of the liver in lymphoid leucosis can take different forms, such as the great enlargement of the liver with visible tumours shown here. C—Haemangiomas appear as dark nodules mostly on the serosal surfaces (gizzard) but can occur elsewhere. (Osteopetrosis is illustrated in Fig. 13.4.)

in the transformed follicles acquire neoplastic characteristics and divide rapidly and encroach upon normal tissue. There is coalescence of adjacent neoplastic follicles into tumours which metastasize. The local and distant growths are composed of the same type of neoplastic lymphoblasts which show many mitotic figures. Both the cortical and medullary portions of the follicles of early bursal lesions show blast cells with a pyroninophilic cytoplasm. Transformed follicles are surrounded by normal ones which contain only a few lymphoblasts and a few pyroninophilic cells. Neoplastic follicles are well circumscribed in the spleen and are situated in close proximity to small arterioles.

The growth of the tumours in the liver may take 2 different forms— discrete or diffuse. The liver in the diffuse form is greatly enlarged with a smooth textured or mottled surface, and grey or red in colour; in the discrete form, it is moderately enlarged and studded with firm, circumscribed greyish-white or cream-coloured tumours of varying sizes. Diffuse and discrete forms may coexist in the same liver. Lymphoid leucosis is essentially extravascular; leukaemia is not common although terminal metastases in the bone marrow, pancreas, thymus and gonads may occur.

Lymphoid leucosis is not the only neoplastic condition initiated by laboratory strains of LLV; osteopetrosis, haemangiomatosis and erythro-blastosis also may develop. The most likely explanation for this is that stocks of LLV contain more than one kind of oncogenic virus, each producing a different type of neoplasm.

The less frequent occurrence of lymphoid leucosis in males and the delay in deaths from lymphoid leucosis until sexual maturity suggests hormone-dependence. Sex differences disappear when males are castrated or when chickens are intravenously inoculated with the blood of birds with lymphoid leucosis. Androgens appear to inhibit the development of lymphoid leucosis although deaths from other causes are increased in number. The influence of sex hormones and castration may possibly be related to the bursal influences since the administration of androgens inhibits the development of the bursa of Fabricius.

Infection of birds with LLV may upset the normal function of other organs and tissues (i.e. the adrenal cortex is enlarged and the level of plasma lactate dehydrogenase is increased in birds with spontaneous lymphoid leucosis). Again, the neoplastic changes of the lymphoid system might be expected to lead to immunological disturbances. In fact, the production of antibodies to some, but not all, antigens is impaired in birds infected with LLV.

13.2.3 LYMPHOID TUMOURS

Tumours are readily obtained by transplantation of cellular material from cases of lymphoid leucosis and transplantable lymphoid tumour strains have been established. When suspensions of tumour cells from these transplantable tumours are injected into young chicks, a tumour appears within a few days at the site of the inoculation and there is rapid and extensive metastasis to the liver where the tumour growth is extravascular. The rapid encroachment of the tumour cells on the host tissues leads to secondary physiological effects such as a reduction in plasma albumin concentration and occasionally a re-duction of the globulins as well. The plasma γ globulin level rises rapidly when the tumour regresses. The β_2 globulin fraction also progressively increases. There is an increase of xanthine dehydrogenase activity in the liver of tumour-bearing birds (Horn *et al* 1974). Studies of the sex chromosome of tumour cells, especially, have been helpful in determining whether trans-planted tumours are virus- or cell-initiated. Chromosome numbers in virus-induced tumours do not appear to differ greatly from the normal number, and are usually diploid or hyperdiploid.

13.2.4 ERYTHROBLASTOSIS

Following the inoculation of erythroblastosis virus (EbV), the first histological changes in the bone marrow are restricted to erythroblastic tissue. Small localized bud-like proliferations of pro-erythroblastic cells form along the sinusoids and ultimately involve their whole surface. The 'tumour' cells that develop from these pro-erythroblastic buds resemble developing erythroid cells and have a strongly basophilic cytoplasm. Within 4 days after inoculation of EbV, all the normal bone marrow is replaced by erythroblastic tissue (Fig. 13.2). Leukaemic cells reach the liver on the 7th day, coinciding with the appearance of a few tumour cells in the peripheral blood. The tumour cells remain intrasinusoidal but their accumulation can lead to pressure atrophy of adjacent liver cells. The earliest quantitative sign of an erythrocytic disturbance in the blood may occur on the day after EbV inoculation when polychromatic erythrocytes increase and then decline in most birds to the normal level of 0·5 per cent. In typical cases, erythroblasts begin to appear by the 3rd or 4th day and are then replaced terminally by tumour cells when large numbers of these cells are found in the blood stream. There are many mitotic figures in the tumour cells and degenerative changes such as vacuolation of the cytoplasm may also occur. Frequent blood sampling will result in thrombocytosis and the appearance of small round cells.

Under our laboratory conditions, birds inoculated with EbV strain R die 9–10 days after inoculation, with a diffusely enlarged, cherry-red liver and spleen. Solid tumours rarely develop although erythroblastomas have been observed. The bone marrow is semiliquid and bright red. Ascites occurs and haemorrhages in the subcutaneous tissue and viscera are common. An anaemic form of erythroblastosis may occur with some strains of EbV in which the visceral organs show extensive accumulations of small, round cells and localized areas of leucostasis.

Attempts to show cell transformation with EbV have been equivocal. Are the erythroblasts in erythroblastosis normal cells produced in response to

---

Fig. 13.2 Changes in bone marrow and liver due to infection with EbV. Tumour cells appear in isolated foci about 3 days after infection and eventually replace the normal bone marrow. A—Normal sinusoid. B—3 days after infection, proliferating tumour cells at upper left. C—3 days after infection, almost complete replacement with tumour cells. D—8 days after infection, very few normal cells left. E—Tumour cells present in liver sinusoid. Sections of bone marrow magnified 500–1000 times.

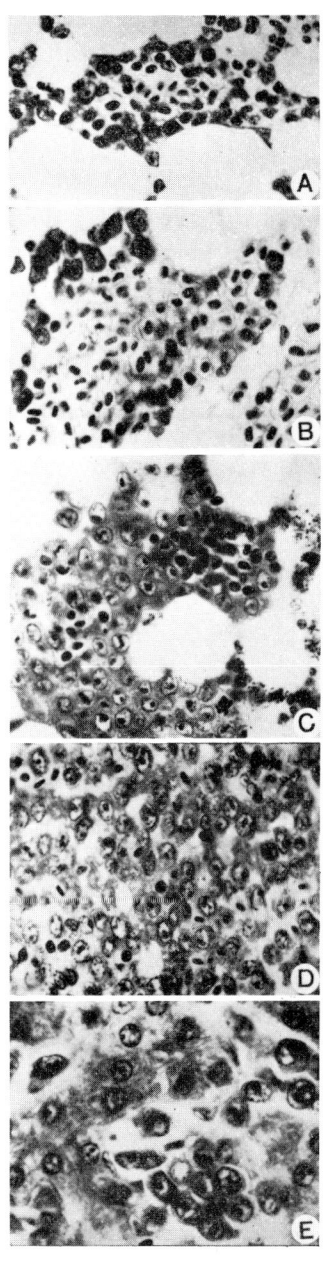

a virus-induced haemolysis? There is, in fact, an increase in plasma haemo-globin and other indications of haemolytic anaemia are present; unfortunately other proofs of red cell destruction have not yet been obtained.

There may be a variable shortening of the life span of red cells in erythro-blastosis but the extremely rapid course of the disease makes results of the red cell survival studies questionable. The circulating red cells in erythroblastosis are more resistant to osmotic lysis than the red cells of normal birds. There is no change in the sensitivity of the red blood cells to saponin and lysoleci-thin, and Coombs tests that have been carried out so far have proved nega-tive. If cell destruction is responsible for the increased liberation into the blood stream of proerythroblasts, it would be pointless to show that the development of erythroblastosis follows a failure to synthesize haemoglobin. However, the incubation of leukaemic blood with radioiron does suggest that iron accumulates in ferritin rather than in haemoglobin.

There are several other terminal plasma changes; those possibly related to the considerable increase in plasma volume and to the impaired plasma clearance, and there are other changes of an unknown origin. The greatly increased plasma volume may explain the apparent level of certain substances, for instance, the lowering of plasma alkaline phosphatase (AP), K^+, Ca^{++} and lipid phosphorus and the free haptoglobin. The expansion of plasma volume leads to an underestimation, by as much as 100 per cent of the true level of plasma components. There are also terminal elevations of haemo-globin and methaemalbumin, bilirubin, plasma lactate dehydrogenase (LDH), total non-haem iron (which has proved to be ferritin) and inorganic phosphorus. Functional impairment of the liver and reticulo-endothelial system may be responsible for the increased levels of some of these substances. Phosphatidyl serine seems to be especially reduced and may lower the electrical charge in α lipoprotein leading to its altered electro-phoretic mobility. The electrophoretic changes of the serum proteins and the fall of plasma AP may be due to the anorexic state of chickens with erythroblastosis.

Many of the systemic effects of avian erythroblastosis may not be directly attributable to the virus. Although other alterations may be of a more specific nature, some of the biochemical changes we have observed are in part due to the nonspecific effects of an anorexia, a slower plasma clearance rate and an increased plasma volume. These changes may appear unimportant but they could follow earlier biochemical alterations in the disease.

Work with leucosis viruses is frequently complicated by the presence of more than one agent in the inoculum and some of the biochemical changes we have observed in erythroblastosis may be due to the presence of other viruses.

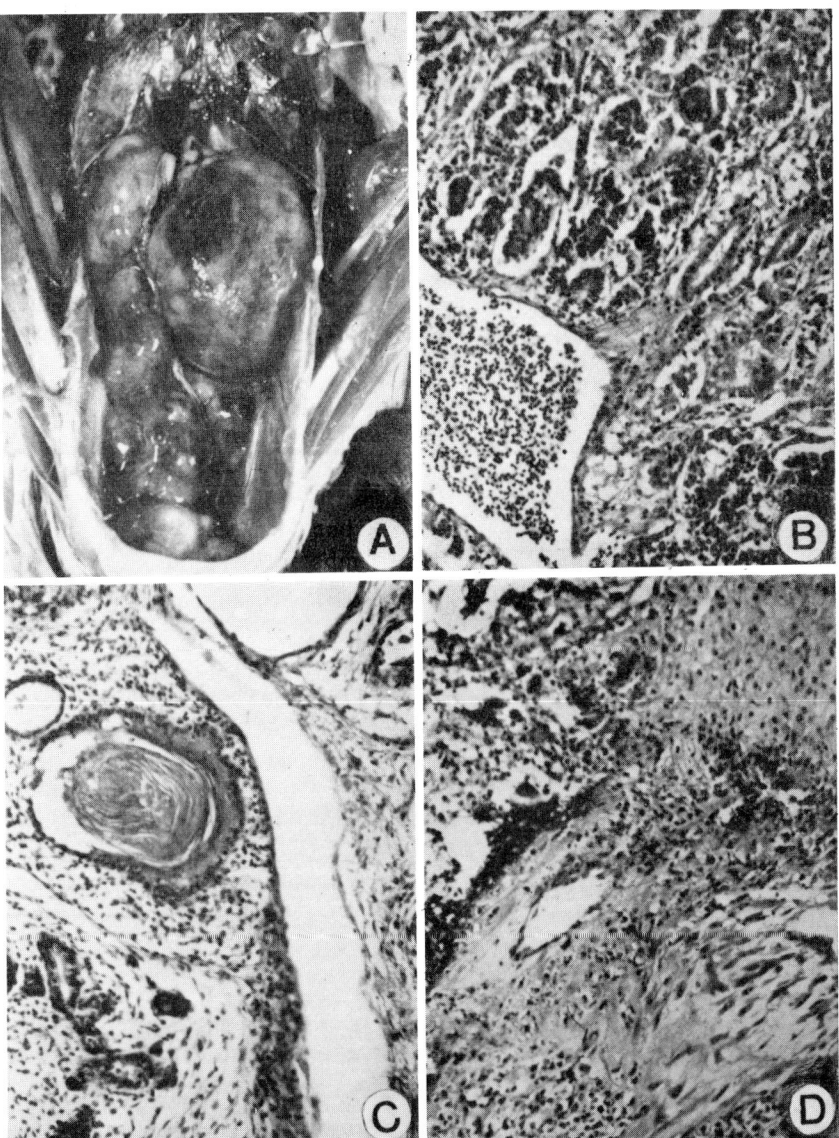

Fig. 13.3 Kidney tumours of birds infected with MbV. A—Kidney tumours at necropsy. B–D—Histology of kidney tumours. B—Embryonic kidney tissue interspersed with connective tissue; blood vessel at lower left contains many leukaemia cells. C—Teratomatous formation, pearl formation and columnar and tubular epithelium. D—Teratomatous formation, bone and cartilage.

13.2.5 MYELOBLASTOSIS (GRANULOBLASTOSIS, DIFFUSE FORM OF MYELOID LEUCOSIS)

Myeloblastosis is characterized terminally by the appearance of myeloblasts and myelocytes in large numbers $(300 \times 10^9/l)$ in the blood stream. Myeloblasts and myelocytes invade the visceral organs and other tissues, and the cells forming these infiltrations continue to divide, producing massive perivascular accumulations around the blood vessels, with replacement of the organ parenchyma. At autopsy the affected organs are usually greatly enlarged and often show greyish mottling of the surface. There is a tendency for the disease to occur along with erythroblastosis. Cases of acute anaemia and kidney tumours of the Wilms type (Fig. 13.3) may occur following infection with myeloblastosis virus (MbV).

Chick embryos inoculated intravenously at 11–12 days of incubation with large doses of MbV develop myeloblastosis within a few days after hatching but with smaller doses of virus, neoplasia may not develop for several months and may take various forms (i.e. kidney tumours, transmissible strains of which are available (Weiler *et al* 1971), myeloblastosis, erythroblastosis, osteopetrosis and lymphoid leucosis). This wide spectrum of tumour types probably means that there is more than one L-S virus present in the laboratory stock. When 3-day-old chicks are used instead of embryonated eggs, very large doses of virus induce only an 80 per cent incidence of myeloblastosis leucosis, and after 3 days of age resistance to the virus increases markedly.

Failure of infected myeloblasts to differentiate normally may lead to an abnormal metabolic behaviour. This could influence cell survival times although studies on this have not been reported. There are alternations in the glucose and lactate concentrations in the plasma. Another secondary effect is the high level of ATPase activity in the plasma. This results from the association of ATPase with virus particles, present in large numbers in leukaemic plasmas. Another feature of the leukaemic myeloblasts that must have secondary effects on the metabolism of the host is their requirement of high concentrations of folic acid.

13.2.6 MYELOCYTOMA

This neoplasm is characterized by friable chalky or yellowish-white masses of tumour tissue. Tumours consisting of compact masses of myeloblasts and myelocytes are often situated on the sternum along the border of the ribs at the costovertebral junction and in the pelvis. The myelocytes show full eosinophil or heterophil granulation. The blood is often anaemic and clots slowly or not at all. Viruses producing myelocytoma have been isolated, one, after intravenous inoculation into young chickens, causes myelocytomas in

3–11 weeks (Bozhkov 1972). Many other types of neoplasms can follow the inoculation of this virus: hepatomas, mesotheliomas of the peritoneum and pericardium, and renal adenocarcinomas, erythroblastosis and lymphoid leucosis.

13.2.7 HAEMANGIOMATOSIS

Haemangiomatosis is sometimes seen in conjunction with erythroblastosis following the inoculation of LLV. The tumours are small, sharply circumscribed raised nodules, dark red in colour on the serosal surfaces of the abdominal viscera, air sacs and peritoneum (Fig. 13.1). They can be classified histologically as well-differentiated capillary and cavernous haemangiomas.

13.2.8 OSTEOPETROSIS

Osteopetrosis is rarely seen in the field but is frequently observed in transmission experiments with LLV. Other L-S virus strains causing osteopetrosis are also available including one which produces the disease before other forms of neoplasia develop. As chickens genetically resistant to 3 of the L-S virus subgroups are susceptible to osteopetrosis virus, the latter may be only distantly related to the former (Fritzsche 1972).

Osteopetrosis is not neoplastic in the sense of the bone-forming tumours of mammals or of the osteochondrosarcoma of chickens. It has also been known as hypertrophic osteitis and diffuse osteoperiostitis and it resembles some human bone diseases.

Birds with osteopetrosis have an anaemic, unthrifty appearance. Many develop leg fractures and the long bones are enlarged but soft and friable. The first alteration seen following experimental infection is an increase in the size and number of cells in the deep layer of the periosteum, the endosteum and in the Haversian canals. These alterations progress rapidly and there is lysis of compact bone (Fig. 13.4). If death from unthriftiness, lameness and secondary infection does not occur, a phase of endochondrial osteogenesis begins. There is mineralization of new cartilage resulting in imperfectly structured bone. Overgrowth and increasing hardness of the diaphysial bone follow and this may lead to the obliteration of the bone marrow.

Changes in other organs may occur. A markedly atrophic and fibrous spleen, and changes in the parathyroids often accompany this disease. It has been assumed that the action of the virus on the skeleton produces a secondary hyperparathyroid response, which is characterized by a rise in blood Ca^{++} and a fall in inorganic phosphorus, leading to secondary demineralization.

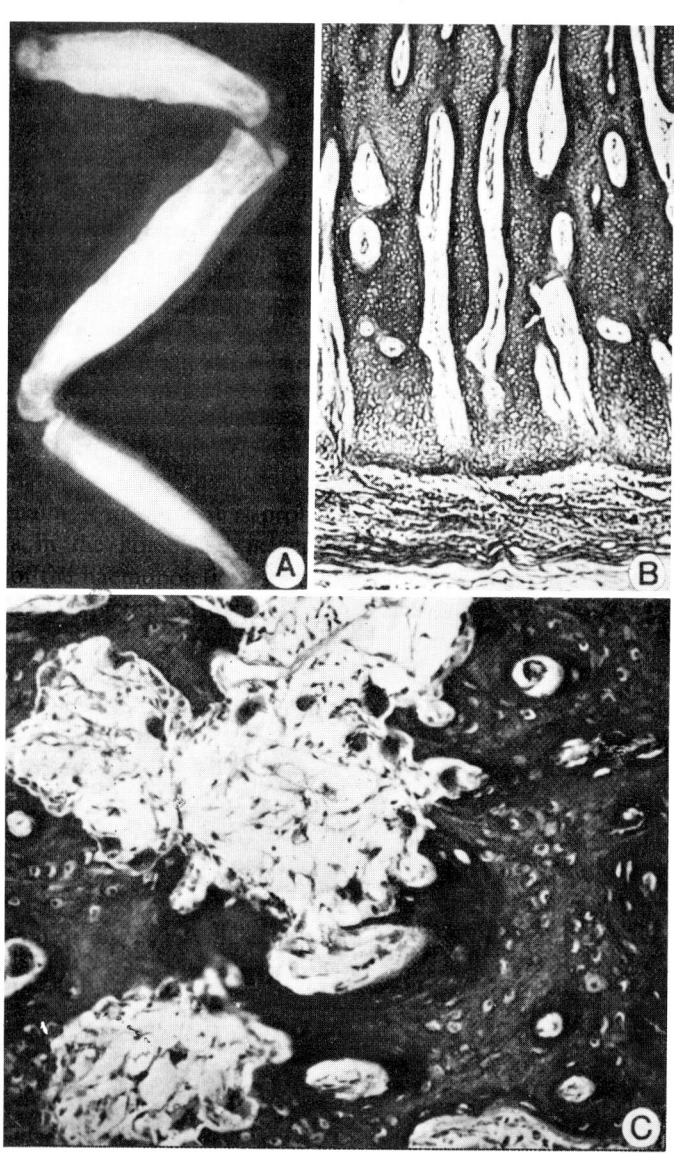

Fig. 13.4 Osteopetrosis. A—X-ray showing complete obliteration of medullary cavity of long bones. B—Trabeculae converging to centre of shaft. C—Area of bone resorption.

13.3   H VIRUS-INDUCED TUMOUR

13.3.1   MAREK'S DISEASE

MD differs between flocks in its manifestations. In some flocks neural involvement predominates, often showing clinically as paralysis of the affected limb; in others, tumours develop in the viscera or skin. Cases of the disease can occur at 6 weeks of age or earlier (i.e. in young broilers) and there may be heavy losses. It has been mentioned that where the neural form of the disease predominates and causes losses of birds between 3 and 5 months of age in up to 30 per cent of the flock, the outbreak is termed classical MD; but when larger numbers of younger birds die with little evidence of neural involvement, the outbreak is said to be due to acute MD. Symptoms are thus determined by the form of the disease. In the neural form the degree of paralysis is variable and the symptoms vary considerably from bird to bird depending on the nerve affected. Where the legs are affected the gait may be impaired at first and only noted when the birds are disturbed. Later, birds may be unable to rise. When other nerves are affected, this may lead to a drooping of one wing and signs of respiratory distress. The birds may also show muscular atrophy and loss of weight, and may appear anaemic. The disease progresses slowly until the bird dies because it can no longer get to food or water. The most noticeable feature of acute MD is a mortality rate that may reach 60 per cent, a generally depressed condition of the birds, and some of the birds developing symptoms similar to classical MD. In experimentally transmitted acute MD, histological lesions are seen in the heart and liver as early as the 3rd day. The initial changes consist of mesenchymal cell proliferation around the adventitia of small veins and capillaries. There is differentiation of these cells into lymphoid cells which form perivascular foci which may become neoplastic or regress (Payne & Roskowski 1972, Payne & Rennie 1973). Cowdry type A nuclear inclusion bodies are occasionally seen, notably in the epithelial cells of the proventriculus (Ratz *et al* 1972, Kardevan *et al* 1973, Sharma *et al* 1973, Frazier 1974). Chromosome breakage has been observed in MD-H virus-induced tumours but this is disputed (Kim *et al* 1972).

The severity of the response seems to depend on whether or not the chicks have maternal antibody. If they have, the lesions are absent or greatly suppressed. Nazerian (1973) has recently reviewed the cellular composition of MD tumours which contain lymphoid cells derived from both the thymus (T) and bursa (B) dependent lymphoid systems. However, the large majority of the cells are T cells (Calnek 1972, Eidison *et al* 1972, Burgoyne & Witter 1973, Hudson & Payne 1973, Rouse *et al* 1973, Doak *et al* 1973). Involvement of cells of the B and T series lowers the immunological responsiveness of MD affected birds to other antigens (Evans & Patterson 1971, 1972, Evans *et al* 1971, Burg *et al* 1971, Jakowski *et al* 1973).

532   *C. le Q. Darcel*

Different effects are exerted by Marek's disease virus on the immunological systems compared with LLV. In susceptible chickens infected with MD, perhaps due to a general debility, there are at least 3 definite changes. The graft versus host reaction is enhanced, homograft rejection is delayed and the antibody response is decreased resulting from the disease process. Specific antibodies to H viruses can be demonstrated in the sera of affected birds.

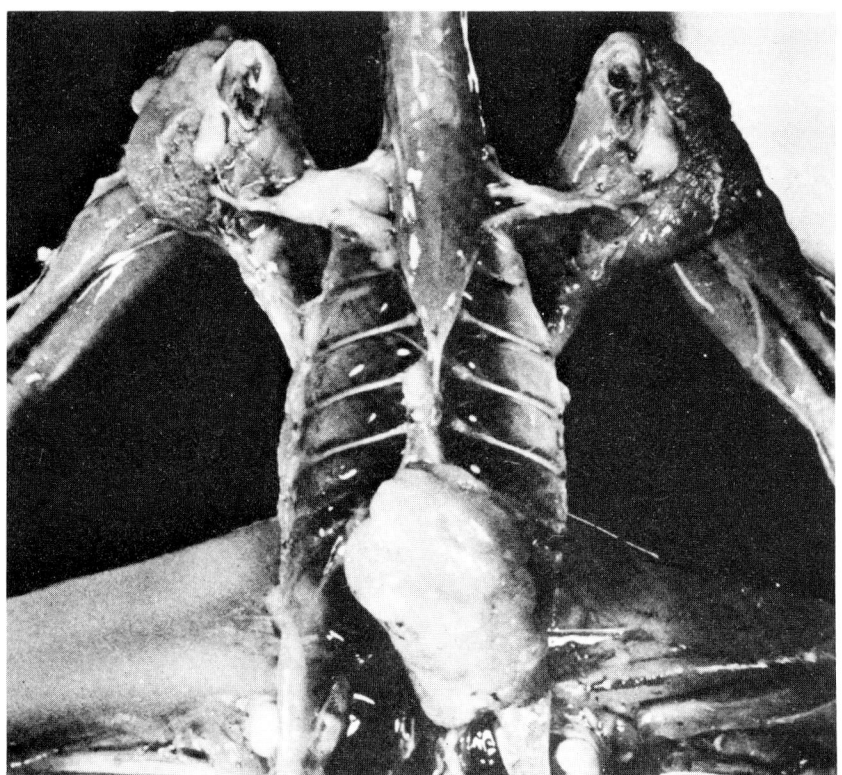

Fig. 13.5 Marek's disease, necropsy appearance, ovarian tumour and involvement of right brachial plexus.

Factors such as influence of age at exposure (Calnek 1973, Witter *et al* 1973), genetic resistance (Sharma & Stone 1972, Grunder *et al* 1972, 1974, Han & Smyth 1973), feed intake and growth, etc. (Han & Smyth, 1972a b) and even haemoglobin type (Washburn *et al* 1971) also affect the number of clinical cases. Unlike lymphoid leucosis, bursectomy has no effect on the development of MD (Fernando & Calnek 1971, Sharma 1974).

When there is neural involvement in MD the nerves lose their glistening white appearance and become more opaque. In the central nervous system, there are perivascular infiltrations with lymphoid cells, although endotheliosis and focal areas of gliosis may also occur. Proliferative lymphoid lesions occur more frequently in the spinal cord and the peripheral nerves than in the brain. The sciatic, vagus and brachial nerves and the dorsal root ganglia are all commonly involved in classical MD (Fig. 13.5). When tumours occur, these are found especially in the gonads and dermis. The reasons for the preferential production of lesions in the ovaries, dermis and peripheral nerves are not clear, as the virus grows well in cells derived from other organs, such as the kidney.

Lymphoid tumours are more frequent in females than in males, possibly because of a predilection for the ovary. The age of the bird also seems to influence the distribution of lesions. Visceral lesions are more common in the acute type of MD which affects younger birds. The thymus and the bursa of Fabricius may be enlarged due to lymphocytic infiltrations but atrophy and degeneration may also occur in these organs. In some birds, however, there is enlargement of the bursa due to lymphocytic infiltrations between the follicles which may become cystic. Studies of hormonal and surgical bursectomy on the incidence of MD have produced conflicting results.

Skin lesions due to MD often occur in broilers affected with MD and may lead to the condemnation of up to 10 per cent of consignments to packing plants (Willemart and Schricke, 1972a b). At about 9 weeks of age in birds developing this condition, the skin becomes thickened with hypertrophy of feather follicles. Most affected birds have fewer than 5 discrete skin lesions (Lapen & Kenzy 1972). Lymphoid cell accumulations, inflammatory in appearance, first develop around the feather follicles; later they become neoplastic in character. Intranuclear eosinophilic inclusion bodies may also be seen in the feather follicles (Lapen *et al* 1971, Sharma *et al* 1972).

The histology of early peripheral nerve lesions is typical of an inflammatory change with cellular infiltrations of lymphocytes, plasma cells, macrophages, heterophils and monocytes. There may be Schwann cell proliferation and myelin sheath degeneration with similar changes in the spinal cord. Electron microscope studies have shown thickening of axons and their fibrils, breakdown of the myelin sheath, increase in collagen fibres and enlargement and degeneration of the Schwann cells. Nerves in MD examined with light electron microscopy show changes essentially similar to the above (Okada & Fujimoto 1971, Doi *et al* 1973, Grundboeck *et al* 1973). The breakdown of the myelin sheath is similar to that in allergic neuritis and it has been suggested that the nerve changes in MD may be the result of a virus-induced autoimmune demyelinating disease (Prineas & Wright 1972).

The proliferative lesions of lymphoid tissue contain small and medium lymphocytes, and other cells encountered in an inflammatory response. The blood is usually normal, although there is evidence of haemopoietic system involvement.

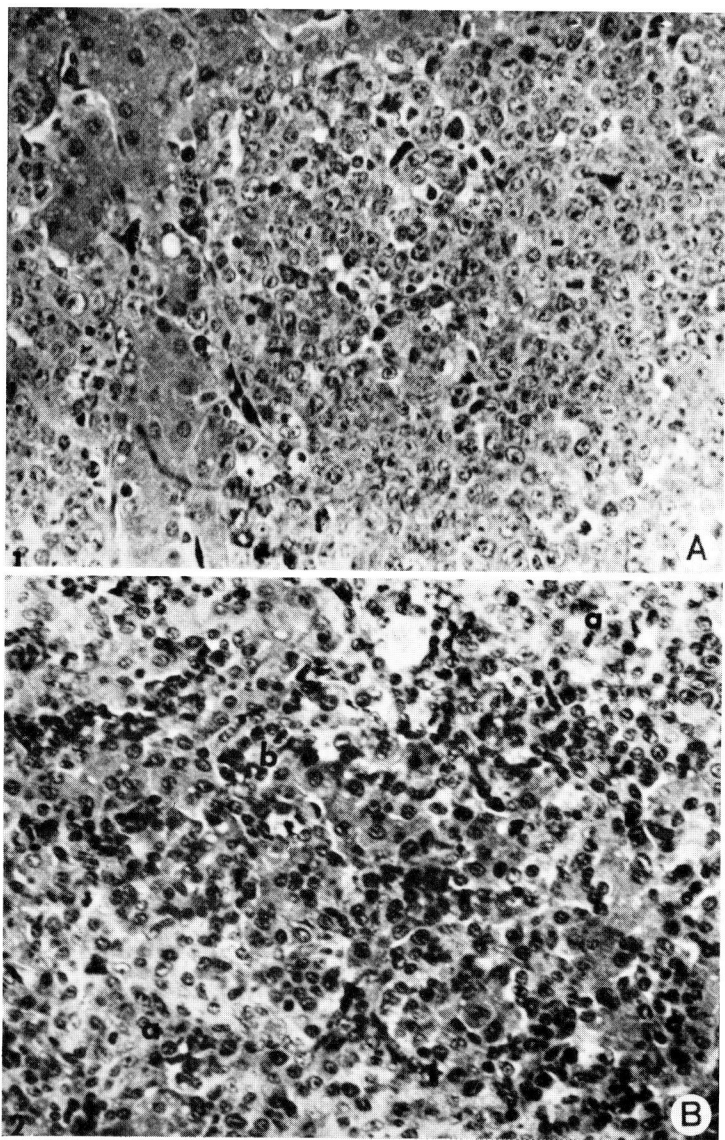

Fig. 13.6 Comparison of histology of liver tumours in lymphoid leucosis (A) and Marek's disease (B). A—Tumour nodules composed of uniform lymphoblasts. B—Infiltrating cells are small, not uniform and more suggestive of an inflammatory lesion.

The heterogeneity of the cell types in MD is characteristic and in marked contrast to that occurring in lymphoid leucosis, where tumour cells are uniformly large lymphoblasts (Fig. 13.6). However, it is often difficult to distinguish MD from lymphoid leucosis on the basis of histopathology, although methyl-green pyronin staining of fixed tissue sections and tumour smears can be helpful. The differential diagnosis of these 2 diseases is discussed by Yamamoto *et al* (1972), Beyer and Urbaneck (1972), Beyer and Vogel (1972), and Purchase and Sharma (1974).

Although it may be extremely difficult to find virus-like particles by electron microscopy of MD tumours, they can be detected in the feather follicles. Circulating lymphocytes from birds with MD can be shown to contain virus by tissue culture procedures.

A start has been made on the biochemistry of the disease. It has been found in vitro that transfer RNA methylase activity of the liver is increased up to 200 per cent compared with that of the liver of unaffected birds. This enzyme is increased in a variety of neoplastic conditions, and it is suggested that oncogenic viruses introduce methylase activities foreign to the host cell and produce an altered pattern of nucleic acid methylation. In MD, as in erythroblastosis, Rous sarcoma and lymphoid leucosis, there is an elevation of plasma LDH, but the Mg^{++} activated DNA polymerase present in lymphoid leucosis is absent in MD tumours (Muto *et al* 1974). Other tissue enzyme changes especially important in MD are increased liver malate dehydrogenase, and ovarian acid phosphatase and decreased liver sorbitol dehydrogenase (Jarajda *et al* 1973). Increased levels of β globulin were found in the sera of MDV-H virus affected birds (Ringen & Dickson 1974). Chromatographic studies of the lipid distribution in affected nerves show a quantitative increase in cholesterol esters and a decrease in triolein components in the acute form of the disease. In more chronic cases of MD there is a total loss of methyl esters and tripalmitin, and in some cases a marked reduction or total disappearance of cholesterol esters and triolein. These changes may be a product of a specific virus-induced demyelination.

13.4 DIAGNOSIS BY IMMUNOLOGICAL METHODS

13.4.1 L-S VIRUSES

All fowl L-S viruses contain group antigens present in the virion cores (Darcel 1973). The activity due to these antigens, of which there are at least 4, can be determined by the complement fixation (COFAL) test using sera obtained from hamsters bearing transplanted Rous sarcomas. Sera giving complement fixation with the COFAL antigen can be produced in other species (i.e. pigeon, where the yield is 100 times more than the hamster (Ayoub & Ebner 1972)). The COFAL test has been very useful for monitoring

C. le Q. Darcel

viral activity in L-S virus infected tissue cultures and egg embryos. Fluorescent antibody tests have been used for demonstrating RSV antibodies, L-S virus infection of tissue cultures and for assaying these viruses (Darcel 1973). Immunohistochemistry may also be a useful new technique in the study of these diseases (Dougherty *et al* 1972, Stefano *et al* 1973).

Recently, more reliable and more sensitive immunological methods using radioisotope labelled reagents have been developed. These newer methods are of such sensitivity that the antigen can be detected in all tissues and cultured cells from leucosis-free chickens but L-S virus infected cells contain 100–1000 times the activity of uninfected cells (Vaheri & Ruoslahti 1973); much less activity being observed in infected embryonal cells (Chen *et al* 1974).

13.4.2   H VIRUSES

The fluorescent antibody, immunodiffusion, indirect haemagglutination and complement fixation tests have all been used to assist diagnosis of the presence of specific antigens in chicken tumours and tissue cultures (Darcel 1973). The most useful of these seems to have been immunodiffusion. Sera from MDHV-infected birds react with extracts of virus infected cells and poultry skin and feathers (Eidson *et al* 1971, Marquardt 1972, Mazurenko *et al* 1972, Casnocha & Salaj 1973). An interesting feature of MD is the presence of delayed skin hypersensitivity reactions (Byerly & Dawe 1972). A recent development is a modified direct complement fixation test for MD (Marquardt & Newman 1972).

13.5   DIAGNOSIS BY TISSUE CULTURE AND EGG EMBRYO INOCULATION TECHNIQUES

13.5.1   L-S VIRUSES

The study and recognition of L-S viruses in tissue culture is complicated by the existence of 'helper' and associated viruses, and genetic variables of the tissue culture cells. Some of the viruses do not transform cells, but their presence can be detected by certain techniques. These include the RIF, COFAL and fluorescent antibody tests (Darcel 1973).

Embryonated chicken eggs inoculated on the chorioallantoic membrane or intravenously have been used for growing certain viruses of this group.

13.5.2   H VIRUSES

The virus produces micro-plaques in tissue cultures of chicken kidney cells and in duck fibroblasts after long periods of incubation, facilitating enumeration assays. MD-H virus can also be assayed in 4-day-old antibody-free chicken embryos by inoculating the test material into the yolk sacs.

14

TECHNICAL METHODS

R. K. ARCHER

Special methods for birds, R. D. Hodges, blood sampling from pigs, P. Imlah and H. S. McTaggart.

14.1 COLLECTION OF BLOOD SAMPLES

Results of examination of a specimen cannot be better than the specimen itself and good results necessitate collecting good samples. Further, if the purpose of bleeding an animal is the diagnosis of disease, then the smallest quantity satisfactory for the tests needed should be the maximum taken. Clearly this is even more important if repeated bleedings are envisaged. Further, speed and precision in the method used are necessary to achieve the best results. Imprecise punctures must be avoided and cleanliness of overlying skin is most necessary. Here the general procedure of taking blood samples will be considered, followed by detailed notes on preferred techniques for most of the species encompassed in this book.

14.1.1 APPARATUS FOR TAKING BLOOD SAMPLES

It is essential that all apparatus used in the collection of blood samples be sterile, clean and dry. Disposable needles which are really sharp are easily available and should be used. Sharpness is far more important than small diameter for painless venepuncture.

Suction apparatus for blood sampling (e.g. 'Vacutainer', Becton Dickinson) has much use, particularly in the field in wet or raining conditions. In some species, notably the horse, the use of this system is not practicable for diagnostic samples since it always leads to appreciable haemolysis of the specimens. Where a degree of haemolysis of the samples is acceptable, in blood group studies for example, suction apparatus is certainly valuable.

14.1.2 GENERAL CONSIDERATIONS AND CONTROL OF THE ANIMAL

PRACTICABLE VOLUMES OF BLOOD TO TAKE IN VARIOUS SPECIES

As a general guide, it is usually quite safe to take about 0·5 ml of blood per kg body weight in all species of the larger mammals, laboratory animals and birds. An indication of the normal circulating blood volume, the recoverable volume when sacrificed by bleeding out and the maximum safe volume to take

Table 14.1 Practicable volumes of blood to take from various animals

Animal	Total blood volume (rounded mean) ml/kg	Available volume when bled out ml/kg	Maximum safe volume at one bleeding during life ml/kg	Practicable volume for diagnostic use in ml from a normal adult
Horse	75	40	8	100
Ox	60	30	7	100
Sheep	60	25	6	20
Goat	70	30	7	20
Pig	65	25	6	10
Dog	90	45	9	2
Cat	75	35	7	1
Rabbit	70	35	7	1
Guinea-pig	75	35	7	0·5
Rat	50	20	5	0·25
Mouse	80	35	7	0·1
Chicken	60	40	9	1

at one bleeding during life are given in Table 14.1. The table also gives an idea of a practicable volume to take easily, and repeatedly, from normal adults of the various species. The figures in this table have been calculated from data of many sources, as well as from the author's own practice in the laboratory, but they can only serve as an approximate guide. In special circumstances much larger volumes of blood may be recovered or taken, but in other circumstances, for example where disease is a factor, the figures given in column 4 may be too high for safety.

The total blood volume measured as ml/kg may vary widely within the same species. Consider, for example, two dogs. One dog may be a Greyhound in training, the other an overfat pet. In the first case the blood volume will be higher than in the second case. Indeed an overall range of about 55 to 135 ml/kg has been quoted for various breeds of dog by various techniques (Altman & Dittmer 1961). As a general rule about one half of the circulating blood can be recovered when an animal is bled out, but clearly this amount cannot always be directly related to the total body weight.

The figures suggested in the last column of Table 14.1 as practicable for diagnostic purposes are based upon two assumptions. The first assumption is that the physiological status of the animal must not be materially affected by the loss of the suggested volumes and the second is that the subject is a normal, healthy adult. In young animals, and especially in the new-born, considerable caution is essential in order to avoid substantial risk.

THE EFFECT OF EXCITATION OF THE SUBJECT

When an animal is frightened or exercised considerable changes in the constitution of the circulating blood occur with great rapidity. In the horse, for example, the mere application of a 'twitch' to control the animal can cause a rise in erythrocyte count of up to 20 per cent within 2 minutes. Unfortunately the effect of even standardized exercise is inconstant. There is some evidence that animals in good athletic training can produce a larger increase when stimulated than other similar animals which have not been trained. No satisfactory tests based upon this observation have yet been described, but the effect must be borne in mind when animals are bled.

PREPARATION OF THE SKIN SITE FOR BLEEDING

The skin area to be used, whether for venepuncture, cardiac puncture or simple penetration with a lancet, should be free of hair or feathers and clean and dry. The more it approaches sterility the better, but this is a difficult goal to achieve. The use of antiseptics is acceptable provided that the skin surface is not actually wet when penetrated. Iodine in alcohol is suitable.

Close clipping with scissors is often preferable to shaving unless the latter is done with a really sharp razor avoiding cutaneous damage and consequent inflammation. Specially made electric clippers are admirable.

The area prepared should be generous. It is often an advantage to wet surrounding unclipped hair with soap and water or dilute antiseptic to avoid contamination of the site by dust or dandruff.

Another precaution, sometimes exceedingly useful, is to inject a small amount of a rapidly acting local anaesthetic intradermally over the proposed site of puncture. Two per cent lignocaine is suitable, in a dose of about 0·2 ml. The manoeuvre is especially useful in nervous, highly strung animals or where the need for large volumes of blood necessitates the use of a large needle.

TRANQUILLISERS

In difficult subjects the administration of tranquillisers before bleeding can be useful, but it has to be accepted that the agent used will to some extent change the constitution of the blood obtained. For instance, acetyl promazine is associated with haemodilution in the horse (see page 191). Where a tranquilliser is used before obtaining a blood sample, the dose and timing will be important in order to enable a correct interpretation of the findings to be attempted.

14.1.2.1 The general technique of venepuncture

The secret of successful venepuncture can be summed up in two phrases: identify the vein and its course and use a correctly sharpened needle of the proper size.

Once the vein has been selected, a sufficient skin area must be properly prepared which lies over it. The vein must be distended both to identify it and to produce an adequate blood flow from the needle when it is punctured. Either a bleeding rope or digital pressure may be used, while in some species special means are necessary. In any event, with the vein distended, identified and with a local injection of anaesthetic if required, the puncture can be made. The needle should be inserted so that it is directed towards the direction of blood flow (i.e. away from the heart) and the needle MUST BE DRY.

It is usually said that the needle should be advanced with a single swift stroke through skin, subcutaneous fascia and vein wall. Certainly this is the preferred method for the expert. The less expert, however, may find the following suggestions helpful. The needle may first be put through skin and into subcutaneous fascia without any attempt to enter the vein, but preferably so that the needle point lies over it. A single swift deliberate movement is required: not a jab and certainly not several insufficient minor jerks. Once the needle point is in the subcutaneous fascia it is largely painless and the next step can be made after due deliberation. The object is to penetrate the vein wall with a second deliberate stroke. The vein can be palpated and the needle aligned correctly before any movement is made. In this way the vein that tends to roll away from the needle may often be successfully punctured. Sometimes the needle may overpenetrate and simple withdrawal a little way may be all that is necessary to achieve a flow of blood.

When the needle is to be withdrawn, a pledget of sterile, dry cotton wool is held over the site and the needle withdrawn from beneath it. A few moments' digital pressure will usually achieve haemostasis of the skin wound. Styptics should be avoided. Collodion may be applied to the larger animals when larger needles have been used.

Neat technique with sharp needles is even more necessary if the same animal is to be bled repeatedly. Any damage to the vein and the perivascular tissue caused by incorrect attempts at puncture will make subsequent efforts far more difficult.

14.1.2.2   The general technique of arterial puncture

Since the arterial wall is highly elastic, it can be punctured with hypodermic needles without subsequent surgical repair of the vessel. It is, however, preferable to use the smallest practicable bore of needle.

Fisher (1956, 1959) has described methods for puncturing the brachial artery of the horse and the ox. A needle of 1·5 to 2 mm diameter and 200 mm long is used. It is inserted at the base of the neck, where pulsation can be felt just slightly lateral to the mid-line. Penetration is at about 5° to the horizontal for 100–180 mm for the horse (Fisher 1959) at 15° for 20–80 mm for the ox (Fisher 1956).

14.1.2.3   The general technique of cardiac puncture

Apart from specialized surgical and research techniques, cardiac puncture is used in rabbits, cats, ferrets etc. The particular heart chamber punctured is not subject to rigid control and there must also be some damage to pleura and lung.

There are 2 main routes used to approach the heart: firstly a lateral approach between the ribs and across the thoracic cavity and secondly beneath the xyphisternum and through the diaphragm. In either case the position of the heart can be identified by careful palpation before attempting puncture. As a general rule the author prefers the first method using lateral approach.

The needle should be advanced slowly, the advance immediately arrested when the heart is punctured. It is important to avoid the great vessels which lie cranial and dorsal to the heart; a true lateral or posterior approach will minimize this hazard.

14.1.2.4   Venous catheterization

When large volumes of blood are to be withdrawn or administered, or when repeated samples are required from one donor over a relatively short period of time, it is often convenient to use an indwelling venous catheter. Polythene or silicone rubber tubes are suitable and there are two main methods of inserting the catheter.

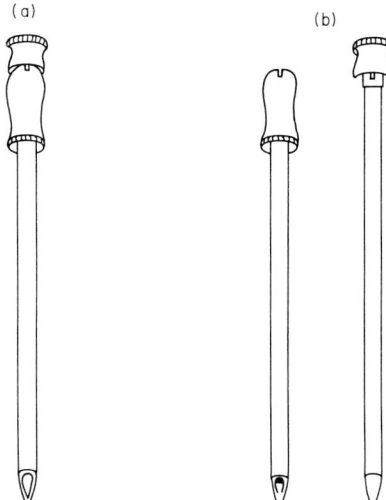

Fig. 14.1 Metal cannula used for venous catheterization. A polythene catheter is inserted into the vein through the cannula after venepuncture. The catheter used is a sliding fit in the cannula. (a) The assembled cannula with stilette, (b) cannula and stilette dismantled.

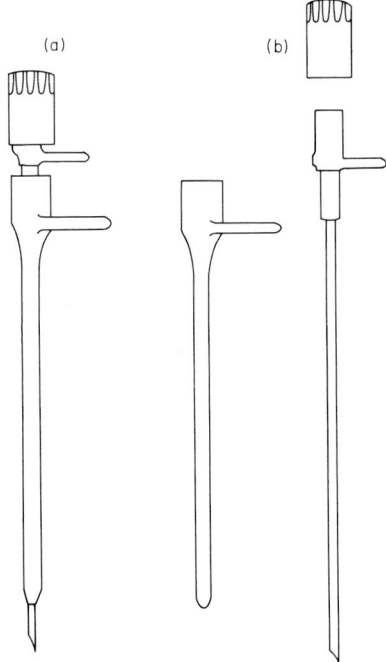

Fig. 14.2 A disposable venous catheter. (a) Assembled for insertion into the vein, (b) 'exploded' view. (Available in various sizes.)

(1) Catheterization by use of a metal cannula (Fig. 14.1). By this technique, a special cannula is inserted into the vein, after surgical exposure if necessary. The cannula must contain a closely fitting stilette which is withdrawn only after the vein is punctured. A suitable catheter, which is a sliding fit within the cannula, is then inserted through the instrument and so into the vein. The cannula is then withdrawn, leaving the catheter only in the vein.

(2) Catheterization by use of disposable apparatus (Fig. 14.2). This method differs from the previous one chiefly in that a fine, metal needle *within* the catheter is used for venepuncture. The needle is then withdrawn and discarded, leaving the catheter in the vein.

VENOUS COLLAPSE

The walls of veins are very insubstantial and some of them also contain valves. If negative pressure is applied to an indwelling needle or catheter, the vein may collapse around it so occluding the flow of blood. If this happens it is worth trying both rotation of the needle so that the bevel lies at a different angle, and reduction of the rate of blood withdrawal. In some cases it is far better to dispense altogether with negative pressure and to rely only on venous pressure to expel blood through the needle. This is particularly true of the wing vein in poultry.

14.1.3   METHODS IN VARIOUS SPECIES

This section consists of notes upon bleeding various species of animals. The preferred route, method and size of needle are considered, together with any particular notes of unusual techniques that have been found useful.

14.1.3.1   Mammalian species

HORSE

The jugular vein, with the use of a rope and bobbin or digital pressure, is the vessel of choice. A site about half way along the course of the jugular furrow is suitable. For small volumes of blood (i.e. up to 20 ml) needles of 1·25 mm diameter and 60 mm long are ideal. Larger volumes are more easily obtained with larger bore needles and those with an expanded mount are best; 3 mm diameter and about 90 mm long is a good size when several litres of blood are to be collected.

Identification of the vein is facilitated if the neck is well extended and turned somewhat away from the operator. The rate of blood flow can be considerably increased by causing the subject to chew, for instance by placing a finger through the interdental space and onto the tongue, such a manipulation to be made by the groom and not by the operator.

With excitable animals, and certainly with the larger needles, the use of an intradermal bleb of lignocaine is a distinct advantage both to horse and to the operator.

A syringe is not necessary to aspirate blood from the jugular vein of the horse and, if a syringe is necessary (for sterile samples or for accurately measured sample volumes) it is usually better to fit it to the needle after a flow of blood has been obtained.

For *new-born foals* a needle of 0·8 mm diameter about 40 mm long is used. In this case the vein is usually raised by digital pressure and a syringe is used to aspirate blood after the vein has been penetrated and digital pressure released.

OX

In general the technique and site is the same as for the horse. Somewhat larger needles are used and those with expanded mounts are preferred. The use of a rope and bobbin to raise the vein is useful. Hole (1953) recommended raising the vein by digital pressure and venepuncture about 12·5 cm below the angle of the jaw. Butler (1962) suggested a needle of 2 mm diameter 80 mm long to which is fixed a metal disc which fits the top of a polythene bottle. The needle is inserted through the cap of the bottle with the plate inside it, and protected by another bottle over the sharpened end. When used, the cap of the receiving bottle is unscrewed slightly to permit the outflow of air displaced by the blood. With this apparatus many blood samples can be collected in the field with minimal trouble. These needles are available from Arnold R. Horwell Ltd. In the *new-born calf* a needle of 1 mm diameter 50 mm long is suitable, using digital pressure to raise the vein. Aspiration with a syringe is frequently advantageous. In cows, puncture of the mammary vein may be a useful alternative to the jugular.

Williams (1966) has recommended puncture of the coccygeal vessels, especially for cattle in standings, but the sample may be arterial, venous or mixed. Using a 20 gauge needle 2·5 cm long on a syringe, puncture is made at right angles to the blood vessels, some 15 cm from the base of the tail.

SHEEP

The jugular vein provides a suitable site for bleeding, but it is necessary carefully to clip and remove the fleece from the site. It is possible to wet the fleece with soapy water and part it to obtain access to the vein, but this method is not recommended unless slight damage to the fleece is quite unacceptable. Stubbs and Boyer (1953) has recommended needles of 2 mm diameter and 80 mm long. Frequently somewhat small needles will suffice, but sheep erythrocytes are particularly prone to lysis if subjected to trauma. It is therefore important not to use needles of small internal diameter and to avoid physical damage to the samples by vigorous aspiration with a syringe.

GOAT

Apart from the fact that the fleece is not a complication, goats can be bled in the same way as sheep. With some breeds the jugular vein may not be easy to identify, but palpation and digital pressure will usually delineate the vessel adequately.

PIG (P. IMLAH and H. S. MCTAGGART)

Samples of less than 10 ml can be obtained from the ear vein. For restraint during bleeding from the ear vein, large pigs are tethered by a sliding noose tether around the snout and small piglets can be held by hand. Bleeding can be by a free flow or closed method. In the former the blood flows either across the surface of the ear after stabbing the vein, or through a needle into an open container. In the latter case the blood flows directly through a needle into a syringe or vacuum tube. There are two main external auricular veins which can be used, one which runs along the caudal edge and the other along the mid-line of the ear. It is essential that the ear is warm and veins are adequately dilated before attempting to bleed. Washing the ear with warm water and

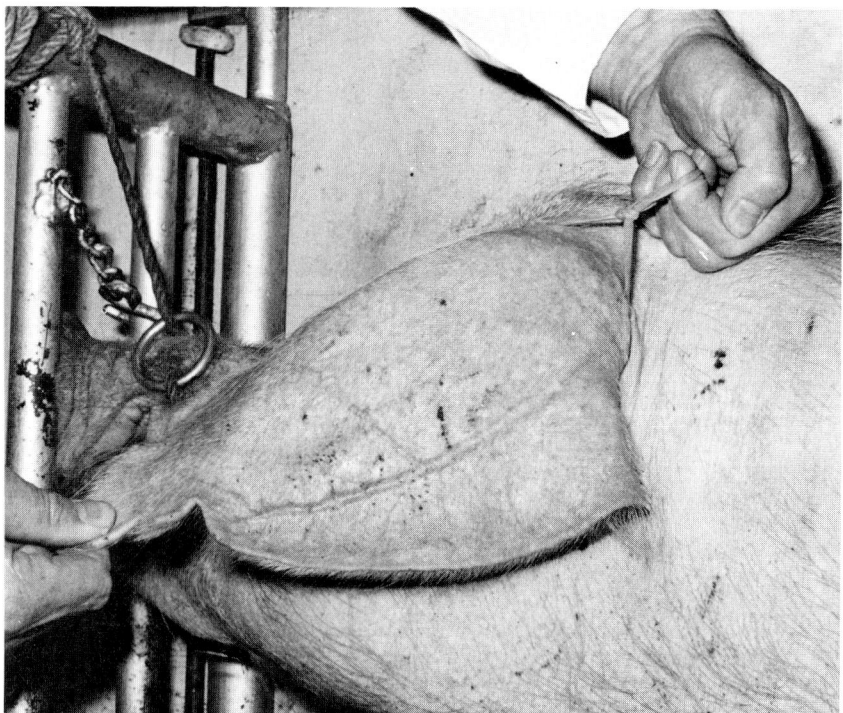

Fig. 14.3 Rubber band tourniquet placed round base of ear to raise external auricular vein.

vigorous drying with a clean towel will help to warm the ear and help vaso-dilatation. Constriction of the vein can be achieved by pressure with the thumb in small pigs and in large pigs by applying one loop of a 10×1 cm rubber band looped in the middle over the base of the ear (see Fig. 14.3). The free loop of the rubber tourniquet can be used to adjust the tension.

When free flow is used it is better to limit the sample to small quantities to avoid the possibility of clotting. Such a method is often adopted with piglets where volumes of 0·1 to 0·5 ml are adequate for haematological work. Aspiration of blood into a Thoma pipette can be achieved in this way. Larger quantities of blood by the free flow method can be obtained by smearing the surface of the skin with silicone grease and collecting blood into an open container from the caudal edge of the ear. Free flow can also be achieved by inserting a siliconized 4 cm $\times$ 1–6 mm needle into the ear vein and allowing blood to flow into a container. A small length of PVC tubing attached to the end of the needle allows the blood to be directed more easily. By the open flow method there is a greater chance of contamination and for this reason a technique employing a closed method is preferable. Drawing blood directly into a sterile disposable syringe or vacuum container using a 4 cm $\times$ 1–1·2 mm needle is recommended. The closed method is more easily carried out in adult pigs from which 10–30 ml quantities of blood can be obtained.

For larger volumes of blood the anterior vena cava may be used. This method was first described by Carle and Dewhirst (1942) and is probably

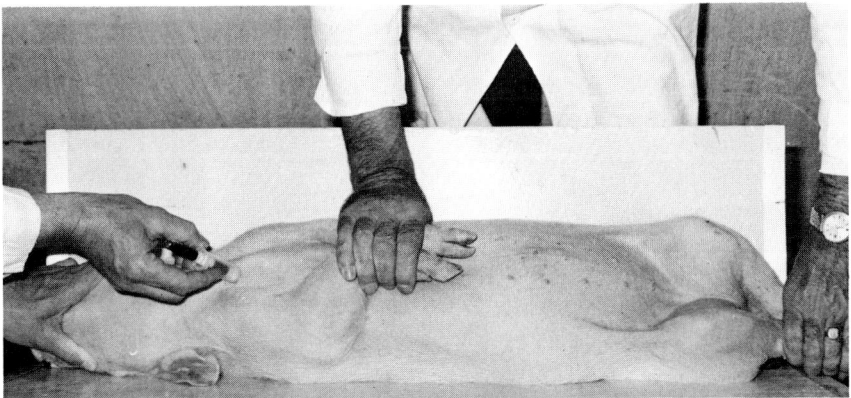

Fig. 14.4 Small pig held in dorsal recumbent position in V-shaped trough while taking blood from anterior vena cava.

superior to other methods. Small pigs up to 60 kg can be restrained by placing on their backs in a V-shaped trough, preferably at a convenient working height and held in the manner shown in Fig. 14.4. Pigs up to 100 kg can be placed on their back, but are obviously more difficult to handle. A sliding noose tether can be used for pigs between 60–100 kg, but is not reliable because the noose is liable to slide off when the tusks of the pig are poorly developed. Beyond 100 kg body weight the pig can be tethered with a noose and bled in the standing position (Hoerlein, Hubbard & Getty 1951). The pig is restrained by passing a 6 mm rope behind the tusks and round the upper jaw, and then to a post, the rope being tied to the latter about 1 metre above ground level. The head is extended upwards. The needles used are 1·25 mm diameter and 115 mm long. A needle is inserted at a point just anterior and slightly lateral to the cariniform cartilage and in a line from the cartilage to the base of the ear. Once inserted, the needle is directed upwards, slightly backwards and medially. In an adult animal, the depth of penetration necessary to reach the anterior vena cava is from 80 to 100 mm. It is important not to penetrate into

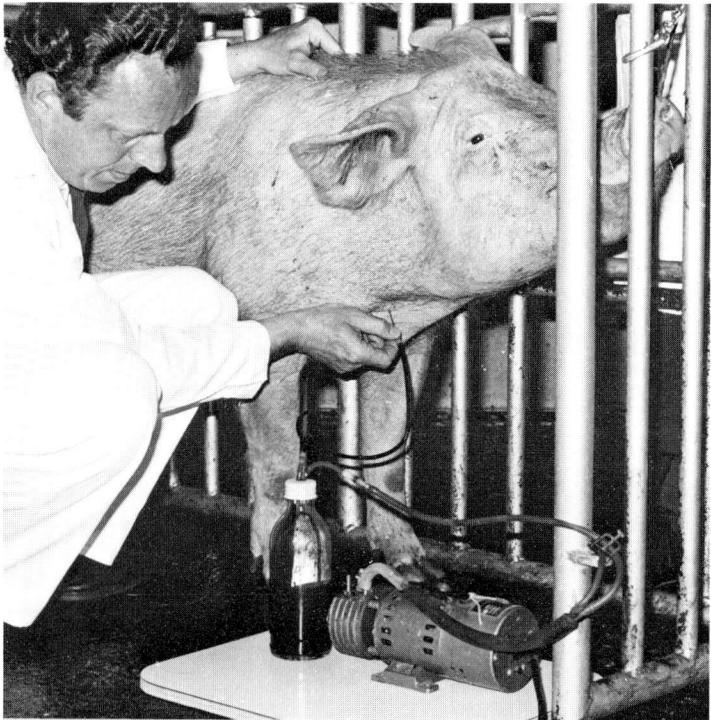

Fig. 14.5 Bleeding from anterior vena cava of large pig directly into 1 pint bottle using vacuum pump with bacterial filter incorporated in the vacuum line.

the space between the first pair of ribs since the pericardial sac may be as far anterior as this.

The anterior vena cava method can be used for pigs of all ages from new-born to adult. It is a closed method in which blood is drawn into a sterile syringe, vacuum container or evacuated vessel. It is the only reliable method in which large volumes of blood can be collected. By using a vacuum line connected via a bacterial filter to an evacuated bottle it is possible to obtain a litre of blood from an adult pig without difficulty (see Fig. 14.5). For smaller volumes from 5 to 50 ml the more usual practice is to use a disposable syringe or vacuum container. The latter has been found to be ideal for this method and can be used successfully in pigs up to 60 kg where a disposable 4 cm × 0·9 mm needle is available. Between 60 and 100 kg a 5–6 cm × 0·9–1·2 mm needle is preferable. In adult pigs over 100 kg bleeding from the anterior vena cava in the standing position can be accomplished by using a 8–10 cm 1·6–1·8 mm needle.

Espartza (1970) has recommended bleeding from the orbital sinus as described by Huhn *et al* (1969) on the lines developed for rats by Halpern *et al* (1951); from the portal vein in piglets by Cimr and Kaspar (1965) and from the median coccygeal artery and vein by Getty and Goshal (1967) who recommended holding the tail in a vertical position and puncture between the 4th and 5th or 5th and 6th coccygeal vertebrae with a 0·9 mm diameter needle inserted at about 45° to the vertical. With pigs weighing less than 100 kg the tail should be kept horizontal to avoid collapse of the vessels. The subcutaneous abdominal vein may also be a useful site in pigs young enough to be turned on their backs.

As with sheep blood, so with pig blood there is a tendency for the erythrocytes to suffer lysis with relatively little physical damage. Care of the specimens obtained is important and thermal, as well as physical, shocks should be avoided.

DOG
The cephalic or tibial veins are usually used, and of those the cephalic vein is recommended. In the dog, the cephalic vein runs along with the ulnar artery: over the upper third of the forearm it is superficial and slightly lateral to the shaft of the radius. At this point it is a relatively simple matter to make a venepuncture.

The dog should lie upon a table in the prone position with the right foreleg extended towards the operator. If an assistant is available, he stands at the left shoulder of the dog, facing the operator. With his left hand the assistant pulls the head of the dog towards himself, and with his right hand he extends the right forelimb of the dog. The assistant's hand should be just beneath and distal to the dog's elbow joint, with his thumb over the limb to occlude and so raise the vein. It is frequently an advantage to rotate the skin overlying the forearm somewhat laterally. With a suitable needle (about 1 mm diameter and 20 mm long) on a syringe with eccentric nozzle the operator can slide the needle through skin and subcutaneous fascia into the vein. If no skilled assistant is available, it is possible satisfactorily to raise the vein with an elastic band and a small ring (ca. 15 mm diameter). The band is passed round the forearm at the elbow joint with the ring attached at one end. The free end is passed through the ring beneath the joint and extended under the limb and so grasped by the operator.

By this technique a large dog, such as a Labrador, can provide 10–20 ml of blood, but if larger volumes are needed either the jugular vein or the heart must be punctured. The tibial vein will provide volumes of blood comparable with that obtainable from the cephalic and can be punctured on the lateral aspect of the hind limb just above the stifle (knee) joint. For this approach the dog should be restrained in lateral recumbency and the vein raised by an assistant grasping the hind limb a little above (proximal) to the site of venepuncture.

The jugular vein of the dog can be punctured by restraining the animal in the supine position or lateral recumbency. The head and neck are fully extended and the jugular veins identified. One of them is raised with thumb pressure and is then punctured with a needle of 1–2 mm diameter, 20 mm long, by approaching from over the thorax and inserting the needle in a cranial direction. Alternatively, the vein can be punctured by an approach alongside the ear towards the heart.

Cardiac puncture may be performed, but it is a hazardous process. The dog is restrained in right lateral recumbency. The heart is palpated through the rib cage and delineated as accurately as possible. If the animal is to be bled out, puncture of the left ventricle is relatively easy with a needle of 1·5–2 mm diameter 90–120 mm long. Some operators prefer puncture of the right heart, made with the dog restrained on its left side. If a large sample, with recovery, is required it is better to attempt puncture of the auricle, but this procedure is dangerous and is not recommended. Jugular venepuncture is safer and is greatly preferred.

Hovell (1968) described a method for jugular puncture with the dog held in the sitting position, head held up and turned slightly right. The vein is occluded with a thumb at the supra-clavicular fossa and the needle and syringe are inserted upwards into the vein using a needle of 0·8 mm diameter. Hendrickson and Marshall (1969) described the use of sealed evacuated glass containers to obtain blood by this method.

CAT

Venepuncture in the cat is not easy. It is usually best to use the cephalic vein by a technique similar to that described for the dog in the previous section. The tibial vein is seldom satisfactory.

Sharp needles are especially important in the cat because this species has particularly tough and very mobile skin. Short needles of small diameter (ca. 0·6 mm) are best.

Hovell *et al* (1970) have used jugular puncture with the cat restrained on its back in a sleeve. The sleeve is made of canvas, 45 cm long and 45 cm circumference with a draw-string at either end. The operator wears the sleeve and inserts the cat into it by grasping the scruff of the cat's neck and sliding the sleeve down from the operator's arm over the animal. The hind legs are inserted into the arm by an assistant, and the draw-strings tied behind the hindquarters and round the neck. The procedure is then similar to that described above for dogs.

Cardiac puncture is satisfactory only for bleeding an animal out, again by the method described for the dog. Jugular puncture can be used and it is possible to obtain substantially larger volumes of blood from this vein than from the cephalic.

Intravenous catheterization is frequently undertaken in the cat. Surgical exposure of the cephalic vein under local anaesthesia followed by insertion of a catheter introducer and, through this, a polythene catheter, is most satisfactory where repeated small blood samples, or intravenous injections, are required.

Small samples may be obtained by lancet wounds of the ear flap. Vallejo-Freire's (1951) technique is also useful—it is described below for the guinea pig.

RABBIT

The classical method of bleeding the rabbit is from the ear veins. Some 20–30 ml can be obtained from a large adult rabbit. There are a number of points which may help to increase the yield of blood and the ease of venepuncture.

The application of a paper clip to the base of the ear assists in dilating the veins. Applying a little xylol to the ear flap causes hyperaemia and improved bleeding, but for some purposes this treatment may be unacceptable. Where a needle is used it should be of about 0·8 mm diameter and no more than 20 mm long. If a syringe is used for aspiration, it is essential that the plunger be withdrawn very slowly since rabbit ear veins are exceedingly thin walled and collapse easily. Frequently it is best to place a ring of petroleum jelly on the ear flap around the proposed site of venepuncture, and then to stab the vein with a needle and allow free haemorrhage from the wound. In this way a surprisingly large volume of blood can be collected but, as with the application of xylol mentioned above, for many purposes such grossly contaminated blood samples as are obtained by this technique would be quite useless.

Jugular venepuncture is also sometimes undertaken in the rabbit by a technique similar to that described for the dog. Transthoracic cardiac puncture is also used, between the ribs at the left side, and appears to be safer in rabbits than it is in cat or dog.

GUINEA PIG, MINK AND FERRET

The techniques of bleeding these three species are similar and can conveniently be considered together. Unhappily some of the techniques used for the smaller animals are decidedly barbaric, but in the absence of better methods some of them must be mentioned.

For small amounts of blood, roughly equivalent to a finger prick in man, scalpel wounds can be made in the foot or the tail. In guinea pigs, the ear can be pricked with a lancet. An ingenious technique has been described by Vallejo-Freire (1951). By this method, a nail is cut through at its insertion and the heat from a 250 watt infra-red lamp is applied from 15 cm for 10 seconds. This causes haemorrhage. In each of these methods, haemorrhage is arrested by pressure from a sterile, dry dressing for a few minutes. Recourse to cautery, whether thermal or chemical, should be avoided if at all possible.

Larger volumes of blood may be obtained by cardiac puncture. Such a technique has been described by Baker and Gorham (1951). For cardiac puncture general anaesthesia may be necessary. I prefer to use ethyl chloride for this purpose, applied to a cardboard cone which is a fit to the face of the subject. Ether may also be used. The animal is placed on its back and the thorax grasped firmly with the left hand. With the right hand, a syringe and needle of 0·9 mm diameter and 30 mm length is advanced towards the xyphisternum. Puncture is made in the midline, just posterior to the xyphoid, and at an angle of about 35°. The heart is reached at a depth of 20–30 mm, and will lie in the midline if the thorax is gently but firmly compressed with the fingers of the operator's left hand. By this technique it is possible to obtain 10–15 ml of blood from large adult guinea pigs, mink or ferrets.

When guinea pigs are to be bled out for maximum blood recovery, the use of the axillary pocket may be useful. The animal is first anaesthetized, or stunned by a blow on the head. It is placed on its back and the axilla incised with a scalpel so that the great vessels of the forelimb are severed at the base of the pocket. Blood is removed from this pocket, as it collects, with a Pasteur pipette.

RAT AND MOUSE

Small amounts of blood can be obtained from lancet wounds of the ear flap or of the foot. Several small samples can also be obtained by progressive amputation of small parts of the tail with a sharp scalpel. In both these techniques there is, of course, contamination by tissue juice which may well be unacceptable. Intravenous injections can be given into the vessels of the tail of the rat if the animal is restrained by allowing it to run head first into a test tube of such size that it cannot turn round. The tail is warmed and illuminated by placing over a low power electric bulb (ca. 15 watts). Bleeding by this technique is almost impossible since the veins are exceedingly small and collapse very easily. None the less Hurwitz (1971) has described a method for puncture of the midventral tail artery with a micro bleeding tube and Plager (1972) has evolved a method for catheterization of a coccygeal vessel in rats.

Cardiac puncture is frequently used and is straightforward. Either the left lateral approach, as described for the dog, or the posterior approach, as described for the guinea pig, may be used. I prefer the lateral approach. It is, however, most important not to penetrate anterior or dorsal to the heart where the great vessels lie.

Kassel and Levitan (1953) have described a method for repeated bleeding of rats and mice from the jugular vein. Their technique is as follows. The animal is grasped by the loose skin of the back and held in the supine position. A piece of surgical gauze about 5×5 cm is held so that some of the threads catch in the upper incisor teeth. This gauze is then pulled so that the neck is fully extended. The hair of the ventral aspect of the neck is removed and the jugular veins can then be seen as dilated, surprisingly large structures. A needle of 0·45 mm diameter and about 15 mm length is attached to a small syringe and moistened with anticoagulant. Puncture is made 1–2 mm lateral to the sterno-clavicular junction.

Rats can be bled from the retro-orbital venous plexus. According to Halpern, Biozzi, Mene and Benaceraff (1951), who modified an idea first proposed by Pettit (1913), a Pasteur pipette can be inserted at the inner canthus, alongside the eyeball and so penetrate the plexus of veins. This method is suitable for repetition on the same subject.

14.1.3.2 Brief notes on bleeding some non-mammalian animals

CHICKEN (R. D. HODGES)

A number of techniques for sampling blood from birds have been described in the literature. The most important of these are:

Cardiac puncture Methods for obtaining arterial blood from the heart via the thoracic wall have been described by Sloan and Wilgus (1930) and Andrews (1944). Entry into the left ventricle is obtained by inserting the needle of a hypodermic syringe between the 5th and 6th ribs close to their junction with the breast bone. Variations of this method are to enter between the 4th and 5th ribs (Genest 1946) or between the sternum and the meta-sternum (Hofstad 1950). Another method, where the needle is inserted between the clavicles close to their point of fusion to enter one of the auricles or the large vessels, has been described by MacArthur (1950). Cardiac puncture is normally used to obtain blood samples from small birds such as quail (Atwal & McFarland 1966) or from chickens under 5 weeks of age, where the superficial veins are too small to permit venepuncture (Fredrickson *et al* 1957), although Nirmalan and Robinson (1971) have used brachial venepuncture in quail. Cardiac puncture can also be used to obtain large samples of blood. A certain risk is involved in this method since, even in experienced hands, a mortality of around 1 per cent is to be expected (Sloan & Wilgus 1930, Andrews 1944). Cardiac puncture is not very suitable for serial sampling due to the risk of mortality or damage to the heart tissue, although Genest (1946) was able to obtain up to 10 samples within 3 days from individual birds using his method.

Venepuncture Venous blood can be obtained from any superficial vein of large enough size; the brachial and jugular veins being normally used. In the case of the brachial vein, lying along the under surface of the upper wing parallel to the humerus, the technique has been described by Fredrickson *et al* (1958). Insertion of the needle peripherally aids collection but considerable care must be taken to prevent subsequent bleeding and haematoma formation which prevents re-use of the vein. Techniques of sampling from the jugular vein have been described by Stevens and Ridgeway (1966). As well as providing large quantities of blood this method can be used for serial sampling since significant leakage of blood does not usually occur (Law 1960). Christie (1970) has used the jugular vein without plucking any feathers.

Collection of blood from an open wound Blood samples can be obtained from lancet wounds of the wing vein (Briles *et al* 1950, Cohen 1967a, Nirmalan & Robinson 1971) or of the comb (Hamre & McHenry 1942). However, care must be taken to prevent the clotting of such samples since they will contain extrinsic thromboplastin from the damaged tissues. Small amounts of arterialized capillary blood can be obtained from superficial comb wounds if the comb has previously been well warmed by the application of pads of cotton wool soaked in hot water. Such blood is identical to arterial blood at least in its acid-base properties (R. D. Hodges, unpublished results).

Sampling of embryos Techniques for obtaining blood from embryos of all ages have been described by Lucas and Jamroz (1961).

Samples of blood are normally collected with a syringe and needle of suitable size. However, Garren (1959) has described a vacuum apparatus by which samples from the heart or a vein can be rapidly and efficiently collected through a needle into a specially prepared tube, and which allows greater ease of handling of the bird. Fredrickson *et al* (1958) devised a simple method of immobilizing chickens so that both hands can be used for sampling.

REPTILES AND FISH
A satisfactory means of bleeding these species is by cardiac puncture. In most, if not all, instances it is necessary to anaesthetize the subject and dissect as may be necessary to reach the heart with a pipette or needle. Clearly this will usually involve sacrifice of the subject. Very small amounts of blood can be

obtained by lancet wounds at any available place, usually the tail. Lizards can be bled by allowing *Rhodnius prolixus* to bite and then pricking the bug (Scorza 1971). Wounds of lizards may bleed fatally.

In the case of fish or aquatic reptiles it is essential to dry the subject carefully in the region to be punctured. Failure to do this will yield samples grossly haemolysed and contaminated. Blaxhall and Daisley (1973) used cardiac puncture about 1 cm behind the apex of the 'V' formed by the gill covers and isthmus after applying anaesthesia as a 1 in 1500 concentration of MS222 (Sandoz) for 2 or 3 minutes.

INVERTEBRATES

Haemolymph is usually obtained by cardiac puncture. I have no personal experience in this field, but it has been stated that in some invertebrates, for example the arthropods, puncture of the main cavity, or section of a leg, can yield about one drop of haemolymph (Bessis 1954). Bessis also states that cardiac puncture can sometimes be used in certain crustaceans, insects, myriapods and molluscs.

Greenwood (1975) punctured the pericardial sinus of lobsters (*Homarus* spp.) by inserting a 0·6 mm diameter needle 4 cm long cranial through the arthrodial membrane between the thoracic carapace and the first abdominal tergum at an angle of 30° to the carapace to a depth of 2 cm.

14.2   ANTICOAGULANTS AND SAMPLING BOTTLES

When a blood sample is taken it may be for any one of a whole variety of purposes. The optimal container, charged with anticoagulant if blood clotting is to be prevented, will vary with the volume and with the intended use of the specimens. One thing, however, is unavoidable since blood, once shed, always changes. Some of these changes can be prevented, but only by introducing other changes. For instance, the coagulation of blood can be prevented by removing ionized calcium.

14.2.1   SAMPLING BOTTLES

GENERAL PRINCIPLE OF PREPARATION OF CONTAINERS

Bottles intended for use as containers of blood must, of course, be clean. Cleanliness should include not only freedom from viable organisms, but also chemical cleanliness. Quite small traces of copper, to take a single example, may produce marked haemolysis.

Sampling bottles must also be quite dry. In the case of liquid anticoagulants (considered below) this does not, of course, apply. Traces of moisture may cause haemolysis and for this reason sterilization of bottles with the autoclave is not acceptable unless they are tightly capped.

GLASS BOTTLES

Glass bottles are still widely used for blood samples. They are probably best where coagulation is to be allowed and serum harvested. Where coagulation is to be prevented it is worth while to coat the bottles with silicone. The use of 'Repelcote' (Hopkins and Williams Ltd) is recommended, but it is necessary to wash and dry the bottles after siliconing and before use. Bottles of such size should be used that the blood sample substantially fills them: avoid a small sample in the bottom of an over-large bottle.

PLASTIC CONTAINERS

A variety of plastics which are non-toxic to blood are now available. These are very satisfactory and are much lighter than glass bottles. Since they are disposable and are formed by precision press methods, they do not normally require any cleaning before use. Non-water-wettable surfaces are available and compare very favourably to silicone-coated glassware.

14.2.2   ANTICOAGULANTS

The anticoagulant now most commonly used, and currently the best for cellular studies, is sequestrene (ethylenediaminetetraacetic acid). The dipotassium salt is preferred since it is very readily soluble in blood, but the disodium salt is also satisfactory. The dilithium salt is useful for certain applications (e.g. assay of blood sodium and potassium) but is more liable to cause morphological changes in the leucocytes.

DIPOTASSIUM SEQUESTRENE (K_2EDTA)

This anticoagulant is used at the rate of 10 mg for 5 ml of blood. It may conveniently be dispensed as an 11 per cent solution in distilled water. 0·1 ml of this, placed in a bijou bottle and evaporated at room temperature or at 50°C (not over 60°C) to dryness will suit 5 ml of blood with a small margin in excess. Plastic phials to hold 2·5 ml of blood and already charged with 5 mg of dipotassium sequestrene are readily available commercially. The dried sequestrene salt dissolves in the added blood within a few seconds.

DISODIUM SEQUESTRENE (Na_2EDTA)

While this is cheaper than the dipotassium salt, its use has generally been dropped because of slightly less rapid solubility. There is some evidence that disodium sequestrene as a liquid anticoagulant is preferable to the dipotassium where cytological studies of leucocytes are required.

DILITHIUM SEQUESTRENE (Li$_2$EDTA)

This material is used as an anticoagulant for the assay of sodium or potassium by some techniques in blood samples. It is only suitable for blood counts if the samples are examined within an hour or so of being drawn from the subject. Suitably charged plastic phials are available.

OXALATE

The classical anticoagulant of Wintrobe consists of a mixture of 4 mg of potassium oxalate and 6 mg of ammonium oxalate for each 5 ml of blood. The use of this mixture has largely been superseded since sequestrene causes less cellular distortion. A 1·34 per cent solution of sodium oxalate is used for some coagulation tests. For use, 1 volume of this solution is mixed with 9 parts of blood.

CITRATE

Trisodium citrate is little used for cellular studies of blood, but it is the anti-coagulant of choice for most coagulation tests. A solution of 3·8 per cent trisodium citrate is used, one part of anticoagulant to nine parts of blood. It is important to note that the trisodium salt of citric acid is used, not the disodium.

Acid citrate dextrose (ACD) is used as an anticoagulant of blood intended for transfusion and also for the preparation of erythrocytes used in serological testing. The material is prepared as follows:

Dextrose	27·3 g
Disodium citrate	23·7 g
Distilled water to	1 litre

Note that in this formulation disodium hydrogen citrate is used, not the tri-sodium salt. The fluid is dispensed as required to the sample bottles and may be autoclaved at 15 lb per square inch pressure for 15 minutes in securely fastened containers. For blood transfusion, the standard plastic units containing ACD anticoagulant suffice for 420 ml of blood: a total volume of 540 ml transfusion fluid. Small samples of blood collected into ACD for laboratory use are usually at 1 part of ACD to 3·5 parts of blood. If ACD is made up in bulk it must be autoclaved to prevent bacterial growth.

HEPARIN

This anticoagulant is only occasionally useful and it is expensive. It can be used at the rate of about 1 mg (approximately 100 i.u.) dry heparin powder per ml of blood. Heparinized blood is usually not suitable for leucocyte studies since the leucocytes may become clumped. It is, however, the only readily available anticoagulant which does not depend upon the chelation of calcium and it is for this reason that it is sometimes of considerable value in the laboratory.

14.2.3 DEFIBRINATION

The effect of defibrination is unique since it yields a suspension of blood cells in *serum*, not plasma. For many purposes this is most useful and it is surprising that, if due care is taken, the leucocyte morphology is exceedingly good. Two main methods are used to take up the fibrin: either glass beads or a glass 'tree'. Where glass beads are used some haemolysis will occur. The method is to add about 1/10th volume of glass beads to an Erlenmeyer flask. For example, for a 250 ml flask about 25 ml of beads would be used. Blood is added directly from a vein to the flask and the latter is gently, but continuously, swirled until all the fibrin threads are formed in and among the mass of beads. The process will take from 10 to 20 minutes, but at no time may swirling be arrested until defibrination is complete since jellification of the specimen would then almost certainly occur.

A better method, especially for smaller volumes, is to use a prepared glass rod for collecting the fibrin. Such a rod may be prepared by heating it to red heat and then pulling out, with forceps, about a dozen spikes ca. 1 cm long. Sometimes odd pieces of glass are fused to these spikes. The 'whisk' is inserted into an Erlenmeyer flask and held somewhat to one side. The blood is added and swirled just as if with glass beads, holding the 'tree' still. Fibrin threads form upon and catch in this 'tree'. There is much less haemolysis by this technique than is the case where glass beads are used and it is highly recommended.

14.2.4 PREPARATION OF PLASMA

Blood plasma is prepared by suitable centrifugation of whole blood which has been taken into an anticoagulant. Usually, freedom from blood cells, other than platelets, can be obtained by centrifuging at 1000 *g* for 20 minutes. If, however, platelet free plasma is required, two centrifugations at 3000 *g* for 20 minutes are necessary. It is a great advantage if centrifugation can be performed at 4°C since at this temperature minimum degradation of blood constituents occurs. Colder temperatures may cause freezing and therefore haemolysis: warmer temperatures do not so effectively delay damage to blood cells.

14.2.5 PREPARATION OF SERUM

Serum is the fluid expressed when blood clots. In the laboratory, clotting is improved if clean glass surfaces are used (*not* siliconed surfaces or plastics). Incubation at 37°C for 4 hours and then at 20°C for 20 hours gives a good yield. Aspiration of the fluid, followed by centrifugation, should yield good serum free of haemoglobin.

Plasma may be clotted to yield a fluid which closely resembles serum, and is free of fibrinogen, but it will be diluted. Blood taken into sequestrene does not yield readily coagulable plasma. For plasma derived from blood taken into ACD the following technique of obtaining 'serum' has been found useful. For each litre of plasma, add 100 ml of molar calcium chloride and incubate at 37°C for 4–8 hours. This incubation must continue until the material clots. The coagulum is then stored at 4°C overnight and, the next day, frozen at −20°C. After 24 hours it is thawed and decanted. About 75 per cent of the volume may be recovered in this way.

14.3 PRESERVATION OF BLOOD SAMPLES

Blood samples can seldom be examined or used as soon as they are taken. Preservation is therefore essential. All forms of blood preservation permit decay to occur, but they delay it or decrease it in degree. Various methods of preservation either of whole blood or of blood fractions can be used. In this section some of these techniques will be considered along with notes of the effects they may produce and the utility of the preserved specimens for different purposes. And it must be emphasized that it is the purpose for which blood is preserved that will determine the method of choice; for best results this necessitates planning ahead.

PRESERVATION OF WHOLE BLOOD IN SEQUESTRENE
If the samples are to be subjected to ordinary haematological cellular examination, samples can be preserved for about 48 hours at room temperature. This presupposes that the samples have been well taken, are kept in properly prepared containers and that sequestrene has been used as the anticoagulant. Somewhat longer preservation can be achieved by conserving the specimens at 4°C. Oxalate is not a satisfactory anticoagulant unless the samples are to be examined at once (Table 14.2).

Transmission of blood samples by post is frequently necessary. In ambient temperatures above 20°C such transmission is seldom practicable since deterioration may occur in much less than 24 hours. Further, in very cold weather satisfactory postal transmission is most difficult since blood cells cannot be counted after they have been disrupted by freezing.

Mechanical shocks can damage blood samples and, indeed, the mechanical fragility of erythrocytes is sometimes measured in the laboratory. For this reason blood samples should ideally be packed in shock-resisting material. Foam polystyrene is particularly recommended as it is both an admirable shock absorber and also a good thermal insulator.

Table 14.2 The useful life of samples of whole blood in an anticoagulant for haematological examinations

Test	Approximate maximum time in hours after sampling that satisfactory tests can be made			
	In sequestrene		In oxalate	
	at 15–20°C	*at* 4°C	*at* 15–20°C	*at* 4°C
Haematocrit or erythrocyte count	36	48	24	36
Haemoglobin	96	150	48	60
Leucocyte count	36	48	4	8
Preparation of blood films	24	36	$\frac{1}{2}$	2

Where blood samples have to be conserved before they can be examined in the surgery or the laboratory, it is best to hold them between 4 and 6°C in a refrigerator. They should be warmed to 20°C before testing especially for such examinations as erythrocyte sedimentation rate.

The longer whole blood is preserved, the greater will be the deterioration. Leucocytes and platelets suffer first, and some of the erythrocytes undergo lysis. Thereafter the samples become of progressively reduced value for haematological tests.

PRESERVATION OF BLOOD SERUM OR PLASMA

Provided blood serum or plasma is separated from the haemic cells, it can be preserved for long periods. The remarks that follow refer only to such cell-free fluids.

In the frozen state, both serum and plasma are well preserved. At temperatures of from 0 to −15°C protein degradation occurs comparatively rapidly, but below −20°C it is almost totally stopped. At −80°C no practicable degeneration occurs. However, there is always some degradation during the cycle of freezing and thawing which cannot be avoided. For serological examinations these effects are not important: for electrophoresis of proteins they should be avoided if at all possible. For most blood coagulation purposes preservation at −20°C or below is acceptable, but it appears that freezing and thawing does have the effect of starting the earliest stage of blood clotting. For blood transfusion, serum and plasma can be stored for at least a year at −20°C, while storage at −80°C appears to be quite satisfactory for almost indefinite periods provided the material is never thawed until it is used.

Frozen serum or plasma may be thawed with the use of heat, but temperatures over 38°C should be avoided. Uneven warming of containers, for example over a flame, is unsatisfactory. A water-bath at 37°C is ideal and much preferred to a 37°C air incubator since the former is much more rapid. A bucket full of water that feels no warmer than tepid to the hand is a satisfactory substitute.

PRESERVATION OF BLOOD FILMS

Properly prepared blood films are surprisingly stable even without fixation. It is essential that they be thoroughly air-dried at room temperature. This may take from half an hour to several hours. Satisfactory blood films cannot be made in very humid conditions or in sub-freezing temperatures. While the films are drying they must be protected from damage by flies etc. and they should not be exposed to the direct rays of the sun.

Films so dried can be stained satisfactorily up to several weeks later provided they are kept dry and protected from humid conditions. If wrapped in clean, dry paper and placed in a sealed container they are suitable for transmission by post.

Blood films can be fixed in a variety of ways. Special staining techniques require different methods. When films are sent to a laboratory for examination it is worth while to send three lots: first, dry but unfixed; second, dried and fixed for 30 seconds in absolute (acetone-free) methanol, and blotted dry only; third, dried and fixed in formol-saline (5 per cent formaldehyde solution in normal saline) for 2 minutes, washed in running tap water for 10 minutes and blotted dry. It is, however, very important to indicate which lot is which since there should be no visible difference between them after these treatments. Of the 3 methods, methanol-fixed films are the most useful for diagnostic purposes.

Fixation of blood films by heat from a naked flame is not satisfactory for haematological purposes since the leucocytes are not sufficiently well preserved for differentiation. This method is best reserved for bacteriological purposes only.

Fixed films are stable practically indefinitely and are proof against humidity. Films, whether fixed or not, are fragile and are very susceptible to damage by scratching. They should be wrapped in fluff-free paper or placed in a dust-proof container for conservation or consignment.

14.4 BASIC HAEMATOLOGICAL TECHNIQUES

In this section the basic techniques used for haematological examinations will be briefly described from a practical viewpoint. A number of more or less specialized techniques, not always in routine use, are considered in section 14.8 below (page 584).

Some routine techniques require special variations for particular species and these have been noted in the descriptions that follow. In general they are all 'common sense' variations, but some of them might not immediately occur to those unfamiliar with handling animal blood.

For routine haematological examination of blood about 2–5 ml is sufficient. Many tests can be performed with much smaller volumes; for example a microhaematocrit requires only about 0·1 ml. Where only drops of blood are available, as from a lancet wound, counts by dilution or the microhaematocrit test can be made directly from the bleeding site. It must, however, be appreciated that such samples of blood are subject to additional variations as compared with venous samples, attributable to the local tissue concerned. For instance, a lancet wound to a hyperaemic (inflamed) area will give different results from a blood sample drawn at a normal site. Bearing such limitations in mind, it is frequently possible to obtain most valuable information from very small blood samples. Use of the microhaematocrit test is particularly recommended for this purpose.

14.4.1 REAGENTS

Certain reagents are required for haematological purposes which either differ from those usually available, or have differing specifications. For instance, glass distilled water is essential for many haematological tests. As a particular example, a trace of copper in the water will affect erythrocyte fragility tests. *Normal saline* is made from sodium chloride (Analar grade) at the rate of 8·5 g/l of water. It should be adjusted to pH 7 with sodium hydroxide solution. *Phosphate buffer* (for use with Leishman stain etc.) is conveniently made from two stock solutions, each M/15.

Table 14.3 Quantities of M/15 solutions required to make phosphate buffer at different pH levels.

pH	Solution (1) ml	Solution (2) ml
6·5	6·82	3·18
6·6	6·30	3·70
6·7	5·66	4·34
6·8	5·08	4·92
6·9	4·48	5·52
7·0	3·89	6·11
7·1	3·34	6·66
7·2	2·80	7·20
7·3	2·32	7·68
7·4	1·92	8·08
7·5	1·59	8·41

Solution (1): Anhydrous KH_2PO_4 9·08 g/l
Solution (2): Anhydrous $Na_2 HPO_4$ 9·47 g/l

These two solutions can be mixed in various proportions to obtain differing pH values. For use with Leishman stain pH 7·2 is recommended, obtained by mixing 2·80 ml of solution (1) with 7·20 ml of solution (2) and glass distilled water to 100 ml. Other pH values may be obtained and these are given in Table 14.3.

Methanol used in Leishman stain must be dry and acetone-free. Commercial grades are not satisfactory. The special solvent methanol prepared by BDH Ltd for Romanowski stains is strongly recommended. Methanol should always be kept in securely stoppered bottles and for this reason it is inadvisable to purchase it in large containers. A number of smaller containers, each convenient to prepare a batch of stain, is better.

Glyoxaline buffer for coagulation work:
  Solution (1) Glyoxaline (imidazole) 680 mg
                    Water   50 ml
  Solution (2) $N/_{10}$ HCl
For pH 7·3, isotonic, use: Solution (1) 25·0 ml
                           Solution (2) 18·6 ml
                           Water   56·4 ml
                           NaCl   0·585 g
Conserve at 4°C in the refrigerator.

PERCENTAGE SOLUTIONS
Given a solution of X per cent, a solution of Y per cent may be readily obtained where $X > Y$.

Take Y vols and dilute to X vols. This gives a solution of Y per cent.

14.4.2 COUNTS BY DILUTION

Blood samples in a suitable anticoagulant must be shaken before dilution counts are prepared from them. Hand shaking for not less than two minutes is satisfactory. There are numerous mechanical blood bottle shakers on the market: such instruments are most useful since they require only 30 seconds to agitate samples and also because they do not occupy the operator. After a blood sample has been shaken it will again begin to settle out. Counts must not be put up more than 1 minute after agitation unless further satisfactory agitation is applied. This is most important if accurate results are to be obtained.

In diluting blood with haematological pipettes, negative pressure is applied from the operator's mouth. It is imperative to use a sufficiently long rubber tube to connect mouthpiece and pipette. I prefer that this tube should not be less than 30 cm, while 45 cm is better. If the tube is too short, the operator cannot observe the pipette adequately for accuracy.

THE COUNTING CHAMBER

Haemocytometers having the improved Neubauer ruling are used exclusively. The chamber depth is 0·1 mm and the ruled area covers 9 mm². If these figures are borne in mind, together with Fig. 14.6 there should never be any difficulty with calculations after counting. For erythrocyte counts the small squares marked 'R' are counted; five upon each side of the chamber, ten in all. Over each of these squares there is 0·004 mm³ of diluted blood. For leucocyte counts the larger corner squares marked 'W' are used, four upon each side of the chamber, eight in all. Over each of the large squares there is 0·1 mm³ of diluted blood.

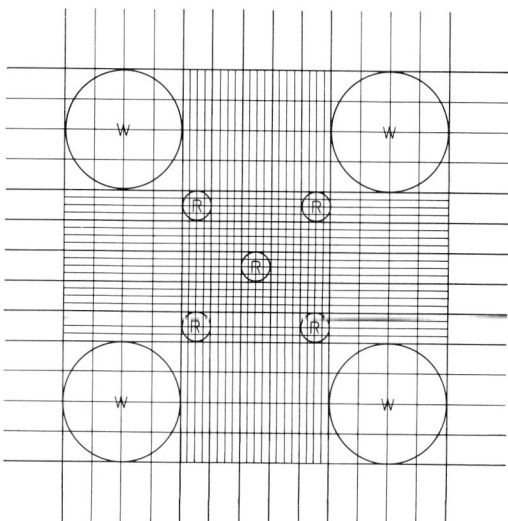

Fig. 14.6 Improved Neubauer ruling of a haemocytometer. The squares containing a W in a circle are used for white cell counts, the squares containing an R in a circle are used for erythrocyte counts.

14.4.3 ELECTRONIC PARTICLE COUNTERS

A number of electronic particle counters, adapted particularly to the solution of problems in cell counting for haematology, are now available. They have the effect that an assay which used to be subjected to large inherent error—the erythrocyte count—has now become the most reliable and repeatable single parameter to measure the red cell status of an individual.

Cost effectiveness will determine whether or not such a machine should be purchased for particular situations, but where absolute accuracy is to be approached as closely as possible an electric counter is mandatory.

Most of the satisfactory machines depend upon the use of some form of venturi or aperture through which a diluted blood sample is forced. At the same time changes in electrical resistance through the aperture are measured and increases are proportional to the *volume* of diluent displaced by a particle.

With any such machine, strict compliance with the instructions of the manufacturer are essential. However, most machines are delivered calibrated to count human erythrocytes assuming a mean cell volume of about 90 fl and a *minimum* cell volume of about 40. This is not acceptable for mammals other than man, where MCV values below 40 are by no means rare and, for example in the goat, may be as small as 20 to 22 fl. It is absolutely necessary, before purchasing any particle counter, to make sure that it is satisfactory and sensitive in the particle volume range to be studied.

Electronic counters need regular standardization. Quality control is not straightforward for non-human mammalian blood since all commercially available preparations are designed to simulate human blood. To detect electronic drift, it is useful to run on a morning the last few samples counted the previous day and check to determine any tendency to rise or fall over a period. A further useful check is to keep 1 or 2 animals of the type to be studied, in normal health, adjacent to the laboratory and run regular samples from them. MCV figures are remarkably constant in a given individual for long periods and any change in the MCV of such subjects, if not attributable to disease or environmental change, will serve as an excellent warning that a drift has taken place.

14.4.4   RED CELL COUNTS

14.4.4.1   The erythrocyte count by dilution and chamber

A red cell pipette is used, giving a final dilution of 1:200. The diluting fluid may be 0.85 per cent saline, but Hayem's solution is preferable:

Sodium chloride	1	g
Sodium sulphate	5	g
Mercuric chloride ($HgCl_2$)	0.5	g
Distilled water	200	ml

Blood is taken from a lancet wound or from a phial into the pipette up to the 0.5 mark. It must not rise above this mark and if it does the pipette must be discarded since 'sucking back' will leave some erythrocytes on the glass walls. The outside of the pipette is wiped clean with a cotton wool pledget and it is then dipped into Hayem's solution: the latter is drawn in until the blood plus diluent reaches the 101 mark. Since the capillary of the pipette

(1 unit) remains filled with diluting fluid, the final dilution of blood in diluent is 0·5 in (101-1) or 1:200.

Where the count is not to be made immediately a pipette containing diluted blood can be closed by passing a broad rubber band round, so sealing both ends. In this state pipettes can be transported from examination room to laboratory for instance, and counts can be made from them up to about 1 hour after dilution.

Animals which have a red count of 8×10^{12} or more (e.g. the horse) require further dilution of blood than the standard 1:200. This dilution is optimal for counts in the range of 3 to 6×10^{12}. Similarly, counts below 3×10^{12} should be derived from blood diluted less than 1:200. It is best to count about 500 cells in the chamber: that is about 50 cells in each small square (Fig. 15.6 squares marked 'R'). An approximate guide to the optimal dilutions for erythrocyte count is given in Table 14.4.

Table 14.4 Optimal dilutions in Hayem's fluid for erythrocyte counts

Anticipated erythrocyte count $\times 10^{12}$ per litre	Dilution to be used for the counts	Mark on the erythrocyte pipette
1 to 3	1:100	1·0
3 to 6	1:200	0·5
over 6	1:500	0·2

Pipettes containing diluted blood must be shaken before filling a haemocytometer so that the erythrocyte suspension is homogeneous. This requires two minutes' agitation in the hand, with a finger over each end of the pipette, or 30 seconds in a mechanical shaker. The haemocytometer must be filled *immediately* after shaking is completed.

The use of erythrocyte dilution pipettes is not essential, though it is recommended. Other methods of diluting blood 1:200 are satisfactory. As an example, the use of an auto zero pipette of 0·05 ml capacity (as used in haemoglobin assay) to wash blood into 10 ml of diluting fluid, produces the same dilution with efficiency. The difficulty which may arise is to produce adequate mixing of the diluted blood, so that the erythrocytes are evenly suspended. Clearly, minor changes in the volumes of diluting fluid used, or of the auto zero pipette, will permit any dilution of blood to be obtained. All counts by dilution can be performed by this method if the usual diluting pipettes are not available.

The haemocytometer to be used is prepared by careful cleaning and drying. The cover glass is put in place after lightly covering the pillars of the chamber with saline. Slight pressure will fix the cover glass in place securely.

Both sides of a haemocytometer should be filled. The pipette, which has been shaken, is picked up and a volume equivalent to at least twice the capillary portion is discarded by blowing it out. The haemocytometer is then filled by touching the tip of the pipette to the space between cover glass and ruling on both sides. The chamber will fill completely and accurately over the ruled areas by capillary attraction provided that it is clean. Over- or under-filled chambers must not be counted—they must be cleaned and refilled correctly. Very slight over-filling is acceptable provided it is at once corrected by briefly touching the region where the pipette was applied with dry filter paper.

If a dilution pipette has not been used, the chambers can conveniently be filled from the vessel containing diluted blood by use of a Pasteur pipette.

Once filled, the haemocytometer should be laid on the bench for about three minutes to allow the cells to settle. After this, it is placed on the microscope and examined with the 16 mm dry objective to make sure that the erythrocytes are evenly spread. If they are not, the haemocytometer may not have been clean and in any case the count must be completely discarded and performed again. It is not satisfactory to fill a second haemocytometer from a previously partly discharged dilution pipette.

If it is available, erythrocyte counts should be made with the 4 mm dry objective. If not, the 16 mm can be used with $\times 8$ eye-pieces. The five small squares marked 'R' in Fig. 14.6 are counted upon both sides of the haemocytometer: ten squares in all. The area of these squares if 0.04 mm^2. When counting the erythrocytes in each square, those touching the upper and left hand boundary lines of each square are excluded, those touching the lower and right hand boundary are included.

Calculation of the count is simple. The general formula is:

$$\frac{\text{Number of cells counted} \times \text{dilution}}{\text{Volume assayed}} \tag{1}$$

For example: assume that a dilution of $1:200$ has been used, 450 cells have been enumerated on 10 small squares. The diluted blood volume counted is therefore (0.04×0.1) mm^3 per square or 0.04 mm^3 over 10 squares. Substituting in the general formula, we have

$$\frac{450 \times 200}{0.04} \quad \text{or} \quad \begin{array}{l} 450 \times 5000 \\ 2{,}250{,}000/\text{mm}^3 \\ \text{or } 2.25 \times 10^{12}/\text{l} \end{array}$$

Many technicians simplify this further to read

$$\frac{\text{Number of erythrocytes counted}}{200} \tag{2}$$

but it must be noted that this will only apply where a dilution of 1:200 is used and a total of 10 small squares are enumerated on an improved Neubauer haemocytometer.

14.4.4.2 The total leucocyte count (standard technique)

This procedure is essentially similar to that described in some detail for the erythrocyte count. Only differences will be noted.

Special leucocyte pipettes are used designed to give dilutions of 1:20 (0·5 mark) or 1:10 (1·0 mark). The 1:20 dilution is normally used. If the anticipated leucocyte count is *below* about $2·5 \times 10^9/l$ then a 1:10 dilution should be prepared. Dilution is made with a fluid designed to stain the leucocytes but lyse the erythrocytes. A suitable formula is as follows:

Acetic acid (glacial)	1·5 ml
Gentian violet 1 per cent aqueous	1·0 ml
Distilled water	97·5 ml

The details of dilution, whether in special pipettes or not, shaking the pipette etc. are similar to the procedure described for the erythrocyte count. Both sides of a haemocytometer are similarly filled after discarding a few drops from the pipette to eliminate the unmixed diluting fluid in the capillary. If the cells are evenly spread, the 4 large corner squares marked 'W' in Fig. 14.6 are counted on both sides, 8 in all. The 16 mm objective is used. The area of each of these squares is 1 mm².

The formula for calculation quoted already is again used. As an example, suppose that 320 leucocytes have been enumerated on 8 large squares in a dilution of 1:20. We have:

$$\frac{\text{Number of cells counted} \times \text{dilution}}{\text{Volume assayed}} \tag{1}$$

$$= \frac{320 \times 20}{8 \times 0·1} = 320 \times 25$$

$$= 8000/\text{mm}^3 \text{ or } 8 \times 10^9/l.$$

This is frequently simplified to read

$$\frac{\text{Number of leucocytes counted}}{40} \tag{3}$$

but equation (3) will only be valid where a dilution of 1:20 is used, 8 mm² are enumerated and the result is expressed as numbers $\times 10^9$ per litre.

Where leucocyte counts are very high it is sometimes convenient to count them as for an erythrocyte count but at 1:20 dilution. Suppose in such a case 100 leucocytes were counted in the 10 *small* squares used for erythrocyte counting, then substituting in equation (1) we have:

$$\frac{100 \times 20}{0\cdot04} = 500,000/\text{mm}^3 \text{ or } 500 \times 10^9/\text{l}$$

since in this example the *volume* assayed will be $0\cdot04/\text{mm}^3$ only as in the erythrocyte count.

14.4.4.3 The total leucocyte count by Randolph and Stanton's technique

An ingenious leucocyte counting technique has been devised by Randolph and Stanton (1945). By this method the leucocytes are to some extent differentially stained. If a 4 mm objective is used it is usually possible to distinguish neutrophils, lymphocytes and eosinophils from one another, but difficulty is likely with monocytes (like large lymphocytes) or basophils (granules not usually visible). With some species this technique is not satisfactory and it is better to use the standard total leucocyte count and a differential count from a stained film (described on page 578).

Randolph and Stanton's technique is as follows:

Two solutions are made up:
  Solution A
    Methylene blue 0·1 per cent in propylene glycol   50 ml
    Distilled water   50 ml
  Solution B
    Phloxine 0·1 per cent in propylene glycol   50 ml
    Distilled water   50 ml

These solutions are stable for some months at 4°C. For use they are mixed usually in equal parts, but for some species variation of from 4–6 parts solution A, solution B up to 10 parts, may give useful improvement. The mixtures of Solutions A and B are not stable and should be discarded after 2 or 3 hours.

Blood is diluted with the mixed Randolph and Stanton solution to 1:20 in the ordinary way. The haemocytometer should not be filled until the diluted blood has stained *in the pipette* for at least 10 minutes.

Pipettes and counting chambers used with propylene glycol should be cleaned at *once* after use. Where this technique is in use it is better to reserve certain diluting pipettes from the general laboratory stock solely for it since they will become stained and less satisfactory for the more usual methods.

14.4.4.4 The eosinophil count

There are several techniques designed to count eosinophils only in diluted blood specimens. The Randolph and Stanton method just described can be used for this purpose sometimes modified by the use of Solution B only, but I prefer the method of Discombe (1946). The diluting fluid used is as follows:

Eosin Y 1 per cent aqueous	5 ml
Acetone	5 ml
Distilled water	90 ml

The solution is stable for some weeks on the bench. Eosinophils take up eosin, the acetone and distilled water cause lysis of other leucocytes and of erythrocytes. Blood is diluted 1:10 in a leucocyte pipette and allowed to stain for at least 5 minutes. It is then spread on a haemocytometer and the cells falling on the whole of the ruled area (i.e. 9 mm² on each side, 18 in all) are enumerated.

Calculation is as follows. If 60 cells have been counted on 18 mm² at a dilution of 1:10 we have:

$$\frac{\text{Number of cells counted} \times \text{dilution}}{\text{Volume assayed}} \tag{1}$$

or, in this case:

$$\frac{60 \times 10}{18 \times 0 \cdot 1} = 60 \times \frac{100}{18}$$
$$= 60 \times 5 \cdot 55/\text{mm}^3$$
$$= 333 \text{ mm}^3 \text{ or } 0 \cdot 33 \times 10^9/\text{l}$$

The formula is commonly simplified to read:

$$\frac{\text{Number of eosinophils counted}}{180} \tag{4}$$

where the blood is diluted 1:10 and the whole ruled area on both sides of the counting chamber is used.

McNary (1958) has recommended the use of bromcresol purple for counting eosinophils. The diluting fluid is as follows:

Bromcresol purple	25 mg
Distilled water	50 ml

This fluid is used in precisely the same way as Discombe's fluid.

None of these techniques for counting eosinophils is satisfactory in the *rabbit* or the *chicken*. In these two species total leucocyte figures should be obtained and used with a differential count made from a stained blood film to derive the eosinophil count. Special staining techniques are necessary for these films, see page 593.

14.4.4.5 The basophil count

The diluting fluid of Moore and James (1953) has been found useful. This is:

Toluidine blue 0·05 per cent in 0·85 per cent saline	40 ml
Ethyl alcohol 95 per cent	11 ml
Saponin, saturated solution in 50 per cent ethyl alcohol	1 ml

Mix and filter. Stable at room temperature for about 3 or 4 months. The blood is diluted 1:10 and must stain in the pipette for 10 minutes before the haemo-cytometer is filled. Basophils appear deep red, but the background is frequently heavily contaminated by cellular debris although this is not meta-chromatic with toluidine blue.

The procedure, and calculation, is the same as for the eosinophil count.

14.4.4.6 The platelet count

Assay of platelets by direct dilution of blood is a method of obtaining reasonably precise results. An approximate guide can be obtained from the stained film but this method has only limited use and is subject to considerable inaccuracy.

An excellent diluting fluid for the platelet count is:

Disodium sequestrene 1 per cent aqueous	10 ml
Saline 0·85 per cent	90 ml

since this fluid tends to prevent platelet clumping.

Blood is diluted in the red cell pipette to 1:200. Platelets are counted on all 25 small squares (5 of them are marked 'R' in Fig. 14.6) on both sides of the haemocytometer—that is a total area of 2 mm². If, as an example, 400 platelets are counted in these conditions, the calculation is as follows:

$$\frac{\text{Number of platelets counted} \times \text{dilution}}{\text{Volume assayed}} \tag{1}$$

or, in this example:

$$\frac{400 \times 200}{2 \times 0 \cdot 1} = 400 \times 1,000$$
$$= 400,000/\text{mm}^3 \text{ or } 400 \times 10^9/\text{l}.$$

This can be simplified to

$$\text{Number of platelets counted} \tag{5}$$

which gives the answer as a number $\times 10^9/\text{l}$ provided that a dilution of 1:200 is adhered to and also that 2 mm² are enumerated.

Counting of platelets on haemocytometers is much facilitated if thin chambers without a ground concavity at the base are used, since this permits phase contrast microscopy by which the platelets are easier to detect.

14.4.4.7 Counting erythrocytes and leucocytes in chickens (R. D. Hodges)

Counting techniques for red and white cells are complicated by the fact that all avian blood cells are nucleated. Consequently standard white cell counting fluids, which lyse the erythrocytes and leave the leucocytes unaffected, reduce avian red cells to almost naked nuclei which are not easily distinguishable from small lymphocytes (Chubb & Rowell 1959). Erythrocytes are easily recognizable in diluting fluids due to their characteristic morphology and can be counted using a dilution of 1 : 200 in a standard red cell pipette and haemocytometer. The diluting fluids recommended are those of Wiseman or Rees-Ecker (Denington & Lucas 1955) or of Natt and Herrick (Chubb & Rowell 1959). To ensure accurate counts both the original blood sample and the diluted sample in the pipette need to be adequately mixed by shaking.

Three methods of counting leucocytes have been discussed by Denington and Lucas (1955)—the direct, semi-indirect and indirect methods. The direct method consists of staining all blood cells with a special diluting fluid and then counting the numbers of cells direct from the haemocytometer chamber. Examples of this are the Rees-Ecker method using brilliant cresyl blue or Natt and Herrick's (1952) method using methyl violet 2B as the dye. Indirect methods, where total white cell numbers are counted from the haemocytometer and then percentage leucocyte counts obtained from a stained smear are used to calculate absolute values for the various cell types, are likely to be less accurate than direct methods since there are two sampling procedures involved, both contributing to the error of the method (Chubb & Rowell 1959). However, the indirect method is the simplest (Lucas & Jamroz 1961).

14.4.5 SOURCES OF ERROR IN COUNTS BY DILUTION

A few notes on some of the sources of error which may occur in blood counts by dilution may be useful.

INHERENT (STATISTICAL) ERROR

Since the distribution of cells in the haemocytometer is random and not subject to control, it follows that there is an inherent error of counts by dilution. The distribution of cells, however, is predictable on a statistical basis. The mathematical random distribution of particles conforms to the Poisson series, and this is well adhered to by blood cells in the haemocytometer. Since the error of this distribution from the theoretical perfect is constant, it follows that replicate counts of similar areas will tend to minimize it. The larger the number of similar areas, or cells, counted, the smaller will be the remaining inherent error of the count.

From a practical point of view, the foregoing paragraph leads to the conclusion that for reasonable accuracy in haematological terms it is necessary so to adjust dilutions of blood that not less than about 300 cells are enumerated over the area assessed.

APPARATUS NOT CLEAN AND DRY

This may cause uneven spreading on the haemocytometer and also counts which tend to be too low.

DILUTIONS PUT UP TOO LONG AFTER AGITATION OF THE BLOOD SAMPLE

Dilutions must be made within 1 minute of adequate shaking. Sedimentation becomes appreciable remarkably quickly.

INCORRECT DILUTIONS

The dilutions should always be standardized and noted. Pipettes must not be left containing blood in the capillary without immediately adding the correct diluent.

PIPETTE OVERFILLED AND RETURNED

If this occurs with blood, the count will be too high because some cells will remain adherent to the capillary wall. If the overfilling occurs with diluent then, obviously, the count will be too low.

PIPETTE INSUFFICIENTLY SHAKEN

By hand, this takes 2 minutes, by machine about 30 seconds. Shorter times do not reliably give uniform suspensions. The shaking must be done *after* the pipette has been laid on the bench for blood cells to stain in those techniques where delay is necessary.

CHAMBER FLOODED OR NOT FULL

Underfilled chambers must be discarded and recleaned before use. Spots of grease (e.g. fingermark) are the usual cause of trouble. Overfilled or flooded chambers can be used if the overfilling is confined to a meniscus slightly bulging over the tables and that this is corrected at once by removing a trace of fluid by aspiration with filter paper or blotting paper. Any degree of over-filling greater than this is unacceptable.

CHAMBER SHOWS UNEVEN SPREAD OF CELLS

Diluted and filled chambers should always be inspected for even distribution of cells before they are counted. Uneven distribution can arise from several causes. The commonest are dirty haemocytometers (greasy fingermarks etc.) and spreading from the pipette without previously discarding the whole of the (unmixed) contents of the capillary.

14.4.6 THE ERYTHROCYTE SEDIMENTATION RATE

There are two techniques commonly in use to measure the erythrocyte sedimentation rate (ESR). All depend upon maintaining a graduated tube of blood vertical. The test depends upon observation for a stated time of the blood column and measurement of the amount of clear plasma appearing above it.

The test is subject to several spurious variations. It is considerably affected

R. K. Archer

by the anticoagulant used, especially if there is any change in erythrocyte volume. Laboratory temperature is another significant variable. It is therefore essential to standardize such matters as these at the outset. I prefer to use disodium or dipotassium sequestrene as the anticoagulant and 20°C as the laboratory temperature.

WINTROBE TUBE METHOD

By this technique, standard Wintrobe haematocrit tubes are used. They are filled with blood to the '0' or '10' mark and placed in a rack which holds the tubes vertical. This is important since falsely fast sedimentation occurs in non-vertical tubes. The tubes are usually examined at 1 hour and the percentage of clear supernatant plasma recorded. In normal animals of some species the ESR is very rapid (e.g. horse), whilst in other species it may be very slow or almost absent (e.g. ox).

WESTERGREN TUBE METHOD

Westergren tubes resemble ordinary graduated laboratory pipettes. These are dipped into a suitable blood sample and blood is sucked up to the '0' graduation. The tubes are placed in a rack similar to that used for the Wintrobe tubes, but with a soft rubber disc at the bottom of each tube so that it is sealed when inserted.

THE MICROTUBE METHOD

It is possible to use the capillaries filled for the microhaematocrit test to obtain a measure of the ESR. In my hands and with animal blood the method has not been very satisfactory.

SPECIAL ESR METHOD FOR CHICKENS (R. D. HODGES)

The erythrocyte sedimentation rate should be performed using standard Wintrobe tubes held at an angle of 45° and read at either 1 or 2 hours. Where possible the tubes should be kept at a standard temperature, preferably 37°C (Sturkie & Textor 1958), although unspecified room temperature has frequently been used (Hunsaker *et al* 1964). When the tubes are held in a vertical position sedimentation is slow and results lower than expected for a given time interval.

MEASUREMENT OF PLASMA VISCOSITY

A method to measure plasma viscosity directly was proposed by Harkness (1971). This was used by Archer and Allen (1970) for plasma from horses, cattle and dogs and gives a very sensitive and reproducible set of figures.

The necessary apparatus is commercially available (Coulter Electronics Ltd) and consists essentially of a glass capillary 0·30 mm diameter and 20 cm long, through which specimens are drawn by a manometer. The results are expressed in centipoises, calibrated by reference to water which has a viscosity of 0·8937 at 25°C.

Some normal figures are given on Table 14.5.

Table 14.5 Some figures for normal plasma viscosity in horses, cattle and dogs

Species	Number	Mean	s.d.	Overall range
Horses	80	1·58	0·076	1·43–1·74
Cattle	12	1·87	—	1·77–2·14
Dogs	8	1·65	—	1·50–2·00

14.4.7 THE PACKED CELL VOLUME (PCV) OR HAEMATOCRIT

The haematocrit is probably the most useful single haematological test. From this one test not only is the packed cell volume obtained, but an idea of the total leucocyte count may be gained from the size of the 'buffy coat' layer and any discoloration (e.g. by bilirubin or haemolysis) of the plasma will be obvious. The microhaematocrit requires only 0·1 to 0·2 ml of blood and can be applied directly to drops of blood from a lancet wound.

THE STANDARD (WINTROBE) METHOD

The same Wintrobe tubes are used as in the ESR method just described. These tubes are filled with a Pasteur pipette exactly to the '0' or '10' mark and they must be entirely free of air bubbles. A centrifuge with a swing-out head is used capable of exerting at least 1500 g on the haematocrit tubes. Centrifugation is at 1500 to 2000 g for at least half an hour. It is not satisfactory to specify the details of centrifugation in rpm only since the relative centrifugal force (RCF) cannot be known from this unless the radius of the head to both top and bottom of the tube is also known. Most commonly instructions are given to centrifuge at 3000 rpm for 30 minutes and this will be satisfactory *only if a sufficient RCF is applied.*

Provided that an RCF of not less than 1500 is used then the application of 45,000 g-min to the haematocrit tubes will suffice. This can be checked by centrifuging again for a further half hour after the tubes have been read to see whether or not there is any more cellular packing. No change should be found.

There will always remain some trapped plasma among the packed cells. Correction can be applied for this. I prefer to standardize, and record, the RCF and time used. Provided this is at least 45,000 g-min at an RCF of not less than 1500, I do not use a correction factor. The plasma which remains trapped in such conditions appears to lie between 1 and 3 per cent.

The RCF of a particular centrifuge and head can be calculated from the formula:

$$RCF = 0.0000284 \times R \times N^2 \qquad (6)$$

where R = the radius in *inches* to the tip of the tube

N = revolutions per minute.

If R is measured in *centimetres* the constant used in (6) is 0.00001118.

It should be noted that the RCF so derived is applicable only to that part of the tube which lies at the radius used.

It will be seen that the haematocrit test can be made on Wintrobe tubes filled and observed for the ESR. Standard practice is to take the tubes from the ESR after 1 hour and centrifuge them to obtain the PCV.

THE MICROHAEMATOCRIT METHOD

Special capillary tubes and a special centrifuge are required. This centrifuge must be capable of exerting a force of 12,000 *g*. Capillary tubes of constant bore are used. Where the microhaematocrit is to be performed on a blood sample in an anticoagulant, an empty capillary is used; where drops of blood from a lancet wound are the source, heparinized capillaries are necessary. In either case the capillary is filled at least three quarters full and sealed by momentarily holding the tip in a flame just sufficiently long to melt and seal the glass, or by inserting the open end into 'Cristaseal' (Gelman-Hawksley Ltd.). After insertion into the head and centrifuging at 12,000 *g* for five minutes (60,000 *g*-min), the microhaematocrit tubes have to be read by means of an instrument since the volume spun is not a constant. A good microhaematocrit reader is marketed by Gelman-Hawksley Ltd.

The microhaematocrit is a remarkably sensitive and useful test. Given a good, special centrifuge it is trouble-free and repeatable. Its use is highly recommended, especially where small volumes of blood are to be examined.

14.4.8 HAEMOGLOBIN

In animals, assay of haemoglobin is complicated by the fact that in many species little or nothing is known about the structure of the molecule. Specifically, the iron content (0.347 g per 100 g anhydrous human haemoglobin) is frequently not known. While colorimetric assay is perfectly feasible, the standards used in the haematology of animals are usually those for man without correction. It must therefore be realized that haemoglobin assay in animals, while giving repeatable and reproducible figures, may be appreciably wrong in absolute value.

Haemoglobinometry should normally be undertaken only by the cyanmethaemoglobin method, but if any other method is used (e.g. oxyhaemoglobin assay) it should be adjusted to be comparable to the standard method.

For this method blood may be diluted with Drabkin's solution 1 in 200. The diluent is:

Potassium ferricyanide	200 mg
Potassium cyanide	50 mg
Potassium dihydrogen phosphate	140 mg
Distilled water to	1 litre

Adjust the pH to 7–7·4. Add 1 ml Nonidet P40 or equivalent colourless surface-active agent.

The resultant solution is measured for optical density in a spectrophotometer reading at 540 nm or at the mercury line, 546 nm. An Ilford filter 625 is suitable.

The colorimeter must be standardized and a calibration curve prepared. This is most easily done using commercially available cyanmethaemoglobin specimens which are checked against the reference standard maintained by the International Committee for Standardization in Haematology (see *British Journal of Haematology*, 1965, **11**, 389) and are usually sent out equivalent to about 10 g/dl of human haemoglobin.

The haemoglobin content of the cyanmethaemoglobin specimen is

$$\frac{\text{Reading of test}}{\text{Reading of standard}} \times \text{Haemoglobin g/dl of standard.}$$

Commercially available variants of Drabkin's solution can be very useful. 'Zap-Oglobin' (Coulter Electronics) for example contains 0·3 g potassium cyanide per 100 ml and a lytic agent. This agent lyses the red cells and their stroma, but leaves leucocytes in suspension and haemoglobin in solution. After the leucocytes have been counted the haemoglobin is measured as cyanmethaemoglobin. All commercial products of this kind must always be used according to the manufacturer's instructions although, for non-human blood, changes in recommended dilutions may have to be worked out.

GREY-WEDGE PHOTOMETER METHOD

Blood is washed into Drabkin's solution as before, at a 1:200 dilution. It is sometimes convenient to wash 0·02 ml into 4 ml, rather than 0·1 ml into 20 ml. The solution is compared in the MRC photometer with a half-field the intensity of which is controlled by a grey wedge. An Ilford No. 625 green filter is used in the instrument, and the result is read off as a percentage. This percentage is based on the assumption that 14·6 g per cent haemoglobin is normal (or 100 per cent) for man.

HAEMOGLOBIN ASSAY IN THE CHICKEN

It is possible to get a repeatable reading from chicken blood by the cyanmethbemoglobin method. The procedure is as described before, with the addition that centrifugation of the solution is essential, before it is placed in the colorimeter. If this is omitted the opacity due to the erythrocyte nuclei is liable to lead to substantial error. How far this method may assay actual chicken haemoglobin cannot at this time be stated. It is, however, quite possible to compare birds by this technique.

14.5   THE BLOOD FILM

The preparation of blood films would appear to be perfectly simple but, to judge by the number which are useless when made, detailed directions are necessary. Examination of well made and properly stained blood films can give much information and it is worth considerable effort to achieve really good preparations.

The preparation of blood films intended to be dried and then subjected to Romanowski staining is considered here. The examination of wet films and a number of special staining methods are described in section 14.8.

14.5.1   PREPARATION OF BLOOD FILMS

It is assumed that blood films are to be made for morphological differentiation of leucocytes after Romanowski staining. Films for other purposes may need to be made differently. The primary requirement of a good blood film is that it be thin enough and that it does not extend more than three quarters of the way along the slide. The slides should be spotlessly clean and free of grease.

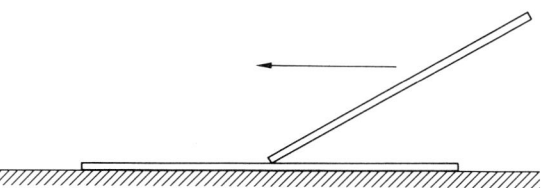

Fig. 14.7   Making a blood film. The spreader slide is moved by hand in the direction of the arrow. This slide should be slightly narrower than standard so that the edges of the blood film are clear of the edges of the slides used.

A drop of blood is placed almost at one end of a clean slide (Fig. 14.7). Another slide is brought towards it at an angle of about 30° to the horizontal until it touches the blood. The drop should spread *at once* along the junction of the two slides (if it does not the slides may not be clean) and the film is made by pulling the drop of blood behind this second slide. If correctly done, the spread film will reach almost, but not quite, to the edges of the slide and not more than three quarters of the way along it. If the 'spreader' slide is held at a more obtuse angle (more towards vertical) the film will be thicker; a more acute angle will give a thinner film. Similarly, more rapid spreading gives a thicker, and therefore shorter, film; the converse also applies.

There is a tendency for leucocytes to collect at the edges and end of blood films. Further, the thickness and quality of these films are variable. Where examinations are directed towards the differentiation of leucocytes it is better to minimize these variables as far as practicable. For this purpose the blood

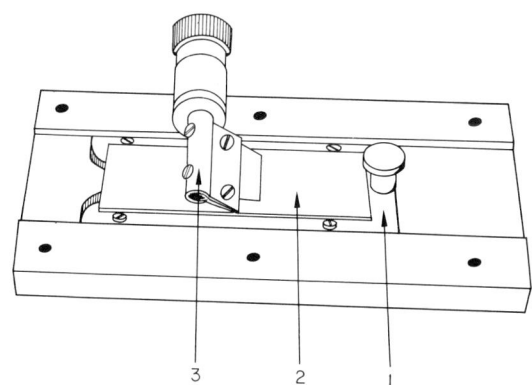

Fig. 14.8 The Marks *et al* blood film machine, a mechanical device used for making blood films. (1) The slide carrying tray, (2) microscope slide, (3) spring loaded blade.

film machine of Marks, Bailey and Gunz (1950) is recommended (Fig. 14.8). The shape of the spreader and the angle at which it is held to the slide are standardized by this instrument, only the speed of spreading remains variable. Since the amount of blood used is small and is placed upon the slide, the spreader of the machine is self-cleaning, in the sense that no blood remains from one specimen to contaminate the next.

Blood films should be air-dried as soon as they are made. This may take half an hour or more, but for the first few minutes the slides should be waved in air quite vigorously to accelerate gross evaporation since this minimizes drying artefacts. Where films are made in the field, it is worth recalling that it is most difficult to produce adequate films in ambient temperatures below freezing point or in very humid conditions.

14.5.2 STAINING BLOOD FILMS FOR LEUCOCYTE DIFFERENTIAL COUNTING

A variety of Romanowsky-type stains may be used, including Giemsa, Leishman or Wright's fluid. I prefer the use of the Leishman stain according to the following schedule, avoiding the use of the stain purchased in the liquid form. It is most important that the methanol used as solvent should be of adequate standard for this particular purpose and that it should be free of acetone.

LEISHMAN STAIN

Prepare and air-dry blood films

Place on a rack, over a sink, film
  uppermost

Fix for 1 minute | Undiluted stock Leishman stain

Stain for 10–15 minutes | Dilute Leishman stain on film with about 2 volumes of phosphate buffer pH 7·2

Wash | Stream of distilled water from a wash-bottle

Blot dry

Examine by oil-immersion without
  mounting

Notes

(1) Preparation of stock Leishman solution:

Leishman stain powder (Hopkins & Williams Ltd)   0·15 g
Methanol (Solvent methanol, BDH Ltd)   100 ml

Place the powder in a mortar. Grind with a little methanol until a smooth suspension is achieved. It is essential that this step be properly done: it cannot be hurried. Complete solution of the stain must be achieved when the remaining methanol is added. The stock so made appears to benefit by storage for a few weeks in a dark glass bottle before it is used.

(2) Phosphate buffer M/15 (see page 562) should be diluted 1:10.

(3) In hot climates the stock stain solution may evaporate on the film during fixation at such a speed that some stain is precipitated. Should this occur, add more stock stain, *not* methanol, during fixation.

(4) When the stain is diluted with buffer, a golden scum should form within about a minute. If it does not, addition of more buffer is usually effective. Diluted Leishman stain is transparent and of a mid-blue colour. The commonest cause of under-staining with Leishman stain is insufficient dilution of the solution with buffer.

(5) Adequate staining of blood films in most species is obtained by this technique. However, in certain cases it fails to some extent. In particular, Leishman stain will not differentiate the eosinophil from the heterophil of the rabbit or the chicken. In the case of the chicken this is of less moment since the heterophils have ovoid granules, and the true eosinophil granules are spheri-

cal. In the rabbit proper differentiation cannot be made from Romanowsky-stained films and a special technique is necessary (see page 593).

WRIGHT'S STAIN

The technique is precisely similar to that described for Leishman stain except that the action of the diluted stain in buffer is sufficient in 5 minutes (not 10 to 15 minutes).

Stock solution of Wright's stain is readily purchased and there seems to be no advantage in making this solution in the laboratory.

GIEMSA'S STAIN

Prepare and air-dry blood films	
Fix for 2 minutes	Absolute methanol
Stain for 5 minutes	Stock Giemsa Solution 1
	Distilled water 2
Wash until film appears pink	Stream of distilled water from a wash-bottle
Blot dry	
Examine by oil-immersion without mounting	

Notes

(1) Giemsa stock solution is readily available. That by Gurr has been found satisfactory.

(2) For most purposes the use of Giemsa stain is less satisfactory than Leishman or Wright's stain where leucocyte morphology is important. In particular, nuclear detail appears to be inferior.

MAY-GRÜNWALD-GIEMSA (MGG) STAIN

Prepare and air-dry blood films	
Fix for 2–10 minutes	Absolute methanol
Stain for 15 minutes in a Coplin jar	May-Grünwald solution 1
	Phosphate buffer pH 7·2 1
Stain for 30 minutes in a Coplin jar	Giemsa stock solution 1
	Phosphate buffer pH 7·2 9
Rinse	Phosphate buffer
Blot dry	

Notes

(1) May-Grünwald and Giemsa stock solutions are used as purchased. Those made by Gurr are satisfactory.

(2) Some haematologists prefer to use a phosphate buffer at pH 6·8. Some variation between 6·8 and 7·2 may be found individually preferable for a particular purpose or species.

(3) The results obtained with the MGG method are excellent. It is, however, much more complex and time consuming than the Leishman technique. Since the latter is almost always adequate for routine purposes I would advise the use of MGG only where particularly well-stained cytoplasmic granules are required, especially in the neutrophil granulocytes.

14.5.3   THE DIFFERENTIAL LEUCOCYTE COUNT

The stained film is examined under an oil-immersion objective. I prefer to use a 3·6 mm fluorite, reserving the 2 mm objective for individual inspection of any doubtful cells. Since the leucocytes do not spread evenly about a film, it is usual to employ a so-called 'battlement' counting technique. Starting at the end (tail) of the film, the cells are differentiated for about 1 mm along the film, 1 mm inwards, along again, outwards and along and so on. By this means the effects of any non-random leucocyte distribution is minimized. At least 200 consecutive leucocytes should be identified.

In conjunction with the total leucocyte count, the differential count can be used to obtain absolute figures. Thus, if the total count is 5×10^9 leucocytes per litre and the differential gives 40 per cent lymphocytes, then there are $(40/100) \times 5 = 2 \times 10^9$ lymphocytes per litre of blood. I prefer to record leucocyte data in this way whenever possible. Eosinophil leucocytes are subject to rather larger errors by this technique since they tend to congregate at the tail of blood films. Where assays of eosinophils are required, counts by direct dilution are recommended (page 569), especially if the counts are low. Somewhat similarly, direct dilution is best for basophil counts.

INDIRECT PLATELET COUNT

It is possible to use the stained film to count platelets or erythrocytes with inclusions such as Howell–Jolly bodies or basophilic stippling. On a stained film the number of platelets seen while a definite number of erythrocytes is passed under the eye of the observer gives a measure of the absolute platelet count. For example, during observation of 1000 erythrocytes on a film, 50 platelets were seen. If the erythrocyte count was $5 \times 10^{12}/l$ then the platelet count is $(5 \times 10^{12})/(1000) \times 50 = 250 \times 10^9/l$. Clearly, this sort of count is subject to substantial error. It has limited use. There are occasions, however, when only one count has been made and a film is available. By extension of this technique it is possible to derive some idea of the leucocyte count where the erythrocyte count is known, or vice versa.

THICK FILM METHOD

On occasion, only thick, badly prepared blood films may be available. There is no way of making a good stained film from bad material, but it is possible to get some information from such films in the following way.

Air-dry the films	
Stain for 5 minutes	Giemsa stock solution 1
	Distilled water 1
Pour off and repeat the staining, 5 minutes	As above
Fix 30 seconds	Leishman stock solution, undiluted
Rinse rapidly	Distilled water
Dry in air without blotting (Care! Film comes away from slide easily)	

The leucocytes are usually too badly spread to permit proper differentiation. Blood parasites are sometimes well shown by this technique.

14.6 CLEANING APPARATUS

It is very important that all haematological glassware be cleaned immediately after use. Haemocytometers and their cover glasses should be washed under a stream of distilled water and dried on fluff-free cloth or soft paper such as 'Kleenex'. Pipettes are dealt with by connection to a suction pump and sucking through, first distilled water, then acetone. It is an advantage if they can be dried overnight at about 37°C. From time to time all pipettes should be soaked overnight in a good cleansing fluid such as 'Hemosol' and then washed again in the morning. Blocked pipettes are best dealt with by treatment with 'Hemosol', but this complication should not arise. Avoid the use of wire, even soft copper wire, to clear blocked pipettes. Monofilament nylon (surgical suture material) is sometimes successful as a probe if such treatment becomes unavoidable.

Microscope slides should be cleaned even though they are new. Good factory-cleaned slides require only a thorough wipe with a 'Kleenex' tissue or chamois leather. If there is any trace of grease, slides should be stored for 24 hours in absolute methanol after vigorous washing with soap and water and thorough rinsing. They are then dried with clean tissue before use.

14.7 CALCULATION OF STANDARD RATIOS

The 3 standard ratios in common use are derived by calculation from the results of haematological tests. These are as follows:

Mean corpuscular haemoglobin (MCH) This is the average haemoglobin content of a single red cell expressed as picograms (10^{-12} g). It is calculated from the formula

$$\text{MCH} = \frac{\text{Haemoglobin in g/dl}}{\text{Erythrocytes per litre}} \times 10^7 \qquad (7)$$

Mean corpuscular volume (MCV)   The average volume of an erythrocyte expressed in cubic microns or femtolitres. It is calculated from the equation:

$$\text{MCV} = \frac{\text{PCV in l/l}}{\text{Erythrocytes per l}} \qquad (8)$$

Mean corpuscular haemoglobin concentration (MCHC)   The concentration of haemoglobin as grams per decilitre of erythrocytes. This is calculated from the formula:

$$\text{MCHC} = \frac{\text{Haemoglobin in g/dl}}{\text{Packed cell volume in l/l}} \times 100 \qquad (9)$$

14.8a   SPECIAL HAEMATOLOGICAL TECHNIQUES

The purpose of this section is to give details of some haematological techniques which have been found useful during the examination of animal blood. These techniques are not in routine use but they are in frequent use.

Clearly the contents of this section could be almost limitless. Some selection of methods to be considered has been essential and it is for this reason that methods of proven use only have been included. Often several techniques have the same object in view: in these instances the selection must of necessity be somewhat personal, and is confined to haematological methods which have been used and found useful in the author's laboratory. Methods for serological tests, including blood group determination and biochemical methods are omitted since both are well covered in the relevant textbooks.

14.8b   SPECIAL CELLULAR TECHNIQUES

In this section staining methods and special microscopic techniques will be noted as well as a test of erythrocyte fragility.

14.8.1   ERYTHROCYTE FRAGILITY TEST

A method after Creed (1938) has proved useful. It depends upon placing erythrocytes in accurately diluted hypotonic saline and is therefore a measure of osmotic fragility. The distilled water used should be glass-distilled and deionized and must be free of copper ions. A standard 1 per cent solution of sodium chloride ('Analar' or equivalent grade) is made in a volumetric flask and stored at 4°C. Twelve test tubes 75 mm × 9·5 mm are set in a rack and prepared with diluted saline by adding drops of 1 per cent saline and of distilled water as shown in Table 14.6.

Table 14.6 Dilutions of saline with water for the Creed (1938) test

Tube No.	Parts saline 1%	Parts water	Final dilution saline %
1	18	7	0·72
2	17	8	0·68
3	16	9	0·64
4	15	10	0·60
5	14	11	0·56
6	13	12	0·52
7	12	13	0·48
8	11	14	0·44
9	10	15	0·40
10	9	16	0·36
11	8	17	0·32
12	7	18	0·28

The preparation of the blood sample is important. Since the degree of oxygenation affects the osmotic fragility of the erythrocytes it is necessary to standardize. This is best done by swirling about 5 ml of blood in the bottom of a 25 or 50 ml wide-mouthed Erlenmeyer flask for about 2 minutes to achieve good oxygenation. The choice of anticoagulant may also affect the test and standardization is important. Sequestrene is commonly used.

The tubes are mixed by inversion, and 1 part of oxygenated blood is added to each. The tubes are again mixed by inversion forthwith and about 10 minutes later. After a further 10 minutes on the bench at about 20°C the tubes are centrifuged.

A standard solution of the subject's haemoglobin is prepared by adding 1 part of blood to 25 parts of distilled water. This is the same dilution as is used in each of the 12 haemolysis tubes for the main test. Haemoglobin assays are then made on the supernatant fluid of all tubes (13 in all) and, from these figures the percentage of haemolysis at a given saline concentration may be calculated.

14.8.2 DEMONSTRATION OF RETICULOCYTES

Reticulocytes can be demonstrated by supravital staining. It must be noted that fixed films cannot be used to show reticulocytes. The methods used all depend upon supravital staining with a suitable dye, usually brilliant cresyl blue.

DRY FILM METHOD

For this technique a 0·3 per cent solution of brilliant cresyl blue is made in absolute alcohol. A drop of this solution is applied about two thirds of the way along an ordinary, but strictly clean, microscope slide. The drop should spread to a circle of about 20 mm diameter. The slides are air-dried and then marked by a cross made with a grease pencil *on the back* of the slide immediately beneath the deposited brilliant cresyl blue. Such prepared slides are stable and can be kept indefinitely if wrapped and stored dry.

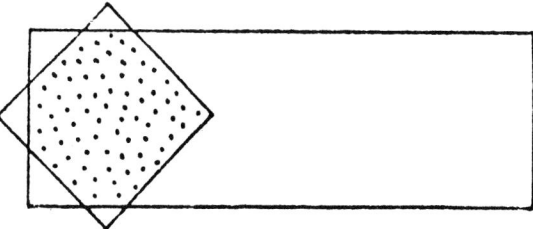

Fig. 14.9 Supravital staining for reticulocytes. A drop of blood is placed under a cover-glass on a prepared slide (see text). The cover-glass is used as a spreader to make a film when staining is complete.

A drop of blood to be examined is placed on the brilliant cresyl blue. A 2·5 × 2·5 cm cover-glass is placed over it crossways (Fig. 14.9). The drop of blood should be of such a size that it just spreads to the edge of the cover-glass. Supravital staining should be allowed to proceed for 2–4 minutes at bench temperature (20°C). Using the cover-glass as a spreader, a film is made on the prepared slide. This film is air-dried, fixed in undiluted Leishman stain for 30 seconds and stained in diluted Leishman stain (see page 580) for 1–2 minutes only. Longer staining in diluted Leishman may make the reticulum less discernible.

It is usual to count 1000 consecutive erythrocytes under the 2 mm objective, noting the number which show any reticular structure. The reticulocytes per cent of the erythrocytes is thus obtained.

DILUTION METHOD

A solution of 0·05 per cent brilliant cresyl blue in 0·85 per cent saline is prepared. The addition of 1 per cent disodium sequestrene is often useful to prevent clumping. Blood is diluted in this fluid 1:10 using a leucocyte counting pipette. Counting may be done on a haemocytometer, but this is extremely difficult unless a special instrument is available (vaccine counting chamber) which is sufficiently thin for use with a 2 mm objective. Counting is more usually made on a wet cover-glass/slide preparation sealed with a paraffin wax or petroleum jelly.

FLUORESCENCE METHOD

Reticulocytes fluoresce well when treated with acridine orange (AO) supravitally. They are not visible on fixed, fluorochromed films. The technique of Vander, Harris and Ellis (1963) has been found useful especially in those species (e.g. the horse) in which reticulocytes are rare and indistinct with brilliant cresyl blue. The diluting fluid is AO in physiological saline. A stock 0·1 per cent AO in 0·85 per cent NaCl is made and kept at 4°C. It is stable for a few weeks. For use, this solution is diluted with 0·85 per cent NaCl to contain 0·01 per cent AO. Blood in sequestrene, or from a lancet wound, is taken into a leucocyte pipette to the 1·0 mark. The pipette is filled with AO solution (i.e. 1:10) and agitated as usual. A drop of cell suspension is placed on a slide, covered with a cover-glass and sealed with paraffin wax. It is best examined about 15 minutes later.

Preparations are illuminated with UV and blue light, excluding wavelengths above 460 mμ. The eye-piece filter should be orange to prevent excessive blue illumination. Suitable exciter filters are Schott BG 12 (6 mm) or BG 12 (2 mm) with UG1 (1·5 mm). Absorption filters should be GG 9 (1 mm) with OG 1 (1·5 mm) or GG 9 (1 mm) alone, the latter with the second exciter filter only. A dark ground or phase contrast condenser should be used with a suitable UV light sources (e.g. Osram HBO 200 w). Reticulocytes stand out clearly as red-fluorescing bodies against a dark blue or black background.

14.8.3 DEMONSTRATION OF ORGANISMS IN BLOOD

The AO method for platelets can be used to demonstrate pyroplasms (Winter 1967). Pyroplasms are also readily seen in routine Romanowsky-stained films, as are trypanosomes. Bartonella stains well with methyl violet by the Gram method. Special methods are generally not needed to detect organisms in blood provided that the Romanowsky preparations are of good quality.

14.8.4 CYTOCHEMISTRY OF LEUCOCYTES

A large number of techniques is available for the cytochemical investigation of leucocytes. Some of the techniques which have either become well established or which appear to be useful in comparative animal haematology are described in this section. For further details, and for proper discussion of the necessary controls of histochemical or cytochemical methods, the reader is referred to the excellent textbooks on this subject already published. For general histochemistry the textbook of Pearse (1972) is recommended; for enzyme histochemistry there is the specialized volume by Burstone (1962).

THE FEULGEN REACTION FOR DNA

This technique is used also to demonstrate nucleoli. The latter are negative, but the perinucleolar ring is strongly Feulgen-positive so that the nucleoli are sharply delineated. This method is useful for the demonstration of chromosomes in mitotic figures.

Use fresh, air-dried films. Films up to 24 hours old may be satisfactory. Films can be used many months, if not years later if they have been fixed.

Fix air-dried films $\frac{1}{2}$–1 minute at 4°C	Formaldehyde 40% 10 ml. Methanol 90 ml. Kept at 4°C

Hydrolyse with N. acid
  2 mins at 20°C
  2 mins at 60°C
  2–4 mins at 20°C
	Hydrochloric acid, normal.

Stain in leucobasic fuchsin $\frac{1}{2}$–2 hours	Schiff's reagent (See note below)
Rinse in 2 or 3 changes of sulphurous acid	Distilled water saturated with SO_2 from a cylinder
Rinse 10–15 mins	Running tap-water
Blot dry	

Result: DNA red.

Films may be mounted directly into DPX, but I prefer to leave them unmounted and examine by oil-immersion.

Preparation of Schiff's reagent Several methods of preparing this reagent are available. I recommend that of Itikawa and Ogura (1954).

Add 1 g of basic fuchsin to 200 ml of distilled water at about 90°C. Shake until dissolved. Cool and filter. Bubble SO_2 from a syphon (BDH Ltd) through the solution until it is saturated. This usually takes about an hour, and the solution should become clear pinkish-yellow in colour. Add 1 g of activated charcoal, shake for a minute or so and filter. Store, well stoppered, at 4°C.

The method of Barger and Delamater (1948) is also recommended. Basic fuchsin is dissolved in hot distilled water as before, filtered and cooled. 1 ml of thionyl chloride ($SOCl_2$) is added, and the mixture stood in the dark overnight. Shake with charcoal and filter. Store at 4°C.

Schiff's reagent should be warmed to 20°C before use.

It should be noted that not all batches of basic fuchsin will form good Schiff's reagent. It is wise to specify the use for which the basic fuchsin is required when it is ordered. In case of difficulty it is worth trying several batches of stain, if possible from more than one supplier.

FLUORESCENT FEULGEN REACTION

This method, after Kasten *et al* (1959), is precisely similar to that just described except for the Schiff's reagent. For the latter is substituted a 0·1 per cent aqueous solution of acriflavine which is treated with SO_2 and extracted with charcoal exactly as in the Itikawa and Ogura method just described. This reagent is stable for about 2 weeks. Examine in UV light as described for reticulocytes (page 587).

Result: DNA fluoresces brilliant orange.

METHYL GREEN–PYRONINE STAIN FOR RNA AND DNA

The method requires exact technique if reproducible and meaningful results are to be obtained. It is a specific technique for RNA if used in conjunction with ribonuclease extraction after Brachet (1942).

Extraction of methyl green. The 2 per cent aqueous solution of methyl green should be shaken up with an equal volume of chloroform in a separating funnel and stood overnight. The process should be repeated until the chloroform does not extract appreciable amounts of violet dye. Washed methyl green is not stable indefinitely and should be replaced at intervals of a few weeks for best results.

Some fixed films are incubated in 0·2 mg/ml ribonuclease in distilled water at 37°C for an hour. When subsequently stained there should be no red-positive material.

Air-dry films and fix ½–1 minute at 4°C	Formalin/methanol, as Feulgen method
Rinse	Phosphate buffer M/15, pH 7
Stain in a Coplin jar ½ hour	Solution A: Aqueous pyronine 5% 1·75 ml Methyl green 2% 1·0 ml (Methyl green must be chloroform-washed to remove methyl violet) Distilled water 25 ml
	Solution B: N/10 acetic acid 80 ml N/10 sodium acetate 120 ml *For use* mix equal parts A and B
Rinse rapidly	Distilled water
Blot dry	

Result: DNA green, RNA red.

ACRIDINE ORANGE FLUORESCENCE METHOD

The method of Bertalanffy (1960) is recommended. It is as follows:

Air-dry films and fix 5 minutes	Absolute methanol	
Pass rapidly through the solutions specified. The whole set should be completed within 90 seconds	1. Alcohol 2. Alcohol 3. Alcohol 4. Distilled water 5. Acetic acid 6. Distilled water	80% 70% 50% 1%
Stain in acridine orange for 3 minutes	Acridine orange 0·1% M/15 phosphate buffer pH 6·0	2 ml 18 ml
Wash at least 1 minute	M/15 phosphate buffer pH 6·0	
Differentiate 1–2 minutes	Calcium chloride 1·1g Distilled water 100 ml	
Rinse	M/15 phosphate buffer pH 6·0	
Mount	in M/15 phosphate buffer pH 6·0	

Result: DNA fluoresces bright green, RNA red, when examined in UV light as described on page 587. Acridine orange staining solution is unstable and should be prepared daily. Stock 0·1 per cent solution is stable at 4°C for a few weeks.

THE PERIODIC ACID SCHIFF REACTION (PAS)

For glycogen and allied compounds.

Air-dry films and fix by a variety of methods, e.g.	(a) Formalin methanol (as Feulgen method) (b) Formalin vapour for 4–5 minutes (as in Sudan black method, below) (c) Methanol 5 minutes
Rinse in water	
Oxidize for 15–20 minutes	1% periodic acid
Drain, immerse in Schiff's Reagent for 15–20 minutes	Schiff reagent as Feulgen method
Rinse several times	Water, saturated with SO_2
Wash 5 minutes	Distilled water
Counterstain, if required 30 to 120 secs	Methyl green 2%
Rinse and blot dry	

Result: glycogen and other PAS-positive materials red.

FLUORESCENT-PAS METHOD
(After Damasio, Montale & Gay 1962.)

Fix air-dried films 10 minutes in a Coplin jar	Osmic acid	1 g
	Distilled water	50 ml
	Phosphate buffer pH 7·4	1 ml
	Stable about 3–4 weeks only	
Oxidize 5–15 minutes	1% periodic acid	
Stain 20 minutes	0·1% acriflavine, saturated with SO_2 as in Fluorescent Feulgen reaction	
Rinse 2 minutes	Acidified alcohol	
Blot dry		
Mount	Entellan (Merck) or phosphate buffer pH 7·4	

Result: PAS-positive materials fluoresce bright orange in UV light. Avoid mounting in glycerol. Most synthetic mountants fluoresce and are useless for this technique, but Entellan is satisfactory.

THE PRUSSIAN BLUE REACTION FOR IRON
(After Pearse (1972) and Hayhoe & Quaglino 1960.)

Fix air dried films	Methanol, formalin or alcohol provided that the pH is neutral. Formalin/methanol as Feulgen reaction is particularly recommended	
Treat in an iron-free Coplin jar for 1 hour at about 20°C	Potassium ferrocyanide 2%	15 ml
	Hydrochloric acid 2%	15 ml
Rinse briefly in distilled water		
Counterstain in nuclear fast red for 4–8 minutes	Nuclear fast red	0·1%
	$Al_2 (SO_4)_3.16H_2O$ in distilled water	7%
Rinse and dry in air		

Result: ferric iron deep Prussian blue.

This test is used to demonstrate haemosiderin or other iron-rich granules in normoblasts or erythrocytes ('siderocytes') and in macrophages which have ingested iron ('siderophage'). The technique may be useful both in bone marrow and peripheral blood films in the investigation of anaemias. Usually, there are less siderocytes than reticulocytes in circulating blood during health.

Films stained previously by Romanowsky techniques, even years before, can successfully be subjected to the Prussian blue reaction. Hayhoe and

Quaglino (1960) recommend decoloration overnight in methanol and then performing the reaction, without further fixation, as described above.

SUDAN BLACK STAINS FOR LIPIDS
(After Hayhoe 1953.)

Fix air-dried films for about 5 minutes in formalin vapour in a closed jar	Paraformaldehyde powder at the bottom of a Coplin jar to a depth of ca. 1 cm
Wash 15 minutes	Running tap water
Stain in Sudan black 30–90 minutes	Solution A
	Phenol (cryst.) 16 g
	Ethanol 30 ml
	Solution B
	$Na_2 HPO_4.12H_2O$ 0·3 g
	distilled water 100 ml
	Solution C
	Sudan Black B 0·3 g
	Ethanol 100 ml
	For use, mix Solution A 20 ml
	Solution B 20 ml
	and add Solution C 60 ml
	This mixture is stable for 6–8 wks in an airtight bottle. Filter by suction before use.
Rinse rapidly	70% alcohol
Wash in water 1 minute	
Counterstain, if desired, 2 minutes	Leishman stock stain solution 1 part
	Phosphate buffer pH 6·8 2 parts
Rinse in water and blot dry	

Result: lipids black.

PEROXIDASE
(After Sato & Sekiya, 1926.)

Air-dried fresh films fixed 30–60 seconds	Copper sulphate 0·5% aqueous solution
Tip off fixative, and without washing stain in benzidene reagent for 2 minutes	Heat 500 ml water to about 80°C and dissolve in it 0·5 g of benzidene. Stand overnight. Filter. Add $\frac{1}{2}$ ml of 6% (20 vols) H_2O_2 and store in a dark bottle
	Stable for some months
Wash well in tap water	

| Counterstain, if desired, 2 minutes | Leishman stock stain solution | 1 part |
| Rinse in water and blot dry | Phosphate buffer pH 8·8 | 2 parts |

Result: sites of peroxidase activity deep blue.

PEROXIDASE

(After Quaglino & Flemans 1958.) This method avoids the use of benzidene by the substitution of O-tolidene. It does not always give satisfactory results with animal blood.

Fix air-dried films 30 seconds	Formaldehyde 40%	10 ml
	Ethanol	90 ml
Wash in tap water and dry in air		
Stain for 7 minutes	O-tolidene	250 mg
	Ethanol	6 ml
	When dissolved, add water	4 ml
	H_2O_2 6% (20 vols)	0·2 ml
	Stable for a few weeks	
Wash in tap water and dry in air		
Counterstain, if required, 2 minutes	Leishman stock stain solution	1 part
	Phosphate buffer pH 6·8	2 parts
Rinse in water and blot dry		

Results: sites of peroxidase activity brownish green.

UNDRITZ MODIFICATION OF THE PEROXIDASE REACTION FOR EOSINOPHILS (1952)

Air-dry films 4 to 5 hours		
Fix 5 minutes	May-Grunwald solution	
Stain in Giemsa with peroxidase reagent for 15–30 minutes with films inverted, resting on match sticks, in a petri dish	Giemsa staining solution	10 parts
	Peroxidase reagent	0·1 part
	Peroxidase reagent: dissolve in 6 ml 96% ethyl alcohol as much benzidene (Merck) as will go on a knife point. Add 4 ml glass distilled water and 0·02 ml H_2O_2 (20 vols)	
	Stable for a few days only	
	Giemsa staining solution:	
	Giemsa stock solution	0·3 ml
	Distilled water to	10 ml
Wash 1 minute	Running tap-water	
Dry in air without blotting		

Result: eosinophils greenish yellow colour; other granulocytes do not react and have a typical Romanowsky-stained, though pale, appearance.

This technique is especially useful in the rabbit and also in the rat and mouse. The benzidene used must be pure or the reaction may fail. Furthermore, films must be dried for some hours: fresh films dried only for a few minutes do not react reliably.

ALKALINE PHOSPHATASE

Two methods of demonstrating this enzyme are given. The first, after Kaplow (1955) is reliable and repeatable; the second, after Burstone (1958) may be more sensitive. Only the incubating solutions used differ, so that the method can be described once and either solution used.

Fix air dried films for 30 seconds at 4°C	Formaldehyde 40%	10 ml
	Methanol	90 ml
Rinse rapidly (ca. 10 seconds)	Distilled water	
Incubate 10–15 minutes in Solution A or B	Solution A:	
	Sodium α naphthyl acid phosphate	35 mg
These solutions are unstable. They are prepared at the last moment and filtered onto the slides	Fast Blue RR	35 mg
	Propanediol buffer	35 ml
	Solution B	
	Naphthol ASBl phosphate	5 mg
	Fast Black B	10 mg
	Propanediol buffer	10 ml
	Propanediol buffer pH 9·75 (1) 2-amino-2-methyl-1,3-	
	propanediol	2·1 g
	Distilled water	100 ml
	(2) 0·1 N.HCl	
	For use, Solution (1)	25 ml
	Solution (2)	5 ml
Wash ca. 20 seconds	Running tap-water	
Counterstain 30 to 120 seconds	Methyl green 2%	
Rinse and dry in air		

Result: sites of alkaline phosphatase activity blue or black according to the stable diazotate and naphthol used.

In Solution A, some authors prefer to use Fast Garnet GBC in place of Fast Blue RR. In Solution B, many different naphthol AS substrates can be used with various stable diazotates. Of the latter, Red-Violet LB has been found useful.

It is convenient to prepare solutions of the naphthol AS phosphates in dimethyl formamide. About 20 mg/ml is suitable, so that 0·25 ml will contain 5 mg.

A useful alternative red counterstain is 0·1 per cent nuclear fast red in 7 per cent $Al_2 (SO_4)_3$. $16H_2O$; 4–8 minutes' staining is sufficient.

A selection of the naphthol AS substrates is available from Nutritional Biochemical Co, and the Sigma Chemical Co.

NON-SPECIFIC ESTERASE
(After Moloney *et al* 1960.)

Fix air dried films at 4°C for 30 seconds	Formaldehyde 40%	10 ml
	Methanol	90 ml
Incubate 30 minutes in the solution	Naphthol AS-D chloro-	
	acetate	10 mg
The solution is unstable and must be	Acetone	0·5 ml
prepared at the last moment and	Add water	5 ml
filtered onto the slides	Buffer	5 ml
	Fast Garnet GBC salt	10 mg
	Buffer pH 7·4	
	Stock solution: sodium	
	acetate trihidrate	9·7 g
	Sodium barbitone	14·7 g
	Water	500 ml
	For use: Stock solution	10 ml
	0·1 N.HCl	10 ml
	Water	26 ml
Rinse in tap water		
Counterstain 5 minutes	Haematoxylin	
Rinse, mount in copolymer without	PVP/VA E-735	1 part
drying	Distilled water	1 part

Result: sites of non-specific esterase activity red.

The copolymer is available from Antara Chemicals, USA, or Fine Dyestuffs and Chemicals, England. It is a valuable water-miscible mountant first recommended by Lamkie and Burstone (1962). Naphthol AS-D chloroacetate is available from the Sigma Chemical Co.

SUMMARY OF CYTOCHEMICAL TECHNIQUES USED IN HAEMATOLOGY
The several techniques described all have one or more particular applications in clinical haematology. Some of these applications are indicated in Table 14.7. These applications are not, of course, exhaustive, but may serve to show how cytochemistry may assist in the investigation of an uncertain cell type or intracellular structure. The remarks made in the table do not necessarily

Table 14.7　Applications of cytochemical tests in clinical haematology

Cytochemical method	Material demonstrated	Some haematological applications
Feulgen	DNA	Nuclear structure. Perinucleolar ring.
Methyl green, pyronine	DNA and RNA	Nature of basophilic inclusions in nucleus or cytoplasm.
PAS	Glycogen and mucopolysaccharides.	Activity, particularly of lymphocytes, altered in certain diseases. Lymphoblasts usually much more active than myeloblasts.
Sudan Black	Lipids	Lipid granules and inclusions.
Peroxidase	Sites of enzyme activity	In granulocytes and some monocytes only.
Alkaline phosphatase	Sites of enzyme activity	Confined almost entirely to mature neutrophils. Activity varies in some diseases.

apply to all species. They do apply, for the most part, to man, horse, dog and the smaller laboratory animals; I have not checked other species by all the techniques mentioned. In the rabbit, the peculiar eosinophil must be remembered, and in the mouse neutrophils are devoid of alkaline phosphatase activity. In the chicken, heterophils are negative for alkaline phosphatase, but contain some acid phosphatase. Whenever a cytochemical abnormality is demonstrated, it is best to confirm the observation with a sufficient number of known normal preparations from the same species taken and treated if possible at the same time and in the same batch as the abnormal specimen.

14.8.5　EXAMINATION OF LIVING CELLS BY PHASE CONTRAST

This method is of value in certain conditions. For example, in haemolytic disease the red cell 'ghosts' are well seen. The use of anticoagulant is mandatory and the examination should be made within about an hour of drawing blood or bone marrow aspirate.

Preparations are made by placing a drop of blood on the centre of a scrupulously clean slide, dropping over this a cover-glass of such size that gentle pressure will cause the material just to reach the edge of the glass. The preparation should be sealed with paraffin wax. Examinations are perfectly satisfactory at 20°C, but for motility studies a warm stage at 37°C should be used.

For haematological purposes the phase contrast microscope need have no low power objective. A dry objective of about ×60 is desirable; a ×100 immersion objective is essential. There appears to be no advantage in using so-called 'negative' phase contrast objectives except for mixed illumination of certain fluorescent specimens.

14.9 BLOOD COAGULATION

Numerous tests of various facets of the blood clotting mechanism have been described. Almost every one of these was proposed for and worked out exclusively with human samples. The study of blood coagulation in animals has been little undertaken and much of the work that has been completed involves the use of non-standard techniques inadequately specified. In this section it is proposed to describe a few well-established methods that are proven for human specimens and have been used satisfactorily for some animal species.

Study of the bleeding time is complicated by the presence of hair or feathers. Depilation is liable to affect the results to a significant extent. At this time I do not know of any satisfactory technique for measuring the bleeding time of hairy animals. I do not consider that scalpel or lancet wounds made upon depilatated areas can as yet yield meaningful results.

For a detailed and lucid exposition of human blood coagulation, the reader is referred to the textbook of Biggs (1972).

THE PLATELET COUNT
This was described above (page 571) but should always be performed whenever possible during coagulation investigations.

14.9.1 WHOLE BLOOD CLOTTING TIME

The method most commonly, and successfully, used is that of Lee and White (1913). It necessitates making the test with a water-bath alongside the subject since whole blood must be incubated at 37°C as soon as possible after it is withdrawn. Glass tubes 70 mm long by 9 mm diameter are used. They must be scrupulously clean and dry and fitted with clean rubber bungs. Blood is taken into a clean and dry syringe, lubricated with a minimal quantity of liquid paraffin, and 1 ml is delivered to each of 2 tubes. A rubber bung is fitted to each, and they are at once immersed in the water-bath. A stop-watch is started at the moment blood enters the syringe. The tubes are inverted under the water at about 30-second intervals until the blood has solidified. The time for each tube is recorded.

The test is reliable but is subject to large variations unless the technique is strictly standardized. In particular, the size of the tubes, the volume of blood, and the temperature of the water-bath should always remain constant and be specified.

A capillary tube method is useful but has proved less accurate. If only capillary blood is available this method is of value, but if venous blood is available the method of Lee and White (1913) just described is greatly preferred. For the capillary method, glass tubes of about 1 mm bore and 200 mm long are used. Such a tube is filled by capillary attraction from drops of blood at a lancet wound. The ends are sealed with plasticine or modelling wax without heating. The whole is immediately immersed in the water-bath for about 3 minutes. Thereafter at 30-second intervals about 5 mm is broken off the capillary tube under water: the end point is reached when a threadlike clot is seen to be formed.

14.9.2   CLOT RETRACTION

The method of Macfarlane (1939) is recommended. Silicone-coated, conical glass centrifuge tubes are used which are graduated to 10 ml. They are fitted with a wire spiral which extends to a loop above the top of the tube. 5 ml of venous blood is placed into the tube (without anticoagulant) and the wire spiral is inserted. Frothing of the blood must be avoided. The whole is incubated in a water-bath at 37°C until it is clotted (about 15 minutes or so). Incubation is continued for one hour. After this, the wire spiral is removed together with the clot, which should be firmly attached to it. The volume of fluid expressed from the clot is read off from the graduated tube. The result is expressed as a percentage of 5 ml. For example, if 2·8 ml is expressed from 5 ml, the clot retraction is 56%.

14.9.3   RECALCIFICATION TIME TEST

This test is of value where circumstances do not allow the performance of a whole blood clotting time determination. Citrated, platelet-poor plasma is used (pages 557 and 558). In a 70×9 mm tube, 0·1 ml plasma is added to 0·1 saline and placed in a water-bath at 37°C. 0·1 ml of M/40 $CaCl_2$ is added and the stop-watch is started. The end point is reached when the mixture coagulates.

14.9.4   ONE STAGE 'PROTHROMBIN' TIME TEST (after Quick (1938))

This test is extensively used in the control of anticoagulant therapy with the coumarin drugs. It is of great value in suspected poisoning with similar agents (e.g. warfarin). The test uses a source of extrinsic thromboplastin.

0·1 ml of citrated platelet-poor plasma is placed in a tube in a water-bath at 37°C and 0·1 ml of thromboplastin at optimal dilution is added. To this mixture 0·1 of M/40 CaCl₂ is added and the stop-watch is started. The tube must be tilted at frequent intervals (ca. once every second) until the material clots.

This test is sensitive to deficiencies of a number of factors in human blood. In animals it appears to be comparable at least in horse and dog. The sensitivity depends greatly upon the source of thromboplastin and it cannot be too strongly emphasized that thromboplastin prepared from the same species as the plasma under investigation should be used. Interspecies experiments are almost impossible to interpret and are only of value at the research level. Brain thromboplastin is commonly used: Russell's viper venom ('Stypven', Burroughs Wellcome & Co) may also serve as a thromboplastic source, but is not satisfactory for the diagnosis of warfarin poisoning or for anticoagulant therapy control. In coumarin treatment or poisoning factor VII is depressed: prothrombin is less affected. In the following table the sensitivities of the one-stage test are set out as they apply to man and horse:

Source of thromboplastin used	Test sensitive to deficiencies of	Test NOT sensitive to deficiencies of:
Brain	V, VII, X	(Prothrombin)
Venom	(V), X, (Prothrombin)	VII

PREPARATION OF BRAIN THROMBOPLASTIN

Fresh brain (not more than 1 hour post mortem) is collected and cleaned of blood clots and meninges. The remainder is cut into lumps of about 1 cm cube with scissors or scalpel and placed in a mortar. It is covered with about 4 volumes of acetone and ground gently for a few minutes until a coarse powder is obtained. The powder is recovered by filtration under negative pressure and the extraction is repeated at least 3 times. An even, buff coloured free running powder should result. This is transferred to a vacuum desiccator containing calcium chloride and left overnight at 4°C. The dried powder is stable in well-stoppered dark glass bottles for about 3 months at 20°C but almost indefinitely at −20°C.

For use, 0·5 g of brain powder is suspended in 10 ml physiological saline and incubated at 37°C for 10–15 minutes with occasional agitation. Any coarse particles settling out to the bottom of the tube are discarded. The remaining fluid is dispensed in 0·5 ml amounts in tubes, capped with 'parafilm' and frozen at −20°C. One tube is thawed when required and diluted to the optimum. The optimal dilution is calculated afresh for each saline extraction by trial undiluted, 1:2, 1:4 and 1:8 with normal plasma in the one-stage test. The dilution giving the shortest time (ca. 15 seconds) is chosen. Diluted brain thromboplastin is stable for 4–6 hours only on the bench.

PREPARATION OF VENOM THROMBOPLASTIN

As mentioned before, this is NOT satisfactory for the diagnosis of poisoning with coumarin-like compounds. Freeze-dried venom of Russell's viper is used at a dilution in saline recommended by the suppliers: usually this is 1:10,000.

Once diluted, it is stable at 20°C for 4 or 5 hours only.

14.9.5 THROMBOPLASTIN GENERATION TEST (TGT)

This test is used in the diagnosis of haemophilia and a number of allied conditions in man. It has been successfully used with systems derived wholly from man, horse or dog respectively. The technique used is that of Biggs and Douglas (1953).

Reagents

(1) Normal citrated plasma.

(2) Subject's citrated plasma.

(3) Subject's plasma treated with aluminium hydroxide. 1 ml of plasma at 37°C in the water-bath is treated with 0·1 ml of $Al(OH)_3$ suspension and incubated for not less than 1 minute. The $Al(OH)_3$ is removed by centrifugation, and the plasma diluted 1:5 with saline for use. $Al(OH)_3$ suspension is prepared by suspending 1 g of wet alumina gel (BDH Ltd) in 4 ml water.

(4) Normal serum diluted 1:10 saline at least 1 hour before use.

(5) Subject's serum diluted 1:10 saline at least 1 hour before use.

(6) Brain extract at optimal dilution. This brain extract is NOT the thromboplastin described in the preceding method. It is made from acetone-dried brain powder by chloroform extraction (Bell & Alton 1954). About 0·5 g of this powder is extracted for 2 hours with 20 ml chloroform, with occasional agitation. The filtrate is recovered after removal of the insoluble debris by filtration under negative pressure. This material is dried in a vacuum desiccator: it is necessary to leave the water pump running for several hours during this procedure. The resulting waxy lipoid material is suspended in 5 ml saline and stored at −20°C in 0·1 ml amounts. For use it is diluted about 1:100 with glyoxaline buffer (page 563) but it is necessary to determine the optimal dilution of each batch by trial in the TGT.

(7) Glyoxaline buffer, isotonic, at pH 7·3. See page 563.

The test: Two stop-watches are required, one to time the incubation mixture and the other to time the several substrate clotting times. 0·3 ml brain lipoid is placed in a tube, and 0·3 ml $Al(OH)_3$ plasma (diluted), 0·3 ml serum (diluted) and 0·3 ml M/40 $CaCl_2$ are added. The first stop-watch is started at the addition of calcium. At intervals of 1 minute, 0·1 ml of this mixture is pipetted into 0·1 ml of normal plasma along with 0·1 ml M/40 CaCl$_2$: the second watch is started with the addition of calcium. The 0·1 ml amounts of plasma are prepared beforehand in each of 6 tubes already in the water-bath. The clotting times of the substrate tubes are recorded. A typical result, obtained with a horse system, is as follows:

Incubation time, in minutes	1	2	3	4	5	6
Clotting time in seconds	55	45	15	11	11	12

The calibration curve: This can be prepared by assuming that, for example, in the above system tube 4 or 5 represents 100% thromboplastin. Such a test is set up and at 4 minutes the *incubation mixture* tube is transferred to melting ice from the water-bath. Various dilutions of this mixture in saline are made and added to substrate plasma. The various clotting times of the latter are recorded. For example:

Thromboplastin %	20	40	60	80	100
Drops of incubation mixture	1	2	3	4	5
Drops saline	4	3	2	1	0
Substrate clotting time (sec)	25	15	12	11	10

From these figures a curve can be prepared (Fig. 14.10) and used to express the results of the TGT as a percentage of thromboplastin developed.

Plan of testing: When investigating a coagulation defect with the TGT a series of tests should be performed. These are summarized in Table 14.8.

In man lines B, C and E are abnormal in haemophilia;
lines B, D and E are abnormal in Christmas disease;
lines B, C, D, E and F if there is circulating anticoagulant;
lines E and F if the later stages only of clotting are concerned.

For animals this scheme can only form a basis for investigation. In horse and dog true haemophilia is readily diagnosed by use of the TGT. Thrombasthenia (platelet functional deficiency) can be diagnosed by substituting the platelets for brain lipoid in line A and comparing normal platelets with those of the subject.

14.9.6 THROMBOPLASTIN SCREENING TEST (TST)

This was proposed by Hicks and Pitney (1957) as a simplified version of the TGT. It has proved useful with animal blood as modified by Hardisty and Margolis (1959) and is sensitive to disorders of those types characterized by a deficiency in thromboplastin generation, but it does not distinguish between them. The plasma used in this test should be 'intact'—i.e. not contacted with glass at any time before testing. Blood is taken into a silicone-coated syringe through a siliconed needle and at once added to sodium

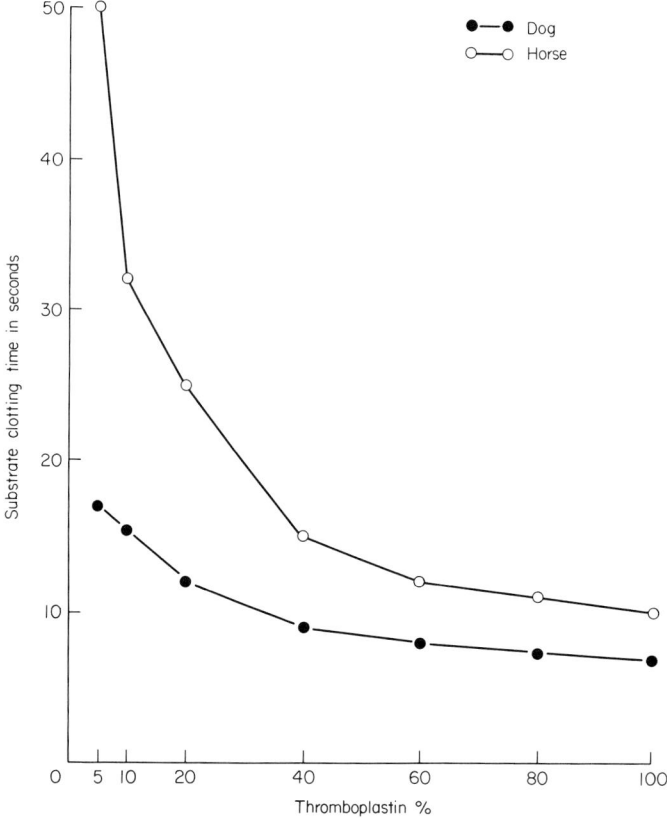

Fig. 14.10 Calibration curves for thromboplastin. The curves relate substrate clotting times to thromboplastin percentage in the thromboplastin generation test: see text.

Table 14.8 Plan of testing, using the TGT

	Source of $Al(OH_3)$ plasma	Source of serum	Source of substrate plasma
A	Normal	Normal	Normal
B	Subject	Subject	Normal
C	Subject	Normal	Normal
D	Normal	Subject	Normal
E	Subject	Subject	Subject
F	Normal	Normal	Subject

citrate in a siliconed glass or a plastic tube placed in melting ice. The mixture is centrifuged at 2000 *g*, preferably in the cold (4°C), for 20 minutes and retained in melting ice till tested.

> Incubation mixture: 0·9 ml glyoxaline buffered saline
> 0·1 ml 'intact' plasma
> 0·1 ml brain lipoid
> 0·1 ml M/40 $CaCl_2$

in a glass tube. A watch is started when the calcium is added and a wooden swab stick is placed in the tube. A clot forms at about 3 minutes and must be removed.

Substrate plasma is normal (not 'intact') citrated plasma placed in 0·1 ml amounts in each of 6 tubes.

As in the TGT so in the TST 0·1 ml amounts of incubation mixture are transferred at intervals to 0·1 ml substrate plasma and 0·1 ml $CaCl_2$ is added at the same moment. Substrate clotting times are recorded at 2 minute intervals. For example, in a horse which was normal the following figures were obtained:

Incubation time, minutes	2	4	6	8	10
Substrate clotting time, seconds	53	29	15	10	12

The figures may vary quite widely and the only valid control is to test in parallel a normal plasma of the same species collected and prepared in the same way. This test cannot be performed on stored plasma.

14.9.7 THE SPECIES SPECIFICITY OF COAGULATION TESTS

In many coagulation tests, for example the one-stage 'prothrombin' time, tissue extracts are used. When such a system is set up, the results obtained often vary considerably with different tissue extracts made from different species. For example, a normal horse plasma gave a one-stage time of 12 seconds with horse brain thromboplastin, but as long as 21 seconds with human brain thromboplastin. This same batch of human thromboplastin gave a time of 11 seconds on normal human plasma. In a similar fashion, very odd results may be obtained from the TGT if an incubation mixture of one species is tested upon substrate plasma of another. From the research point of view such findings may have considerable interest and even importance. Where clinical veterinary medicine is concerned, I strongly urge that all coagulation investigations should be confined absolutely and entirely to the species under investigation. Since dried brain powder can easily be preserved (see page 600) and since substrate plasma may also be kept at a temperature of −20°C or colder, I suggest that such an ideal is well within practicable possibilities. If, for any reason, it is not done, then a note to that effect should always form a part of any report based upon the results of laboratory coagulation tests.

14.10　ASPIRATION BIOPSY

Whenever a blood sample is taken, an aspiration biopsy has in reality been made since blood is a fluid organ. The term 'aspiration biopsy' is more usually used to indicate a method of sampling solid or semi-solid organs during life and it is in this sense that it is used here. For practical purposes only the bone marrow is commonly subjected to aspiration biopsy. While techniques for liver biopsy exist—indeed many organs can be sampled—such methods are outside the scope of this book. Biopsy of lymph nodes is sometimes undertaken by simple direct puncture, but this is only practicable in pathological

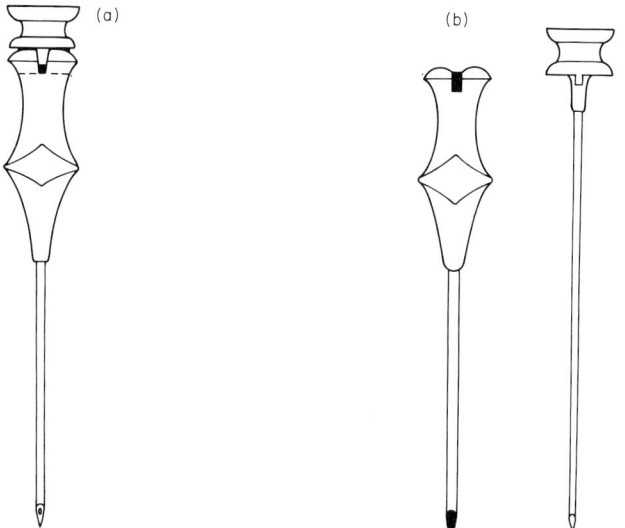

Fig. 14.11 Human type Salah needle for bone marrow biopsy. The guard has been removed. The needles are about 90 mm overall length and 2 mm overall diameter of the shaft. (a) Ready for use, (b) stilette removed.

nodes since it is virtually impossible to identify normal nodes without surgical interference during the life of the animal. Frank tumours are also sometimes subjected to aspiration biopsy.

In this section a description of some apparatus for aspiration biopsy is set out, followed by a description of bone marrow biopsy in several species. Treatment of the aspirated material occupies sections 14.10.4–6.

14.10.1 APPARATUS FOR BONE MARROW BIOPSY

In the smaller laboratory animals (rat, mouse etc.) an ordinary hypodermic needle of about 1–1·25 mm diameter and 15–25 mm long can sometimes be used. With larger mammals (cat, dog, pig etc.) a human-size Salah needle is satisfactory (Fig. 14.11). These needles, with closely fitting stilette, are readily available from instrument houses.

For the largest domesticated mammals (horse, ox) larger needles of the Salah type are recommended. One design which has been found useful is illustrated in Fig. 14.12 (Archer 1964). These needles are available from Down Bros Mayer and Phelps Ltd.

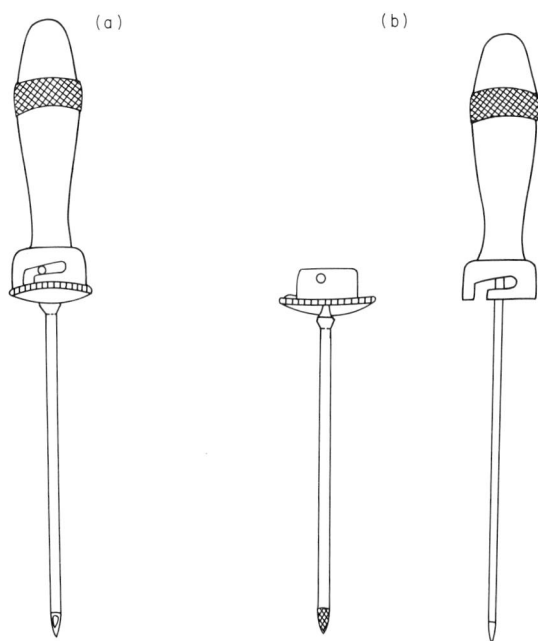

Fig. 14.12 Large bone marrow biopsy needle. The needles are 150 mm overall, shaft 75 mm in length and 2–3 mm diameter. (a) Ready for use, (b) stilette, which is integral with the handle, removed. Available from Down Bros Mayer and Phelps Ltd.

A great variety of other instruments have been used including twist drills and bone trephines. Such methods have not become established for routine use and are not considered here.

14.10.2 GENERAL TECHNIQUE OF BONE MARROW BIOPSY

A bone must be selected for puncture which contains active haemopoietic (red) marrow. In older animals this may present considerable difficulty.

If fatty (yellow) marrow is punctured in error, the sample will consist only of blood and a few fat droplets. Such a sample is, of course, quite valueless for haematological assessment.

The site for skin puncture overlying the bone concerned should be clipped, shaved and thoroughly cleansed. Since the operation of bone marrow biopsy involves deep tissue penetration, full surgical asepsis is essential. Local anaesthesia is induced in the skin with about 0·1 ml of lignocaine intra-dermally or 0·5 ml subcutaneously. The needle is advanced deeper into the tissue and a further injection of about 0·5 ml made into or at least nearby the highly sensitive periosteum.

The site is again cleansed and, with surgical aseptic techniques, a suitable biopsy needle is inserted through skin, subcutaneous tissue and periosteum

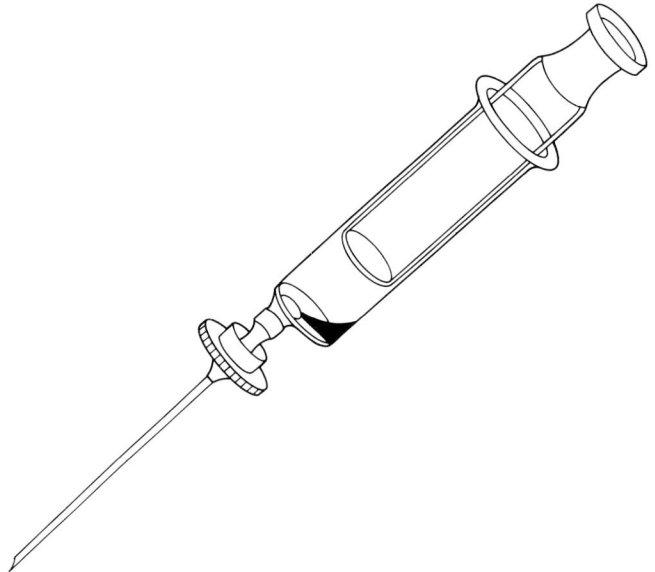

Fig. 14.13 Position of syringe for aspiration biopsy. A syringe with eccentric nozzle is used so that aspirated material drops into the barrel. When the suction is released, the sample will remain within the syringe.

to the bone. It is advanced further slowly, and with a rotating motion, into the bone only far enough to enter the red marrow. At this point the advance is halted, the stilette removed, and aspiration applied from a hypodermic syringe. The method of application of this aspiration is very important. I prefer to use a 20 ml syringe with a metal eccentric nozzle. Plastic disposable syringes are usually unsatisfactory for aspiration. The syringe is attached to the needle mount with nozzle uppermost (Fig. 14.13) and the plunger abruptly withdrawn about half way and held there. This suction may cause minor, brief pain to the subject. If the needle is correctly placed, fragments of marrow with some blood will spurt irregularly into the syringe and drop to the bottom. When about 0·5 ml has been collected (much smaller volumes in small animals), pressure is released and the syringe detached. The marrow sample will remain in the syringe provided the nozzle is kept at the top.

The smallest practicable volume should be aspirated, since larger volumes are inevitably increasingly contaminated with blood. It should always be remembered that the red bone marrow has such an extensive blood supply that it is literally possible to give intravenous injections by the intramedullary route.

14.10.3 SPECIAL TECHNIQUES FOR VARIOUS SPECIES

In many species I have no personal experience of marrow biopsy and in this section emphasis is placed on methods known to be satisfactory. There should be no insurmountable difficulty in other species by extension from the notes that follow.

HORSE

The site used is the external angle of the ileum. Puncture is made at the middle third of the coxal tuber in the direction of the hip joint of the *opposite side*. In animals up to 2 years old, it is usually enough to penetrate about 1 cm into the bone. Five-year-olds may require 4 or 5 cm penetration. Older horses usually cannot be sampled from the coxal tuber without considerable penetration.

Occasionally a rib has been used, but it seems hazardous for the subject and difficult for the operator. The rib is best penetrated by open surgery to the bone and then a twist drill

The sternum is a satisfactory site in the adult horse for bone marrow biopsy. A lateral approach, avoiding the cartilaginous keel, is practicable in standing animals.

OX

The external angle of the ileum has been used as in the horse. Wilde (1961) recommends the 3rd or 4th sternebrae. This technique is as follows: the ox is cast on the right side and the left fore-leg extended forwards to expose the sternum. After suitable preparation and anaesthesia of the site a human-type Salah needle 40 mm long is inserted into the centre of the body of the 3rd or 4th sternebra as near as possible to the midline.

SHEEP

Grunsell (1951) has sampled sternal marrow with success in this species.

Puncture of the 3rd sternebra is recommended. The sheep is restrained in the sitting position by an assistant behind it who holds one of its forelegs in each of his hands. The 3rd sternebra is identified by following the 3rd rib and it is penetrated with a human type Salah needle in the midline. About 0·5 cm of bone penetration is required: beyond 2·5 cm into the bone risks thoracic puncture and is dangerous. The 2nd or 4th sternebrae are also satisfactory sources of bone marrow in the sheep.

PIG

Cartwright *et al* (1949) have used sternal biopsy in the pig by aspiration with a standard (human) 16 gauge sternal puncture needle. The region of the sternum which was penetrated was not specified.

DOG

Bone marrow may be aspirated from the external angle of the ileum with a human-type Salah needle. The sternum can also be used, but it is more hazardous to the subject and is not recommended. An ingenious method has been proposed by Spranger and Hime (1961). This technique uses femoral marrow. A Salah type needle is inserted at the proximal end of the femur exactly as if inserting an intramedullary pin: that is the needle is inserted midway between the head of the femur and the great trochanter into the fossa. It is then advanced into the marrow cavity by careful alignment of needle and femur. Marrow is aspirated from the middle third of the femur and penetration to this depth is ascertained by measurement of a suitable needle along the bone of the subject before the operation is begun. Spranger and Hime remark that their method is satisfactory on day-old puppies and also on the smaller breeds of dog.

CAT

Aspiration from the iliac crest is sometimes satisfactory. The method of Spranger and Hime (1961), described for the dog, may also be useful but I have no experience of it in the cat.

RABBIT, GUINEA PIG, RAT, MOUSE, CHICKEN, ETC

Apart from delicate research techniques requiring extensive experience, there is no simple and satisfactory method of bone marrow *biopsy* in these species. In the rabbit the femoral aspiration method of Spranger and Hime (1961) for the dog can be adapted. Apart from this, bone marrow can be obtained at post mortem examination or under deep anaesthesia. It is usually convenient to dissect out rapidly the whole of one femur and split it longitudinally with bone scissors. Samples of marrow can then be taken with a Volkman spoon or a spatula. Where possible such marrow samples should be collected within 15 minutes of cardiac arrest, if they are to be satisfactory for detailed cellular study.

14.10.4 HANDLING THE ASPIRATED BIOPSY MATERIAL

In the case of all bone marrow aspirates speed and care in handling are of the utmost importance. The large nucleated cells are very fragile and particularly susceptible to mechanical damage. Aspirated marrow clots very readily, perhaps because of its high fat content, and anticoagulants, if used, must be both potent and properly mixed into the specimens.

In many cases, the preparation of *fresh films* will be required. These should be thin and are best made by hand as described on page 578. They should be air-dried at once.

Sequestrene is a suitable *anticoagulant*. About 10 mg is enough for 1 ml of marrow. The plastic phials of 2·5 ml capacity intended for blood samples are satisfactory. They contain 5 mg di-K sequestrene and are suitable for 0·5 ml samples of marrow (see page 556). Samples in sequestrene can be used for differential counting only if films are prepared within an hour, preferably within half an hour.

The greatest use for marrow samples in sequestrene is for the preparation of *fractions of the marrow*. Centrifuging at about 300 g for 5 minutes will give a large buffy coat layer which contains most of the nucleated cells. This is a most useful technique with samples of low nucleated cellularity.

Another use for marrow in sequestrene is the isolation and handling of *marrow fragments*. In some samples, flecks of marrow can be found floating in blood. If the sample is placed in a watch-glass it is possible to suck off most of the blood with filter paper, leaving marrow particles. The latter are used to make films.

Films can be made from marrow fragments by gentle squashing between 2 cover-glasses and then sliding them apart. Marrow from different animals varies widely and optimal techniques for making films must be found by experiment.

14.10.5 COUNTS BY DILUTION

Cellular counts on aspirated marrow are made by ordinary techniques (page 565). Total nucleated cells often approximate to $250 \times 10^9/l$ and it is convenient to count them by the modified method for high counts given on page 568. Counts of eosinophils or basophils are made in the ordinary way (pages 569, 570) although higher dilutions may be needed.

14.10.6 COUNTS FROM FIXED FILMS

Differential nucleated cell counts are made from not less than 500 consecutive cells using an objective of at least 63x. The staining techniques described earlier for blood are suitable. When very high counts of nucleated cells occur, it is better to prolong the staining time recommended on page 580 for diluted Leishman's fluid from 15 to 30 minutes.

14.10.7   POST MORTEM MATERIAL

It is usually valueless to attempt to make bone marrow films from any cadaver which has been dead for more than a few hours. In ideal conditions, periods up to 12 hours may sometimes be acceptable. Marrow should be obtained by open dissection and removal of a portion with a scoop or Volkman spoon. This material should be *very gently* dispersed and suspended in about 5 times its own volume of serum (from the same species) or of 30% bovine plasma albumin. Saline will NOT do. Films are carefully made by hand from this suspension.

15

NORMAL HAEMATOLOGICAL VALUES IN RATS, MICE AND MARMOSETS

ENID ECCLESTON

15.1   INTRODUCTION

There is surprisingly little knowledge about the clinical haematology of small laboratory animals, although colonies with particular inherited disorders have been evolved (Bannerman & Edwards 1976). These latter conditions are really outside the intended compass of this book; however, the provision of reliable figures from known normal colonies may be useful.

The haematology of all animals is affected by breeding, environment, health status and exertion. This is particularly important where small laboratory animals are concerned since widely differing figures for supposed normal haematological parameters are quoted in the literature (Altman & Dittmer 1974) usually without adequate control values. A particular strain of rats may show normal values quite markedly different from the mean values for the common rats and yet there be no indication of poor health. The temperature or humidity of the animal houses also exerts an effect on the blood. The ability, or lack of it, of the housed small animals to relax affects the supposed 'resting' values, even more than the undoubted diurnal variations.

Meaningful haematological figures from blood samples out of laboratory animals require standardization as to time of bleeding, conditions of the animal house, before or after feeding and so on. The method of bleeding (see Chapter 14, pp. 551–3) should also be standardized as to site, needle size, syringe, anticoagulant, etc. Attention to such details will materially improve the quality and reproducibility of the results.

Problems in counting erythrocytes from small laboratory animals on automated electronic equipment may arise since the MCV is, in general, lower than that of man. Most automated equipment is installed to count human erythrocytes (MCV of about 78–94 f l) which will not count all of the smaller red blood cells of the laboratory animals. Mice, for instance, have an MCV around 54; rats about 65 (up to about 75 in rats under 6 months), guinea pigs about 67 and marmosets about 72 f l.

There follow tables, prepared by Miss Eccleston, of normal values which she has obtained in the Alderley Park colonies of mice, rats and marmosets using the methods enumerated below.

THE EDITORS

15.2 METHODS

WBC and RBC	Coulter Counter Model ZF
Platelets	Coulter Thrombocounter
Haemoglobin	Coulter Haemoglobinometer—cyanmethaemoglobin method
PCV	Micromethod—Hawkesley microhaemotocrit centrifuge
Wright's stain	Using Ames' Hema-tek slide stainer,
Prothrombin time	Quick's one stage—Human thromboplastin
PTTK	Diagen PTTK reagent
Reticulocytes	Brilliant Cresyl Blue

15.3 HAEMATOLOGICAL PARAMETERS

It has not been possible to write a full chapter on the clinical haematology of laboratory animals but the following normal figures are presented as reference values for rats, mice and marmosets.

(a) Haematological parameters	1. SPF Albino rats—Tables 1 and 2
	2. SPF Albino Swiss mice—Table 3
	3. Marmosets—Table 4
(b) Coagulation	1. Prothrombin and partial thromboplastin time in rats, mice and marmosets—Table 5

(c) Clinical Chemistry   1. SPF Albino rats—Table 6
                            2. SPF Albino Swiss mice—Table 7
                            3. Marmosets—Table 8

Table 15.1   Comparison of haematology values in tail and heart blood in 200 male SPF Albino rats

	5–6 weeks*	6–7 weeks†
Hb g/dl	13·5	14·6
	11·9–15·6	13·0–16·4
RBC $\times 10^{12}$/l	5·6	6·4
	4·3–6·9	4·7–8·1
PCV	0·41	0·45
	0·37–0·45	0·41–0·50
Reticulocytes %	10·7	5·3
	7·0–16·5	2·6–12·7
Platelets $\times 10^9$/l	720	636
	450–995	500–885
WBC $\times 10^9$/l	10·2	5·7
	5·0–17·4	3·5–11·2
Neutrophils %	25·1	19·3
	9–47	7–49
Lymphocytes %	73·5	79·3
	52–90	48–93
Eosinophils %	0·8	0·4
	0–3	0–2
Monocytes %	0·6	1·0
	0–2	0–4
Basophils %	0	0

* Tail blood.
† Cardiac blood.

Enid Eccleston

Table 15.2 Mean and 95 per cent confidence limits of haematology values in Alderley Park SPF albino rats

Age	No. of rats	Sex	Hb g/dl	RBC $\times 10^{12}/l$	PCV	Reticulocytes %	Platelets $\times 10^9/l$
5–6 weeks	200	♂	13·5 11·9–15·6	5·6 4·3–6·8	0·41 0·37–0·45	10·7 7·0–16·5	720 450–995
	200	♀	13·9 12·2–16·2	5·8 4·5–7·4	0·41 0·37–0·47	5·3 2·1–13·0	783 555–1065
10–32 weeks	100	♂	16·0 14·7–17·2	7·0 5·3–8·3	0·47 0·42–0·52	2·0 0·4–4·0	656 511–927
	100	♀	15·6 14·2–16·9	6·4 4·9–7·9	0·45 0·41–0·50	1·1 0·3–3·3	673 506–987
12 months	20	♂	15·7 14·5–17·5	8·0 6·9–8·9	0·46 0·42–0·50	—	719 485–994
	20	♀	15·7 14·7–16·8	7·6 6·3–8·6	0·45 0·41–0·48	—	682 524–857
18 months to 2 years	26	♂	15·6 13·3–17·1	—	0·46 0·38–0·52	—	769 412–1082
	23	♀	15·3 13·5–16·8	—	0·45 0·40–0·53	—	782 541–1060

Table 15.2   (contd)

Age	No. of rats	Sex	WBC ×10⁹/l	N %	L %	E %	M %	B %
5–6 weeks	200	♂	10·2 (5·0–17·4)	25·1 (9–47)	73·5 (52–90)	0·8 (0–3)	0·6 (0–2)	0 (0)
	200	♀	9·3 (4·1–15·8)	20·3 (8–40)	78·3 (58–90)	1·0 (0–3)	0·4 (0–2)	0 (0)
10–32 weeks	100	♂	11·6 (6·3–17·8)	18·6 (7–36)	79·9 (62–90)	0·9 (0–3)	0·6 (0–3)	0 (0)
	100	♀	9·7 (5·3–15·9)	19·4 (9–35)	78·9 (63–91)	1·2 (0–3)	0·5 (0–2)	0 (0)
12 months	20	♂	11·7 (6·0–20·3)	28·5 (16–41)	69·3 (56–82)	1·5 (0–6)	0·7 (0–3)	0 (0)
	20	♀	7·5 (5·0–12·0)	27·9 (13–39)	70·2 (59–85)	1·1 (0–3)	0·8 (0–3)	0 (0)
18 months to 2 years	26	♂	13·9 (7·8–30·8)	42·5 (19–72)	54·4 (24–78)	2·0 (0–4)	1·1 (0–4)	0 (0)
	23	♀	8·6 (4·4–26·4)	43·5 (19–69)	54·2 (27–80)	1·7 (0–5)	0·6 (0–3)	0 (0)

Table 15.3 Mean and 95 per cent confidence limits of haematology values in 60 male and 60 female SPF Albino Swiss mice, Alderley Park Strain 1

	60 *male* (7–8 *wks*)	60 *female* (9–10 *wks*)
Hb g/dl	17·2	16·8
	15·4–19·2	15·7–18·1
RBC × 10^{12}/l	9·1	9·1
	7·9–10·3	8·1–10·1
PCV	0·49	0·49
	0·45–0·54	0·46–0·53
Reticulocytes %	4·6	3·0
	1·3–6·8	1·0–7·0
Platelets × 10^9/l	928	752
	716–1314	604–933
WBC × 10^9/l	11·4	8·5
	5·0–16·7	5·2–13·7
Neutrophils %	13·5	11·0
	5–28	4–27
Lymphocytes %	85·8	87·5
	72–95	71–95
Eosinophils %	0·6	1·3
	0–3	0–6
Monocytes %	0·1	0·2
	0–1	0–1
Basophils %	0	0

Table 15.4   Mean and 95 per cent confidence limits of haematology values in 97 male and 99 female marmosets (*Callithrix jacchus*) 7–17 months of age

	97 *male*	99 *female*
Hb g/dl	15·5	15·5
	12·3–18·1	12·7–17·7
RBC × 10^{12}/l	6·8	6·6
	5·2–7·9	5·4–8·1
PCV	0·48	0·48
	0·41–0·56	0·41–0·54
Reticulocytes %	5·3	4·6
	2·5–10·0	2·0–8·5
Platelets × 10^9/l	401	394
	183–585	215–693
WBC × 10^9/l	10·0	10·1
	5·5–16·0	5·8–16·6
Neutrophils %	36·4	38·5
	15–74	14–72
Lymphocytes %	60·7	59·1
	23–83	25–84
Eosinophils %	1·0	0·8
	0–4	0–3
Monocytes %	1·7	1·5
	0–5	0–4
Basophils %	0·2	0·1
	0–1	0–1

15.4   COAGULATION. PROTHROMBIN AND PARTIAL THROMBOPLASTIN TIME IN RATS, MICE AND MARMOSETS, TABLE 15.5

Table 15.5   Normal range for the prothrombin time and the partial thromboplastin time (PTTK) with kaolin for rats, mice and marmosets

Species	*No. of animals*	*Sex*	*Prothrombin time— seconds*		*PTTK—seconds*	
			mean	*range*	*mean*	*range*
Mice	30	♂	10·7	9·5–11·6	25·2	20·0–28·9
	30	♀	10·4	9·5–11·1	22·9	20·4–26·4
Rats	50	♂	12·9	11·5–14·3	18·0	15·6–22·2
	50	♀	12·4	11·6–14·2	17·8	15·4–22·0
Marmosets	30	♂	5·7	5·0–6·4	35·7	30·1–43·7
	30	♀	5·6	5·0–6·5	36·3	31·9–41·0

15.5 CLINICAL CHEMISTRY

Table 15.6 Mean and 95 per cent confidence limits of some clinical chemistry tests in the blood of male and female Alderley Park albino rats

Test	Units	Sex	No. of values	Mean	95% Confidence limits	
					minimum	maximum
Sugar	mmol/l	♂	220	10·3	4·4	23·2
		♀	179	9·1	3·8	20·0
Urea	mmol/l	♂	223	7·9	4·8	13·2
		♀	181	9·4	5·1	29·2
Total protein	g/l	♂	116	70·4	61	78
		♀	99	73·8	64	85
Albumin	g/l	♂	223	34·7	29	40
		♀	180	37·6	30	48
Total bilirubin	μmol/l	♂	117	2·5	1	6
		♀	95	2·7	1	6
Alkaline phosphatase (AP)	iu/l	♂	117	145·9	73	248
		♀	99	97·5	42	183
Alanine aminotrans-ferase (ALAT)	iu/l	♂	223	41·2	24	71
		♀	175	38·7	22	75
Aspartate amino-transferase (AAT)	iu/l	♂	222	115·3	56	221
		♀	174	130·0	51	281
Sodium (Na^+)	mmol/l	♂	117	142·6	136	149
		♀	97	141·6	135	147
Potassium (K^+)	mmol/l	♂	115	5·6	4·3	7·4
		♀	93	5·4	3·4	8·3

Table 15.7 Mean and 95 per cent confidence limits of clinical chemistry tests in the blood of male and female SPF Albino Swiss mice, Alderley Park strain 1

Test	Sex	No.	Mean	Min.	Max.
AP	♂	30	86·1	55	143
i.u./l	♀	30	114·6	74	159
Sugar	♂	30	14·3	9·3	18·9
mmol/l	♀	30	15·4	11·5	19
Urea	♂	30	9·9	7·5	13·3
mmol/l	♀	30	8·2	6·5	10·6
Albumin	♂	30	29·5	25	32
g/l	♀	30	33·4	30	36
ALAT	♂	30	33·7	19	69
i.u./l	♀	30	23·4	15	31
AAT	♂	30	80·6	47	145
i.u./l	♀	30	92·3	51	202
Na	♂	28	155·7	150	161
mmol/l	♀	30	154·4	150	161
K	♂	28	7·2	5·0	10·0
mmol/l	♀	30	7·0	5·7	8·8

Table 15.8 Mean and 95 per cent confidence limits of some clinical chemistry tests in the blood of marmosets (*Callithrix jacchus*)

Test	No.	Sex	Mean	Min.	Max.
Sugar	25	♂	6·5	3·4	13·1
mmol/l	31	♀	6·9	4·1	17·8
Urea	25	♂	6·5	4·1	10·6
mmol/l	27	♀	5·9	2·9	9·0
TP	22	♂	70	56	82
g/l	22	♀	73	60	82
Albumin	25	♂	41·6	35	48
g/l	27	♀	41·6	34	57
AP	21	♂	203·7	87	332
i.u./l	18	♀	195	73	335
ALAT	23	♂	9·0	4	22
i.u./l	38	♀	9·8	5	22
AAT	24	♂	134·4	78	147
i.u./l	38	♀	104·9	63	221
Na	16	♂	153·8	149	160
mmol/l	21	♀	153·8	145	160
K	16	♂	5·3	3·3	7·5
mmol/l	21	♀	5·3	3·7	6·4
Total	15	♂	14·0	7	21
bilirubin	13	♀	10·0	3	21
μmol/l					

REFERENCES

ABBRECHT P.H. & MALVIN R.L. (1966) Renal production of erythropoietin in the dog. *Am. J. Physiol.* **210**, 237.

ABDEL-HAMEED M.F. & NEAT H.J. (1972) A study of erythrocyte cell volume and number in normal adult and triploid intersex chickens. *Poult. Sci.* **51**, 1376–82.

ABDEL-HAMEED M.F., NEAT H.J. & BRILES W.E. (1971) Differences in erythrocyte measurements of intersex and normal chickens. *Poult. Sci.* **50**, 1847–54.

ABEL H.H. & SCHNEIDER B. (1973) Einige 'Normwerte' des Blutes für den Hunde-auszuchtstamm Brack: Beagle (Beagle/Brackwede). *Z. Versuchstierk* **15**, 160.

ABILDGAARD C.F., HARRISON J. & JOHNSON C.A. (1971) Comparative study of blood coagulation in non-human primates. *J. appl. Physiol.* **30**, 400.

ABOU-ASHOUR A.M. & EDWARDS H.M. (1972) Hematological changes in laying hens receiving Sterculia foetida oil supplements. *Poult. Sci.* **51**, 300–5.

ABRAMOVA E.N., KONDRATEV V.S. & SYTINSKII I.A. (1974) The biochemistry of leucosis in cattle. *Vet. Bull.* **44**, 689–711.

ABT D.A., IPSEN J., HARE W.C.D., MARSHAK R.R. & SAHL J. (1966) Circadian and seasonal variations in the hemogram of mature dairy cattle. *Cornell Vet.* **56**, 479–520.

ADAVAL S.C. & GANGWAR P.C. (1972) Blood coagulation in buffaloes. *Indian vet. J.* **49**, 670–2.

ADELSON E., RHEINGOLD J.J., PARKER O., BUENAVENTURA A. & CROSBY W.H. (1961) Platelet and fibrinogen survival in normal and abnormal states of coagulation. *Blood* **17**, 267.

AFANAS'EV V.P. (1963) Seasonal changes in protein and blood picture of Reindeer. *Trudȳ mosk. vet. Akad.* **47**, 329–39. (Russian).

AFONSKY D. (1954) Folic acid deficiency in the dog. *Science* **120**, 803.

AFONSKY D. (1955) Blood picture in normal dogs. *Am. J. Physiol.* **180**, 456.

AHMED S.U. & RAHMAN M.M. (1973) Studies on total leucocyte and differential counts for Bangladesh goat. *J. Anim. Morph. Physiol.* **20**, 106–16.

AKROYD P. (1967) Acrylamide gel slab electrophoresis in a simple glass cell for improved resolution and comparison of serum proteins. *Analyt. Biochem.* **19**, 399–410.

AKROYD P. (1968) Pig serum protein phenotyping by electrophoresis in thin acrylamide gel slabs. *XIth European Conference on Animal Blood Groups and Biochemical Polymorphism, Warsaw*, pp. 311–14. PWN—Polish Scientific Publishers.

ALBRECHT A., LIMA E. DE GARCIA, GELDERMANN H., MITSCHERLICH E. & SCHMIDT W. (1974) Epidemiology of bovine leucosis and the efficacy of a control programme in Lower Saxony. *Zentbl. VetMed.* **B21**, 520–39.

ALBRITTON E.C. (1952) *Standard values in blood.* W.B. Saunders, Philadelphia, USA.

ALDOUS H.M.J. (1970) Hematology of foals. *Proc. 16th A. Conv. Am. Ass. equine Pract.*, 37–41.

ALENCAR R.A. DE FO, PENHA A.M. & CINTRA L.C. (1971) Blood picture of acclimatised Dutch red and white cattle. *Biológico* **37**, 272–5.

ALEXANDER F. & ASH R.W. (1955) The effect of emotion and hormones on the concentration of glucose and eosinophils in horse blood. *J. Physiol.* **130**, 703–10.

ALEXANDER F. & DAVIES M.E. (1969) Studies on vitamin B_{12} in the horse. *Br. vet. J.* **125**, 169–76.

ALEYAS N.M. & RAJAMANI S. (1972) Haematological studies. I. Normal haemogram of adult she-buffaloes. *Kerala J. vet. Sci.* **3**, 164–8.

ALKJAERSIG N., FLETCHER A.P. & SHERRY

S. (1959) The mechanism of clot dissolution by plasmin. *J. clin. Invest.* **38**, 1086.

ALLAN G.S., WATSON A.D.J., DUFF B.C. & HOWLETT C.R. (1974) Disseminated mastocytoma and mastocytemia in a dog. *J. Am. vet. med. Ass.* **165**, 346.

ALLEN B.V. (1976) Personal communication.

ALLEN B.V. & ARCHER R.K. (1971) Haptoglobins in the horse. *Vet. Rec.* **89**, 106–9.

ALLEN B.V. & ARCHER R.K. (1972) A blood coagulation test (Normotest) as another measure of liver function in the horse. *Equine vet. J.* **4**, 217–22.

ALLEN B.V. & ARCHER R.K. (1973) Studies with normal erythrocytes of the English Thoroughbred horse. *Equine vet. J.* **5**, 135–6.

ALLEN B.V. & ARCHER R.K. (1976) Some haematological values in English Thoroughbred horses. *Vet. Rec.* **98**, 195–6.

ALLEN D.W. & SARMA P.S. (1972) Identification and localization of avian leukosis group-specific antigen within 'leukosis-free' chick embryos. *Virology* **48**, 624–6.

ALLEN J.R. & CARSTENS L.A. (1965) Haematologic alterations observed in newly acquired monkeys during a period of their isolation. *Lab. anim. care* **15**, 103.

ALLEN J.R. & SEIGFRIED L.M. (1966) Haematologic alterations in pregnant rhesus monkeys. *Lab. anim. care* **16**, 465.

ALLEN R.L. (1971) The properties and biosynthesis of the haemoglobins. In: Bell D.J. & Freeman B.M. (Eds) *Physiology and biochemistry of the domestic fowl*, pp. 873–81. Academic Press, London.

ALLEN W. M., BERRETT S. & PATTERSON D.S.P. (1967) A haematological study of clinical cases of Johne's disease and the assessment of an intravenous Johnin diagnostic test. *J. comp. Path.* **77**, 71–9.

ALLISON A.C. & REES W. (1957) The binding of haemoglobin by plasma proteins (haptoglobins). *Br. med. J.*, **2**, 1137.

ALTMAN N.H. (1974) Intraerythrocytic chrystalloid bodies in cats and their comparison with haemaglobinopathies of man, *Ann. N.Y. Acad. Sci.* **241**, 589–93.

ALTMAN P.L. & DITTMER D.S. (1961) Blood and other body fluids. *Fed. Amer. Soc. Exper. Biol.* Washington, D.C.

ALTMANN P.L. & DITTMER D.S. (1974) *Biology data book*, Vol. 3, p. 1782. Federation of American Societies for Experimental Biology.

ALUJA A.S. DE (1970) *Lantana camara* poisoning in cattle in Mexico. *Vet. Rec.* **86**, 628.

AMERICA ASSOCIATION OF EQUINE PRACTITIONERS (1975) *Proceedings of First International Symposium on Equine Hematology*, Michigan, USA.

ANANTHAKRISHNAN R. & WALTER H. (1973) Electrophoretic variation of adenosine deaminase in pigs. *Z. Saugetierk.* **38**, 318–20.

ANDERSEN S. (1966) The physiological range of the formed elements in the peripheral blood of the harbour porpoise, *Phocaena phocaena* in captivity. *Nord. VetMed.* **18**, 51.

ANDERSEN A.C. & GEE W. (1958) Normal blood values in the Beagle. *Vet. Med.* **53**, 135.

ANDERSEN A.C. & GOLDMAN M. (1970) Growth and Development. In: Andersen A.C. (Ed.) *The Beagle as an experimental dog*, p. 43. Iowa State University Press, Ames, Iowa, USA.

ANDERSEN A.C. & SCHALM O.W. (1970) Hematology. In: Andersen A.C. (Ed.) *The Beagle as an experimental dog*, p. 261. Iowa State University Press, Ames, Iowa, USA.

ANDERSON G.F. & BARNHART M.I. (1964) Prothrombin synthesis in the dog. *Am. J. Physiol.* **206**, 929.

ANDERSON A.E., MEDIN D.E. & BOWDEN D.C. (1970) Erythrocytes and leukocytes in a Colorado mule deer population. *J. Wildl. Mgmt.* **34**, 389–406.

ANDERSON A.E., MEDIN D.E. & BOWDEN D.C. (1972a) Total serum protein in a population of mule deer. *J. Mammal.* **53**, 384–7.

ANDERSON A.E., MEDIN D.E. & BOWDEN D.C. (1972b) Blood serum electrolytes in a Colorado mule deer population. *J. Wildl. Dis.* **8**, 183–90.

ANDERSON S. & NIELSEN R. (1973) Pathology of isoimmune purpura thrombocytopenica in piglets. *Nord. VetMed.* **25**, 211–19.

ANDERSON L., WILSON R. & HAY D. (1971) Haematological values in normal cats from four weeks to one year of age. *Res. vet. Sci.* **12**, 579–83.

ANDERSON L.J., JARRETT W.F.H., JARRETT O. & LAIRD H.M. (1971) Feline leukemia-virus infection of kittens: mortality associated with atrophy of the thymus and lymphoid depletion. *J. natn. Cancer Inst.* **47**, 807–17.

ANDRADE S.O., PEREGRINO C.J.B. & AGUIAR A.A. (1971) Studies on *Brachiaria* spp. (Tanner grass). I and II. *Arq. Inst. biol.*, *S. Paulo* **38**, 135–50 and 151–61.

ANDRADE S.O., RETZL L. & MARMO C.O. (1971) Studies on *Brachiaria* spp. (Tanner grass). III. *Arq. Inst. biol.*, *S. Paulo* **38**, 239–52.

ANDREANI E. & SCARANO C. (1973) On an outbreak of bovine and swine acute leptospirosis in Sardinia. *Atti Soc. ital. Sci. vet.* **27**, 649–52.

ANDREASSEN M. (1943) Haemofili I Danmark, En Klinisk, Haematologisk og Arvebiologisk Undersøgelse af 63 Haemofilislaegter. *Opera ex Domo Biol. Hered. Humanae Univ. Hafniensis* (Copenhagen) **6**, 57.

ANDRESEN E. (1963) *A study of blood groups of the pig*. Munksgaard, Copenhagen.

ANDRESEN E. (1970a) Linkage between the H and 6-PGD loci in pigs. *Acta vet. scand.* **11**, 136–7.

ANDRESEN E. (1970b) Close linkage between the locus for phosphohexose isomerase (PHI) and the H blood group locus of pigs. *Anim. Blood Grps. biochem. Genet.* **1**, 171–2.

ANDRESEN E. & BAKER L.N. (1963) Haemolytic disease in pigs caused by anti Ba. *J. Anim. Sci.* **22**, 720–5.

ANDRESEN E. & BAKER L.N. (1964) The C blood group system in pigs and the detection and estimation of linkage between the C and J systems. *Genetics* **49**, 379–86.

ANDREWS F.N. (1944) An improved method of obtaining blood from the chicken heart. *Poult. Sci.* **23**, 542–4.

ANGER H.O. & VAN DYKE D. (1964) Human bone marrow distribution shown in vitro by iron-52 and the positron scintillation camera. *Science* **144**, 1587–9.

ANNAU E., CORNER A.M., MAGWOOD S.E. & JERICHO K. (1964) Electrophoretic and chemical studies on sera of swine following the feeding of toxic groundnut meal. *Can. J. comp. Med.* **28**, 264–9.

ANSAY M. (1973) Thesis—University of Liege, Faculty of Veterinary Medicine.

ANSTALL H.B. & HUNTSMAN R.G. (1960) Influence of temperature upon blood coagulation in a cold and a warm blooded animal. *Nature (London)* **186**, 726.

ARCHER R.K. (1954) Sequestrene (E.D.T.A.) as an anticoagulant for equine blood. *Vet. Rec.* **66**, 447.

ARCHER R.K. (1954) Bone marrow biopsy in the horse. *Vet. Rec.* **66**, 261–4.

ARCHER R.K. (1956) Studies upon the blood picture of Equidae. PhD thesis, Univ. of Cambridge, pp. 33–54.

ARCHER R.K. (1959) The normal haemograms and coagulograms of the English Thoroughbred horse. *J. comp. Path.* **69**, 390–9.

ARCHER R.K. (1960a) The biology of the eosinophil leucocyte. *Vet. Rec.* **72**, 155–8.

ARCHER R.K. (1960b) Studies on the coagulation defect produced by sodium warfarin in the horse. *Proc. 7th. Cong. Europ. Soc. Haemat.*, London (1959) pp. 867–70.

ARCHER R.K. (1961) True haemophilia (Haemophilia A) in a thoroughbred foal. *Vet. Rec.* **73**, 338–40.

ARCHER R.K. (1963) *The eosinophil leucocytes*. Blackwell, Oxford.

ARCHER R.K. (1964) A new type of needle for bone marrow biopsy in the larger animals. *Vet. Rec.* **76**, 465–6.

ARCHER R.K. (1969) Symposium on haematology—Cellular aspects of blood. *Equine vet. J.* **1**, 187–90.

ARCHER R.K. (1971) Blood coagulation. In: Bell D.J. & Freeman B.M. (Eds) *Physiology and biochemistry of the domestic fowl*, pp. 897–911. Academic Press, London.

ARCHER R.K. (1974a) Haematology in relation to performance and potential. 1. A general review. *Jl S. Afr. vet. Ass.* **45**, 273–7.

ARCHER R.K. (1974b) Personal communication.

ARCHER R.K. & ALLEN B.V. (1970) The viscosity of equine blood plasma: A new non-specific test. *Vet. Rec.* **86**, 360–3.

ARCHER R.K. & ALLEN B.V. (1972) True haemophilia in horses. *Vet. Rec.* **85**, 655–6.

ARCHER R.K. & BOWDEN R.S.T. (1959) A case of true haemophilia in a Labrador dog. *Vet. Rec.* **71**, 560.

ARCHER R.K. & CLABBY J. (1965) The effect of excitation and exertion on the circulating blood of horses. *Vet. Rec.* **77**, 689–90.

ARCHER R.K. & FRANKS D. (1961) Blood transfusion in veterinary practice. *Vet. Rec.* **73**, 657–61.

ARCHER R.K. & MILLER W.C. (1959) The interpretation of haematological examinations in Thoroughbred horses. *Vet. Rec.* **71**, 273–7.

ARCHER R.K. & MILLER W.C. (1965) A case of idiopathic hypoplastic anaemia in a two-year-old thoroughbred filly. *Vet. Rec.* **77**, 538–41.

ARCHER R.K. & POYNTER D. (1957) Anaemia and eosinophilia associated with helminthiasis in young horses. *J. comp. Path.* **67**, 196–207.

AREEKUL S. & TIPAYAMONTRI U. (1974) Experimental infection of *Ancylostoma braziliense* in dogs and cats in Thailand. I. Morphology, route of infection, worm burden and egg output. *S.E. Asian J. trop. Med. publ. Hlth* **5**, 31.

ARMBRECHT B.H., GELETA J.N., SHALKOP W.T. & DURBIN C.G. (1971) A subacute exposure of Beagle dogs to Aflatoxin. *Toxic. appl. Pharmac.* **18**, 579.

ASHTON G.C. (1960) Thread protein and β-globulin polymorphism in the serum protein of pigs. *Nature* **186**, 991–2.

ASHTON G.C. (1965) Serum amylase (thread protein) polymorphism in cattle. *Genetics* **51**, 431–7.

ASHWORTH B. (1973) The frequency of animal poisoning by warfarin. *Vet. Rec.* **93**, 50.

ASTRUP T. & BULUK K. (1963) Thromboplastic and fibrinolytic activities in vessels of animals. *Circulation Res.* **13**, 253.

ATIVAL O.S. & McFARLAND L.Z. (1967) Histochemical study of the distribution of alkaline phosphatase in leukocytes of the horse, cow, sheep, dog and cat. *Am. J. vet. Res.* **28**, 971–74.

ATWAL O.S., McFARLAND L.Z. & WILSON W.O. (1964) Hematology of *Coturnix* from birth to maturity. *Poult. Sci.* **43**, 1392–401.

ATWAL O.S. & McFARLAND L.Z. (1966) A morphologic and cytochemical study of erythrocytes and leukocytes of *Coturnix coturnix japonica*. *Am. J. vet. Res.* **27**, 1059–65.

AUFDERHEIDE W.M., SKINNER S.F. & KANEKO J.J. (1975) Clearance of cryoprecipitated factor VIII in canine hemophilia A. *Am. J. vet. Res.* **36**, 367–70.

AUGUSTINSSON, K.-B. & OLSSON B. (1961) Genetic control of arylesterase in the pig. *Hereditas* **47**, 1–22.

AUSTIN F.H. (1964) Bracken poisoning. A review. *Ir. vet. J.* **18**, 22–8.

AVOLT M.D., LUND J.E. & PICKETT J.C. (1973) Autoimmune hemolytic anemia in a dog. *J. Am. vet. med. Ass.* **162**, 45.

AYOUB N.N.K. & EBNER D. (1972) Significance of the COFAL test with pigeon antiserum. *Mh. Vet.Med.* **27**, 806–9.

AZZIE M.A.J. (1973) Personal communication.

BAARS J.C. (1971) Haemoglobin level and P.C.V. in calves *Tijdschr. Diergeneesk.* **96**, 1488–1500.

BACH L.G. & RICKETTS S.W. (1974) Paracentesis as an aid to the diagnosis of abdominal disease in the horse. *Equine vet. J.* **6**, 116–21.

BACK N., WILKENS H., BARLOW B. & CZARNECKI J. (1968) Fibrinolytic studies with biguanide derivatives. *Ann. N.Y. Acad. Sci.* **148**, 691.

BÄCKGREN A.W. & JÖNSSON G. (1969) Blood and bone marrow studies in cattle feeding on *Brassica* species. *Acta vet. scand.* **10**, 309–18.

BAETZ A.L. & MENGELING W.L. (1971) Blood constituents of fasted swine. *Am. J. vet. Res.* **32**, 1491–9.

BAILEY W.S., HOERLEIN B.F. & HORNE R.D. (1968) Metazoal Infections. In: Catcott E.J. (Ed.) *Canine medicine*, First Catcott Edn, p. 187. American Veterinary Publications Inc., Wheaton, Illinois, USA.

BAILLIE A.J. & SIM A.K. (1971) Activation of the fibrinolytic enzyme system in laboratory animals and man—a comparative study. *Thromb. Diath. haemorrh.* **25**, 499–506.

BAIN A.D. & McTAGGART H.S. (1974) Unpublished data.

BAINTON D.F. (1975) Annotation: neutrophil granules. *Br. J. Haemat.* **29**, 17–22.

BAKER L.N. (1968) New allele in the transferrin system of pigs, Tf^E Ames, an apparent mutation. *Vox Sang.* **14**, 446–51.

BAKER N.F. & DOUGLAS J.R. (1957) Pathogenesis of *Trichostrongyloid* parasites. II. Ferrokinetic studies in ruminants. *Am. J. vet. Res.* **18**, 295–302.

BAKER, G. A. & GORHAM J.R. (1951) A technique for bleeding ferrets and mink. *Cornell Vet.* **41**, 235–6.

BALL S., HAWKEY C.M., HIME J.M., KEYMER I.F. & BRAMBELL M.R. (1976) Red cell sickling in genets. *Comp. Biochem. Physiol.* 54A, 49–54.

BALMACIDA R.H. & BOTTARI C.V. (1974) Serum gammaglobulin fraction of various breeds of cattle. *Revta. Med. vet., B. Aires* **55**, 1–6. Source ref. *Vet. Bull.* **44**, (1974).

BALUDA M.A. (1972) Widespread presence, in chickens, of DNA complementary to the RNA genome of avian leukosis viruses. *Proc. natn. Acad. Sci. USA.* **69**, 576–80.

BANAS D.A. (1974) Experiences with the nitroblue tetrazolium test in four domestic species. *Bull. Am. Soc. vet. clin. Path.* **3**, 17.

BANDY P.J., KITTS W.D., WOOD A.J. & COWAN I. McT. (1957) The effect of age and the plane of nutrition on the blood chemistry of the Columbian black-tailed deer (*Odocoileus hemionus columbianus*). B. Blood glucose, non-protein nitrogen, total plasma protein, plasma albumin, globulin and fibrinogen. *Can. J. Zool.* **35**, 283–9.

BANGHAM A.D. (1961) A correlation between surface charge and coagulant action of phospholipids. *Nature (London)* **192**, 1197.

BANNERMAN R.M., EDWARDS J.A. & PINKERTON P.H. (1973) Hereditary disorders of the red cell in animals. In: Brown E.B. (Ed.) *Progress in haematology*, Vol. VIII, p. 131. Grune and Stratton, New York,

BANNERMAN R.M. & EDWARDS J.A. (1976) Hereditary anaemias in laboratory animals. *Br. J. Haemat.* **32**, 299–307.

BARANOV O.K. (1970) An immunological study of protein polymorphism in haemolysates of pigs and cattle. *Biochem. Genet.* **4**, 549–64.

BARBER R.S., BRAUDE R. & MITCHELL K.G. (1968) The effects of feeding toxic groundnut meal to growing pigs and its interaction with high-copper diets. *Br. J. Nutr.* **22**, 535–54.

BARBIER M., MANUEL Y., VUILLARD P. & DESCOTES J. (1973) Étude de la formation du complexe haptoglobine-hémoglobine dans le sérum du chien a l'état normal et en cours d'expérimentation. *Path. Biol.* **21**, 359.

BARGER J.D. & DeLAMATER E.D. (1948) The use of thionyl chloride in the preparation of Schiff's reagent. *Science* **108**, 121–2.

BARKER I.K. (1973) A study of the pathogenesis of Trichostrongylus colubriformis infection in lambs with observations on the contribution of gastrointestinal plasma loss. *Int. J. Parasitol.* **3**, 743–57.

BARKER R.W., HOCH A.L., BUCKNER R.G. & HAIR J.A. (1973). Hematological changes in white-tailed deer fawns, *Odocoileus virginianus*, infested with *Theileria*-infected lone star ticks. *J. Parasit.* **59**, 1091–8.

BARKHAN P., TOMLIN S.C. & ARCHER R.K. (1957) Comparative coagulation studies on horse and human blood. *J. comp. Path.*, **67**, 358–68.

BARNETT S.F. (1968) In: Weinman D. & Ristic M. (Eds) *Infectious blood diseases of man and animals*, Vol. 2, p. 309. Academic Press, New York and London.

BARNHART M.I., CRESS D.C., HENRY R.L. & RIDDLE J.M. (1967) Influence of fibrinogen split products on platelets. *Thromb. Diath. haemorrh.* **17,** 78.

BARNICOT N.A. & COHEN P. (1970) Red cell enzymes of primates (Anthropoidea). *Biochem. genet.* **4,** 41–57.

BARNICOT N.A. & HEWETT-EMMETT D. (1971) Red cell and serum proteins of Talapoin, Patas and Vervet monkeys. *Folia Primat.* **15,** 65.

BARNICOT N.A. & JOLLY C.J. (1966) Haemoglobin polymorphism in the orangutan and an animal with four major haemoglobins. *Nature (London)* **210,** 640–2.

BARNICOT N.A., JOLLY C.J. & WADE P.T. (1967) Protein variations and Primatology. *Am. J. phys. Anthrop.* **27,** 343.

BARON D.N., BROUGHTON P.M.G., COHEN M., LANGLEY T.S., LEWIS S.M. & SHINTON N.K. (1974) The use of SI units in reporting results obtained in hospital laboratories. *Ann. clin. Biochem.*, **11,** 194–202.

BARTELS H., HILPERT P., BARBEY K., BETKE K., REIGEL K., LANG E.M. & METCALFE J. (1963) Respiratory functions of blood of the yak, llama, camel, Dybowski deer, and African elephant. *Am. J. Physiol.* **205,** 331–6.

BARTHEL C.H. (1974) Acute myelomonocytic leukemia in a dog. *Vet. Path.* **11,** 79.

BAUMGARTNER H.R. & BORN G.V.R. (1968) 5-hydroxytryptamine in rabbit platelets and their aggregation. *J. Physiol.* **194,** 92P.

BEALL G.N., BENFIELD J.R., KRUGER S.R. & BYFIELD P.E. (1974) Canine lymphocytes that form rosettes with human red blood cells. *J. surg. Res.* **17,** 330.

BECKETT S.D., BURNS M.J. & CLARK C.H. (1964) A study of blood glucose, serum transaminases and electrophoretic patterns of dogs with infectious canine hepatitis. *Am. J. vet. Res.* **25,** 1186.

BEDRAK E. (1965) Effect of muscular exercise in a hot environment on canine fibrinolytic activity. *J. appl. Physiol.* **20,** 1307.

BEGOVIĆ S., KADIĆ M. & TAFRO A. (1972) [Experimental basophilia in dogs, sheep and rabbits.] *Veterinaria, Saraj.* **21,** 447.

BEHNKE O. (1970) A comparative study of microtubules in disk-shaped blood cells. *J. Ultrastruct. Res.* **31,** 61–75.

BELL D.J. (1957) The distribution of glucose between the plasma water and the erythrocyte water in hen's blood. *Q. Jl. exp. Physiol.* **42,** 410–16.

BELL D.J., BIRD T.P. & McINDOE W.M. (1965) Changes in erythrocyte levels and mean corpuscular haemoglobin concentration in hens during the laying cycle. *Comp. Biochem. Physiol.* **14,** 83–100.

BELL J.T. (1964) Enzyme histochemical techniques in veterinary haematology. *Am. J. vet. Res.* **25,** 230.

BELL K. (1972) Blood groups in cattle. *Refresher course for veterinarians on blood disorders.* Proc. No. 17—Postgraduate Committee on Veterinary Science, University of Sydney.

BELL W.N. & ALTON H.G. (1954) A brain extract and substitute for platelet suspensions in the thromboplastin generation test. *Nature* **174,** 880–1.

BELL W.N., TOMLIN S.C. & ARCHER R.K. (1955) The coagulation mechanism of the blood of the horse with particular reference to its 'haemophiloid' status. *J. comp. Path.* **65,** 255–61.

BELLARS A.R.M. (1969) Hereditary disease in British Antarctic sledge dogs. *Vet. Rec.* **85,** 600.

BELLEVILLE J., THOUVEREZ J.-P., MIKAELOFF, PH. & DESCOTES J. (1966) Étude des principaux tests de l'hémostase chez le chien normal. *Path. Biol. (Paris)* **14,** 41.

BENDIXEN H.J. (1960) Untersuchungen über die Rinderleukose in Dänemark. *Dt. tierärztl. Wschr.* **67,** 57–63.

BENDIXEN H.J. (1965) Bovine enzootic leukosis. *Adv. vet. Sci.* **10,** 129–204.

BENNETT B. (1974) Annotation: Antihaemophilic factor, normal and abnormal. *Br. J. Haemat.* **26.** 1–7.

BENNETTS H.W. & CHAPMAN F.E. (1937) Copper deficiency in sheep in Western Australia: a preliminary account of the aetiology of enzootic ataxia of lambs and an anaemia of ewes. *Aust. vet. J.* **13**, 138–49.

BENTINCK-SMITH J. (1969) Hematology. In: Medway W., Prier J.E. & Wilkinson J.S. (Eds) *Textbook of veterinary clinical pathology*, p. 205. Williams & Wilkins, Baltimore, USA.

BERENBAUM M.C. (1956) The use of bovine albumin in the preparation of marrow and blood films. *J. clin. Path.* **9**, 381.

BERGENTZ S.E. & NILSSON I.M. (1961) Effect of trauma on coagulation and fibrinolysis in dogs. *Acta. chir. scand.* **122**, 21.

BERITIĆ T. (1965) Studies on Schmauch bodies. I. The incidence in normal cats (Felis domestica) and the morphologic relationship to Heinz bodies. *Blood* **25**, 999–1008.

BERLIN N.I., WALDMANN T.A. & WEISSMAN S.M. (1959) Life span of red blood cells. *Physiol. Rev.* **39**, 577.

BERNSTAD S., LJUNGBERG O. & HUGOSON G. (1971) A comparative study on the frequency of lymphocytosis and leucosis within herds in a region with low leucosis frequency. *Nord. VetMed.* **23**, 91–8.

BERTALANFFY F.D. (1960) Cytodiagnosis of cancer using acridine orange with fluorescence microscopy. *C.A. Bull (Amer. Cancer Soc.)* **10**, 118–23.

BERTH D. & SCHAICH K. (1973) Untersuchungen zur experimentellen Fasciolose bei Reh- (*Capreolus capreolus*) und Rotwild (*Cervus elaphus*). *Z. Jagdwiss.* **19**, 183–97.

BESSIS M. (1954) *Traitè de cytologie sanguine*. Masson, Paris.

BESSIS M. (1973) *Living blood cells and their ultrastructure*. Springer-Verlag, Berlin, New York.

BEUTLER E. (1968) (Ed.) *Hereditary disorders of erythrocyte metabolism*. Grune and Stratton, New York.

BEYER J. & URBANECK D. (1972) Pathological classification and differential diagnosis of Marek's disease and lymphoid leucosis. *Mh. VetMed.* **27**, 672–7.

BEYER J. & VOGEL K. (1972) Diagnosis and differential diagnosis of Marek's disease. 2. Pathological and histological criteria. *Mh. VetMed.* **27**, 72–4.

BIANCA W. (1970) Effects of dehydration, rehydration and overhydration on the blood and urine of oxen. *Br. vet. J.* **126**, 121–33.

BIANCA W., FINDLAY J.D. & McLEAN J.A. (1965) Responses of steers to water restriction. *Res. vet. Sci.* **6**, 38–55.

BIELY J. & PALMER E.E. (1935) Studies of total erythrocyte and leucocyte counts of fowls. III. Variation in number of blood cells of normal fowl. *Can. J. Res.* D, **13**, 61–71.

BIGGS P.M. (1973) Marek's disease. In: Kaplan A.S. (Ed.) *The herpesviruses*, p. 557–94. Academic Press, London and New York.

BIGGS R. (1972, 1976) (Ed.) *Human blood coagulation, haemostasis and thrombosis*. Blackwell Scientific Publications, Oxford.

BIGGS R. & DOUGLAS A.S. (1953) The thromboplastin generation test. *J. clin. Path.* **6**, 23–9.

BIGGS R. & DOUGLAS A.S. (1953) The measurement of prothrombin in plasma: a case of prothrombin deficiency. *J. clin. Path* **6**, 15.

BIGGS R., DOUGLAS A.S. & MACFARLANE R.G. (1953) The formation of thromboplastin in human blood. *J. Physiol.* **119**, 89.

BIGGS R. & MACFARLANE R.G. (1962) *Human blood coagulation and its disorders*. Blackwell Scientific Publications, Oxford.

BIGGS R., MACFARLANE R.G. & PILLING J. (1947) Observations on fibrinolysis. Experimental production by exercise or adrenaline. *Lancet* **i**, 402.

BIGLAND C.H. & TRIANTAPHYLLOPOULOS D.C. (1960) A re-evaluation of the clotting time of chicken blood. *Nature (London)* **186**, 644.

BILD C.E. (1965) The capillary hematocrit value and erythrocyte sedimentation rate in examination and treatment of the young dog. *J. Am. vet. med. Ass.* **147**, 1419–23.

BLAXHALL P.C. & DAISLEY K.W. (1973) Routine haematological methods for use with fresh blood. *J. Fish Biol.* **5**, 771–81.

BLAXTER K.L., KAY R.N.B., SHARMAN G.A.M., CUNNINGHAM J.M.M. & HAMIL-

TON W.J. (1974) *Farming the Red Deer.* H.M.S.O.

BLECHER T.E. & GUNSTONE M.J. (1969) Fibrinolysis, coagulation and haematological findings in normal Large White/Wessex cross pigs. *Brit. vet. J.* **125**, 74–81.

BLENDIS L.M., BANKS D.C., RAMBOER C. & WILLIAMS R. (1970) Spleen blood flow and splanchnic haemodynamics in blood dyscrasia and other splenomegalies. *Clin. Sci.* **38**, 73–84.

BLEVINS D.I., GLENN M.W., HAMDY A.H., BRODASKY T.F. & EVANS R.A. (1969) Mycotoxicosis associated with haemorrhagic enterocolitis and abortion in swine. *J. Am. vet. med. Ass.* **154**, 1043–50.

BLOOM F. & MEYER L.M. (1944) The morphology of the bone marrow cells in normal dogs. *Cornell Vet.* **34**, 13.

BLOUNT W.P. (1939) Thrombocyte formation in the domestic hen. *Vet. J.* **95**, 195–8.

BLOWEY R.W., WOOD D.W. & DAVIS JENNIFER R. (1973) A nutritional monitoring system for dairy herds based on blood glucose, urea and albumin levels. *Vet. Rec.* **92**, 691–6.

BLUNT M.H., HUISMAN T.H.J. & LEWIS J.P. (1969) The production of haemoglobin C in adult sheep and goats. *Aust. J. exp. Biol. med. Sci.* **47**, 601–11.

BOCCADORO B., DEPELCHIN A. & LIEGEOIS, F. (1957) Polyglobulies compensatrices au cours des cardiopneumopathies du chien. *Ann. Méd. vét.* **101**, 123.

BOGART R. & MUHRER M.E. (1942) The inheritance of a hemophilia-like condition in swine. *J. Hered.* **33**, 59–64.

BOGGS D.R., CARTWRIGHT G.E. & WINTROBE M.M. (1966) Neutrophilia-inducing activity in plasma of dogs recovering from drug-induced myelotoxicity. *Am. J. Physiol.* **211**, 51.

BOITI C. & GROSSO G. (1972) La protrombina nei bovini. *Atti Soc. ital. Sci. vet.* **26**, 194–9.

BOKELMAN D.L., BAGDON R.D. & ZWICKEY R.E. (1972) Aspirin: three-month oral toxicity studies in dogs and rats. *Toxic. appl. Pharmac.* **22**, 333.

BOKORI J. (1974) Contribution to the haemograms of the buffalo and of the camel. *Acta vet. hung.* **24**, 73–6.

BORGESE T.A. & BERTLES F.J. (1964) Differential synthesis of hemoglobin in the White Pekin duck. *Fedn. Proc. Fedn. Am. Socs Exp. Biol.* **23**, 500.

BORGESE T.A. & BERTLES J.F. (1965) Ontogeny of duck hemoglobins. *Fedn. Proc. Fedn. Am. Socs exp. Biol.* **24**, 721.

BORN G.V.R. (1972) In: Biggs R. (Ed.) *Human blood coagulation, haemostasis and thrombosis.* Blackwell Scientific Publications, Oxford.

BORN G.V.R. & WRIGHT H.P. (1968) Diminished platelet aggregation in experimental scurvy. *J. Physiol.* **197**, 27P.

BOST J. & MAGAT A. (1975) Répartition du glucose sanguin entre le plasma et les globules chez quelques espèces animales (étude critique). *Bull. Soc. Sci. vét. Méd. comp. Lyon* **77**, 109.

BOSTEDT H., WAGENSEIL F. & GARHAMMER M. (1974) Studies on iron and copper content and the erythrocyte picture in the blood of cows during pregnancy and the puerperal period. *Zuchthyg, Fortpfl-Stör, Besam, Haustiere.* **9**, 49–57.

BOTHWELL T.H. & CHARLTON R.W. (1970) Absorption of iron. *A. Rev. Med.* **21**, 145–56.

BOTROS B.A.M., MOCH R.W. & BARSOUM I.S. (1975) Some observations on experimentally induced infection of dogs with *Babesia gibsoni. Am. J. vet. Res.* **36**, 293.

BOTTIGER L. (1967) Erythrocyte sedimentation rate and protein-bound carbohydrates in domestic animals. *Acta vet. scand.* **8**, 279.

BOWDLER A.J., BULL R.W., DRIES C., SLATING R. & SWISHER S.N. (1973) Representation of the ABH blood group system in the dog. *Vox. Sang.* (Basel) **24**, 228.

BOWDLER A.J. (1975) The spleen and haemolytic disorders. *Clin. Haematol.* **4**, 231–46.

BOWIE E.J.W., OWEN C.A. JR., ZOLLMAN P.E., THOMPSON J.W. & FASS D.N. (1973) Tests of hemostasis in swine: normal values and values in pigs affected with von Willebrand's disease. *Am. J. vet. Res.* **34**, 1405–7.

BOWLES C.A., WHITE G.S. & LUCAS D.

(1975) Rosette formation by canine peripheral blood lymphocytes. *J. Immun.* **114**, 399.

BOZHKOV S. (1972) Relationships between myelocytes and reticular cells in myelocytomatosis in chickens. *Izv. Inst. srav. Patol. dom. Zhiv. Sof.* **14**, 39–42.

BRACE K. & ALTLAND P.D. (1956) Life span of the duck and chicken erythrocyte as determined with C¹⁴. *Proc. Soc. exp. Biol. Med.* **92**, 615–17.

BRACHET J. (1942) La localisation des acides pentosenucleques dans les tissus animaux et les oefs d'amphibiens en voie development. *Archs. Biol. (Liège)* **53**, 207–57.

BRAÇO F.J.M. DA C., DURÃO J.F. DA C., LAGE M.C.D. DA & TEIXEIRA F.A. DA S. (1972a) Basis of prophylaxis of bovine leucosis in Portugal. Preliminary note. *Anais Esc. sup. Med. vet., Lisb.* **14**, 101–15.

BRAÇO F.J.M. DA C., DURÃO J.F. DA C., LAGE M.C.D. DA & TEIXEIRA F.A. DA S. (1972b) Bovine leucosis—histology. *Anais Esc. sup. Med. vet., Lisb.* **14**, 117–37.

BRADLEY O.C. & GRAHAME T. (1960) *The structure of the fowl.* Oliver & Boyd, Edinburgh.

BRADLEY W.B., EPPSON H.F. & BEATH O.A. (1940) Methylene blue as an antidote for poisoning by oat hay and other plants containing nitrates. *J. Am. vet. med. Ass.* **96**, 41–2.

BRAEND M. (1962) Studies on blood and serum groups in the elk (*Alces alces*). *Ann. N.Y. Acad. Sci.* **97**, 296–305.

BRAEND M. (1964) Genetic studies on serum transferrins in reindeer. *Hereditas* **52**, 181–8.

BRAEND M. (1973) Genetic variation in equine blood plasma. *Proc. 3rd Int. Conf. Equine Infectious Diseases, Paris,* pp. 394–406. Karger, Basel.

BRAGANZA C.M., STATHOPOULOS G., DAVIES A.J.S., ELLIOTT E.V., KERBEL R.S., PAPAMICHAIL M. & HOLBORROW E.J. (1975) Lymphocyte:erythrocyte (L.E.) rosettes as indicators of the heterogeneity of lymphocytes in a variety of mammalian species. *Cell* **4**, 103.

BRAIN M.C. (1970) Microangiopathic hemolytic anemia. *A. Rev. Med.* **21**, 133–44.

BRAIN M.C. (1971) The red cell and haemolytic anaemia. In: Goldberg A. & Brain M.C. (Eds) *Recent advances in haematology,* pp. 146–93. Churchill Livingstone, Edinburgh and London.

BRECHER G. & CRONKITE E.P. (1964) Estimation of the number of platelets by phase microscopy. In: Tocantins L.M. & Kazal L.A. (Eds). *Blood coagulation hemorrhage and thrombosis,* p. 52. Grune and Stratton, New York.

BREEUWSMA A.J. (1968) A case of XXY sex chromosome constitution in an intersex pig. *J. Reprod. Fert.* **16**, 119–20.

BREEUWSMA A.J. (1970) Genetic and cytogenetic studies in porcine intersexes. *Giessener Beitr. Erbpath. Zuchthyg.* Suppl. **1**, 151–5.

BREMNER K.C. (1966a) The reticulocyte response in calves made anaemic by phlebotomy. *Aust. J. exp. Biol. med. Sci.* **44**, 251–8.

BREMNER K.C. (1966b) Variations with age in the plasma iron and total iron-binding capacity in dairy calves. *Aust. J. exp. Biol. med. Sci.* **44**, 259–70.

BREUKINK H.J., WENSING TH & SCHOTMAN A.J.H. (1974) Variations in the composition of the blood in veal calves solely fed on a milk replacer during a fattening period of eighteen weeks. *Tijdschr. Diergeneesk.* **99**, 1219–34.

BREWER N.R. (1968) Radiation Injury. In: Catcott E.J. (Ed.) *Canine medicine,* First Catcott Edn, p. 264. American Veterinary Publications, Wheaton, Illinois, USA.

BRILES W.E., McGIBBON W.H. & IRWIN M.R. (1950) On multiple alleles effecting certain cellular antigens in the chicken. *Genetics* **35**, 633–53.

BRINKHOUS K.M., DAVIS P.D., GRAHAM J.B. & DODDS W.J. (1973) Expression and linkage of genes for x-linked hemophilias A and B in the dog. *Blood* **41**, 577.

BRION A. (1949) Vivi l'ictère hémolytique du poulain nouveau-né. *Rev. de Med. Vet.* **100**, 229–35.

BRITTON C.J.C. (1969) In: Whitby, L.E.H.

& Britton C.K. *Disorders of the blood*, 10th Edn, p. 1. J. & A. Churchill, London.

BROCK W.E., BUCKNER R.G., HAMPTON J.W., BIRD R.M. & WULZ C.E. (1963) Canine hemophilia: establishment of a new colony. *Arch. Path.* **76**, 464.

BRODEY R.S. (1964) Clinico-Pathologic Conference. *J. Am. vet. med. Ass.* **144**, 628–36.

BRODEY R.S. & SCHALM O.W. (1963) Hemobartonellosis and thrombocytopenic purpura in a dog. *J. Am. vet. med. Ass.* **143**, 1231–6.

BROOKS C.C. & DAVIS J.W. (1969) Changes in hematology of the perinatal pig. *J. Anim. Sci.* **28**, 517–22.

BROOKSBANK N.H. (1954) Anaemia in piglets associated with a copper deficiency *Vet. Rec.* **66**, 322–4.

BROWMAN L.G. & SEARS H.S. (1955) Erythrocyte values, and alimentary canal pH values in the mule deer. *J. Mammal.* **36**, 474–6.

BROWN J.M., KINGREY B.W. & ROSENQUIST B.D. (1959) The hematology of chronic bovine reticuloperitonitis. *Am. J. vet. Res.* **20**, 255–64.

BROWN R.V. & TENG Y.-S. (1975) Studies of inherited pyruvate kinase deficiency in the Basenji. *J. Am. Anim. Hosp. Assn.* **11**, 362.

BRUERE A.N., FIELDEN E.D. & HUTCHINGS H. (1968) XX/XY mosaicism in lymphocyte cultures from a pig with freemartin characteristics. *N.Z. vet. J.* **16**, 31–8.

BRUMMERSTEDT-HANSEN E. (1967) *The serum proteins of the pig*. Thesis. Munksgaard, Copenhagen.

BRUNK R.R. (1969) Standard values in the beagle dog. Haematology and clinical chemistry. *Fd. Cosmet. Toxicol.* **7**, 141.

BRUNS G.A.P. & INGRAM V.M. (1973) The erythroid cells and haemoglobins of the chick embryo. *Phil. Trans. R. Soc. B* **266**, 225–305.

BRYANS J.T., DOLL E.R., CROWE M.E.W. & McCOLLUM W.H. (1957) The blood picture and thermal reactions in experimental viral arteritis of horses. *Cornell Vet.* **47**, 42–52.

BUCK W.B., RAMSAY F.K. & DUNCAN J.R. (1968) Diseases caused by physical and chemical agents. In: Catcott E.J. (Ed.) *Canine medicine*, First Catcott Edn, p. 229. American Veterinary Publications, Wheaton, Illinois, USA.

BUCKELL M.B. (1958) The effect of citrate on euglobulin methods of estimating fibrinolytic activity. *J. clin. Path.* **11**, 403.

BUCKNER R.G., HAMPTON J.M., BIRD R.M. & BROCK W.E. (1967) Hemophilia in the Vizla. *J. small Anim. Pract.* **8**, 511.

BUHLES W.C. JR., HUXSOLL D.L. & RISTIC M. (1974) Tropical canine pancytopenia: clinical, hematologic, and serologic response of dogs to *Ehrlichia canis* infection, tetracycline therapy, and challenge inoculation. *J. infect. Dis.* **130**, 357.

BUHLES W.C. JR., HUXSOLL D.L. & HILDEBRANDT P.K. (1975) Tropical canine pancytopenia: role of aplastic anaemia in the pathogenesis of severe disease. *J. comp. Path.* **85**, 511–21.

BULGIN M.S., MUNN S.L. & GEE W. (1970) Hematologic changes to $4\frac{1}{2}$ years of age in clinically normal Beagles. *J. Am. vet. med. Ass.* **157**, 1064–70.

BULL R.W., SCHIRMER R. & BOWDLER A.J. (1971) Autoimmune hemolytic disease in the dog. *J. Am. vet. med. Ass.* **159**, 880.

BUNCE S.A. (1954) Observations on the blood sedimentation rate and packed cell volume of some domestic farm animals. *Brit. vet. J.* **110**, 322–8.

BUONACCORSI A., CARDINI G. & TESSARI E. (1973) Su alcuni aspetti del ricambio idrocarbonato delle emazie di cani sani ed ammalati. *Atti Soc. ital. Sci. vet.* **27**, 317.

BURG R.W., FELDBUSH T., MORRIS C.A. & MAAG T.A. (1971) Depression of thymus- and bursa-dependent immune systems of chicks with Marek's disease. *Avian Dis.* **15**, 662–71.

BURGOYNE G.H. & WITTER R.L. (1973) Effect of passively transferred immunoglobulins on Marek's disease. *Avian Dis.* **17**, 824–37.

BURMESTER B.R. & WITTER R.L. (1966) *An outline of the diseases of the avian leukosis complex*. Rep. U.S. Dep. Agric. **94**, 2–8.

BURSTONE M.S. (1958) The relationship between fixation and techniques for the histochemical localisation of hydrolytic enzymes. *J. Histochem. Cytochem.* **6,** 322–39.

BURSTONE M.S. (1962) *Enzyme histochemistry.* Academic Press, New York.

BURTON R.R., BESCH E.L. & SMITH A.H. (1966) The erythrocyte sedimentation rate test in the domestic fowl (chicken). *Poult. Sci.* **45,** 1222–30.

BURTON R.R. & HARRISON J.S. (1969) The relative differential leucocyte count of the newly hatched chick. *Poult. Sci.* **48,** 451–3.

BURTON R.R., SAHARA R. & SMITH A.H. (1967) The use of radio-iodinated (I^{131}) serum albumin in determining whole body blood volumes in the chicken. *Poult. Sci.* **46,** 1395–7.

BUSHBY S.R.M. (1970) Haematological studies during toxicity tests. In: Paget G.E. (Ed.) *Methods in toxicology,* p. 338. Blackwell Scientific Publications, Oxford.

BUTKUS A., EHRHART L.A., LEWIS L.A. & McCULLAGH K.G. (1974) Changes in erythrocyte lipid composition and osmotic fragility in dogs fed an atherogenic diet. *Artery* **1,** 46.

BUTLER E.J. (1962) Apparatus for collecting blood samples for copper estimation. *Vet. Rec.* **74,** 1178–9.

BYERLY J.L. & DAWE D.L. (1972) Delayed hypersensitivity reactions in Marek's disease virus-infected chickens. *Am. J. vet. Res.* **33,** 2267–73.

CADE J.F. & ROBINSON T.F. (1975) Coagulation and fibrinolysis in the dog. *Can. J. comp. Med.* **39,** 296.

CAILLARD B., DEVANT J. & KLEPPING J. (1962) Etude comparative de la coagulabilité sanguine chez l'homme et quelques espèces animales. *C.R. Soc. Biol.* **156,** 1813.

CALHOUN M.L. (1954) A cytological study of costal marrow. I. The adult horse. *Am. J. vet. Res.* **15,** 181.

CALKINS J., LANE K.P., LoSASSO B. & THURBER L.E. (1974) Comparative study of platelet aggregation in various species. *J. Med.* **5,** 292.

CALNEK B.W. (1972) Effects of passive antibody on early pathogenesis of Marek's disease. *Infec. Immunity* **6,** 193–8.

CALNEK B.W. (1973) Influence of age and exposure on the pathogenesis of Marek's disease. *J. natn. Cancer Inst.* **51,** 929–39.

CALVO W., FLIEDNER T.M., HERBST E.W. & FACHE I. (1975) Regeneration of blood-forming organs after autologous leukocyte transfusion in lethally irradiated dogs. I. Distribution and cellularity of the bone marrow in normal dogs. *Blood,* **46,** 453–57.

CAMERON R.D. & LUICK J.R. (1972) Seasonal changes in total body water, extracellular fluid, and blood volume in grazing reindeer. *Can. J. Zool.* **50,** 107–16.

CAMPBELL A. (1972) A method to determine the proportion of sheep blood monocytes which replicates DNA in culture. *J. Physiol., Lond.* **226,** 36–7P.

CAMPBELL E.A. (1957) The use of paper electrophoresis as an aid to diagnosis. *J. comp. Path.* **67,** 345–53.

CAMPBELL F. (1967) Fine structure of the bone marrow of the chicken and pigeon. *J. Morph.* **123,** 405–39.

CAPEL-EDWARDS K. & HALL D.E. (1968) Factor VII deficiency in the beagle dog. *Lab. Anim.* **2,** 105.

CAPEL-EDWARDS K. & HALL D.E. (1970) Haematological observations on the Squirrel monkey. *Folia primatol.* **12,** 142.

CAPEL-EDWARDS K., HALL D.E., FELLOWES K.P., VALLANCE D.K., DAVIES M.J., LAMB D. & ROBERTSON W.B. (1973) Long term administration of progesterone to the female beagle dog. *Toxic. appl. Pharmac.* **24,** 474.

CAPEL-EDWARDS K., HALL D.E. & SANSOM A.G. (1971) Hematological changes observed in female beagle dogs given ethynylestradiol. *Toxic. appl. Pharmac.* **20,** 319.

CARLE B.N. & DEWHIRST W.H. (1942) A method of bleeding swine. *J. Am. vet. med. Ass.* **101,** 495–6.

CARLSON H.C. & ALLEN J.R. (1969) The acute inflammatory reaction in chicken skin: blood cellular response. *Avian Dis.* **13,** 817–33.

CARLSON H.C. & HACKING M.A. (1972) Distribution of mast cells in chicken, turkey, pheasant and quail and their differentiation from basophils. *Avian Dis.* **16**, 574–7.

CARLSON H.C., SWEENY P.R. & TOKARYK J.M. (1968) Demonstration of phagocytic and trephocytic activities of chicken thrombocytes by microscopy and vital staining techniques. *Avian Dis.* **12**, 700–15.

CARPER H.A. & HOFFMANN P.L. (1966) The intravascular survival of transfused canine Pelger-Huet neutrophils and eosinophils. *Blood* **27**, 739–43.

CARROLL E.J., SCHALM O.W. & WHEAT J.D. (1965) Endotoxemia in a horse. *J. Am. vet. med. Ass.* **146**, 1300–3.

CARTER G.B., SEAMER J. & SNAPE T. (1971) Diagnosis of tropical canine pancytopenia (*Ehrlichia canis* infection) by immunofluorescence. *Res. vet. Sci.* **12**, 318–22.

CARTWRIGHT G.E. & DEISS A. (1975) Sideroblasts, siderocytes and sideroblastic anemia. *New Engl. J. Med.* **292**, 185–93.

CARTWRIGHT G.E., LAURITSEN M.A., HUMPHREYS S., JONES P.J., MERRILL I.M. & WINTROBE M.M. (1946) The anaemia associated with chronic infection. *Science* **103**, 72.

CARTWRIGHT G.E., SMITH E.L., BROWN D.M. & WINTROBE M.M. (1948) Electrophoretic analyses of sera of normal and hypoproteinaemic swine. *J. biol. Chem.* **176**, 585–9.

CARTWRIGHT G.E., TATTING B., ASHENBRUCKER H. & WINTROBE M.M. (1949) Experimental production of a nutritional macrocytic anaemia in swine. *Blood*, **4**, 301–23.

CARTWRIGHT G.E. & WINTROBE M.M. (1948) Studies on free erythrocyte protoporphyrin, plasma copper and plasma iron in protein deficient and iron deficient swine. *J. biol. Chem.* **176**, 571–83.

CASE A.A. (1957) Some aspects of nitrate intoxication in livestock. *J. Am. vet. med. Ass.* **130**, 323–9.

CASE M.T. & SIMON J. (1972) Whole-body gamma irradiation of newborn pigs: hematologic changes. *Am. J. vet. Res.* **33**, 1217–22.

CASNOCHA E. & SALAJ J. (1973) Detection of precipitation antigen in poultry skin and feathers for diagnosing Marek's disease. *Vet. Med., Praha* **18**, 491–8.

CATLING S.J. (1975) Studies on haematology of exertion in horses. *Br. J. Haemat.* **30**, 123.

CATLING S.J. (1976) Personal communication.

CATLING S.J. & JEFFCOTT L.B. (1975) Personal communication.

CATOVSKY D., PETTIT J.E., GALTON D.A., SPIERS A.S.D. & HARRISON C.V. (1974) Leukaemic reticuloendotheliosis ('Hairy' cell leukaemia): A distinct clinicopathological entity. *Br. J. Haemat.* **26**, 9–27.

CELANDER E. & CELANDER D.R. (1968) Comparison of *in vivo* effects on components of the canine fibrinolytic enzyme system of AMCHA fed at varying dose levels. *Thromb. Diath. haemorrh.* **20**, 574.

CHAFFEE V.W., EDDS G.T., HIMES J.A. & NEAL F.C. (1969) Aflatoxicosis in dogs. *Am. J. vet. Res.* **30**, 1737–49.

CHANARIN I. (1969) *The megaloblastic anaemias.* Blackwell Scientific Publications, Oxford.

CHANDER S. (1972) Mechanisms of lymphocytosis in some leukosis herds. *Diss. Abstr. Int.* **33B**, 488–9.

CHANDER S. & GILMAN J.P.W. (1974a) Bovine leukosis. I. Seasonal influences on lymphocytosis. *Can. J. comp. Med.* **38**, 168–72.

CHANDER S. & GILMAN J.P.W. (1974b) Bovine leukosis. II. Comparison of hematological classification with DNA synthesis between herds. *Can. J. comp. Med.* **38**, 173–8.

CHANDER S. & GILMAN J.P.W. (1975) Trypanosomiasis, lymphocytosis and DNA synthesis. *Can. J. comp. Med.* **39**, 94–100.

CHANDLER F.W., JR., PRASSE K.W. & CALLAWAY C.S. (1975) Surface ultrastructure of pyruvate kinase-deficient erythrocytes in the Basenji dog. *Am. J. vet. Res.* **36**, 1477–80.

CHAPPUIS G. & TERRÉ J. (1970) [Blood

groups and blood transfusion in the dog.] *Recl. Méd. vet.* **146**, 671.

CHARGAFF E., BENDICH A. & COHEN S.S. (1944) The thromboplastic protein; structure, properties, disintegration. *J. Biol. Chem.* **156**, 161.

CHEN J.H. & HANAFUSA H. (1974) Detection of a protein of avian leukoviruses in uninfected chick cells by radioimmunoassay. *Virology* **13**, 340–46.

CHEN J.H., HAYWARD W.S. & HANAFUSA H. (1974) Avian tumor virus proteins and RNA in uninfected chicken embryo cells. *J. Virol.* **14**, 1419–29.

CHEVILLE N.F. (1975) The Gray Collie Syndrome (cyclic neutropenia). *J. Am. Anim. Hosp. Assn.* **11**, 350.

CHEVRIER L. & GAYOT G. (1972) Contribution à l'étude de la numération leucocytaire du bovin Holstein. *Bull. Acad. vét. Fr.* **45**, 93–102.

CHIEN S., DELLENBACK R.J., USAMI S. & GREGERSEN M.I. (1965) Plasma trapping in hematocrit determinations. *Proc. Soc. exp. Biol. Med.* **119**, 1155–58.

CHIU T. (1974) Studies on estrogen-induced proliferative disorders of hemopoietic tissue in dogs. *Diss. Abstr. Int.* **35B**, Part 6, 3104.

CHO D.Y., FREY R.A., GUFFY M.M. & LEIPOLD H.W. (1975) Hypervitaminosis A in the dog. *Am. J. vet. Res.* **36**, 1597–603.

CHRISTIE D.W. (1970) A technique for blood sampling the chicken from the jugular vein. *Vet. Rec.* **86**, 521.

CHUBB L.G. & ROWELL J.G. (1959) Counting blood cells of chickens. *J. agric. Sci., Camb.* **52**, 263–72.

CHUSID M.J., BUJAK J.S. & DALE D.C. (1975) Defective polymorphonuclear leukocyte metabolism and function in canine cyclic neutropenia. *Blood* **46**, 921.

CIBA FOUNDATION SYMPOSIA (1976) *Congenital disorders of erythropoiesis.* **No. 37** (new series) Elsevier/Excerpta Medica/North Holland.

CIMR J. & KASPAR F. (1965) Method of repeated collection of blood from the portal vein of piglets. *Vet. Med. Praha* **10**, 173–5.

CLAGUE D.C. & GRANZIEN CORINNE K.

(1966) Enzootic bovine leucosis in S.E. Queensland. *Aust. vet. J.* **42**, 177–82.

CLARK R. (1942) Eperythrozoon felis in a cat. *Jl. S. Afr. vet. med. Ass.* **13**, 15–16.

CLARK W.T. & HALLIWELL R.E.W. (1963) The treatment with Vitamin K preparations of Warfarin poisoning in dogs. *Vet. Rec.* **75**, 1210.

CLARKE E.G.C. & CLARKE M.L. (1967) *Veterinary toxicology*, pp. 145–9. Ballière, Tindall & Cassell, London.

CLAWSON C.C., COOPER M.D. & GOOD R.A. (1967) Lymphocyte fine structure in the bursa of Fabricius, the thymus and the germinal centres. *Lab. Invest.* **16**, 407–21.

CLEGG F.G. & EVANS R.K. (1962) Haemoglobinaemia of cattle associated with the feeding of *Brassicae* species. *Vet. Rec.* **74**, 1169–76.

CLEVENGER A.B., MARSH W.L. & PEERY T.M. (1971) Clinical laboratory studies on the gorilla, chimpanzee and orangutan. *Am. J. clin. Path.* **55**, 479.

CLIFFTON E.E. & CANNAMELA D.A. (1951) Variations in proteolytic activity of serum of animals including man. *Proc. Soc. exp. Biol. Med.* **77**, 305.

CLINE M.J. (1974) Granulocytes in human disease. *Ann. intern. Med.* **81**, 801–16.

CLINE H.J. (1975) *White cells.* Harvard University Press, Cambridge, Massachusetts.

COATES V. & MARCH B.E. (1966) Reticulocyte counts in the chicken. *Poult. Sci.* **45**, 1302–5.

COBURN R.F. & KANE P.B. (1968) Maximal erythrocyte and hemoglobin catabolism. *J. clin Invest.* **47**, 1435.

COGGINS L., NORCROSS N.L. & NUSBAUM S.R. (1972) Diagnosis of equine infectious anemia by immuno-diffusion test. *Am. J. vet. Res.* **33**, 11–18.

COHEN H., CHAPMAN A.L., BOPP W.J., SCHMIDT C.E., PRZYBYLSKI C.E. & MCPHEE M.S. (1974) Pathogenesis of a transplanted canine lymphocyte leukemia. *Cancer*, **33**, 1313.

COHEN R.R. (1967a) Anticoagulation, centrifugation time and sample replicate number in the microhematocrit method for avian blood. *Poult. Sci.* **46**, 214–18.

COHEN R.R. (1967b) An estimation of percentage trapped plasma in normal chicken microhematocrit, using Cr^{51}. *Poult. Sci.* **46**, 219–23.

COHEN R.R. (1967c) Total circulating erythrocyte and plasma volumes of ducks measured simultaneously with Cr^{51}. *Poult. Sci.* **46**, 1539–44.

COLDMAN M.F., GENT M. & GOOD W. (1969) The osmotic fragility of mammalian erythrocytes in hypotonic solutions of sodium chloride. *Comp. Biochem. Physiol.* **31**, 605.

COLLETTE W.L. & MERIWETHER W.F. (1965) Some changes in the peripheral blood of dogs after administration of certain tranquilizers and narcotics. *Vet. Med/ Small Anim. Clin.* **60**, 1223.

COMMON R.H., BOLTON W. & RUTLEDGE W.A. (1948) The influence of gonadal hormones on the composition of the blood and liver of the domestic fowl. *J. Endocr.* **5**, 263.

CONBOY H.J. & POWERS R.D. (1971) Equine malignant lymphoma. *J. Am. vet. med. Ass.* **159**, 53–4.

COOK W.R. (1968) The clinical features of guttural pouch mycosis in the horse. *Vet. Rec.* **83**, 336–45.

COOK W.R. (1974) Epistaxis in the racehorse. *Equine vet. J.* **6**, 45–58.

COOK W.R. & LITTLEWORT M.C.G. (1974) Progressive haematoma of the ethmoid region in the horse. *Equine vet. J.* **6**, 101–8.

COOMBS R.R.A., MOURANT A.E. & RACE R.R. (1945) A new test for detection of weak and 'incomplete' Rh agglutinins. *Br. J. exp. Path.* **26**, 255–66.

COOMBS R.R.A., MOURANT A.E. & RACE R.R. (1946) In vivo iso-sensitisation of red cells in babies with haemolytic disease. *Lancet* **i**, 264–6.

COOMBS R.R.A., CROWHURST R.C., DAY F.T., HEARD D.H., HINDE I.T., HOOGSTRATEN J. & PARRY H.B. (1948) Haemolytic disease of newborn foals due to Iso-Immunization of pregnancy. *J. Hyg.* **46**, 403–18.

COOPER A.C.D. (1974) Haematology of normal native cattle in Botswana. *Trop. Anim. Hlth. & Prod.* **6**, 53–4.

COOPER B.J. & WATSON A.D.J. (1975) Myeloid neoplasia in a dog. *Aust. vet. J.* **51**, 150–54.

COOPER H.A., BOWIE E.J.W. & OWEN C.A. JR. (1973) Chronic induced intravascular coagulation in dogs. *Am. J. Physiol.* **225**, 1355.

COOPER M.D., GABRIELSON A.E. & GOOD R.A. (1967) Role of the thymus and other central lymphoid tissues in immunological diseases. *A. Rev. Med.* **18**, 113–38.

COPLAND J.W. (1974) Canine pneumonia caused by *Pneumocystis carinii*. *Aust. vet. J.* **50**, 515–18.

COPLEY A.L. & LALICH J.J. (1941) Bleeding time in men. *Am. J. Physiol.* **133**, 246–7.

CORBIN J.E., LEHRER W.P. JR., NEWBERNE P.M., VISEK W.J. & WIESE H.F. (1972) Nutrient requirements of dogs. *Nutrient requirements of domestic animals*, No. 8. Nat. Acad. Sci., Washington D.C.

CORNELIUS C.E. (1970) Liver Function. In: Kaneko J.J. & Cornelius C.E. (Eds) *Clinical biochemistry of domestic animals*, 2nd Edn, Vol. I, p. 161. Academic Press, New York.

CORNELIUS C.E., BISHOP J., SWITZER J. & RHODE E.A. (1959) Serum and tissue transminase activities in domestic animals. *Cornell, Vet.* **49**, 116–26.

CORNELIUS C.E., GOODBARY R.F. & KENNEDY P.C. (1959) Plasma cell myelomatosis in a horse. *Cornell Vet.* **49**, 478–93.

CORNELIUS C.E., KANEKO J.J. & BENSON D.C. (1959) Erythrocyte survival studies in the mule deer, Aoudad sheep, and springbok antelope, using glucine-2-C^{14}. *Am. J. vet. Res.* **20**, 917–20.

CORNELIUS C.E., KANEKO J., BENSON D.C. & WHEAT J.D. (1960a) Erythrocyte survival studies in the horse, using glycine-2-C^{14}. *Am. J. vet. Res.* **21**, 1123–4.

CORNELIUS C.E., KILGORE W.W. & WHEAT J.D. (1960b) Chromatographic identification of bile pigments in several species. *Cornell Vet.* **50**, 47–53.

CORNELL C.N. & MUHRER M.E. (1964) Coagulation factors in normal and hemophiliac-type swine. *Am. J. Physiol.* **206**, 926–8.

COSGROVE J.S. (1969) The practical application of haematology—1. *Equine vet. J.* **1**, 194–8.

COTCHIN E. (1960) Tumours of farm animals. *Vet. Rec.* **72**, 816–22.

COTTER P.F., COLLINS W.M., DUNLOP W.R. & CORBETT A.C. (1973) Host age dependency of regression of Rous sarcomas of chickens. *Cancer Res.* **33**, 3310–11.

COTTER S.M., HARDY W.D. & ESSEX M. (1975) Association of the feline leukemia virus with lymphosarcoma and other disorders. *J. Am. vet. med. Ass.* **166**, 449–54.

COULON J. (1973) Transfusion de sang A negatif conservé chez le chien: Place actuelle de la transfusion sanguine en clinique canine. *Revue Med. vet.* **124**, 1515.

COWAN I.McT. & BANDY P.J. (1969) Observations on the haematology of several races of black-tailed deer (*Odocoileus hemionus*). *Can. J. Zool.* **47**, 1021–4.

CRADDOCK C.G., ADAMS W.S., PERRY S. & LAWRENCE J.S. (1955) The dynamics of platelet production as carried out by a depletion technic in normal and irradiated dogs. *J. Lab. Clin. med.* **45**, 906–19.

CRADDOCK C.G., PERRY S. & LAWRENCE J.S. (1963) Control of the steady state of proliferation of leukocytes. In: Stohlman F. (Ed.) The Kinetics of Cellular Proliferation, p. 242. Grune and Stratton, New York.

CRADDOCK C.G., LONGMIRE R. & McMILLAN R. (1971) Medical Progress: Lymphocytes and the immune response (second of two parts). *New Engl. J. Med.* **285**, 378–84.

CREED E.F.F. (1938) The estimation of the fragility of red blood corpuscles. *J. Path. Bact.* **46**, 331–40.

CRONIN M.T.I. (1953) Exchange transfusion in the foal. *Vet. Rec.* **65**, 120–2.

CRONIN M.T.I. (1955) Haemolytic disease of newborn foals. *Vet. Rec.* **67**, 479–84.

CROOKSHANK H.R., SMALLEY H.E. & STEEL E. (1975) Hematological parameters of American-Essex Swine. *J. Anim. Sci.* **40**, 190.

CROSSMAN P.J., WIJERATNE W.V.S., IMLAH P., BUCKNER D.R.P. & GOULD C.M.

(1973) Experimental evidence of sire effect on piglet mortality. *Br. vet. J.* **129**, 58–62.

CRUZ W.O. & BAUMGARTEN A. (1957) Susceptibility of the red blood cell of the dog to haemolysis in alkaline media. *Br. J. Haemat.* **3**, 359–65.

CRUZ W.O., HAHN P.F., BALE W.F. & BALFOUR W.M. (1941) The effect of age on the susceptibility of the erythrocyte to hypotonic salt solutions. Radioactive iron as a means of tagging the red blood cell. *Am. J. med. Sci.* **202**, 157.

CUMMING M. (1853) On puerperal Red Water in cows. *Trans. Highld agric. Soc. Scotl.* pp. 9–36.

CYPRESS R.H., WALLER J.H., REDMOND C.K., TASHJIAN R.J. & HURVITZ A.I. (1974) Epidemiologic and pedigree study of the occurrence of lymphosarcoma from 1953–71 in a closed herd of Jersey cows. *Am. J. Epidem.* **99**, 37–43.

DACIE J.V. (1960) *The haemolytic anaemias, congenital and acquired*: Vol. I: *The congenital anaemias*, 2nd Edn. Churchill Livingstone, Edinburgh and London.

DACIE J.V. (1962) *The haemolytic anaemias: congenital and acquired.* Vol II: *The autoimmune haemolytic anaemias*, 2nd Edn. Churchill Livingstone, Edinburgh and London.

DACIE J.V. & LEWIS S.M. (1972) Paroxysmal nocturnal haemoglobinuria: clinical manifestations and nature of the disease. *Ser. Haemat.* **5** (3), 3–23.

DACIE J.V. & LEWIS S.M. (1975) *Practical haematology*, 5th Edn. Churchill Livingstone, Edinburgh and London.

DACIE J.V. & WORLLEDGE S.M. (1969) Auto-immune hemolytic anemias. *Prog. Hemat.*, **6**, 82–120.

DAGG J.H., CUMMING R.L.C. & GOLDBERG A. (1971) Disorders of iron metabolism. In: Goldberg A. & Brain M.C. (Eds) *Recent advances in haematology*, pp. 77–145. Churchill Livingstone, Edinburgh and London.

DALTON R.G. (1964) The effects of batyl alcohol on the haematology of cattle poisoned with bracken. *Vet. Rec.* **76**, 411–16.

DALTON R.G. (1967) Variations in calf plasma with age. *Br. vet. J.* **123**, 48–52.

DALTON R.G. (1968) Renal function in neonatal calves. *Br. vet. J.* **124**, 371–81.

DALTON R.G., FISHER E.W. & MCINTYRE W.I.M. (1965) Changes in blood chemistry, body weight and haematocrit of calves affected with neonatal diarrhoea. *Br. vet. J.* **121**, 34–41.

DAMASIO E., MONTALE P. & GAY A. (1962) Nuove possibilità d'impiego in isto-chemica della microscopia in fluorescenza: techniche per la visualizzazione dell' A.D.N. e delle sostanze PAS-positive. *L'informatore Medico* **17**, 1–24.

DARCEL C. LE Q. (1973) *Tumor viruses of the fowl*. Information Division, Agriculture Canada Monograph No. **8**.

D'ARCY P.F. & HOWARD E.M. (1962) The acute toxicity of ferrous salts administered to dogs by mouth. *J. Path. Bact.* **83**, 65–72.

DARGIE J.D. & PRESTON J.M. (1974) Patho-physiology of ovine schistosomiasis. VI Onset and development of anaemia in sheep experimentally infected with Schistosoma mattheei—ferrokinetic studies. *J. comp. Path. Ther.* **84**, 83–91.

DAVIDSON E. & TOMLIN S. (1963) The levels of plasma coagulation factors after trauma and childbirth. *J. clin. Path.* **16**, 112.

DAVIDSON W.M. (1968) Inherited variations in leukocytes. *Semin. Hematol.* **5**, 255–74.

DAVIES E. (1971) The production of Vitamin B_{12} in the horse. *Br. vet. J.* **127**, 34–6.

DAVIES R.F. & REINERT H. (1965) Arteriosclerosis in the young dog. *J. Atheroscler. Res.* **5**, 181.

DAVIS J.W. & LIBKE K.G. (1968) Hematologic studies in pigs fed clay pigeon targets. *J. Am. vet. med. Ass.* **152**, 382–4.

DAWES R.L.F. (1967) A Romanowsky-type stain for canine blood; phloxine and rose bengal used in place of eosin. *Stain Technol.* **42**, 30–32.

DEATON J.W., REECE F.N. & TARNER W.J. (1969) Hematocrit, hemoglobin and plasma-protein levels of broilers reared under constant temperatures. *Poult. Sci.* **48**, 1993–6.

DEAVERS S., SMITH E.L. & HUGGIN R.A. (1971) Changes in red cell volume, venous hematocrit and haemoglobin concentration in growing Beagles. *Proc. Soc. exp. Biol. Med.* **137**, 299.

DEBBIE J.G., ROWSELL H.C., KARSTAD L.H. & DITCHFIELD J. (1965) An approach to the pathogenesis of viral hemorrhagic disease of deer. *Trans. N. Am. Wildl. Conf.* **30**, 196–204.

DEBELAK-FEHIR K.M., CATCHATOURIAN R. & EPSTEIN R.B. (1975) Hemopoietic colony forming units in fresh and cryo-preserved peripheral blood cells of canines and man. *Exp. Hematol.* **3**, 109.

DENICOLA P. (1953) Factor VII (SPCA): its physiopathologic significance. *Blood* **8**, 947–54.

DENICOLA P., CAPPELLETTI G. & SARTORI S. (1957a) Studio comparativo dei reperti trombelastografici ed emocoagulativi nell-uomo e in varie specie animali. *Haematologica* **42**, 179.

DENICOLA P., CAPPELLETTI, G. & SARTORI S. (1957b) Untersuchungen über die Artspezifität der Blutgerinnung bei einigen Säugetieren. *Schweiz. med. Wschr.* **39**, 1223.

DENINGTON E.M. & LUCAS A.M. (1955) Blood techniques for chickens. *Poult. Sci.* **34**, 360–8.

DENNIS R.A., O'HARA P.J., YOUNG M.F. & DORRIS K.D. (1970) Neonatal immuno-hemolytic anaemia and icterus of calves. *J. Am. vet. med. Ass.* **156**, 1861–9.

DENSON K.W. (1961) Levels of blood coagulation factors during anticoagulant therapy with phenindione. *Brit. med. J.* **i**, 1205.

DENSON K.W. (1961) The specific assay of Prower Stuart factor and factor VII. *Acta haemat.* **25**, 105–20.

DENSON K.W.E. (1972) In: Biggs R. (Ed.) *Human blood coagulation, haemostasis and thrombosis*, p. 587. Blackwell Scientific Publications, Oxford.

DENSON K.W.E., BORRETT R. & BIGGS R. (1971) The specific assay of prothrombin using the Taipan snake venom. *Br. J. Haemat.* **21**, 219–26.

DENVER REPORT (1960) A proposed standard system of nomenclature of human mitotic chromosomes. *Lancet*, **i**, 1063–5.

DEPELCHIN A. (1956) Hématologie animale. II. Le myélogramme normal des espèces bovine, ovine et canine. *Annls Méd. vét.* **100**, 325–45.

DESHAW J.R., BROWN S.O. & SZABUNIEWICZ M. (1969) Hematology of the developing juvenile Spanish goat. *SWest. Vet.* **22**, 287–92.

DE SHAZER J.A. & WEISS H.S. (1963) A comparison among variations in the dye dilution procedure for determining blood volume. *Poult. Sci.* **42**, 778–80.

DETWEILER D.K. & PATTERSON D.F. (1965) The prevalence and types of cardiovascular disease in dogs. *Ann. N.Y. Acad. Sci.* **127**, 481.

DETWEILER D.K., PATTERSON D.F., LUGINBÜHL H., Rhodes W.H., BUCHANAN J.W., KNIGHT D.H. & HILL J.D. (1968) Diseases of the cardiovascular system. In: Catcott E.J. (Ed.), *Canine medicine*, First Catcott Edn, p. 589. American Veterinary Publications, Wheaton, Illinois, USA.

DEUBELBEISS K.A., DANCEY J.T., HARKER L.A., CHENEY B. & FINCH C.A. (1975a) Marrow erythroid and neutrophil cellularity in the dog. *J. clin. Invest.* **55**, 825.

DEUBELBEISS K.A., DANCEY J.T., HARKER L.A. & FINCH C.A. (1975b) Neutrophil kinetics in the dog. *J. clin. Invest.* **55**, 833.

DEVI C.S., REDDY C.N., DEVI S.L., SUBRAHMANYAM Y.R., BHATT H.V., SUVARNAKUMARI G., MURTHY D.P. & REDDY C.R.R.M. (1970) Defibrination syndrome due to scorpion venom poisoning. *Br. med. J.* **1**, 345–47.

DHILLON K.S., PAUL B.S. & GARG B.D. (1970) Some haematological aspects in *Lantana camara* poisoning in buffalo calves. *J. Res. Ludhiana* **7**, 262–5.

DHINDSA D.S., HOVERSLAND A.S. & TEMPLETON J.W. (1972) Postnatal changes in oxygen affinity and concentrations of 2,3, diphosphoglycerate in dog blood. *Biology of the Neonate* **20**, 226.

DHINGRA L.D., PARRISH W.B. & VENZKE W.G. (1969) Electron microscopy of granular leukocytes of chicken (*Gallus domesticus*). *Am. J. vet. Res.* **30**, 637–42.

DICK A.T. (1953) The control of copper storage in the liver of sheep by inorganic sulphate and molybdenum. *Aust. vet. J.* **29**, 233–9.

DIDISHEIM P. & BUNTING D.L. (1964) Canine hemophilia. *Thromb. Diath. haemorrh.* **12**, 377.

DIDISHEIM P., HATTORI K. & LEWIS J.H. (1959) Hematologic and coagulation studies in various animal species. *J. Lab. clin. Med.* **53**, 866–75.

DIESEM C.D., VENZKE W.G. & MOORE E.N. (1958) The haemogram of chickens. *Am. J. vet. Res.* **19**, 719–24.

DIETERICH R.A. (1970) Hematologic values of some Arctic mammals. *J. Am. vet. med. Ass.* **157**, 604–6.

DIETERICH R.A. & LUICK J.R. (1971) Reindeer in biomedical research. *Lab. Anim. Sci.* **21**, 817–24.

DINKLAGE H. (1970) The alkaline phosphatase system in the pig. *Proc. 11th Eur. Conf. Anim. Blood Grps Biochem. Polymorphism* (Warsaw, 1968); 329–30.

DISCHE F.E. & BENFIELD V. (1959) Congenital factor VII deficiency. Haematological and genetic aspects. *Acta haemat.* **21**, 257.

DISCOMBE G. (1946) Criteria of eosinophilia. *Lancet*, **1**, 195–6.

DITCHFIELD W.J.B. (1968) Mycotic Diseases In: Catcott E.J. (Ed.) *Canine medicine*, First Catcott Edn, p. 170. American Veterinary Publications Inc., Wheaton, Illinois, USA.

DIXON J.B. & ARCHER R.K. (1975) Interpretation of equine anaemias. *Vet. A.* **15**, 185–91.

DIXON J.M. & TORBERT B.J. (1958) Posthatching changes in the hemoglobin and erythrocytes of the chick. *Poult. Sci.* **37**, 1198–9.

DOAK R.L., MUNNELL J.F. & RAGLAND W.L. (1973) Ultrastructure of tumour cells in Marek's disease virus-infected chickens. *Am. J. vet. Res.*, **34**, 1063–9.

DODDS W.J. (1966) Familial canine thrombocytopathy. *Blood* **28**, 1013–14.

DODDS W.J. (1967) Familial canine thrombocytopathy. Platelets: their role in hemostasis and thrombosis. *Thromb. Diath. haemorrh.* Supp. **26**, 241.

DODDS W.J. (1968) Current concepts of hereditary coagulation disorders in dogs. *Exp. Anim.* **1**, 243.

DODDS W.J. (1970a) Congenital thrombopathies and related coagulation disorders in dogs. Proceedings of Colloquium No. 924 of Centre National de la Recherche Scientifique. *Les Mutants Pathologiques Chez L'Animal*, p. 317. Orléans-la-Source, France, April 1969. Éditions C.N.R.S. (Paris).

DODDS W.J. (1970b) Canine von Willebrand's disease. *J. Lab. clin. Med.* **76**, 713–21.

DODDS W.J. (1971) Hemorrhagic disorders. In: Kirk R.W. (Ed.) *Current veterinary therapy*, 4th Edn, p. 247. W.B. Saunders Co., Philadelphia, USA.

DODDS W.J. (1973) Canine factor X (Stuart-Prower factor) deficiency. *J. Lab. clin. Med.* **82**, 560–6.

DODDS W.J. (1974a) Blood Coagulation: Hemostasis and Thrombosis. In: Melby E.C., Jr. & Altman N.H. (Eds) *Handbook of laboratory animal science*, Vol. II, p. 87. C.R.C. Press, Cleveland, Ohio, USA.

DODDS W.J. (1974b) Hereditary and acquired hemorrhagic disorders in animals. In: Spaet T.H. (Ed.) *Progress in hemostasis and thrombosis*, Vol. II, p. 215. Grune and Stratton, New York.

DODDS W.J. (1975) Further studies of canine von Willebrand's disease. *Blood* **45**, 221–30.

DODDS W.J. & KANEKO J.J. (1971) Hemostasis and Blood Coagulation. In: Kaneko J.J. & Cornelius C.E. (Eds) *Clinical biochemistry of domestic animals*, 2nd Edn, Vol. II, p. 179. Academic Press, New York.

DODDS W.J. & KULL J.E. (1971) Canine factor XI (plasma thromboplastin antecedent) deficiency. *J. Lab. clin. Med.* **78**, 746–52.

DODDS W.J., PACKHAM M.A., ROWSELL H.C. & MUSTARD J.F. (1967) Factor VII survival and turnover in dogs. *Am. J. Physiol.* **213**, 36.

DOETTL K. & RIPKE O. (1938) *Medicine in its chemical aspects*, Vol. 3. Bayer, Leverkusen, Germany.

DOI K., KOJIMA A., NAITO M. & KATO S. (1973) Histopathological changes occasionally found in the peripheral nerve of chickens free from Marek's disease. *Natn. Inst. Anim. Hlth Q., Tokyo* **13**, 227–8.

DOMM L.V. & TABER E. (1946) Endocrine factors controlling erythrocyte concentration in the blood of the domestic fowl. *Physiol. Zool.* **19**, 258–81.

DOMMERT A.R., TUMBLESON M.E., WESCOTT R.B., MURPHY D.A. & KORSCHGEN L.J. (1968) Hematologic values for dieldrin-treated white-tailed deer (*Odocoileus virginianus*) in Missouri. *Am. J. vet. clin. Path.* **2**, 181–4.

DONATIEN A. & LESTOQUARD F. (1926) Etiologie des anémies du mouton et de la chèvre. IV. Anémie pernicieuse de mouton et de la chèvre. *Revue vét. Toulouse* **78**, 675–94.

DONNER L. & HOUSKOVA J. (1972) Some properties of blood platelets in animal species. *Folia haemat.* **98**, 296.

DORN C.R., TAYLOR D.O.N. & HIBBARD H.A. (1967) Epizootiologic characteristics of canine and feline leukemia and lymphoma. *Am. J. vet. Res.* **28**, 993–1001.

DORN C.R., TAYLOR D.O.N., SCHNEIDER R., HIBBARD H.H. & KLAUBER M.R. (1968) Survey of animal neoplasms in Alameda and Contra-Costa Counties, California. II. Cancer morbidity in dogs and cats from Alameda county. *J. natn. Cancer Inst.* **40**, 307–18.

DORNER J.L. & BASS V.D. (1974) Normal prothrombin times and partial thromboplastin times for horse, cow and goat. *Vet. Med.* **69**, 647–8.

DOSNE A-M., JOSSO F., SOULIER J.P., LAVERGNE J.M. & MALMEJAC J. (1968) Injection d'extraits tissulaires et d'hémolysats autologuez le chien. Effets sur les facteurs de l'hémostase. *Nouv. Revue. fr. Hèmat.* **8**, 21–34.

DOUGHERTY J.H. & ROSENBLATT L.S. (1965) Changes in the hemogram of the beagle with age. *J. Geront.* **20**, 131.

DOUGHERTY R.W., SHUMAN R.D., MULLENAX C.H., WITZEL D.A., BUCK W.B.,

WOOD R.L. & COOK H.M. (1965) Physiopathological studies of erysipelas in pigs. *Cornell Vet.* **55**, 87–109.

DOUGHERTY R.M., MARUCCI A.A. & DISTEFANO H.S. (1972) Application of immunohistochemistry to study of avian leukosis virus. *Jnl gen. Virol.* **15**, 149–62.

DOUGLAS A.S. (1962) *Anticoagulant therapy.* Blackwell Scientific Publications, Oxford.

DOUGLAS A.S. (1973) (Ed) Blood coagulation and fibrinolysis in clinical practice. *Clin. Haematol.* **2**, 1–239.

DOW C. (1957) The cystic hyperplasia-pyometra complex in the bitch. *Vet. Rec.* **69**, 1409–14.

DOXEY D.L. (1966a) Cellular changes in the blood as an aid to diagnosis. *J. small Anim. Pract.* **7**, 77.

DOXEY D.L. (1966b) Some conditions associated with variations in circulating oestrogens—blood picture alterations. *J. small Anim. Pract.* **7**, 375.

DOXEY D.L. (1971) *Veterinary clinical pathology*, p. 79. Baillière Tindall, London.

DRESCHER-KADEN U. (1974) Vergleichende hämatologische Untersuchungen an wildlebenden Wiederkäuern (Rotwild, Rehe, Gemsen, Rentiere). 3. Mitteilung: Der Gehalt an Calcium, Magnesium, anorganisch gebundenem Phosphor sowie die Aktivität der alkalischen Phosphatase im Plasma. *Z. Jagdwiss.* **20**, 192–201.

DRESCHER-KADEN U. & HOPPE P. (1972) Verleichende hämatologische Untersuchungen an wildlebenden Wiederkäuern (Rehe, Rotwild, Gemsen, Rentiere). 1. Mitteilung: Erythrozytenzahl, Erythozytendurchmesser, Hämoglobingehalt und Hämatokrit. *Z. Jagdwiss.* **18**, 121–32.

DRESCHER-KADEN U. & HOPPE P. (1973) Vergleichende hämatologische Untersuchungen an wildlebenden Wiederkäuern (Rehe, Rotwild, Gemsen, Rentiere). 2. Mitteilung: Das weisse Blutbild (Zahl der gesamten und der eosinophilen Leucozyten, Differentialblutbild). *Z. Jagdwiss.* **19**, 65–76.

DRESLER S.L., RUNKEL D., STENZEL P., BRIMHALL B. & JONES R.T. (1974) Multiplicity of the hemoglobin α chains in dogs and variations among related species. *Ann. N.Y. Acad. Sci.* **241**, 411.

DREVEMO S., GROOTENHUIS J.G. & KARSTAD L. (1974) Blood parameters in wild ruminants in Kenya. *J. Wildl. Dis.* **10**, 327.

DREVEMO S. & KARSTAD L. (1974) The effect of xylazine and xylazine-etorphine-acepromazine combination on some clinical and haematological parameters in impala and eland. *J. Wildl. Dis.* **10**, 377.

DREW R.A. & GREATOREX J.C. (1974) Vertebral plasma cell myeloma causing posterior paralysis in a horse. *Equine vet. J.* **6**, 131–4.

DRILL V.A. & IVY A.C. (1944) Comparative value of bromsulphalein, serum phosphatase, prothrombin time and intravenous galactose tolerance tests in detecting hepatic damage produced by carbon tetrachloride. *J. clin. Invest.* **23**, 209.

DUDOT DE WIT C., COENEGRACHT N.A.C.J., POLL P.H.A. & LINDE J.D. (1967) The practical importance of blood groups in dogs. *J. small Anim. Pract.* **8**, 285.

DUIVEDI S.K., SHIVNANI G.A. & JOSHI H.C. (1971) Clinical and biochemical studies in *Lantana* poisoning in ruminants. *Indian J. Anim. Sci.* **41**, 948–53.

DUKE K.L. (1963) Erythrocyte diameter in *Tragulus javanicus*, the chevrotain or mouse deer. *Anat. Rec.* **147**, 239.

DUKE W.W. (1910) The relation of blood platelets to hemorrhagic diseases. *J. Am. med. Ass.* **55**, 1185–92.

DUNBAR G.M. & CHAMBERS T.A.M. (1963) Suspected kale poisoning in dairy cattle. *Vet. Rec.* **75**, 566–7.

DUNNE H.W. (1961) The diagnosis of hog cholera. *Proc. 65th Ann. Meet. U.S. Livestock San. Assoc., Minneapolis*, 478–84.

DUNNE H.W. (1963) Field and laboratory diagnosis of hog cholera. *Vet. Med.* **58**, 222–39.

DVOŘÁK M. (1969) Eosinophil levels in the blood of piglets with normal and retarded development. *Doc. vet. Brno* **7**, 199–206.

EADIE G.S., SMITH W.W. & BROWN I.W. (1960) The use of DFP^{32} as a red cell tag with and without simultaneous tagging with chromium[51] in certain animals in the presence or absence of random destruction. *J. gen. Physiol.* **43**, 825–39.

EARL F.L., MELVEGER B.E. & WILSON R.L. (1973) The hemogram and bone marrow profile of normal, neonatal and weanling beagle dogs. *Lab. Anim. Sci.* **23**, 690.

EBERT R.H. & FLOREY H.W. (1939) The extravascular development of the monocyte observed *in vivo*. *Br. J. exp. Path.* **20**, 342–56.

EDERSTROM H.E. & DE BOER B. (1946) Changes in the blood of the dog with age. *Anat. Rec.* **94**, 663.

EDGAR J.T. & THIN I.M. (1968) Plant poisoning involving male fern. *Vet. Rec.* **82**, 33–4.

EGEBERG O. (1961) Assay of antihaemophilic A, B & C factors by one-stage cephalin systems. *Scand. J. clin. Lab. Invest.* **13**, 140.

EGEBERG O. (1963) The effect of exercise on the blood clotting system. *Scand. J. clin. Lab. Invest.* **15**, 8.

EGEBERG O. (1966) Blood factor XI after fat-rich meals. *Thromb. Diath. haemorrh.* **15**, 390.

EGOROVA V.D. (1974) Observations by indirect immunofluorescence of surface antigens of the leucocytes of cattle with leucosis. *Dokl. vses. Akad. sel'.-khoz. Nauk*, No. 8, 30–1.

EIDSON C.S., FLETCHER O.J., KLEVEN S.H. & ANDERSON D.P. (1971) Detection of Marek's disease antigen in feather follicle epithelium of chickens vaccinated against Marek's disease. *J. natn. Cancer Inst.* **47**, 113–20.

EIDSON C.S., KLEVEN S.H., LACROIX V.M. & ANDERSON D.P. (1972) Maternal transfer of resistance against development of Marek's disease tumors. *Avian Dis.* **16**, 139–52.

EIKMEIER H. & MANZ D. (1966) Research into eosinophilia in dogs. III. Occurrence of eosinophilia in digestive disturbances. *Berl. Münch. tierärztl Wschr.* **79**, 329.

EIKMEIER H. & MAYER H. (1965) Untersuchungen zum weissen Blutbild des Schweines. *Berl. Münch. tierärztl. Wschr.* **78**, 289–90.

EISEN V. (1964) The kinin system. *Brit. med. Bull.* **20**, 205.

EISENBRANDT D.L. & SMITH J.E. (1974) Effects of various additives on *in vitro* parameters related to viability and function of stored canine blood. *Res. vet. Sci.* **17**, 231–5.

EK N. (1972) The quantitative determination of fibrinogen in normal bovine plasma and in cows with inflammatory conditions. *Acta vet. scand.* **13**, 175–84.

EL-HINDAWY M.R. (1948) Studies on the blood of dogs. III. Haematological findings in some physiological states— (a) Pregnancy (b) Post-Partum and lactation. *Vet. J.* **104**, 194.

EL-LATIF, K. ABD. & AWAD F.I. (1964) Haemoglobinuria of buffaloes associated with the excessive feeding of *Tripholium alexandrinum* (barseem). *J. vet. Sci. U.A.R.* **1**, 69–74.

ELLERMAN V. (1922) *The leucosis of fowls and leucaemia problems.* Glydendal, London.

ENBERGS H. (1973a) Die Feinstruktur der eosinophilen Granulozyten der Hausente (*Anas* platyrhynchos dom.). *Zentbl. Vet Med.*, Reihe A **20**, 47–55.

ENBERGS H. (1973b) Die Feinstruktur der Leukozyten der Ente (*Anas platyrhynchos dom.*). *Berl. Münch. tierärztl. Wschr.* **86**, 285–9.

ENBERGS H. & BEARDI B. (1971) Zur Feinstruktur der eosinophilen Granulozyten der Hausgans (*Anser anser dom.*). *Z. Zellforsch. mikrosk. Anat.* **122**, 520–7.

ENBERGS H. & KRIESTEN K. (1968a) Zytoplasmatische Feinstrukturen der Thrombozyten des Haushuhns. *Experientia* **24**, 597–8.

ENBERGS H. & KRIESTEN K. (1968b) Die weissen Blutzellen des Haushuhns im elektronenmikroskopischen Bild. *Dt. tierärztl. Wschr.* **75**, 271–5.

ENBERGS H. & KRIESTEN K. (1969) Zur Feinstruktur der Blutmonozyten des Haushuhns. *Z. Zellforsch. mikrosk. Anat.* **97**, 377–82.

ENBERGS H. & KRIESTEN K. (1970) Zur zytoplasmatischen Feinstruktur der eosinophilen Granulozyten des Hühnerbluts. *Zentbl. VetMed. A.* **17**, 430–9.

ENDE N. & AUDITORE J.V. (1964) Activation of the fibrinolytic system in a dog with mast cell tumour. *Am. J. Physiol.* **206**, 567.

ENGEL R.R., BRACHO M., SCHWARTZ S. & RODKEY F. LEE (1973) Carboxyhemoglobin and fecal urobilinogen in bovine erythropoietic porphyria. *Am. J. vet. Res.* **34**, 743–6.

ENGELBERT V.E. & YOUNG A.D. (1970) Erythropoiesis in peripheral blood of seven species of New Zealand and one species of Canadian birds. *Can. J. Zool.* **48**, 227–30.

ENGEN M.H., WEIRICH W.E. & LUND J.E. (1974) Fibrinolysis in a dog with diaphragmatic hernia. *J. Am. vet. med. Ass.* **164**, 152–3.

ENGLE R.L. & WOODS K.R. (1960) Comparative biochemistry and embryology. In: Putnam F. (Ed.) *The plasma proteins*, Vol. 2, pp. 184–266. Academic Press, New York.

ENZYME NOMENCLATURE (1972) Recommendation (1972) of the International Union of Pure and Applied Chemistry and the International Union of Biochemistry. Elsevier, Amsterdam and New York.

EPSTEIN M.A., HUNT R.D. & RABIN H. (1973a) Pilot experiments with EB virus in owl monkeys (*Aotus trivirgatus*). I. Reticuloproliferative disease in an inoculated animal. *Int. J. Cancer* **12**, 309.

EPSTEIN M.A., RABIN H., BALL G., DICKINSON A.B., JARVIS J. & MENDÉLEZ L.V. (1973b). Pilot experiment with EB virus in owl monkeys (*Aotus trivirgatus*). II. EB virus in a cell line from an animal with reticuloproliferative disease. *Int. J. Cancer* **12**, 319.

ERBSLOH J.K.E. (1975) Babesiosis in the newborn foal. In: 'Equine Reproduction'. *J. Reprod. Fert. Suppl.* **23**, 725–6.

ERICSSON J.L.E. & NAIR M.K. (1973) Electron microscopic demonstration of acid phosphatase activity in the developing and mature heterophils of the chicken. *Histochemie* **37**, 97–105.

ERNST R.A., COLEMAN T.H., KULENKAMP

A.W., RINGER R.K. & PANGBORN S. (1971) The packed cell volume and differential leucocyte count of Bobwhite quail (*Colinus virginianus*). *Poult. Sci.* **50**, 389–92.

ESNOUF M.P. (1972) In Biggs R. (Ed.) Human Blood Coagulation, Haemostasis and Thrombosis. Blackwell Scientific Publications, Oxford.

ESPARTZA M. (1970) Collection of blood samples. *Vet. Rec.* **86**, 758.

ESPINASSE J., BONEU B. & CABANIE P. (1973) Observations et commentaires sur un syndrome hemorragique du veau de boucherie en allaitement artificiel. *Revue méd. vét.* **124**, 1503–13.

ESSEX M., COTTER S.M., HARDY W.D., HESS P., JARRETT W., JARRETT O., MACKEY L., LAIRD H., PERRYMAN L., OLSEN R.G. & YOHN D.S. (1975) Feline oncornavirus-associated cell membrane antigen. IV. Antibody titres in cats with naturally occurring leukemia, lymphoma, and other diseases. *J. natn. Cancer Inst.* **55**, 463–7.

ESSEX M., COTTER S.M. & CARPENTER J.L. (1975) Feline oncornavirus-associated cell membrane antigen. II. Antibody titres in healthy cats from pet households and laboratory colony environments. *J. natn. Cancer Inst.* **54**, 631–5.

EVANS D.L., BEASLEY J.N. & PATTERSON L.T. (1971) Correlation of immunological competence with lesions in selected lymphoid tissues from chickens with Marek's disease. *Avian Dis.* **15**, 680–7.

EVANS D.L. & PATTERSON L.T. (1971) Correlation of immunological responsiveness with lymphocyte changes in chickens infected with Marek's disease. *Infect. Immun.* **4**, 567–74.

EVANS D.L. & PATTERSON L.T. (1972) Changes in serum proteins associated with two immunosuppressive effects of acute leucosis (Marek's disease). *J. Reticuloendothel Soc.* **11**, 325–42.

EVANS E.T.R., EVANS W.C. & ROBERTS H.E. (1951) Studies on bracken poisoning in the horse. Part 2. *Br. vet. J.* **107**, 399–411.

EVANS W.C., EVANS I.A., THOMAS A.J.,

WATKINS J.E. & CHAMBERLAIN A.G. (1958) Studies on bracken poisoning in cattle. Part IV. *Br. vet. J.* **114**, 180–98.

EVANS I.A., JONES R.S. & MAINWARING-BURTON, R. (1972) Passage of bracken fern toxicity into milk. *Nature* **237**, 107–8.

EVANS J.V. & WHITLOCK J.H. (1964) Genetic relationships between maximum haematocrit values and haemoglobin type in sheep. *Science, N.Y.* **145**, 1318.

EVELETH D.F. (1937) Comparison of the distribution of magnesium in blood cells and plasma of animals. *J. biol. Chem.* **119**, 289–92.

EVELETH D.F. & SCHWARTE L.H. (1939) Chemical changes in the blood of swine infected with Hog Cholera. *J. Am. vet. med. Ass.* **94**, 411–17.

EVELETH D.F., SCHWARTE L.H. & MILLEN T.W. (1941) Chemical changes in the blood of swine infected with hog cholera. II. The serum bases and whole blood haemoglobin and glutathion. *Vet. Med.* **36**, 510–13.

EWING G.O. (1969) Familial nonspherocytic hemolytic anaemia of Basenji dogs. *J. Am. vet. med. Ass.* **154**, 503–7.

EWING G.O., SATER P.F. & BAILEY C.S. (1974) Hepatic insufficiency associated with congenital anomalies of the portal vein in dogs. *J. Am. Anim. Hosp. Assoc.* **10**, 463.

EWING G.O., SCHALM O.W. & SMITH R.S. (1972) Hematologic values of normal Basenji dogs. *J. Am. vet. med. Ass.* **161**, 1661–4.

EWING S.A. (1963) Observations on leukocytic inclusion bodies from dogs infected with *Babesia canis*. *J. Am. vet. med. Ass.* **143**, 503–6.

FAGAN J.A. (1965) Water intoxication of calves. *Ir. vet. J.* **19**, 209–10.

FANTL P. & WARD H.A. (1957) Comparison of blood clotting in marsupials and man. *Aust. J. exp. Biol. med. Sci.* **33**, 209.

FANTL P. & WARD H.A. (1960) Clotting activity of maternal and foetal sheep blood. *J. Physiol., Lond.* **150**, 607–20.

FARKAS M.C. & FARKAS J.N. (1974) Hemolytic anemia due to ingestion of onions in a dog. *J. Am. Anim. Hosp. Ass.* **10**, 65.

FARNES P., POVAR M.L., FIESCHKO J. & BARKER B.E. (1972) N.B.T. tests in dog neutrophils. *Lancet* **i**, 47.

FARRELL R.K. (1968) Rickettsial diseases. In: *Canine medicine* Catcott E.J. (Ed.) 1st ed. p. 164. American Veterinary Publications Inc., Wheaton, Illinois, USA.

FARRELLY B.T., BELONJE C.W.A. & CRONIN M.T.I. (1950) The technique of exchange transfusion in the newborn foal. *Vet. Rec.* **62**, 403–4.

FARRELLY B.T., COLLINS J.D. & COLLINS J.M. (1966) Autoimmune haemolytic anaemia (AHA) in the horse. *Ir. vet. J.* **20**, 42–5.

FEARNLEY G.R. (1965) *Fibrinolysis*, p. 30. Edward Arnold, London.

FEARNLEY G.R., BALMFORTH G. & FEARNLEY E. (1957) Evidence of a diurnal fibrinolytic rhythm; with a simple method of measuring natural fibrinolysis. *Clin. Sci.* **16**, 645.

FEIDER B. (1971) Die Thrombozytenzahl beim Schwein in Abhängigkeit vom Tag-Nacht-Rhythmus, von Köroperlicher und von psychischer Belastung. *Inaug. Diss., Hannover.*

FELDMAN W.H. (1932) *Neoplasms of domesticated animals.* W.B. Saunders & Co., Philadelphia.

FERGUSON T.M., GOLAN F.A., TRAMMEL J., SMITH E., OMAR E. & COUCH J.R. (1964) Hematological data and blood pressure for male Broad Breasted Bronze turkeys. *Poult. Sci.* **43**, 1318.

FERNANDO W.W.D. & CALNEK B.W. (1971) Influence of bursa of Fabricius on infection and pathological response of chickens exposed to Marek's disease herpesvirus. *Avian Dis.* **15**, 467–76.

FERRER J.F. & BHATT D. (1973) Occurrence of fluorescent and precipitin antibodies to the bovine C-type virus (BLV) among the cattle population. *Proc. Am. Ass. Cancer Res.* **14**, 118.

FERRER J.F., ABT D.A., BHATT DIANE M. & MARSHAK R.R. (1974) Studies on the relationship between infection with bovine C-type virus, leukaemia and persistent lymphocytosis in cattle. *Cancer Res.* **34**, 893–900.

FIELD H.I. (1957) Observations on copper deficiency in cattle in East Anglia. *Vet. Rec.* **69**, 788–95 and 832–9.

FIELD R.A., RICKARD C.G. & HUTT F.B. (1946) Haemophilia in a family of dogs. *Cornell Vet.* **36**, 285.

FIENNES R.N.T.-W. (1952) Diurnal variation in the blood picture of cattle. *Nature (London)* **170**, 934.

FIENNES R.N.T.-W. (1954) Haematological studies in trypanosomiasis of cattle. *Vet. Rec.* **66**, 423–34.

FINCH C.A., DEUBELBEISS K., COOK J.D., ESCHBACH J.W., HARKER L.A., FUNK D.D., MARSAGLIA G., HILLMAN R.S. SLICHTER S., ADAMSON J.W., GANZONI A. & GIBLETT E.R. (1970) Ferrokinetics in man. *Medicine (Baltimore)* **49**, 17–53.

FINCO D.R. & LOW D.G. (1968) Fibrinogen content and fibrinolytic activity of plasma from dogs infected with *Leptospira canicola*. *Am. J. vet. Res.* **29**, 2037.

FINLAYSON R. (1965) Spontaneous arterial disease in exotic animals. *J. zool.* **147**, 239.

FINOCCHIO E.J., COFFMAN J.R. & OSBALD-ISTON G.W. (1970) Platelet counts in horses. *Cornell Vet.* **60**, 518–27.

FISH P.A. & HAYDEN C.E. (1926) A comparison of the blood of a normal and two castrated billy goats. *Cornell Vet.* **16**, 82–7.

FISHER E.W. (1956) Arterial puncture in cattle. *Vet. Rec.* **68**, 691–2.

FISHER E.W. (1959) Arterial puncture in horses. *Vet. Rec.* **71**, 514.

FISHER J.W. (1968) (Ed.) Erythropoietin. *Ann. N.Y. Acad. Sci.* **149**, 1–583.

FLAHERTY J.T., FERRANS V.J., PIERCE J.E., CAREW T.E. & FRY D.L. (1972) Localizing factors in experimental atherosclerosis. In: Likoff W., Segal B.L., Insull W. Jr. & Moyer J.H. (Eds) *Atherosclerosis and coronary heart disease*, 24th Hahnemann Symposium, p. 40. Grune & Stratton, New York.

FLETCH S.M., PINKERTON P.H. & BRUECK-NER P.J. (1975) The Alaskan Malamute chondrodysplasia (dwarfism-anemia) syndrome—in review. *J. Am. Anim. Hosp. Ass.* **11**, 353.

FLUHARTY D.M. & UHLER S.P. (1975) Aspiration of bone marrow using EDTA fortified serum. *Bull. Am. Soc. vet. clin. Path.* **4**, 1, 14.

FLUTE P.T. (1959) Fibrinolytic factors as demonstrated by electrophoresis of human blood. *Proc. 7th European Congr. Haemat. (London)*. Part III, p. 894.

FLYNN R.J. (1973) *Parasites of Laboratory animals*. Iowa State Univ. Press, Ames, Iowa.

FOGGIE A. & NISBET D.I. (1964) Studies on Eperythrozoon infection in sheep. *J. comp. Path. Ther.* **74**, 45–61.

FOLLIS T.B. (1972) *Reproduction and hematology of the cache elk herd*. Ph.D. Thesis, Utah State University.

FORBES C.D., THOMSON C., PRENTICE C.R.M. McNICOL G.P. & McEWEN A.D. (1973) Experimental warfarin poisoning in the dog. Platelet function, coagulation and fibrinolysis. *J. comp. Path.* **83**, 173–80.

FOREYT W. & TRAINER D.O. (1970) Experimental haemonchosis in white-tailed deer. *J. Wildl. Dis.* **6**, 35–42.

FORGACS J. & CARLL W.T. (1962) Mycotoxicoses. *Adv. vet. Sci.* **7**, 273–382.

FORGET B.G. (1974) The molecular basis of thalassemia. *CRC Crit. Rev. Biochem.* **2**, 311–42.

FOSTER S.J. (1967) Blood transfusion techniques in practice. *J. small Anim. Pract.* **8**, 587.

FOWLER E.H., WILSON G.P., ROENIGK W.J. & KOESTNER A. (1966) Mast cell leukemia in three dogs. *J. Am. vet. med. Ass.* **149**, 281–5.

FOWLER M.E., CORNELIUS C.E. & BAKER N.F. (1964) Clinical and erythrokinetic studies on a case of bovine polycythemia vera. *Cornell Vet.* **54**, 151–60.

FOY H., KONDI A. & MBAYA V. (1965) Haematologic and biochemical indices in the East African baboon. *Blood* **26**, 682–6.

FRANK J.F. (1948) The toxicity of sodium chorate herbicides. *Can. J. comp. Med.* **12**, 216–8.

FRANKEL H.M., YOUSEF R., BAYER R. & DILL D.B. (1972) Blood composition in normothermic and hyperthermic kangaroo rats, *Dipodomys merriami*, and laboratory rats, *Rattus norvegicus. Comp. Biochem. Physiol.* **43A**, 733.

FRANKEL W.J. & GROUPE V. (1971) Interactions between Marek's disease herpesvirus and avian leucosis virus in tissue culture. *Nat. New Biol.* **234**, 125–6.

FRANKLIN E.C. (1973) (Ed.) Immunoglobulin diseases. *Semin. Hemat.* 1–177.

FRANKS D. (1962) Horse blood groups and hemolytic disease of the newborn foal. *Ann. N.Y. Acad. Sci.* **97**, 235–50.

FRASER A.C. (1929–30) A study of the blood of cattle and sheep in health and disease. *Univ. Cambridge Inst. Anim. Pathol. Report of the Director.* No. 1, 114–204.

FRASER A.C. (1938) A study of the blood of pigs. *Vet. J.* **94**, 3–21.

FRAZIER J.A. (1974) Ultrastructure of lymphoid tissue from chicks infected with Marek's disease virus. *J. natn. Cancer Inst.* **52**, 829–37.

FREDRICKSON T.N., CHUTE H.L. & O'MEARA D.C. (1957) Preliminary investigations on the hematology of broiler flocks. *Avian Dis.* **1**, 67–74.

FREEMAN B.M. (1971) The corpuscles and the physical characteristics of blood. In: Bell D.J. & Freeman B.M. (Eds) *Physiology and biochemistry of the domestic fowl*, pp. 841–52. Academic Press, London.

FRIESEN S.R., HARSHA W.M. & MCCROSKEY C.H. (1952) Massive generalized wound bleeding during operation with clinical and experimental evidence of blood transfusion reactions. *Surgery*, **32**, 620.

FRITSCHEN R.D., PEO E.R. JR., LUCAS L.E. & GRACE O.D. (1970) Nutritionally induced hemophilia in swine. *J. Anim. Sci.* **31**, 199–200.

FRITZ T.E., NORRIS W.P. & TOLLE D.V. (1973) Myelogenous leukemia and related myeloproliferative disorders in beagles continuously exposed to ^{60}Co γ radiation. *Biblthca. haemat. (Basel)*, **39**, 170.

FRITZSCHE K. (1972) Experimental studies on the susceptibility of leucosis-resistant chicks to osteopetrosis virus. *Zentbl. VetMed.* **19B**, 832–9.

FRYMUS T. (1974) Immunoelectrophoretic analysis of the blood serum of cattle with leucosis. *Medycyna wet.* **30**, 109–11.

FURUGOURI K. (1971) Normal values and physiological variations of plasma iron and total iron-binding capacity in pigs. *J. Anim. Sci.* **32**, 667–72.

GABRIEL B., LYHS L. & SCHÜLKE B. (1965) Zum Tagesrhythmus der eosinophilen Granulozyten beim Schwein. *Mschr. VetMed.* **20**, 911–16.

GÁBRIŠ J. (1973) Rozdiely v krvnom obraze ciciakov, medzi pohlaviami, v lete a v zime. *Folia vet.* **17**, 303–13.

GAHNE B. (1970) The genetic control of arylesterase activity in pig serum. *Anim. Blood Grps biochem. Genet.* **1**, 33–42.

GAHNE B. & RENDEL J. (1961) Blood and serum groups in reindeer compared with those in cattle. *Nature (London)* **192**, 529–30.

GAJEWSKI J. (1971) Blood coagulation values of sheep. *Am. J. vet. Res.* **32**, 405–9.

GALLAGHER C.H. (1963) Studies on trichostrongylosis of sheep: plasma volume, haemoglobin concentration, and blood cell count. *Aust. J. agric. Res.* **14**, 349–63.

GALLIMORE M.J., NULKAR M.V. & SHAW J.T.B. (1965) A comparative study of the inhibitors of fibrinolysis in human, dog and rabbit blood. *Thromb. Diath. haemorrh.* **14**, 145.

GALTON D.A.G. (Ed.) (1977) The chronic leukaemias. *Clin. Haematol.* **6**, 1–274.

GARDIKAS C., KALLINKOU M. & KALLINIKOS G. (1965) Observations on horse blood coagulation. *Scand. J. Haemat.* **2**, 31–5.

GARDNER M.B. (1971) Current information on feline and canine cancers and relationship or lack of relationship to human cancer. *J. natn. Cancer Inst.* **46**, 281–90.

GARLICK N.L. (1975) The management of canine dirofilariasis. *Canine Pract.* **2**, 1, 22.

GARNER R., CHATER B.V. & BROWN D.L. (1974) The role of complement in endotoxin shock and disseminated intravascular coagulation: experimental observations in the dog. *Br. J. Haemat.* **28**, 393–401.

GARNER R. & CONNING D.M. (1970) The assay of human factor VII by means of modified factor VII deficient dog plasma. *Br. J. Haemat.* **18**, 57–66.

GARNER R. & EVENSEN S.A. (1974) Endotoxin-induced intravascular coagulation and shock in dogs: the role of factor VII. *Br. J. Haemat.* **27**, 655–68.

GARNER R., HERMOSO-PEREZ C. & CONNING D.M. (1967) Factor VII deficiency in beagle dog plasma and its use in the assay of human factor VII. *Nature (London)* **216**, 1130.

GARREN H.W. (1959) An improved method for obtaining blood from chickens. *Poult. Sci.* **38**, 916–18.

GARTNER R.J.W., RYLEY J.W. & BEATTIE A.W. (1965) The influence of degree of excitation on certain blood constituents in beef cattle. *Aust. J. exp. Biol. med. Sci.* **43**, 713–24.

GAWIENOWSKI A.M., MAYER D.T. & LASLEY J.F. (1955) The serum protein-bound iodine of swine as a measure of growth potentialities. *J. Anim. Sci.* **14**, 3–6.

GENEST P. (1946) A technique of heart puncture in the chicken for obtaining blood. *J. Am. vet. med. Ass.* **108**, 239–41.

GENTRY P.A., CRANE S. & LOTZ F. (1975) Factor XI (plasma thromboplastin antecedent) deficiency in cattle. *Can. vet. J.* **16**, 160–3.

GEORGIEV S., KONSTANTINOV P., RADO-SLAVOV V. & GEORGIEVA R. (1973) Dynamics of total proteins and protein fractions in the blood serum of sheep and goats during oestrus, pregnancy and the postpartum period. *Vet-Med. Nauk.* **10**, 53–8.

GERACI J.R. & MEDWAY W. (1973) Simulated field blood studies in the bottle-nosed dolphin, *Tursiops truncatus*. *J. Wildl. Dis.* **9**, 29.

GERBER J.D. & BROWN A.L. (1974) Effect of development and aging on the response of canine lymphocytes to phytohemagglutinin. *Infect. Immunity* **10**, 695.

GETTY R. & GHOSAL N.G. (1967) Applied anatomy of the sacrococcygeal region of the pig as related to tail-bleeding. *Vet. Med./Small Anim. Clin.* **62**, 361–7.

GIBBS H.C. (1960) Some haematological values for the barren-ground caribou. *Can. J. comp. Med.* **24**, 150–2.

GIBSON Q.H., KREUZER F., MEDA E. & ROUGHTON F.J.W. (1955) The kinetics of human haemoglobin in solution and in the red cell at 37°C. *J. Physiol.* **129**, 65.

GIBSON J.G., SELIGMAN A.M., PEACOCK W.C., AUB J.C., FINE J. & EVANS R.D. (1946) The distribution of red cells and plasma in large and minute vessels of the normal dog, determined by radioactive isotopes of iron and iodine. *J. clin. Invest.* **30**, 848.

GIDDENS W.E., LABBE R.F., SWANGEO L.J. & PADGETT G.A. (1975) Feline congenital erythropoietic porphyria associated with severe anemia and renal disease. *Am. J. Path.* **80**, 367–86.

GILBERT A.B. (1962) Sedimentation rate of erythrocytes in the domesticated cock. *Poult. Sci.* **41**, 784–8.

GILBERT A.B. (1963) The effect of estrogen and thyroxine on the blood volume of the domestic cock. *J. Endocr.* **26**, 41–7.

GILBERT A.B. (1965) Sex differences in the erythrocyte of the adult domestic fowl. *Res. vet. Sci.* **6**, 114–6.

GILBERT A.B. (1966) Effect of oestrogen on the blood volume of the domestic cock. *Proc. R. phys. Soc., Edinb.* **29**, 89–94.

GILBERT A.B. (1968) The relationship between the erythrocyte sedimentation rate and packed cell volume in the domestic fowl. *Br. Poult. Sci.* **9**, 297–9.

GILBERT A.B. (1969) The erythrocyte sedimentation rate and packed cell volume with respect to age and sex. *Br. Poult. Sci.* **10**, 109–13.

GILBERT C.F. (1966) Effects of staphylococcal enterotoxin B on the coagulation mechanisms and leucocyte response in Beagle dogs—a preliminary study. *Thromb. Diath. haemorrh.* **16**, 697.

GILES R.C., HILDEBRANDT P.K. & MONTGOMERY C.A. (1974) Carcinoid tumor in the small intestine of the dog. *Vet. Path.* **11**, 340–49.

GILLES H.M., MAEGRAITH B.G. & ANDREWS W.H.H. (1953) The liver in *Babesia canis* infection. *Ann. trop. med. Parasit.* **47**, 426.

GILLESPIE J.H. & CARMICHAEL L.E. (1968) Distemper and infectious hepatitis. In: Catcott E.J. (Ed.) *Canine medicine*, 1st ed. p. 111. American Veterinary Publications Inc, Wheaton, Illinois, USA.

GILMORE C.E., GILMORE V.H. & JONES T.C. (1964) Bone marrow and peripheral blood of cats: technique and normal values. *Path. vet.* **1**, 18–40.

GLENN B.L., GLENN H.G. & OMTVEDT I.T. (1968) Congenital porphyria in the domestic cat (felis catus): preliminary investigations on the inheritance pattern. *Am. J. vet. Res.* **29**, 1653–7.

GOLDBERG A. (1971) Porphyrins and Porphyrias, in Goldberg A. & Brain M.C. (Eds) *Recent advances in haematology*, pp. 302–36. Churchill Livingstone, Edinburgh and London.

GOLDMAN M. & ROSENBERG A.S. (1974) Immunofluorescence studies of the small *Babesia* spp. of cattle from different geographical areas. *Res. vet. Sci.* **16**, 351–4.

GONZAGA A.C. & DE GUZMAN V.A. (1964) Observation on the blood sugar, iron and haemoglobin of Philippine native goats. *Nutr. Abstr. Rev.* **34**, 103.

GOODMAN M., MOORE G.W. & MATSUDA G. (1975) Darwinian evolution in the geneology of haemoglobin. *Nature (London)* **253**, 603–8.

GOODWIN R.F.W. (1956) The distribution of sugar between red cells and plasma: variations associated with age and species. *J. Physiol.* **134**, 88–101.

GOODWIN R.F.W. (1957) The relationship between concentration of blood sugar and some vital body functions in the newborn pig. *J. Physiol.* **136**, 208–17.

GOODWIN R.F.W., HEARD D.H., HAYWARD B.H.G. & ROBERTS G.F. (1956) Haemolytic disease of the newborn piglet. *J. Hyg.* **54**, 153–71.

GORDON A.S. (1970a) (Ed.) *Regulation of hematopoiesis*. Vol. 1: *Red cell production*. Appleton-Century-Crofts, New York.

GORDON A.S. (1970b) (Ed.) *Regulation of haematopoiesis*. Vol. 2: *White cell and platelet production*. Appleton-Century-Crofts, New York.

GORDON A.S. (1971) Annotation: The current status of erythropoietin. *Br. J. Haemat.* **21**, 611–6.

GORDON E.S., BROWNLEE A., WILSON D.R., & MACLEOD J. (1962) The epizootiology of louping-ill and tick-borne fever with observations on the control of these sheep disease. *Symp. zool. Soc. Lond.* No. 6, 1–27.

GORDON-SMITH E.C. & WHITE J.M. (1974) Annotation: Oxidative haemolysis and Heinz body haemolytic anaemia. *Br. J. Haemat.* **26**, 513–7.

GORHAM J.R., BOE N. & BAKER G.A. (1951) Experimental 'yellow fat' disease in pigs. *Cornell Vet.* **41**, 332–8.

GORHAM J.R., LEADER R.W., PADGETT G.A., BURGER D. & HENSON J.B. (1965) Some observations on the natural occurrence of Aleutian disease. In: Gajdusek D.C., Gibbs C.J. & Alpers M. (Eds) *Slow, latent and temperate virus infections*, p. 279. National Institute of Neurological Diseases & Blindness, Washington, D.C.

GORIŠEK J. & MARŽAN B. (1965) Veränderungen des Blutbildes und der Blutgerinnung bei mit Adlerfarn (*Pteridium aquilinum*) vergifteten Kälbern. *Wien. tierärztl. Mschr.* **52**, 530–8.

GORODETSKII V.K. (1959a) Changes in the blood of the reindeer due to aging. *Dokl. Akad. Nauk SSSR* **124**, 234–6.

GORODETSKII V.K. (1959b) A picture of the blood of reindeer. *Zhivotnovodstvo* **2**, 74–6. (Russian.)

GORODETSKII V.K. (1962) Ecological and physiological peculiarities of blood in northern stag. *Trudȳ Inst. Morf. Zhivot.* **41**, 47–90. (Russian.)

GÖTZE R., ROSENBERGER G. & ZIEGENHAGEN G. (1954) Leucosis in cattle. Haematological and clinical diagnosis. *Mh. VetMed.* **23**, 517–26.

GOWER SMITH S. (1944) Evidence that the physiologic normal haemoglobin value for adult dog blood is 18 grams per 100 cc. *Am. J. Physiol.* **142**, 476.

GRAHAM R., SAMPSON J. & HESTER H.R. (1941) 1. Acute hypoglycaemia in newly born pigs (So-called baby pig disease). *Proc. Soc. exp. Biol. Med.* **47**, 338–9.

GRAHAM J.B., BUCKWALTER J.A., HARTLEY L.J. & BRINKHOUS K.M. (1949) Canine hemophilia, observations on the course, the clotting anomaly, and the effect of blood transfusions. *J. exp. Med.* **90**, 97.

GRAHAM E.A., RAINEY R., KUHLMAN R.E., HOUGHTON E.H. & MOYER C.A. (1962) Biochemical investigations of deer antler growth. Part 1. Alterations of deer blood chemistry resulting from antlerogenesis. *J. Bone Jt Surg.* **44A**, 482–8.

GRAHAM J.B., LANGDELL R.D. & BRINKHOUS K.M. (1964) Estimation of the rate of prothrombin utilization. In: Tocantins L.M. & Kazal L.A. (Eds) *Blood coagulation, hemorrhage and thrombosis*, p. 165. Grune and Stratton, New York.

GRANCIU I., DUICA S., CUREU I. & MILOVAN E. (1973) Blood group and biochemical polymorphism studies in *Bos bubalus*. *Anim. Blood Grps. biochem. Genet.* **4**, 11–14.

GRANT C.A., HOLTENIUS P., JÖNSSON G. & THORELL C.B. (1968) Kale anaemia in ruminants. I. Survey of the literature and experimental induction of kale anaemia in lactating cows. *Acta vet. scand.* **9**, 126–40.

GRAY J.E., SNOEYENBOS G.H. & REYNOLDS I.M. (1954) The hemorrhagic syndrome of chickens. *J. Am. vet. med. Ass.*, **125**, 144–51.

GRAY M.L. & KILLINGER A.H. (1966) Listeria monocytogenes and Listeric infections. *Bact. Rev.* **30**, 309–82.

GREATOREX J.C. (1954) Studies on the haematology of calves from birth to one year of age. *Br. vet. J.* **110**, 120–33.

GREATOREX J.C. (1957) Observations on the haematology of calves and various breeds of adult dairy cattle. *Br. vet. J.* **113**, 469–81.

GREEN R.A., MONLUX A.W. & RANDOLPH T.C. (1973) Blood porphyrin determination. A rapid field test for lead poisoning in cattle. *The Bovine Practitioner* No. 8, 30–5.

GREENBERG M.L., ATKINS H.L. & SCHIFFER L.M. (1966) Erythropoietic and reticuloendothelial function in bone marrow in dogs. *Science* **152**, 526–28.

GREENHALGH J.F.D. (1969) Kale anaemia. *Proc. Natr. Soc.* **28**, 178–83.

GREENHALGH J.F.D., SHARMAN G.A.M. & AITKEN J.N. (1969) Kale anaemia. I. The toxicity to various species of animal of three types of kale. *Res. vet. Sci.* **10**, 64–72.

GREENLEE J.C. & CARPER H.A. (1968) Blood coagulation. III. Hemophilia A. *Am. J. vet. clin. Path.* **2**, 27.

GREENWOOD B. (1968) The motility of sheep, human and pig blood eosinophil leucocytes *in vitro*. *J. Physiol., Lond.* **196**, 108–9P.

GREENWOOD B. (1969a) The motility of blood eosinophils on glass. *Br. J. Derm.* **81**, Suppl. 3, 36–7.

GREENWOOD B. (1969b) The mitosis of cultured blood monocytes from the sheep. *J. Physiol., Lond.* **202**, 92–3P.

GREENWOOD B. (1971) The stimulation of sheep monocyte mitosis *in vitro* by autologous plasma taken after implanting a Teflon chamber into the sheep. *J. Physiol., Lond.* **215**, 25–6P.

GREENWOOD B. (1972) A constituent of sheep plasma capable of promoting mitosis of cultured sheep blood monocytes. *J. Physiol., Lond.* **224**, 47–8P.

GREENWOOD B. (1973) The mitosis of sheep blood monocytes in tissue culture. *Q. Jl exp. Physiol.* **58**, 369–77.

GREENWOOD A.P. (1975) A simple technique for bleeding the lobster. *Vet. Rec.* **97**, 476.

GRIBBLE D.H. (1969) Equine ehrlichiosis. *J. Am. vet. med. Ass.* **155**, 462–9.

GRIMINGER P. (1965) Blood coagulation. In Sturkie P.D. (Ed.) *Avian physiology*, 2nd Edn, pp. 21–31. Baillière, Tindall & Cassell, London.

GROSS W.B. (1961) Blood cultures, blood counts and temperature records in an experimentally produced 'air sac disease' and uncomplicated *Escherichia coli* infection of chickens. *Poult. Sci.* **41**, 691–700.

GROTH A.H., BAILEY W.S. & WALKER D.F. (1960) Bovine mastocytoma. *J. Am. vet. med. Ass.* **137**, 241–4.

GROULADE P. (1972) Syndrome mononucléosique infectieux chez le chien. *Bull. Acad. vet. Fr.* **45**, 269.

GROULADE P. & LAURIAN D. (1957) Contribution à l'étude de l'eosinophilie sanguine dans diverses formes d'eczéma chez le chien. *Bull. Acad. vét. Fr.* **30**, 103.

GRUHZIT O.M. (1931a) Anemia of dogs produced by feeding of the whole onions and of onion fractions. *Am. J. med. Sci.* **181**, 812–5.

GRUHZIT O.M. (1931b) Anemia in dogs produced by feeding disulphide compounds. *Am. J. med. Sci.* **181**, 815–20.

GRUNDBOECK M. & WILCZYNSKA-CIEMIEGA K. (1971) Cellular infiltrations in irises of chickens infected experimentally with Marek's disease virus, strain HPRS-16. *Bull. Vet. Inst. Pulawy* **15**, 92–5.

GRUNDBOECK M., WILCZYNSKA-CIEMIEGA K. & JAROSZ A. (1973) Histopathological changes in the nervous system of chickens affected with Marek's disease. *Polskie Archwm. wet.* 509–19.

GRUNDER A.A., JEFFERS T.K., SPENCER J.L., ROBERTSON A. & SPECKMANN G.W. (1972) Resistance of strains of chickens to Marek's disease. *Can. J. Anim. Sci.* **52**, 1–10.

GRUNDER A.A., SPENCER J.L., ROBERTSON A., SPECKMANN G.W. & GOWE R.S. (1974) Resistance of Marek's disease observed among sire families and inbred lines. *Br. Poult. Sci.* **15**, 165–75.

GRUNDER A.A. & KRISTJANSSON F.K. (1974) Genetic control of serum esterases in day-old pigs. *Anim. Blood Grps. biochem. Genet* **5**, 143–52.

GRUNSELL C.S. (1951) Bone marrow biopsy in sheep. 1. Normal. *Brit. vet. J.* **107**, 16–23.

GRUNSELL C.S. (1955a) The marrow cells of normal sheep. *J. comp. Path. Ther.* **65**, 8–16.

GRUNSELL C.S. (1955) Seasonal variation in the blood and bone marrow of Scottish hill sheep. *J. comp. Path. Ther.* **65**, 93.

GUELFI J.F., LESCURE F. & FLORIO R. (1972) Les syndromes d'hypocoagulabilite sanguine chez le chien. *Revue Méd. vét.* **123**, 1205.

GUILLEMAIN B., LEVY D., CHEVRIER L., MARCHAND A. & PARODI A.L. (1975) Leucosis in French cattle. III. *Recl. Méd. vét. Éc. Alfort* **151**, 179–82.

GULLIVER G. (1840) Observations on the blood corpuscles of certain species of the genus *Cervus*. *Lond. Edinb. Dubl. Phil. Mag.* **17**, 327–30.

GULLIVER G. (1840) Observations on the blood corpuscles or red disks of the mammeriferous mammals. *Lond. Edinb. Dubl. Phil. Mag.* **17**, 327–30.

GULLIVER G. (1845) On the size of the red corpuscles of the blood in the vertebrata, with copious tables of measurement. *Proc. zool. Soc. Lond.* **1845**, 93–102.

GULLIVER G. (1848) Additional measurements of the red blood corpuscles of the blood of vertebrata. No. 4. *Proc. zool. Soc. Lond.* **1848**, 36–40.

GULLIVER G. (1875) Observations on the sizes and shapes of the red corpuscles of the blood of vertebrates, with drawings of them to a uniform scale, and extended and revised tables of measurements. *Proc. zool. Soc. Lond.* **1875**, 474–95.

GUNZ F. & BAIKIE A.G. (1974) *Leukaemia*, 3rd Edn. Grune & Stratton, New York.

GUPTA P.P. (1973) Normal haematological and biochemical parameters of Indian pigs (Sus scrofa domestica). *Indian vet. J.* **50**, 406–9.

GYNN T.N., MESSMORE H.L. & FRIEDMAN I.A. (1972) Drug-induced thrombocytopenia. *Med. Clins. N. Am.* **56**, 65.

HAARANEN S. (1960) Some blood components of growing pigs. *Nord. VetMed.* **12**, 239–44.

HADEN R.L. (1934) The mechanism of the increased fragility of the erythrocytes in congenital hemolytic jaundice. *Am. J. med. Sci.* **188**, 441.

HADWEN S. & BRUCE E.A. (1933) The poisoning of horses by the common bracken. *Vet. J.* **89**, 120–8.

HALL B.E. (1929) The morphology of the cellular elements of the blood of the monkey, *Macaca rhesus*. *Folia haemat.* **38**, 30.

HALL D.E. (1970a) Sensitivity of different thromboplastin reagents to factor VII deficiency in the blood of beagle dogs. *Lab. Animals* **4**, 55.

HALL D.E. (1970b) A naturally occurring red-cell antigen antibody system in Beagle dogs. *J. small Anim. Pract.* **11**, 543.

HALL D.E. (1972) *Blood coagulation and its disorders in the dog.* Baillière Tindall, London.

HALL D.E. & FOLLETT A.J. (1972) Red cell osmotic fragility in the beagle dog. Normal values and diagnostic application. *Vet. Rec.* **91**, 263.

HALL J.G. (1959) Blood grouping in domestic animals. *Vet. Rec.* **17**, 1062–70.

HALL J.G. (1963) Cattle blood groups. *Occasional Paper No.* 18, *Royal Anthropological Inst.* 25–33.

HALL J.G. (1969) Blood groups and reproduction. *A.B.R.O. Report*, January, 1969.

HALL S.A., REST J.R., LINKLATER K.A. & McTAGGART H.S. (1972) Concurrent haemolytic disease of the newborn and thrombocytopenic purpura in piglets without artificial immunisation of the dam. *Vet. Rec.* **91**, 677–8.

HALLETT J.W. JR. & WILSON J.W. (1973) Nitroblue tetrazolium reduction by neutrophils in experimental hemorrhagic shock. *Am. J. Path.* **73**, 173.

HALPERN B.N., BIOZZI G., MENE G. & BENACERAFF B. (1951) Étude quantitative de l'activité granulopexique du système reticulo-endothelial par l'injection intraveneuse d'encre de Chine chez les diverses espèces animales. *Ann. Inst. Pasteur.* **80**, 582–604.

HAMILTON L.H. & HORVATH S.M. (1954) Comparison of blood cell counts from major vessels in the dog. *Proc. Soc. exp. Biol. Med.* **86**, 360.

HAMILTON FAIRLEY G. (1974) (Ed.) Leukemia and lymphoma. *Semin. Hemat.* **11**, 1–227.

HAMMOND P.B. & ARONSON A.L. (1964) Lead poisoning in cattle and horses in the vicinity of a smelter. *Ann. N.Y. Acad. Sci.* **111**, 595–611.

HAMPTON J.W., BUCKNER R.G., GUNN C.G., MILLER L.R. & MAYES J.W. (1973) Canine hemophilia in Beagles: genetics, site of factor VIII synthesis and attempts at experimental therapy. In: Ala F. & Denson K.W.E. (Eds) *Proc.*

VII Congr. Wld Fed. Haemophilia, May 17–20 (1971) p. 26. Excerpta medica, Tehran, Iran.

HAMRE C.J. & McHENRY J.T. (1942) Methods of obtaining blood of fowl for complete blood examination. *Poult. Sci.* **21**, 30–4.

HAN P.F.S. & SMYTH J.R. (1972a) The influence of growth rate on the development of Marek's disease in chickens. *Poult. Sci.* **51**, 975–85.

HAN P.F.S. & SMYTH J.R. (1972b) The influence of restricted feed intake on the response of chickens to Marek's disease. *Poult. Sci.* **51**, 986–91.

HAN P.F.S. & SMYTH J.R. JR. (1973) The influence of maternal effects on the response of fast and slow growing chickens to a Marek's disease virus. *Poult. Sci.* **52**, 909–15.

HANNAN J. (1965) Water intoxication of calves. *Ir. vet. J.* **19**, 211–4.

HANNAN J. (1971) Recent advances in our knowledge of iron deficiency anaemia in piglets. *Vet. Rec.* **88**, 181–90.

HANSEN M.F., TODD A.C., KELLEY G.W. & HULL F.E. (1950a) Studies on the hematology of the Thoroughbred horse. 1. Mares in foal. *Am. J. vet. Res.* **11**, 296–300.

HANSEN M.F., TODD A.C., KELLEY G.W., CAWEIN M. & McGEE W.R. (1950b) Studies on the hematology of the Thoroughbred horse. 2. Weanlings. *Am. J. vet. Res.* **11**, 393–6.

HANSEN M.F., TODD A.C., CAWEIN M. & McGEE W.R. (1950c) Studies on the hematology of the Thoroughbred horse. 3. Stallions. *Am. J. vet. Res.* **11**, 397–9.

HANSEN M.F., TODD A.C. & McGEE W.R. (1950d) Blood pictures of lactating and non-lactating Thoroughbred mares. *Vet. Med.* **45**, 228–30.

HANSEN M.F. & TODD A.C. (1951) Preliminary report on the blood picture of the Arabian horse. *J. Am. vet. med. Ass.* **118**, 26–7.

HANSEN M.F., TODD A.C., KELLEY G.W. & CAWEIN M. (1951) Studies on the hematology of the Thoroughbred horse. 4. Barren mares. *Am. J. vet. Res.* **12**, 31–4.

HARDAWAY R.M. (1966) *Syndromes of disseminated intravascular coagulation.* Charles C. Thomas, Springfield, Ill.

HARDISTY R.M. (1969) Haemorrhagic disorders due to functional abnormalities of platelets. *Jl R. Coll. Physicians (London)*, **3**, 182.

HARDISTY R.M. (1972) In: Biggs R. (Ed.) *Human blood coagulation, haemostasis and thrombosis.* Blackwell Scientific Publications, Oxford.

HARDISTY R.M. & HUTTON R.A. (1965) The kaolin clotting time of platelet-rich plasma: a test of platelet factor 3 availability. *Brit. J. Haemat.* **11**, 258–68.

HARDISTY R.M. & HUTTON R.A. (1966) Platelet aggregation and the availability of platelet factor 3. *Brit. J. Haemat.* **12**, 764.

HARDISTY R.M. & HUTTON R.A. (1967) Bleeding tendency associated with a 'new' abnormality of platelet behaviour. *Lancet*, **i**, 983–85.

HARDISTY R.M. & INGRAM G.I.C. (1965) *Bleeding disorders. Investigation and management*, pp. 44, 58 and 293. Blackwell Scientific Publications, Oxford.

HARDISTY R.M. & MARGOLIS J. (1959) The role of Hageman factor in the initiation of blood coagulation. *Brit. J. Haemat.* **5**, 203–11.

HARDISTY R.M. & WEATHERALL D.J. (1975) *Blood and its Disorders.* Blackwell Scientific Publications, Oxford.

HARDY J. (1970) Enzymes in pig red cell typing. *XIth European Conference on Animal Blood Groups and Biochemical Polymorphism-Warsaw.* pp. 317–20. PWN—Polish Scientific Publishers.

HARDY W.D., OLD L.J., HESS P.W., ESSEX M. & COTTER S.M. (1973) Horizontal transmission of feline leukaemia virus. *Nature* **244**, 266–9.

HAREMSKI T., KASZUBKIEWICZ C. & MADEJ I.A. (1973) Occurrence of leucosis and tuberculosis in cattle. *Medycyna wet.* **29**, 96–8.

HARI R., SHIVNANI G.A. & JOSHI H.C. (1973) Therapeutic efficacy in *Lantana* poisoning in buffalo calves in relation to clinical and haematological studies. *Indian vet. J.* **50**, 764–70.

HARKNESS D.R., PONCE J. & GRAYSON V. (1969) A comparative study on the phospho-glyceric acid cycle in mammalian erythrocytes. *Comp. Biochem. Physiol.* **28**, 129–38.

HARKNESS J. (1971) The viscosity of human blood plasma: its measurement in health and disease. *Biorheology* **8**, 171.

HARRINGTON W.J., SPRAGUE C.S., MINNICH V., MOORE C.V., AULVIN R.C. & DUBACH R. (1953) Immunologic mechanisms in idiopathic neonatal thrombocytopenic purpura. *Ann. intern. Med.* **38**, 433–69.

HARRIS J.R. (1971) The ultrastructure of the erythrocyte. In: Bell D.J. & Freeman B.M. (Eds) *Physiology and biochemistry of the domestic fowl*, pp. 853–62. Academic Press, London.

HARRIS J.R. & BROWN J.N. (1971a) Fractionation of the avian erythrocyte: an ultrastructural study. *J. Ultrastruct. Res.* **36**, 8–23.

HARRIS J.R. & BROWN J.N. (1971b) The preparation of nucleated erythrocyte ghosts from avian erythrocytes. *Br. Poult. Sci.* **12**, 95–9.

HARRIS M.J., HUISMAN T.H.J. & HAYES F.A. (1973) Geographic distribution of hemoglobin variants in the white-tailed deer. *J. Mammal.* **54**, 270–4.

HARRIS M.J., WILSON J.B. & HUISMAN T.H.J. (1972) Structural studies of hemoglobin α chains from Virginia white-tailed deer. *Archs Biochem. Biophys.* **151**, 540–8.

HARVEY D.G. (1967) Some laboratory aspects in the assessment of liver function. *J. small Anim. Pract.* **8**, 473.

HARVEY J.W. & KANEKO J.J. (1974) Interactions between methylene blue and erythrocytes of several mammalian species. *Proc. Soc. exp. Biol. med.* **147**, 245.

HARVEY M.J.A. (1968) A male pig with an XXY/XXXY sex chromosome complement. *J. Reprod. Fert.* **17**, 319–24.

HARWIG J. & MUNRO I.C. (1975) Myotoxins of possible importance in diseases of Canadian farm animals. *Can. vet. J.* **16**, 125–38.

HATHAWAY W.E., HATHAWAY H.S. & BELHASEN L.P. (1964) Coagulation factors in newborn animals. *J. Lab. clin. Med.* **63,** 784–90.

HATHAWAY W.E., BELHANSEN L.P. & HATHAWAY H.S. (1965) Evidence for a new plasma thromboplastin factor. I. Case report, coagulation studies and physico-chemical properties. *Blood* **26,** 521–32.

HATTERSLEY P.G. & HAYSE D. (1970) Fletcher factor deficiency: a report of three unrelated cases. *Brit. J. Haemat.* **18,** 411–6.

HAWKEY C.M. (1966) Coagulation of primate blood by Russell's viper venom. *Nature (London)* **210,** 141–2.

HAWKEY C.M. (1970) Fibrinolysis in Animals. In: Macfarlane R.G. (Ed.) *The haemostatic mechanism in man and other animals*, p. 133. Symposia of the Zoological Society of London, No. 27. Academic Press, London.

HAWKEY C.M. (1972) Coagulation, fibrinolysis and platelet function. In: Fiennes R.N.T.-W. (Ed.) *Pathology of simian primates*, Part I, p. 318. S. Karger, Basel.

HAWKEY C.M. (1974) The relationship between blood coagulation and thrombosis and atherosclerosis in man, monkeys and carnivores. *Thromb. Diath. haemorrh.* **31,** 103–18.

HAWKEY C.M. (1975) *Comparative mammalian haematology: cellular components and blood coagulation of captive wild animals*, p. 93. Heinemann Medical Books, London.

HAWKEY C.M. & DEAN S. (1976) The effect of anaesthetic and tranquillizing drugs on the blood picture of the patas monkey (*Erythrocebus patas*). (In preparation).

HAWKEY C.M. & JORDAN P. (1967) Sickle-cell erythrocytes in the mongoose, *Herpestes sanguineus*. *Trans. R. Soc. trop. Med. Hyg.* **61,** 180.

HAWKEY C.M. & STAFFORD J.L. (1961) Influence of serum factors on the species specificity of tissue thromboplastin. *Nature (London)* **191,** 920.

HAWKEY C.M. & SYMONS C. (1968) Variation in ADP-induced platelet aggregation in Primates as a result of differences in plasma ADP-inhibitor levels. *Thromb. Diath. haemorrh.* **19,** 29–35.

HAWKINS W.B. & JOHNSON A.C. (1939) Bile pigment and haemoglobin interrelation in anemic dogs. *Am. J. Physiol.* **126,** 326.

HAXTON J.A., SCHNEIDER M.D. & KAYE M.P. (1974) Blood volume of the male Holstein-Friesian calf. *Am. J. vet. Res.* **35,** 835–7.

HAYDEN D.W. & VAN KRUININGEN H.J. (1975) Experimentally induced canine toxocariasis: laboratory examinations and pathologic changes, with emphasis on the gastro-intestinal tract. *Am. J. vet. Res.* **36,** 1605–14.

HAYES K.C. (1974) Haemolytic anaemia in monkeys deficient in vitamin E. *Am. J. Path.* **77,** 123.

HAYHOE F.G.J. (1953) Cytological demonstration of lipids in blood and bone marrow cells. *J. Path. Bact.* **65,** 413–21.

HAYHOE F.G.J. & QUAGLINO D. (1960) Refractory sideroblastic anaemia and erythraemic myelosis: possible relationship and cytochemical observations. *Brit. J. Haemat.* **6,** 381–7.

HAYHOE F.G.J. & FLEMANS R.J. (1969) *An atlas of haematological cytology.* Wolfe Medical Books, London.

HEAD K.W., CAMPBELL J.G., IMLAH P., LAING A.H., LINKLATER K.A. & McTAGGART H.S. (1974) Hereditary lymphosarcoma in a herd of pigs. *Vet. Rec.* **95,** 523–7.

HEDLIN A.M., MONKHOUSE F.C. & MILOJEVIC S.M. (1972) A comparative study of fibrinolytic activity in human, rat, rabbit and dog blood. *Can. J. Physiol. Pharmac.* **50,** 11.

HEENE D., HOFFMANN-FEZER G., HOFFMAN R., WEISS E., MÜLLER-BERGHAUS G. & LASCH H.B. (1971) (Coagulation disorders in acute swine fever). *Beitr. Path.* **144,** 259–71 (VB 72, 3336).

HEGREBERG G.A. (1975) Animal model: Ehlers-Danlos syndrome in dogs and mink, canine cutaneous asthenia. *Am. J. Path.* **79,** 383.

HEGREBERG G.A., PADGETT G.A., GORHAM J.R. & HENSON J.B. (1969) A connective tissue disease of dogs and mink resembling the Ehlers-Danlos syndrome of man. II. Mode of inheritance. *J. Hered.* **60,** 249.

HEGREBERG G.A., PADGETT G.A. & HENSON J.B. (1970) Connective tissue disease of dogs and mink resembling the Ehlers-Danlos syndrome of man. *Archs. Path.* **90,** 159.

HEILMEYER L. & BEGEMANN H. (1955) *Atlas der klinischen hämatologie und cytologie.* Springer-Verlag, Berlin.

HEINSEN (1930) Quoted by Schermer (1958).

HELLEM A.J. (1960) The adhesiveness of human blood platelets *in vitro. Scand. J. clin. Lab. Invest.* **12,** Suppl. 51.

HELLEMANS J., VORLAT M. & VERSTRAETE M. (1963) Survival time of prothrombin and factors VII, IX and X after completely synthesis blocking doses of coumarin derivatives. *Br. J. Haemat.* **9,** 506.

HENDRICKSON C.C. & MARSHALL P.M. (1969) Large scale collection of blood specimen in dogs by jugular puncture. *Vet. Rec.* **84,** 290–1.

HENRICSON B. & BÄCKSTRÖM L. (1964) Translocation heterozygosity in a boar. *Hereditas,* **52,** 166–70.

HENSON J.B., McGUIRE T.C., KOBAYASHI K. & GORHAM J.B. (1967) The diagnosis of equine infectious anemia using the complement-fixation test, siderocyte counts, hepatic biopsies and serum protein alterations. *J. Am. vet. med. Ass.* **151,** 1830–9.

HENSON J.B. & McGUIRE T.C. (1972) Equine infectious anaemia. In: Catcott E.J. & Smithcors J.F. (Eds) *Equine medicine and surgery,* 2nd Ed., pp. 35–43. American Veterinary Publications, Wheaton, Illinois, USA.

HERBERT V. (1965) Folic acid. In: *Annual Review of Medicine* **16,** 359–70. Annual Reviews Inc. USA.

HERBERT V. (1970) (Ed.) Symposium on Vitamin B$_{12}$ and folate. *Am. J. Med.* **48,** 539–617.

HERCZEG B., MÁRTONFFY K. & KÁNTOR J. (1974) Änderungen des Plasmavolumens bei experimenteller Darmokklusion. *Acta Chir. Acad. Sci. Hung.* **15,** 155.

HERIN R.A. (1968) Physiological studies

in the Rocky Mountain elk. *J. Mammal.* **49,** 762–4.

HERTZ A., THEILEN G.H., SCHALM O.W. & MUNN R.J. (1970) C-type virus in bone marrow cells of cats with myeloproliferative disorders. *J. natn. Cancer Inst.* **44,** 339–48.

HESSELHOLT M. (1963) Haptoglobin polymorphism in pigs. *Acta vet. scand.* **4,** 238–46.

HESSELHOLT M., LARSEN B. & NEILSEN P.B. (1966) Studies on serum amylase systems in swine, horses and cattle. *Royal vet. and agric. Coll. Yearbook,* pp. 78–90.

HEVESY G. & OTTESEN J. (1945) Life cycle of the red corpuscles of the hen. *Nature* **156,** 534.

HEWETT C. (1974) On the causes and effects of variations in the blood profile of Swedish dairy cattle. *Acta vet. scand.,* Suppl. **50,** 1–152.

HEWITT E.A. (1931–32) Certain chemical and morphologic phases of the blood of normal and cholera-infected swine. 1. The concentration of certain chemical constituents. *Iowa State College, J. of Sci.* **VI,** 143–226.

HEYNS H. (1971) The effect of breed on the composition of blood. *J. agric. Sci., Camb.* **76,** 563–5.

HIBBS J.W., CONRAD H.R., VANDERSALL J.H. & GALE C. (1963) Occurrence of iron deficiency anemia in dairy calves at birth and its alleviation by iron dextran injection. *J. Dairy Sci.* **46,** 1118–24.

HICKS N.D. & PITNEY W.R. (1957) A rapid screening test for disorders of thromboplastin generation. *Brit. J. Haemat.* **3,** 227–37.

HILLIARD E.P., POOLE D.B.R. & COLLINS J.D. (1973) Accidental lead intoxication of cattle. Further evidence of an interference in heme biosynthesis. *Br. vet. J.* **129,** lxxxii.

HILLMAN R.S. & FINCH C.A. (1969) The misused reticulocyte. *Br. J. Haemat.* **17,** 313–5.

HIME J.M. (1963) An attempt to simulate the 'fading syndrome' in puppies by means of an experimentally-produced haemolytic disease of the new born. *Vet. Rec.* **75,** 692.

HINES J.D. & GRASSO J.A. (1970) The sideroblastic anemias. *Semin. Hemat.* **7,** 86–106.

HIPPE E. & SCHWARTZ M. (1971) Intrinsic factor activity of stomach preparations from various animal species. *Scand. J. Haemat.* **8,** 276–81.

HIRSH J. & DOEVY J.C.G. (1971) Platelet function in health and disease. *Prog. Haemat.* **7,** 185–234.

HIRUMI H., FRANKEL J.W., PRICKETT C.O. & MARAMOROSCH K. (1974) Coexistence of particles resembling herpesvirus and type-C virus in feather follicle epithelium of chickens. *J. natn. Cancer Inst.* **52,** 303–6.

HOCK R.J. (1966) Analysis of the blood of the American black bear. *Comp. Biochem. Physiol.* **19,** 285.

HODGES R.D. (1974) *The histology of the fowl.* Academic Press, London.

HODGETTS V.E. (1961) The dynamic red cell storage system in sheep. III. Relationship to determination of blood volume, total red cell volume, and plasma volume. *Aust. J. exp. Biol. med. Sci.* **39,** 187–96.

HODSON H.H., LEE B.D., WISECUP W.G. & FINEG J. (1967) Baseline blood values of the chimpanzee. I. The relationship of age and sex and haematological values. *Folia Primatol.* **7,** 1.

HOE C.M. (1969) Liver function tests. In: Medway W., Prier J.E. & Wilkinson J.S. (Eds) *Veterinary clinical pathology,* p. 61. Williams & Wilkins, Baltimore.

HOEKSTRA W.G., LEWIS P.K. JR., PHILLIPS P.H. & GRUMMER R.H. (1956) The relationship of parakeratosis, supplemental calcium and zinc to the zinc content of certain body components of swine. *J. Anim. Sci.* **15,** 752–64.

HOEKSTRA W.G., POPE A.L. & PHILLIPS P.H. (1952) Response of cobalt-deficient sheep to intravenously administered Vitamin B_{12}. *J. Nutr.* **48,** 431–41.

HOERLEIN A.B., HUBBARD E.D. & GETTY R. (1951) The procurement and handling of swine blood samples on the farm. *J. Am. vet. med. Ass.* **119,** 357–62.

HOFFBRAND A.V. (1971) The megaloblastic anaemia. In: Goldberg A. & Brain M.C. (Eds) *Recent advances in haematology,* pp. 1–76. Churchill Livingstone, Edinburgh and London.

HOFFBRAND A.V. (1975) Synthesis and breakdown of natural folates (folate polyglutamates). *Prog. Hemat.* **9,** 85–105.

HOFFBRAND A.V. (Ed.) (1976) Megaloblastic anaemia. *Clin. Haematol.* **5,** 471–769.

HOFFBRAND A.V. & LEWIS S.M. (1972) *Tutorials in postgraduate medicine: haematology.* Heinemann Medical Books London.

HOFFMAN VON R. (1973) Verbrauchskoagulopathie bei spontaner Panleukopenie der Haus- und Wildkatzen. *Berl. Munch. tierärztl. Wschr.* **86,** 72–4.

HOFMANN W., HOFFMANN R. & HOFFMANN-FEZER G. (1974) Untersuchungen über die chronische Furazolidon-Vergiftung beim Kalb. 1. Mitteilung. Klinische, hamatologische und morphologische Untersuchungen. *Dtsch. tierärztl. Wschr.* **81,** 53–8.

HOFFMANN-FEZER G., HOFFMANN R. & HOFMANN W. (1974) Untersuchungen über die chronische Furazolidon-Vergiftung beim Kalb. 2. Mitteilung. Verlaufsuntersuchungen am Knochenmask. *Dtsch. tierärztl. Wschr.* **81,** 59–63.

HOFSTAD M.S. (1950) A method of bleeding chickens from the heart. *J. Am. vet. med. Ass.* **116,** 353–4.

HOGAN A.G., MUHRER M.E. & BOGART R. (1941) A hemophilia-like disease in swine. *Proc. Soc. exp. Biol. Med.* **48,** 217–9.

HOJNY J. (1974) H blood group genotypes and expression of A and O antigens in pigs. *Anim. Blood Grps biochem. Genet.* **5,** 3–10.

HÓJOVCOVA M. (1971) Bilirubin in the blood serum of pigs under various physiological and pathological conditions. *Acta vet. Brno* **40,** 415–21.

HOLBROOK A.A., FRERICHS W.M. & ALLEN P.C. (1973) Laboratory diagnosis of equine piroplasmosis. In: Bryans J.T. & Gerber H. (Eds) *Equine infectious diseases* **3,** 467–75. S. Karger, Basel.

HOLE N.H. (1953) Blood sampling large numbers of cattle. *Vet. Rec.* **65**, 279.

HOLEMANS R. (1965) Enhancement of fibrinolysis in the dog by injection of vasoactive drugs. *Am. J. Physiol.* **208**, 511.

HOLLAND J.A. (1969) Discussion of disseminated intravascular coagulation in decompression sickness. *U.S. Naval Submarine Medical Center Report No.* 585, Groton, Connecticut, USA.

HOLMAN H.H. (1944) Studies on the haematology of sheep. 1. The blood picture of healthy sheep. *J. comp. Path. Ther.* **54**, 26–40.

HOLMAN H.H. (1945a) Studies on the haematology of sheep. IV. Erythrocytic and thrombocytic pictures, and variations in physical attributes. *J. comp. Path. Ther.* **55**, 146–57.

HOLMAN H.H. (1945b) Studies on the haematology of sheep. V. A survey of blood pictures in sheep diseases. *J. comp. Path. Ther.* **55**, 229–42.

HOLMAN H.H. (1955) The blood picture of the cow. *Br. vet. J.* **111**, 440–57.

HOLMAN H.H. (1956) Changes associated with age in the blood picture of calves and heifers. *Br. vet. J.* **112**, 91–104.

HOLMAN H.H. & DEW S.M. (1963) The blood picture of the goat. I. The two-year-old female goat. *Res. vet. Sci.* **4**, 121–30.

HOLMAN H.H. & DEW S.M. (1964) The blood picture of the goat. II. Changes in erythrocyte shape, size and number associated with age. *Res. vet. Sci.* **5**, 274–85.

HOLMAN H.H. & DEW S.M. (1965a) The blood picture of the goat. III. Changes in haemoglobin concentration and physical measurements occurring with age. *Res. vet. Sci.* **6**, 245–53.

HOLMAN H.H. & DEW S.M. (1965b) The blood picture of the goat. IV. Changes in coagulation times, platelet counts and leucocyte numbers associated with age. *Res. vet. Sci.* **6**, 510–21.

HOLMAN H.H. & DEW S.M. (1966a) The blood picture of the goat. V. Variations due to season, sex and reproduction. *Res. vet Sci.* **7**, 276–86.

HOLMAN H.H. & DEW S.M. (1966b) Effect of an injection of iron-dextran complex on blood constituents and body weight of young kids. *Vet. Rec.* **78**, 772–6.

HOLMES P.H., DARGIE J.D., MACLEAN J.M. & MULLIGAN W. (1968) Albumin and globulin turnover in chronic ovine fascioliasis. *Vet. Rec.* **83**, 227–8.

HOLMES P.H. & DARGIE J.D. (1975) Pathophysiological mechanisms in ovine anaemias. In Blunt M.H. (Ed.) *The blood of sheep.* Springer-Verlag, Berlin, Heidelberg, New York.

HOLZWORTH J. (1956) Anemia in the cat. *J. Am. vet. med. Ass.* **128**, 471–88.

HOLZWORTH J. & MEIER H. (1957) Reticulum cell myeloma in a cat. *Cornell Vet.* **47**, 301–16.

HOOVER E.A., KOCIBA G.J., HARDY W.D. & YOHN D.S. (1974) Erythroid hypoplasia in cats inoculated with feline leukemia virus. *J. natn. Cancer Inst.* **53**, 1271–6.

HOOVER E.A., McCULLOUGH C.B. & GRIESEMER R.A. (1972) Intranasal transmission of feline leukemia. *J. natn. Cancer Inst.* **48**, 973–83.

HORAK I.G., CLARK R. & GRAY R.S. (1968) The pathological physiology of helminth infestations. III. Trichostrongylus colubriformis. *Onderstepoort J. vet. Res.* **35**, 195–224.

HORN G.W., CHANDLER F.W., JR. & FLETCHER O.J., JR. (1974) Hepatic xanthine dehydrogenase activity and plasma uric acid concentration of chicks with lymphoid tumor-induced anemia. *Am. J. vet. Res.* **35**, 981–3.

HOROWITZ H.I., COHEN B.D., MARTINEZ P. & PAPAYOANOU M.F. (1967) Defective ADP-induced platelet factor 3 activation in uraemia. *Blood* **30**, 331–40.

HOTTENDORF G.H. & HIRTH R.S. (1974) Lesions of spontaneous subclinical disease in Beagle dogs. *Vet. Path.* **11**, 240–58.

HOUCHIN O.B., GRAHAM W.R., PETERSON V.E. & TURNER C.W. (1939) The chemical composition of the blood of the dairy goat. *J. Dairy Sci.* **22**, 241–50.

HOUSTON D.B. (1969) A note on the blood chemistry of the Shiras moose. *J. Mammal.* **50**, 826.

Hove E., Elvehjem C.A. & Hart E.B. (1940) The relation of zinc to carbonic anhydrase. *J. biol. Chem.* **136**, 425–34.

Hove K. & Jacobsen E. (1975) Renal excretion of urea in reindeer. Effect of nutrition. *Acta vet. scand.* **16**, 513–19.

Hovell G.J.R. (1968) Jugular puncture in the dog. *Vet. Rec.* **83**, 289–90.

Hovell G.J.R., O'Reilly K.J., Calder H.A.M. & Pover R.C. (1970) A method of vein puncture in the cat. *Vet. Rec.* **87**, 184–5.

Hovig T., Rowsell H.C., Dodds W.J., Jørgensen L. & Mustard J.F. (1967) Experimental hemostasis in normal dogs and dogs with congenital disorders of blood coagulation. *Blood*, **30**, 636–68.

Howard D.A. (1970) The effects of cobalt and copper treatment on the weight gains and blood constituents of cattle in Kenya. *Vet. Rec.* **87**, 771–4.

Howell J.McC. & Lambert P.S. (1964) A case of Haemophilia A in the dog. *Vet. Rec.* **76**, 1103–4.

Howell R.M. & Evans I.A. (1967) Chromatographic characteristics of fibrinogen and seromucoid in bovine bracken poisoning. *J. comp. Path.* **77**, 117–28.

Hruban V., Simon M. & Hradecký J. (1974) Histocompatibility studies in pigs from outbred and semi-inbred families. *Anim. Blood Grps. biochem. Genet.* **5**, 171–6.

Hruban V., Simon M. & Hradecký J. (1972) Alloantigens common to erythrocytes and leucocytes in pigs. *Anim. Blood Grps biochem. Genet.* **3**, 157–62.

Huang L.H., Lalezari P. & Swisher S.N. (1974) An automated technique for canine blood typing. *Immunology* **26**, 1059–60.

Hubbert W.T. & Hollen Eric J. (1971) Cellular blood elements in the developing bovine fetus. *Am. J. vet. Res.* **32**, 1213–19.

Hudgins P.C., Whorton C.M., Tomoyoshi T. & Riopelle A.J. (1966). Comparison of the molecular structure of myoglobin of fourteen primate species. *Nature (London)* **212**, 693–5.

Hudson A.E.A. & Osborn J.C. (1954) A note on certain blood values of adult sheep. *Vet. Med.* **49**, 423.

Hudson G. (1970) Ultrastructure of eosinophil leucocyte granules in the dog. *Acta. anat.* **77**, 62.

Hudson L. & Payne L.N. (1973) An analysis of the T and B cells of Marek's disease lymphomas of the chicken. *Nat. New Biol.* **241**, 52–3.

Huehns E.R. (1970) Diseases due to the abnormalities of hemoglobin structure. *A. Rev. Med.* **21**, 157–78.

Hugoson G. (1967) Juvenile bovine leukosis. *Acta vet. scand.* Suppl. **22**, 1–106.

Huhn R.G., Osweiler G.D. & Switzer W.P. (1969) Application of the orbital sinus bleeding technique to swine. *Lab. Anim. Care.* **19**, 403–5.

Huhrer M.E., Hogan A.G. & Bogart R. (1942) A defect in the coagulation mechanism of swine blood. *Am. J. Physiol.* **136**, 355–9.

Huisman T.H.J., Dozy A.M., Blunt M.H. & Hayes F.A. (1968) The hemoglobin heterogeneity of the Virginia white-tailed deer: a possible genetic explanation. *Archs Biochem. Biophys.* **127**, 711–17.

Humphrey J.H. & Toh C.C. (1954) Absorption of serotonin (5-hydroxytryptamine) and histamine by dog platelets. *J. Physiol.* **124**, 300.

Hunsaker W.G. (1968) Blood volume of geese treated with androgen and estrogen. *Poult. Sci.* **47**, 371–6.

Hunsaker W.G. (1969a) Effect of centrifugal force on packed cell volume and trapped plasma in avian blood. *Poult. Sci.* **48**, 705–11.

Hunsaker W.G. (1969b) Species and sex differences in the percentage of plasma trapped in packed cell volume determinations on avian blood. *Poult. Sci.* **48**, 907–9.

Hunsaker W.G., Hunt J.R. & Aitken J.R. (1964) Physiology of the growing and adult goose. I. Physical characteristics of blood. *Br. Poult. Sci.* **5**, 249–56.

Hunt T.E. & Hunt E.A. (1959) Blood basophils of cockerels before and after intravenous injection of compound 48/80. *Anat. Rec.* **133**, 19–33.

HUNTER V.E., LESPERANCE A.L. & PAPEZ N.J. (1972) Plasma inorganic phosphorus levels in Nevada mule deer. *J. Anim. Sci.* **35**, 230.

HURWITZ A. (1971) A single method for obtaining blood samples from rats. *J. Lab. clin. Med.* **78**, 172–4.

HUSER H.J. (1964) *The haematology of non-human primates*, p. 1. Proc. 10th Congr. Intern. Soc. Haematol., Stockholm.

HUSER H.J. (1970) *Atlas of comparative primate haematology*. Academic Press, New York.

HUSTON T.M. (1960) The effects of high environmental temperatures upon blood constituents and thyroid activity of domestic fowl. *Poult. Sci.* **39**, 1260.

HUSTON T.M. (1965) The influence of different environmental temperatures on immature fowl. *Poult. Sci.* **44**, 1032–6.

HUTCHINS D.R., LEPHERD E.E. & CROOK I.G. (1967) A case of haemophilia. *Aust. vet. J.* **43**, 83–7.

HUTT F.B., RICKARD C.G. & FIELD R.A. (1948) Sex-linked hemophilia in dogs. *J. Hered.* **39**, 3.

HUXSOLL D.L., HILDEBRANDT P.K., NIMS R.M. & WALKER J.S. (1970) Tropical canine pancytopenia. *J. Am. vet. med. Ass.* **157**, 1627–32.

HWANG S.W. & WOSILAIT W.D. (1970) Comparative and developmental studies on blood coagulation. *Comp. Biochem. Physiol.* **37**, 595.

HYDE J.L., KING J.M. & BENTINCK-SMITH J. (1958) A case of bovine myelogenous leukaemia. *Cornell Vet.* **48**, 264–76.

HYLDGAARD-JENSEN J., PALLUDAN B., PANIC B. & VALENTA M. (1969) Plasma enzymes of hepatic origin. A study of changes in plasma LDH activity and isoenzymes, GLDH, GOT and AP during experimentally produced liver injury in pigs. *Araskr. K. Vet. Landbohjsk.*, pp. 117–40. Arsskrift den Kongelige Veterinser-ag Landbokjskole.

HYSLOP N.ST.G. (1966) Equine infectious anaemia (Swamp fever): A review. *Vet. Rec.* **78**, 858–64.

HYVÄRINEN H. & HELLE T. (1974) The effects of winter conditions and winter nutrition on some blood parameters in the reindeer, *Rangifer tarandustarandus*, in Finland. *First International Theriological Congres, Transactions* **1**, 225–6.

HYVÄRINEN H., HELLE T., NIEMINEN M., VÄYRYNEN P. & VÄYRYNEN R. (1976) Some effects of handling reindeer during gatherings on the composition of their blood. *Anim. Prod.* **22**, 105–114.

HYVÄRINEN H., HELLE T., VÄYRYNEN R. & VÄYRYNEN P. (1975) Seasonal and nutritional effects on serum proteins and urea concentration in the reindeer (*Rangifer tarandus tarandus* L.). *Br. J. Nutr.* **33**, 63–72.

IAMPIETRO P.F., BURR M.J., FIORICA V., MCKENZIE J.M. & HIGGINS E.A. (1967) pH-Dependent lysis of canine erythrocytes. *J. appl. Physiol.* **23**, 505.

IATRIDIS S.G. & FERGUSON J.H. (1963) Effects of physical exercise on blood clotting and fibrinolysis. *J. appl. Physiol.* **18**, 337.

IKKALA E., MYLLYLA G. & SARAJAS H. (1963) Haemostatic changes associated with exercise. *Nature (London)*, **199**, 459–61.

IMLAH P. (1963) *Blood Groups of pigs*. Thesis, Edinburgh.

IMLAH P. (1964) Inherited variants in serum caeruloplasmins of the pig. *Nature (London)* **203**, 658–9.

IMLAH P. (1965) A study of blood groups in pigs. In: Matoušek J. (Ed.) *Blood groups of animals*, pp. 109–22. Publishing House of the Czechoslovak Academy of Sciences, Prague.

IMLAH P. (1970a) Ontogenic and familial variation in serum alkaline phosphatase of pigs. *XIth European Conference on Animal Blood groups and Biochemical Polymorphism*, Warsaw.

IMLAH P. (1970b) Evidence for the Tf locus being associated with an early lethal factor in a strain of pigs. *Anim. Blood Grps biochem. Genet.* **1**, 5–13.

IMLAH P. (1972) Application of blood group loci in studies on pre-natal and post-natal survival of piglets. *Anim. Blood Grps biochem. Genet.* **3**, Suppl. 1, 80.

IMLAH P. (1974) Blood group genotype effect on litter size at birth and at three weeks of age. *Anim. Blood Grps biochem. Genet.* **5,** Suppl. 1, 37–8.

INGRAM M. & COOPERSMITH A. (1969) Reticulated platelets following acute blood loss. *Br. J. Haemat.* **17,** 225–9.

INGRAM V.M. (1957) Gene mutations in human haemoglobin: the chemical difference between normal and sickle cell haemoglobin. *Nature (London),* **180,** 326–8.

INTERNATIONAL COMMITTEE FOR STANDARDIZATION IN HAEMATOLOGY OF THE EUROPEAN SOCIETY OF HAEMATOLOGY (1965) Recommendations and requirements for haemoglobinometry in human blood. *Brit. J. Haemat.* **11,** 389–91.

INTERNATIONAL COMMITTEE FOR STANDARDIZATION IN HEMATOLOGY (1971) Recommended methods for radioisotope red-cell survival studies. *Br. J. Haemat.* **21,** 241–50.

IRFAN M. (1961) Studies on the peripheral blood picture of the normal dog. *Ir. vet. J.* **15,** 65, 86 & 110.

IRFAN M. (1967) The electrophoretic pattern of serum proteins in normal animals. *Res. vet. Sci.* **8,** 137–42.

IRFAN M. (1968) Fibrinolytic activity in animals of different species. *Q. Jl. exp. Physiol.* **53,** 374–80.

IRFAN M. (1971) The peripheral blood picture in myositosis and atrophy of head muscles in dogs. *Ir. vet. J.* **25,** 189.

IRSIGLER K., LECHNER K. & DEUTSCH E. (1965) Studies on tissue thromboplastin: species specificity. *Thromb. Diath. haemorrh.* **14,** 18.

IRVINE C.G.H. (1958) The blood picture in the race-horse. 1. The normal erythrocyte and hemoglobin status—a dynamic concept. *J. Am. vet. med. Ass.* **133,** 97–101.

IRZHAK L.I. (1964) Contribution to the physiology of the blood in elks. *Trudy Pechoro-Ilychskogo Gos. za Povednika* **11,** 61–6. (Russian.)

IRZHAK L.I. (1973) Types of hemoglobin in ontogensis of the reindeer *Rangifer tarandus. J. Evol. Biochem & Physiol.* **9,** 341–5. (Russian.)

IRZHAK L.I., KACHMARCHIK E.V. & MONGALEV N.P. (1973) Types of hemo-globin in the early embryogenesis of reindeer. *Zh. obshch. Biol.* **34,** 777–81. (Russian.)

IRZHAK L.I. & KAHMARIK E.V. (1971) Hemoglobin types in growing elks. *Zh. obshch. Biol.* **32,** 377–80. (Russian.)

ISARD P.F. (1974) Contribution à l'etude des coagulations intravasculaires disseminées. L'envénimation ophidienne par les Vipéridae chez le chien. *Thèse Ecole Nat. Vet. Lyon.* 58 pp.

ISHMAEL J., GOPINATH C. & HOWELL J.McC. (1972) Experimental chronic copper toxicity in sheep. *Res. vet. Sci.* **13,** 22–9.

ITIKAWA O. & OGURA Y. (1954) Simplified manufacture and histochemical use of the Schiff reagent. *Stain Technol.* **29,** 9–11.

IVANOV V.L. (1973) Detection of specific antigen in organs of leucotic cattle. *Veterinariya Moscow* No. 1, 47–9.

IVES M. & DACK G.M. (1956) 'Alarm reaction' and normal blood picture in *Macaca mulatta. J. Lab. clin. Med.* **47,** 723.

JACKSON D.E., LOAN R.W., DALE H.E. (1971) Canine A red blood cell isoantigen. *Missouri Vet.* **21,** 7.

JACOBS A. & WORWOOD M. (1974) (Eds) *Iron in biochemistry and medicine.* Academic Press, London and New York.

JAFFE P. (1960) Differences in numbers of erythrocytes between inbred lines of chickens. *Nature (London),* **186,** 978–9.

JAIN N.C. (1967) Alkaline phosphatase activity in the canine and feline granulocytes. *Vet. Rec.* **81,** 266.

JAIN N.C. (1972) Osmotic fragility of erythrocytes of dogs and cats in health and in certain haematological disorders. *Cornell Vet.* **63,** 411–23.

JAIN N.C. (1975) A scanning electron microscopic study of platelets of certain animal species. *Thromb. Diath. haemorrh.* **33,** 501–7.

JAIN N.C. & SCHALM O.W. (1966) Influence of corticosteroids on total and differential blood leukocyte counts. *Calif. Vet.* **20,** 28–31.

JAIN N.C. & KEETON K.S. (1973) Scanning

electron-microscopic features of haemobartonella felis. *Am. J. vet. Res.* **34,** 697–700.

JAIN N.C. & KONO C.S. (1975) Erythrocyte sedimentation rate in the dog and cat: comparison of two methods and influence of packed cell volume, temperature and storage of blood. *J. small Anim. Pract.* **16,** 671.

JAKOWSKI R.M., FREDRICKSON T.N. & LUGINBUHL R. (1973) Immunoglobulin response in experimental infection with cell-free and cell-associated Marek's disease virus. *J. Immun.* **111,** 238–48.

JAMIESON A. (1966) The application of a blood group formula. *Xth European Conference on Animal Blood Groups and Biochemical Polymorphisms, Paris,* pp. 461–4. Institut National de la Recherche Agronomique.

JARAJDA V., NAPRAVNIK A. & JURAJDOYA J. (1973) Enzyme studies in Marek's disease tumors. *Acta vet. Brno* **42,** 29–33.

JARRETT W.F.H. (1976) Cat leukaemia and its viruses. *Adv. vet. Sci. & comp. Med.* **19,** 165–93.

JARRETT W.F.H., CRIGHTON G.W. & DALTON R.G. (1966) Leukaemia and lymphosarcoma in animals and man. *Vet. Rec.* **79,** 693–9.

JARRETT W.F.H., MARTIN W.B., CRIGHTON G.W., DALTON R.G. & STEWART M.F. (1964) Transmission experiments with leukaemia (lymphosarcoma). *Nature,* **202,** 566–7.

JARRETT W.F.H. & MACKEY L.J. (1974) International histological classification of tumours of domestic animals. Neoplastic diseases of the haematopoietic and lymphoid tissues. *Bull. Wld. Hlth. Org.* **50,** 21–34.

JASPER D.E. & JAIN N.C. (1965a) Effects of lipemia upon erythrocyte fragility, sedimentation rate and plasma refractometer indexes in the dog. *Am. J. vet. Res.* **26,** 332–8.

JASPER D.E. & JAIN N.C. (1965b) The influence of adrenocorticotropic hormone and prednisolone upon marrow and circulating leucocytes in the dog. *Am. J. vet. Res.* **26,** 844–50.

JATKAR P.R. & KREIER J.P. (1967) Relationship between severity of anemia and plasma erythropoietin titer in anaplasma-infected calves and sheep. *Am. J. vet. Res.* **28,** 107–113.

JAYASOORIYAN M.S. & NAIR S.G. (1971) Serum enzyme levels in dogs during regeneration of blood. *J. Anim. Morph. Physiol.* **18,** 164.

JEFFCOTT L.B. (1969) Haemolytic disease of the newborn foal. *Equine vet. J.* **1,** 165–70.

JEFFCOTT L.B. (1971) Perinatal studies in equidae with special reference to passive transfer of immunity. PhD. thesis, Univ. of London.

JEFFCOTT L.B. (1974) Haematology in relation to performance and potential. 2. Some specific aspects. *Jl S. Afr. vet. Ass.* **45,** 278–86.

JEFFCOTT L.B., BETTS A.O. & HARVEY D.G. (1967) Nephritis in sows. *Vet. Rec.* **81,** 446–7.

JENNINGS A.R. & SEAMER J. (1956) A new blood parasite in British pigs. *Nature* **178,** 153–4.

JENSEN E.L., SMITH C., BAKER L.N. & COX D.F. (1968) Quantitative studies on blood group and serum protein systems in pigs. II. Effects on production and reproduction. *J. Anim. Sci.* **27,** 856–62.

JEPSON J.H. & LOWENSTEIN L. (1967) The effect of testosterone, adrenal steroids and prolactin on erythropoiesis. *Acta Haemat. (Basel)* **38,** 292–9.

JOHNSON H.E., YOUATT W.G., FAY L.D., HARTE H.D. & ULLREY D.E. (1968) Hematological values of Michigan white-tailed deer. *J. Mammal.* **49,** 749–54.

JOHNSON J.L. & TUMBLESON M.E. (1971) Serum biochemic values in piglets exhibiting diarrhoea. *SWest. Vet.* **24,** 297–9.

JONES B. (1974) Some screening tests to investigate hemorrhagic disorders in dogs. *Proc. 12th Nordic Vet. Congr. Reykjavic,* 7–10 Aug. 1974. Mortensen, Copenhagen, Denmark, 287.

JONES D.M. (1976) Personal communication.

JONES D.M. (1976) The husbandry and veterinary care of wild horses in captivity. *Equine vet. J.* **8,** 140–6.

JONES D.R.E. & DARKE P.G.G. (1975) Use of papain for the detection of incomplete erythrocyte autoantibodies in autoimmune haemolytic anaemia of the dog and cat. *J. small Anim. Pract.* **16**, 273.

JONES D.R.E. & HILL F.W.G. (1974) Suspected thrombasthenia in a Shetland Sheepdog. *Vet. Rec.* **94**, 558.

JONES D.R. & JOHANSEN K. (1972) The blood vascular system of birds. In: Farner D.S. & King J.R. (Eds) *Avian Biology* II, pp. 157–285. Academic Press, London.

JONES E.W., KLIEWER I.O., NORMAN B.B. & BROCK W.E. (1968) *Anaplasma marginale* infection in young and aged cattle. *Am. J. vet. Res.* **29**, 535–44.

JONES J.B., LANGE R.D. & JONES E.S. (1975a) Cyclic hematopoiesis in a colony of dogs. *J. Am. vet. med. Ass.* **106**, 365–7.

JONES J.B., YANG T.J., DALE J.B. & LANGE R.D. (1975b) Canine cyclic haematopoiesis: marrow transplantation between littermates. *Br. J. Haemat.* **30**, 215–23.

JORDAN H.E. (1935) The significance of the lymphoid nodule. *Am. J. Anat.* **57**, 1–37.

JORDAN H.E. (1936) The relation of lymphoid tissue to the process of blood production in avian bone marrow. *Am. J. Anat.* **59**, 249–97.

JONES R.F. & PARIS R. (1963) The greyhound eosinophil. *J. small Anim. Pract.* **4**, 29–33.

JOYSEY V.C., GOODWIN R.F.W. & COOMBS R.R.A. (1959a) The blood groups of the pig. VI. Red cell antigens other than the A-O system. *J. comp. Path.* **69**, 29–44.

JOYSEY V.C., GOODWIN R.F.W. & COOMBS R.R.A. (1959b) The blood groups of the pig. VII. The distribution of twelve red cell antigens in seven breeds. *J. comp. Path.* **69**, 292–9.

KAKKUK T.J. & CONNOR G.H. (1970) Experimental canine herpesvirus in the gnotobiotic dog. *Lab. Anim. Care* **20**, 69.

KALETA E.F. & BERNHARDT D. (1968) Beitrag zur Hämatologie der Gans. I. Morphologische Untersuchung des Gänseblutes. *Arch. Geflügelk.* **32**, 84–90.

KAMMERMANN-LÜSCHER B. (1970) Uber Thrombozytenzahlen beim Hund. *Schweizer. Arch. Tierheilk.* **112**, 588.

KAMMERMANN-LÜSCHER B., GMÜR, J. & STÜNZI H. (1971) A fibrinogenämie beim Hund. *Zentbl. VetMed. A.* **18**, 192.

KAMMERMANN-LÜSCHER B. (1974a) Die Interpretation des Weissen Blutbildes beim Hund (1). *Tierärztl. prax* **2**, 215.

KAMMERMANN-LÜSCHER B. (1974b) Die Interpretation des weissen Blutbildes beim Hund (2). *Tierärztl. prax.* **2**, 307.

KANEKO J.J. (1974) Comparative erythrocyte metabolism. In: Brandly C.A. & Cornelius C.E. (Eds). *Advances in veterinary science and comparative Medicine*, **18**, p. 117. Academic Press, New York.

KANEKO J.J., CORDY D.R. & CARLSON G. (1967) Canine hemophilia resembling classic hemophilia A. *J. Am. vet. med. Ass.* **150**, 15–21.

KANEKO J.J. & MILLS R. (1970) Hematological and blood chemical observations in neonatal normal and porphyric calves in early life. *Cornell Vet.* **60**, 52–60.

KANEKO J.J., ZINKL J., TENNANT B.C. & MATTHEEUWS D.R.G. (1968) Iron metabolism in familial polycythemia of Jersey calves. *Am. J. vet. Res.* **29**, 949–52.

KANEKO J.J., ZINKL J.G. & KEETON K.S. (1971) Erythrocyte porphyrin and erythrocyte survival in bovine erythropoietic porphyria. *Am. J. vet. Res.* **32**, 1981–5.

KAPLOW L.S. (1955) A histochemical procedure for localising and evaluating leucocyte alkaline phosphatase activity in smears of blood and marrow. *Blood* **10**, 1023–9.

KARDEVAN A., THAKUR H.N., MASZTIS S. & TOTH B. (1973) Pathogenesis and epidemiology of Marek's disease. II. Histogenesis. *Magy. Allatorv. Lap.* **28**, 234–40.

KARG H. (1955) Das Verhalten der Bluteosinophilen als Belastungsprobe bei Rind und Schwein. *Zbtl. VetMed.* **2**, 682–92.

KARSTAD L., WINTER A. & TRAINER D.O. (1961) Pathology of epizootic hemorrhagic disease of deer. *Am. J. vet. Res.* **22**, 227–35.

KARVONEN M.J. (1954) The diameter of

foetal sheep erythrocytes. *Acta anat.* **20,** 53–61.

KAŠE F. (1972) [Comparison of some coagulation tests in man and four mammal species (rabbit, dog, cow and pig.)] *Veterinární Med.* **17,** 495.

KASHIWABARA T. (1964) Size of sperm head and of red blood cells in the domestic fowl. *Poult. Sci.* **43,** 411–4.

KASSEL R. & LEVITAN S. (1953) A jugular technique for the repeated bleeding of small animals. *Science* **118,** 563–4.

KASTEN F.H., BURTON V. & GLOVER P. (1959) Fluorescent Schiff-type reagents of cytochemical detection of polyaldehyde moieties in sections and smears. *Nature (London),* **184,** 1797–8.

KAUFMAN R.M., AIRO R., POLLACK S., CROSBY W.H. & DOBERNECK R. (1965) Origin of pulmonary megakaryocytes. *Blood,* **25,** 767–75.

KELÉNYI G. & NÉMETH Á. (1969) Comparative histochemistry and electron microscopy of the eosinophil leucocytes of vertebrates. *Acta biol. hung.* **20,** 405–22.

KELLER C. (1933) Vergleichende Zellen- und Kernmessungen bei grossen und kleinen Hühnerrassen zur Prüfung der genetisch begingten Wuchsunterschiede Zugleich ein Beitrag zur Frage des rhythmischen Wachstums der Kerne. *Z. Zellforsch. mikrosk. Anat.* **19,** 510–36.

KELLY D.F. & DARKE P.G.G. (1976) Cushing's syndrome in the dog. *Vet. Rec.* **98,** 28.

KELLY J.W. & DEARSTYNE R.S. (1935) Haematology of the fowl. A. Studies on normal chick and normal adult blood. *N. Carol. Agric. Exp. Sta. Tech. Bull.* No. 50.

KELLY D.F. & HILL F.W.G. (1975) Intestinal malabsorption in the dog. In: Grunsell C.S.G. & Hill F.W.G. (Eds) *Veterinary annual,* 15th Edn, p. 238. Wright Scientechnica, Bristol.

KELLY J.D. & FARROW B.R.H. (1970) Auto-immune haemolytic anaemia in a dog. *Aust. vet. J.* **46,** 475–9.

KERNKAMP H.C.H. (1941) Diseases of swine due to nutritive deficiencies. *J. Am. vet. med. Ass.* **99,** 373–81.

KERNOHAN J.C. (1961) Kinetics of the reactions of two sheep haemoglobins with oxygen and carbon monoxide. *J. Physiol., Lond.* **155,** 580–8.

KERRY P.J. (1976) The isolation of ovine lymphocytes and granulocytes from whole blood using hydroxyethylcellulose. *Res. vet. Sci.* **21,** 356–7.

KETZ H.A., VOGEL G. & WESTPHAL W. (1956) Vergleichende Untersuchungen über die Steuerung des weissen Blutbildes in Abhängigkeit von der Alkalireserve des Blutes. I. Der Einfluss verschiedener Fütterung, des Hungers und der Wieder-fütterung auf Alkalireserve und weisses Blutbild bei Pferd, Hund und Schwein. *Zbtl. VetMed.* **3,** 44–54.

KHAN P.M. & BLANER H. (1972) Polymorphic enzymes in rhesus monkeys. *medical primatology. Proc. 3rd Conf. exp. med. surg. Primates,* Lyon 1972, Pt. 1, p. 363. Karger, Basel.

KHANNA N.D., CHET RAM, TANDON K.N. & PRABHU S.S. (1970) Studies on biochemical polymorphism in bovines. I. Haemoglobin variations in Hariana breed of cattle. *J. Genet.* **60,** 159–63.

KIM S.N., YOON J.W., OLMSTED J. & KENYON A.J. (1972) Chromosome studies of lymphoblastic leukemia of domestic fowl, JM-V. *Fedn Proc. Fedn Am. Socs exp. Biol.* **31,** 620.

KINCADE P.W., LAWTON A.R. & COOPER M.D. (1971) Restriction of surface immunoglobulin determinants to lymphocytes of the plasma cell line. *J. Immun.* **106,** 1421–3.

KING W.E. & WILSON R.H. (1910) Studies in hog cholera preventive treatment. II. Hematological studies. *Kans. State agric. exp. Sta. Bull.* **171,** 139.

KIREV T. (1972) Morphological studies on the central nervous system in chickens with experimentally induced myelocytomatosis. *Izv. Inst. obshcha srav. Patol. dom. Zhiv., Sof.* **14,** 43–50.

KIRKHAM W.W., GUTTRIDGE H., BOWDEN J. & EDDS E.T. (1971) Hematopoietic response to hematinics in horses. *J. Am. vet. med. Ass.* **159,** 1316–8.

KIRSNER J.B. & FORD H. (1955) Phenyl-butazone (Butazolidin)—effect on basal gastric secretion and production of gastroduodenal ulcerations in dogs. *Gastroenterology*, 29, 18.

KISS M. & KÓMÁR J.G. (1967) Pelger-Huet'sche Kernanomalie der Leukozyten bei einem Hunde. *Berl. Münch. tierärztl. Wschr.* 80, 474.

KITCHEN H. (1974) Animal haemoglobin heterogeneity. *Ann. N.Y. Acad. Sci.* 241, 12.

KITCHEN A. & BRETT I. (1974) Embryonic and fetal hemoglobin in animals. *Ann. N.Y. Acad. Sci.* 241, 653.

KITCHEN H. & BUNN H.F. (1971) Oxygen transport and adaptation in the fetus and newborn foal. *Proc. 17th. A. Conv. Am. Ass. equine Pract.* 81–8.

KITCHEN H. & BUNN H.F. (1975) Ontogeny of equine haemoglobins. *J. Reprod. Fert.*, Suppl. 23, 595–8.

KITCHEN H., JACKSON W.F. & TAYLOR W.J. (1965) Hemoglobin and hemodynamics in the horse during physical training. *Proc. 11th. A. Conv. Am. Ass. equine Pract.* 97–110.

KITCHEN H., PUTNAM F.W. & TAYLOR W.J. (1964) Hemoglobin polymorphism: its relation to sickling of erythrocytes in white-tailed deer. *Science, N.Y.* 144, 1237–9.

KITCHEN H., PUTNAM F.W. & TAYLOR W.J. (1966) The structural basis for the polymorphic hemoglobins of white-tailed deer (*Odocoileus virginianus*): a comparison of the hemoglobins associated with sickled and nonsickled erythrocytes. In: Polychronakos D.J. (Ed.) *International symposium on comparative hemoglobin structure*, pp. 73–82. M. Triantafylou & sons, Thessaloniki.

KITCHEN H., PUTNAM F.W. & TAYLOR W.J. (1967) Hemoglobin polymorphism in white-tailed deer: subunit basis. *Blood* 29, 867–77.

KITCHEN H., EASLEY C.W., PUTNAM F.W. & TAYLOR W.J. (1968) Structural comparison of polymorphic hemoglobins of deer with those of sheep and other species. *J. biol. Chem.* 243, 1204–11.

KITTS W.D., BANDY P.J., WOOD A.J. & COWAN I.McT. (1956) Effect of age and plane of nutrition on the blood chemistry

of the Columbian black-tailed deer (*Odocoileus hemionus columbianus*). *Can. J. Zool.* 34, 477–84.

KLOSTER G., LARSEN B. & NIELSEN P.B. (1970) Carbonic anhydrase polymorphism in cattle and swine. *Acta vet. scand.* II, 318–21.

KNIGHT H.D. & BURAU R.G. (1973) Chronic lead poisoning in horses. *J. Am. vet. med. Ass.* 162, 781–6.

KNILL L.M., McCONAUGHY M.S., CAMARENA B.S. & DAY M. (1969) Hemogram of the Arabian horse. *Am. J. vet. Res.* 30, 295–8.

KNISELEY R.M. (1972) Marrow studies with radiocolloids. *Semin. Nucl. Med.* 2, 71–85.

KNOLL W. (1932) Das morphologische Blutbild der Säugetiere. I. Allgemeine und spezielle Morphologie der kernhaltigen Blutzellen der Säugetiere. *Z. mikrosk.-anat. Forsch.* 30, 116–50.

KOCIBA G.J. & HATHAWAY J.E. (1974) Disseminated intravascular coagulation associated with heartworm disease in the dog. *J. Am. Anim. Hosp. Ass.* 10, 373.

KOCIBA G.J., RATNOFF O.D., LOEB W.F., WALL R.L. & HEIDER L.E. (1969) Bovine plasma thromboplastin antecedent (Factor XI) deficiency. *J. Lab. clin. Med.* 74, 37–41.

KÖHLER H. (1956) Knochenmark und Blutbild des Ferkels. I. Das gesunde Ferkel. *Zbtl. VetMed.* 3, 359–95.

KONNO S., FUJIWARA H., ISHIHARA T. & USHIMI C. (1971) Panmyelopathia in pastured cattle. *Natn. Inst. Anim. Hlth. Q. Tokyo* 11, 201–10.

KONTTINEN Y.P. (1968) *Fibrinolysis, Chemistry, Pathology and Clinics.* Pub. Oy Star Ab, Finland.

KOSTROMITINOV N.M., MOLCHANAV V.P. & NIKOLSKII V.K. (1972) Role of heredity in the aetiology of leucosis. Quoted by Abramova *et al.* (1974) *Vet. Bull.* 44, 690.

KOTULA A.W. & HELBACKA N.V. (1966) Blood volume of live chickens and influence of slaughter technique on blood loss. *Poult. Sci.* 45, 684–8.

KOTULA A.W. & HELBACKA N.V. (1968) Chicken blood volume: the hematocrit and comparison of I^{131} and Evans Blue methods. *Poult. Sci.* 47, 26–31.

KOWALSKI E., BUDZYŃSKI A.Z., KOPÉC M., LATALLO Z.S., LIPINSKI B. & WEGRZYNOWICZ Z. (1964) Studies on the molecular pathology and pathogenesis of bleeding in severe fibrinolytic states in dogs. *Thromb. Diath. haemorr.* **12**, 69.

KOZMA C.K., WEISBROTH S.H., STRATMAN S.L. & CONEJEROS M. (1969) Normal biological values for Long-Evans rats. *Lab. Anim. Care* **19**, 746.

KRAMER D.V. & LEWIS R.N. (1972) Reticulocyte response in the cat. *J. Am. vet. med. Ass.* **160**, 61–7.

KRANTZ S.B. (1973) Pure red cell aplasia. *Br. J. Haemat.* **25**, 1–6.

KRAVCHENKO D.N. & KRAVCHENKO R.S. (1971) Polymorphous systems of blood serum proteins in *Cervus elaphus* L. *Tsitol. Genet.* **5**, 311–5. (Russian.)

KREIER J.P. & RISTIC M. (1963) Morphologic, antigenic and pathogenic characteristics of Eperythrozoon ovis and Eperythrozoon wenyoni. *Am. J. vet. Res.* **24**, 488–500.

KREIER J.P., RISTIC M. & SCHROEDER W. (1964) Anaplasmosis. XVI. Pathogenesis of anaemia produced by infection with *Anaplasma. Am. J. vet. Res.* **25**, 343–52.

KRIESTEN K. & ENBERGS H. (1970) Elektronmikroskopische Untersuchungen zur Feinstruktur der basophilen Granulozyten des Haushuhns. *Blut,* **20**, 282–7.

KRISTJANSSON F.K. (1960) Genetic control of two blood serum proteins in swine. *Can. J. Genet. Cytol.* **2**, 295–300.

KRISTJANSSON F.K. (1961) Genetic control of three haptoglobins in pigs. *Genetics,* **46**, 907–10.

KRISTJANSSON F.K. (1963) Genetic control of two prealbumins in pigs. *Genetics* **48**, 1059–63.

KRISTJANSSON F.K. (1966) Fractionation of serum albumin and genetic control of two albumin fractions in pigs. *Genetics,* **53**, 675–9.

KROGER L.M. (1956) Onion poisoning in cattle. *J. Am. vet. med. Ass.* **129**, 75.

KRZYWANEK H. & WITTE G. (1970) Parameter des energiestoffwechsels und des Sauerstofftranports bei vollblutrennpferden un Perioden unterschiedlicher Trainingsintensitaat. *Int. Z. angew. Physiol.* **28**, 228.

KUBA N., ONO Y. & FUKUSHIMA T. (1963) Histopathological studies of so-called Kuwazu disease (cobalt deficiency) in cattle in Japan. *Jap. J. vet. Sci.* **25**, 363–74.

KUBASEK F.O.T., LEAT W.M.F. & BUTTRESS N. (1974) Plasma lipoproteins of the suckling lamb compared with adult sheep. *Proc. Nutr. Soc.* **33**, 47–8A.

KÚBEK A. (1968a) A study on postalbumins in pigs. *European conference on animal blood groups and biochemical polymorphism,* Warsaw, pp. 315–16. PWN—Polish Scientific Publishers.

KUBEK A. (1968b) Electrophoretical study of the Esterases in Pig Serum. *XIth European conference on animal blood groups and biochemical polymorphism,* Warsaw, pp. 355–8. PWN—Polish Scientific Publishers.

KUKAINE R.A., NAGAYEWA L.I., TSCHAPENKO S.V., BRATTSSLAVSKAYA O.I., ALEXANDROWA M.A., USTINCOWA E.M., RUNTZIS A.Y., KUDELEWA G.O., SCHITOVA T.F. & SCHASHINA S.S. (1973) Detection of C-type oncornaviruses of cattle with spontaneous and with experimentally induced lymphatic leucosis. *Arch. Geschwulstforsch.* **42**, 263–73.

KUKSOVA M.I. (1960) Seasonal and diurnal fluctuations in the red blood cells of monkeys. In: Utkin I.A. (Ed.) *Theoretical and practical problems of medicine and biology in experiments on monkeys,* p. 123. Pergamon Press, Oxford.

KURKCUOGLU N. & MCELFRESH A.E. (1960) The Hageman factor: determinations of its concentration during the neonatal period and presentation of a case of Hageman factor deficiency. *J. Pediat.* **56**, 61.

KURUMA I., OKADA T., KATAOKA K. & SORIMACHI M. (1970) Ultrastructural observation of 5-hydroxytryptamine-storing granules in the domestic fowl thrombocytes. *Z. Zellforsch. mikrosk. Anat.* **108**, 268–81.

KVITKIN YU (1957) Seasonal changes in blood picture of reindeer. *Trudȳ gos. Inst. éksp. Vet.* **20**, 294–305. (Russian.)

LAAKE K., VENNERÖD A.M., HAUGEN G. & GJÖNNAESS H. (1974) Cold-promoted activation of factor VII in human plasma: studies on the associated acyl-arginine esterase activity. *Thromb. Res.* **4**, 769.

LABER J., PERMAN V. & STEVENS J.B. (1974) Polychromasia or reticulocytes—an assessment of the dog. *J. Am. Anim. Hosp. Ass.* **10**, 399.

LACROIX J.A. & PULLEY L.T. (1974) Primary cholangiohepatitis in a dog. *J. Am. Anim. Hosp. Ass.* **10**, 55.

LAHEY M.E., GUBLER C.J., CHASE M.S., CARTWRIGHT G.E. & WINTROBE M.M. (1952) Studies on Copper Metabolism. II. Hematologic manifestations of copper deficiency in swine. *Blood* **7**, 1053–74.

LAJTHA L.J. (1965) Cellular mechanism of red cell production. *Ser. Haemat.* (first series) **2**, 26–33.

LALA P.K., PATT H.M. & MALONEY M.A. (1966) An evaluation of erythropoiesis in canine marrow. *Acta haemat.* **35**, 311–8.

LAMKIE N.J. & BURSTONE M.S. (1962) Vinylpyrrolidone-vinyl acetate copolymers as mounting media for azo and other dyes. *Stain Technol.* **37**, 109–10.

LANDSTEINER K. (1901) Uber Agglutinationserscheinungen normalen menschlichen Blutes. *Wien. klin. Wschr.* **14**, 1132–4.

LANE A.G. & CAMPBELL J.R. (1969) Relationship of hematocrit values to selected physiological conditions in dairy cattle. *J. Anim. Sci.* **28**, 508–11.

LANG B.G. (1968) Globulin allotyping in pigs using iso-precipitins. *XIth European conference on animal blood groups and biochemical polymorphism*, Warsaw, pp. 301–6. PWN—Polish Scientific Publishers.

LANGE W. (1919) Untersuchungen über den Hämoglobingehalt, die Zahl und die Grösse der roten Blutkörperchen. *Zool. Jber. Neapel.* **36**, 657–98.

LANGFORD G., KNOTT S.G., DIMMOCK C.K. & DERRINGTON P. (1971) Haemolytic disease of newborn calves in a dairy herd in Queensland. *Aust. vet. J.* **47**, 1–4.

LAPEN R.F., KENZY S.G., PIPER R.C. & SHARMA J.M. (1971) Pathogenesis of cutaneous Marek's disease in chickens. *J. natn. Cancer Inst.* **47**, 389–99.

LAPEN R.F. & KENZY S.G. (1972) Distribution of gross cutaneous Marek's disease lesions. *Poult. Sci.* **51**, 334–6.

LAPIN B.A., YAKOLEVA L.A., INDZHIIA L.V., AGRBA V.Z., TSIRIPOVA G.S., VOEVODIN A.F., IVANOV M.T. & DJATCHENKO A.G. (1975) Transmission of human leukaemia to non-human primates. *Proc. R. Soc. Med.* **68**, 141.

LARKIN E.C., SIMMONDS R.C., ULVEDAL F. & WILLIAMS W.T. (1972) Responses of some haematological parameters of active and hibernating squirrels (*Spermophilus mexicanus*) upon exposure to hypobaric and isobaric hyperoxia. *Comp. Biochem. Physiol.* **43A**, 757.

LAUFENSTEIN-DUFFY H. (1971) The daily variation of the resting packed cell volume in the racing thoroughbred and the difficulty in evaluating the effectiveness of hematinic drugs. *Proc. 17th A. Conv. Am. Ass. equine Pract.* 151–4.

LAWRENCE J.A. & BERLIN N.I. (1952) Relative polycythemia—the polycythemia of stress. *Yale J. Biol. Med.* **24**, 498–505.

LAZARUS A.E. & RAJAMANI S. (1968) Poisoning due to onion spoilage in cattle. *Indian vet. J.* **45**, 877–80.

LEBLOND P.F. (1973) Étude, au microscope électronique a balayage, de la migration des cellules sanguines a travers les parois des sinusoïdes spléniques et médullaires chez le rat. *Nouv. Revue fr. Hemat.* **13**, 771–88.

LECRONE C.N. (1970) Absence of special fetal hemoglobin in Beagle dogs. *Blood* **35**, 451.

LEE C.K., ODELL G.V., ELIOT F.P., ANDERSON I.L. & JONES E.W. (1971) Postnatal loss of bovine fetal haemoglobin. *Am. J. vet. Res.* **32**, 1039–44.

LEE K.M., TAKAHASHI R. & GILLESPIE J.H. (1970) Virus-like particles associated with buffy coat cells of a cow with lymphosarcoma. *Cornell Vet.* **60**, 139–42.

LEE R.I. & WHITE P.D. (1913) A clinical study of the coagulation time of blood. *Am. J. med. Sci.* **145**, 495–503.

LEHMANN H. & HUNTSMAN R.G. (1974) *Man's haemoglobins*. North Holland Publishing Co., Amsterdam.

LEHNER N.D.M., BULLOCK B.C. & CLARKson T.B. (1968) Ascorbic acid deficiency in the squirrel monkey. *Proc. Soc. exp. Biol. Med.* **128,** 512–4.

Leibetseder J., Kment A., Skalicky M. & Niedermüller H. (1972) Uber den Zinkstoffwechsel beim Schwein. 4. Mitteilung: Verteilung und Dynamik im Blut. *Wien. tierärztl. Mschr.* **59,** 209–11.

LeResche R.E., Seal U.S., Karns P.D. & Franzmann A.W. (1974) A review of blood chemistry of moose and other cervidae with emphasis on nutritional assessment. *Naturaliste can.* **101,** 263–90.

Lessard J.L. & Taketa F. (1969) Multiple haemoglobins in foetal, newborn and adult cats. *Biochim. biophys. Acta.* **175,** 441–4.

Lewis E.F. & Holman H.H. (1951) Haemophilia in a St Bernard dog. *Vet. Rec.* **63,** 666.

Lewis I.N. & McLean J.G. (1975) Physiological variations in levels of 2,3-diphosphoglycerate in horse erythrocytes. *Res. vet. Sci.* **18,** 186–9.

Lewis P.A. & Shope R.E. (1929) The study of the cells of the blood as an aid to the diagnosis of hog cholera. *J. Am. vet. med. Ass.* **74,** 145–52.

Lewis R.M. (1965) Clinical evaluation of the lupus erythematosus cell phenomenon in dogs. *J. Am. vet. med. Ass.* **147,** 939.

Lewis R.M., Henry W.B. Jr., Thornton G.W. & Gilmore C.E. (1963) A syndrome of autoimmune hemolytic anemia and thrombocytopenia in dogs. *Scientific Proceedings*, 100th *Meeting American Veterinary Medical Association* **1,** 140.

Lewis R.M. & Schwartz R.S. (1971) Canine systemic lupus erythematosus—genetic analysis of an established breeding colony. *J. exp. Med.* **134,** 417–38.

Lewis R.M., Schwartz R.S. & Gilmore C.E. (1965a) Autoimmune diseases in domestic animals. *Ann. N.Y. Acad. Sci.* **124,** 178.

Lewis R.M., Schwartz R. & Henry W.B. (1965b) Canine systemic lupus erythematosus. *Blood* **25,** 143–60.

Lewis S.M. (1971) Aplastic anaemia. *Br. J. Hosp. Med.* **6,** 593–604.

Lewis S.M., Osborn J.S. & Stuart P.R. (1968) Demonstration of an internal structure within the red blood cell by ion etching and scanning electron microscopy. *Nature* **220,** 614–6.

Lewis S.M., Szur L. & Hoffbrand A.V. (1972) Thrombocythaemia. *Clin. Haematol.* **1,** 339–57.

Lewis S.M. & Verwilghen R.L. (1973) Dyserythropoiesis and dyserythropoietic anemias. *Prog. Hemat.* **8,** 99–129.

Lewis S.M. & Verwilghen R.L. (1977) *Dyserythropoiesis.* Academic Press, London.

Lichtman (Ed.) (1975) Granulocyte and monocyte abnormalities. *Clin. Haematol.* **4,** 483–725.

Lie H. (1966) The Complexity of Platelet Antigens in Pig. *Xth European conference on animal blood groups and biochemical polymorphisms, Paris.* pp. 181–4. Institut National de la Recherche Agronomique.

Lie H. (1968) Thrombocytes, leucocytes and packed red cell volume in piglets during the first two weeks of life. *Acta. vet. scand.* **9,** 105–11.

Liegeois A. & Monaco A.P. (1973) Une nouvelle technique de préparation de moelle osseuse chez le chien vivant. *Biomed. Express* **19,** 200.

Lima E. Garcia de & Mitscherlich E. (1973) Studies on the number of B and T lymphocytes in the circulating blood of healthy leucosis suspected and leucosis affected cattle of the German black and white breed. *Zentbl. VetMed.* **B20,** 665–84.

Lindblad G. & Bäckgren A.W. (1964) Megakaryocytes, thrombocytes and blood clotting time in dogs with experimental hepatitis contagiosa canis. *Acta vet. scand.* **5,** 370.

Lindsay S., Chaikoff I.L. & Gilmore J.W. (1952) Arteriosclerosis in the dog. I. Spontaneous lesions in the aorta and coronary arteries. *Archs Path.* **53,** 281.

Link K.P. (1944) The anticoagulant from spoiled sweet clover hay. *Harvey Lectures* **39,** 162. The Science Press Printing Co., Lancaster, Pennsylvania, USA.

Link R.P. (1970) Toxic plants, rodenticides, herbicides, lead and yellow fat diseases. In: Dunne H.W. (Ed.) *Diseases of swine*, 3rd Ed, pp. 780–98. Iowa State Univ. Press, Ames.

LINKLATER K.A. (1968) Iso-immunisation in the Parturient Sow by Foetal Red Cells. *Vet. Rec.* **83**, 203–4.

LINKLATER K.A. (1971) A study of some blood cellular antigenic factors and iso-immunisation in the pig, p. 153. Thesis, Edinburgh.

LINKLATER K.A. & MCTAGGART H.S. (1971) Unpublished data.

LINKLATER K.A. & MCTAGGART H.S. (1972) Unpublished data.

LINKLATER K.A., MCTAGGART H.S. & IMLAH P. (1973) Haemolytic disease of the newborn, thrombocytopenic purpura and neutropenia occurring concurrently in a litter of piglets. *Br. vet. J.* **129**, 36–46.

LINKLATER K.A. & IMLAH P. (1974b) Serological techniques for the detection of antibodies to porcine thrombocytes. 2. The complement fixation and anti-globulin consumption techniques. *Anim. Blood Grps biochem. Genet.* **5**, 41–52.

LITTLE W. (1974) An effect of the stage of lactation on the concentration of albumin in the serum of dairy cattle. *Res. vet. Sci.* **17**, 193–9.

LITTLEJOHN A. (1968) PCV, Hb and plasma electrolyte studies in horses. 1. Mean values in clinically normal horses. *Br. vet. J.* **124**, 529–39.

LITTLEJOHNS I.R. (1960) Eperythrozoonosis in sheep. *Aust. vet. J.* **36**, 260–5.

LIU S.K. & CARB A.V. (1968) Erythroblastic leukemia in a dog. *J. Am. vet. med. Ass.* **152**, 1511–6.

LOBUE J. & GORDON A.S. (1967) (Ed.) Dynamics of hematopoiesis. *Semin. Hematol.* **4**, 289–461.

LOEB W. (1969) Diseases of the blood. In: Medway W., Prier J.E. & Wilkinson J.S. (Eds) *A textbook of veterinary clinical pathology*, p. 316. Williams & Wilkins, Baltimore, USA.

LOEB W.F. (1972) Blood and blood-forming organs. In: Catcott E.J. & Smithcors J.F. (Eds) *Equine medicine and surgery*, 2nd Edn, pp. 349–57. American Veterinary Publications, Illinois.

LOEB W.F. & MACKEY B. (1973) A com-parative study of platelet aggregation in Primates. *J. med. Primat.* **2**, 195.

LÖLIGER C.H. & SCHUBERT H.J. (1967) Der Hämatokritwert von gesunden und kranken Hühnen verschiedener Alters-gruppen und sein diagnosticher Anwend-ungsbereich. *Berl. Münch. tierärztl. Wschr* **80**, 171–6.

LOOSMORE R.M., HARDING J.D.J. & LEWIS G. (1967) Mercury poisoning in pigs. *Vet. Rec.* **81**, 268–9.

LORAND L. (1964) Assays for the fibrin stabilizing factor (FSF). In: Tocantins L.M. & Kazal L.A. (Eds) *Blood coagula-tion, hemorrhage and thrombosis*, p. 239. Grune & Stratton, New York.

LORD G.H., TODD A.C. & KABAT C. (1954) The blood picture of the muskrat under pentobarbital sodium. *Am. J. vet. Res.* **15**, 79–81.

LORTHIOIR F. (1968) Iconographie des cellules sanguines du chien normal. *Cah. Méd. vét.* **37**, 159.

LOTZ F., CRANE S. & DOWNIE H.G. (1972) A study of a specific congenital platelet functional abnormality in dogs. *Pro-ceedings of 3rd Congress of Int. Soc. on thrombosis and haemostasis*, Abstr. p. 220. Washington D.C.

LOZZIO B.B. (1973) Regulators of cell division. *Exp. Hemat.* **1**, 309–39.

LUCAS A.M. (1959) A discussion of synonymy in avian and mammalian hematological nomenclature. *Am. J. vet. Res.* **20**, 887–97.

LUCAS A.M. & JAMROZ C. (1961) *Atlas of avian haematology*. Agriculture Mono-graph No. 25. Washington, U.S. Dept. of Agriculture.

LUDWIG H.J. (1956) Das Blutbild trans-portmüder Schweine. Inaug. Diss., Berlin.

LUECKE R.W., HOEFER J.A., BRAMMEL W.S & SCHMIDT D.A. (1957) Calcium and zinc in parakeratosis of swine. *J. Anim. Sci.* 16, 3–11.

LUGINBÜHL H. & DETWEILER D.K. (1965) Cardiovascular lesions in dogs. *Ann. N.Y. Acad. Sci.* **127**, 517.

LUKE D. (1953b) The effect of adrenocorti-cotrophic hormone and adrenal cortical extract on the differential white cell count in the pig. *Br. vet. J.* **109**, 434–6.

LUKE D. (1953a) The reaction of the white blood cells at parturition in the sow. *Br. vet. J.*, **109**, 241–4.

LUND J.F. (1974) Hemoglobin crystals in canine blood. *Am. J. vet. Res.* **35**, 575.

LUND J.E. & AVOLT M.D. (1972) Erythrocyte aplasia in a dog. *J. Am. vet. med. Ass.* **160**, 1500–3.

LUNDEVALL J. (1958) Serological studies of human blood platelets. Thesis. *Scand. J. clin. Lab. Invest.* **10** (suppl.).

LYUBASHENKO S.Y. & NOVIKOVA L.S. (1947) Equine Leptospirosis. *Veterinariya* **24**, 11–15.

MACARTHUR F.X. (1950) Simplified heart puncture in poultry diagnosis. *J. Am. vet. med. Ass.* **116**, 38–9.

MCARTHUR W.P., CARSWELL E.A. & THORBECKE G.J. (1972) Brief communication: growth of Rous sarcomas in bursectomized chickens. *J. natn. Cancer Inst.* **49**, 907–9.

MCCANDLESS E.L. & DYE J.A. (1950) Physiological changes in intermediary metabolism of various species of ruminants incident to functional development of rumen. *Am. J. Physiol.* **162**, 434–46.

MCCARTHY K. & TOSOLINI F.A. (1975) A review of primate herpes viruses. *Proc. R., Soc. Med.* **68**, 145.

MCCARTNEY M.G. (1952) Total blood and corpuscular volume in turkey hens. *Poult. Sci.* **31**, 184–5.

MCCLELLAN R.O., VOGT G.S. & RAGAN H.A. (1966) Age-related changes in hematological and serum biochemical parameters in miniature swine. In: Bustad L.K., McClellan R.O. & Burns M.P. (Eds) *Swine in biochemical research*, pp. 597–610. Battell-Northwest, Richland, Washington.

MCCLUGAGE S.G., MCCLUSKEY R.S. & MEINEKE H.A. (1971) Microscopy of living bone marrow in situ. II. Influence of the microenvironment on hemopoiesis. *Blood* **38**, 96–107.

MCCULLOCH E.C. & MURER H.K. (1939) Sodium chlorate poisoning. *J. Am. vet. med. Ass.* **95**, 675–82.

MCDERMID E.M., AGAR N.S. & CHAI C.K.

(1975) Electrophoretic variation in red cell enzyme systems. *Anim. Blood Grps biochem. Genet.* **6**, 127–74.

MCDONALD G.A., DODDS T.C. & CRUICKSHANK B. (1968) *Atlas of haematology*, 2nd Edn. Edinburgh, Livingstone.

MCDONALD G.A., DODDS T.C. & CRUICKSHANK B. (1970) *Atlas of haematology*, 3rd Edn. Churchill Livingstone, Edinburgh and London.

MCDOUGALL E.I. & LOWE V.P.W. (1968) Transferrin polymorphism and serum proteins of some British deer. *J. Zool.* **155**, 131–40.

MCEWAN E.H. (1968) Hematological studies of barren-ground caribou. *Can. J. Zool.* **46**, 1031–6.

MCEWAN E.H. & WHITEHEAD P.E. (1969) Changes in the blood constituents of reindeer and caribous occurring with age. *Can. J. Zool.* **47**, 557–62.

MACEWEN E.G., DRAZNER F.H., MCCLELLAND A.J. & WILKINS R.J. (1975) Treatment of basophilic leukemia in a dog. *J. Am. vet. med. Ass.* **166**, 376–80.

MACFARLANE R.G. (1939) A simple method for measuring clot retraction. *Lancet*, **1**, 1199–201.

MACFARLANE R.G. (1972) Haemostasis. In: Biggs R. (Ed.) *Human blood coagulation, haemostasis and thrombosis*, p. 543. Blackwell Scientific Publications, Oxford.

MACFARLANE R.G. & ASH R.J. (1964) The activation and consumption of factor X in recalcified plasma. The effect of added factor VIII and Russell's viper venom. *Brit. J. Haemat.* **10**, 217.

MCFEE, A.F., KNIGHT M. & BANNER M.W. (1966) An intersex pig with XX/XY leucocyte mosaicism. *Can. J. genet. Cytol.* **8**, 502–5.

MCFEELY R.A. & HARE W.C.D. (1966) Cytogenic studies of the domestic pig. In: Bustad L.K., McClellan R.O. & Burns M.P. (Eds) *Swine in biomedical research*, pp. 13–23. Battel-Northwest, Richland, Washington.

MCGAVIN M.D., RANBY P.D. & TAMMEMAGI L. (1962) Demyelination associated with low liver copper levels in pigs. *Aust. vet. J.* **38**, 8–14.

McGrath C.J. (1974) Polycythemia vera in dogs. *J. Am. vet. med. Ass.* **164**, 1117.

McGuire T.C. & Henson J.B. (1968) The diagnosis of equine anemias. *Proc. 14th A. Conv. Am. Ass. equine Pract.* 31–8.

McGuire T.C., Henson J.B. & Quist S.E. (1969) Impaired bone marrow response in equine infectious anemia. *Am. J. vet. Res.* **30**, 2099–104.

McGuire T.C., Poppie M.J. & Banks K.L. (1974) Combined (B- and T-lymphocyte) immunodeficiency: a fatal genetic disease in Arabian foals. *J. Am. vet. med. Ass.* **164**, 70–6.

McKay D.G., Hardaway R.M. III, Wahle G.H., Jr., Edelstein R. & Tartock D.E. (1955) Alterations in blood coagulation mechanism after incompatible blood transfusion. *Am. J. Surg.* **89**, 583.

McKenna P.B., McPherson W.B. & Falconer G.J. (1975) Fatal ancylostomiasis in a dog. *N.Z. vet. J.* **23**, 151.

Mackenzie A. (1959) Studies on lungworm infection of pigs. III. The progressive pathology of experimental infections. *Vet. Rec.* **71**, 209–14.

Mackenzie C.P. (1969) Idiopathic (acquired) haemolytic anaemia in the dog. *Vet. Rec.* **85**, 356–61.

Mackey L.J. (1975) Feline leukaemia virus and its clinical effects in cats. *Vet. Rec.* **96**, 5–11.

Mackey L.J. & Jarrett W.F.H. (1972) Pathogenesis of lymphoid neoplasia in cats and its relationship to immunologic cells pathways. I. Morphologic aspects. *J. natn. Cancer Inst.* **49**, 853–65.

Mackey L.J., Jarrett W.F.H., Jarrett O. & Laird H.M. (1972) An experimental study of virus leukemia in cats. *J. natn. Cancer Inst.* **48**, 1663–70.

Mackey L.J., Jarrett W.F.H., Jarrett O. & Laird H.M. (1975a) Anemia associated with feline leukemia virus infection in cats. *J. natn. Cancer Inst.* **54**, 209–17.

Mackey L.J., Jarrett W.F.H., Jarrett O. & Wilson L. (1975b) B and T cells in a cat with thymic lymphosarcoma. *J. natn. Cancer Inst.* **54**, 1483–7.

Mackey L.J., Jarrett W.F.H. & Lauder I.M. (1975c) Monocytic leukaemia in the dog. *Vet. Rec.* **96**, 27.

Mackey L.J., Jarrett W.F.H. & Coombs R.R.A. (1975d) Two populations of lymphocytes in the cat. *Vet. Rec.* **96**, 41.

McKinna W.R. (1936) Haemophilia. *Vet. J.* **92**, 370.

MacKinney A.A. & Cline W.S. (1974) Annotation: Infectious mononucleosis. *Br. J. Haemat.* **27**, 367–72.

MacLean C.W. (1968) The thin sow problem. *Vet. Rec.* **83**, 308–16.

MacLeod J., Ponder E., Aitken G.J. & Brown R.B. (1947) The blood picture of the Thoroughbred horse. *Cornell Vet.* **37**, 305–13.

Macmillan D.C. & Sim A.K. (1970) A comparative study of platelet aggregation in man and laboratory animals. *Thromb. Diath. haemorrh.* **24**, 385–94.

McNary W.F. (1958) A new diluting fluid for eosiniphils, using bromocresol purple. *Am. J. clin. Path.* **30**, 373–4.

McPherson E.A. (1975) Personal communication.

MacRae E.K. & Spitznagel J.K. (1975) Ultrastructural localization of cationic proteins in cytoplasmic granules of chicken and rabbit polymorphonuclear leukocytes. *J. cell Sci.* **17**, 79–94.

McSherry B.J., Roe C.K. & Milne F.J. (1966) The hematology of phenothiazine poisoning in horses. *Can. vet. J.* **7**, 3–12.

McTaggart H.S. (1975) Lymphocytosis in normal young pigs. *Br. vet. J.* **131**, 574–9.

McTaggart H.S. (1976) Unpublished data.

McTaggart H.S. & Rowntree P.G.M. (1969) The haematology of 'minimal disease' bacon pigs: a comparison with genetically-related conventionally-reared pigs. *Br. vet. J.* **125**, 240–7.

Maegraith B., Gilles H.M. & Devakul K. (1957) Pathological processes in *Babesia canis* infections. *Z. Tropenmed. Parasit.* **8**, 485.

Magath T.B. & Higgins G.M. (1934) The blood of the normal duck. *Folia haemat.* **51**, 230–41.

MALASEZ. Quoted by Sturkie (1965).

MALHERBE W.D. (1969) Blood Parasites. In: Medway W., Prier J.E. & Wilkinson J.S. (Eds) *A Textbook of Veterinary Clinical Pathology*, p. 352. Williams & Wilkins, Baltimore, USA.

MALHERBE W.D. (1970) A clinico-pathological study of bilharziasis in sheep. *Onderstepoort J. vet. Res.* **37**, 37–44.

MALIK J.K., CHAND N., SINGH R.V., SINGH P.P., BAGHA H.S. & SUD S.C. (1974) Haematology of male buffalo calves. *Indian vet. J.* **51**, 95–9.

MALIK K.S. & GAUTAM O.P. (1971) Haemoglobinuria in buffaloes. *Haryana agric. Univ. J. Res.* **1**, 109–13.

MALONEY M.A., LUND J.E. & PATT H.M. (1974) Modification of canine cyclic hematopoiesis by endotoxin. *Proc. Soc. exp. Biol. Med.* **147**, 205.

MALONEY M.A., WEBER C.L. & PATT H.M. (1963) Ineffective granulopoiesis. *Nature* **197**, 150–2.

MAMMERICKX M. (1971a) Enquete sur la leucose bovine dans le cheptel de la commune d'Eynatten. *An. Méd. Vét.* **115**, 41–53.

MAMMERICKX M. (1971b) Sur l'utilisation des clés pour le diagnostic de la leucose bovine. *An. Méd. Vét.* **115**, 111–8.

MANDEL E.E. & GERHOLD W.M. (1969) Plasma fibrin-stabilizing factor: acquired deficiency in various disorders. *Am. J. clin. Path.* **52**, 547.

MANN F.D. & HURN M. (1952) Species specificity of thromboplastin. *Proc. Soc. exp. Biol. Med.* **79**, 19.

MÄNNEL K. (1966) A haematological study of the Black Australorp in relation to certain economic characteristics. II. Haemoglobin. *S. Afr. J. agric. Sci.* **9**, 835–48.

MÄNNEL K. (1967) A haematological study of the Black Australorp in relation to certain economic characteristic. III. Number of erythrocytes. *S. Afr. J. agric. Sci.* **10**, 19–30.

MANSTON R., RUSSELL A.M., DEW S.M. & PAYNE J.M. (1975) The influence of dietary protein upon blood composition in dairy cows. *Vet. Rec.* **96**, 497–502.

MANWELL C., BAKER C.M.A., ROSKLANSKY J.D. & FOGHT M. (1963) Molecular genetics of avian proteins. II. Control genes and structural genes for embryonic and adult haemoglobin. *Proc. natn. Acad. Sci. USA.* **49**, 496–503.

MANYAN D.R., ARIMURA G.K. & YUNIS A.A. (1972) Chloramphenicol induced erythroid suppression and bone marrow ferrochelatase activity in dogs. *J. Lab. clin. Med.* **79**, 137.

MARCH B.E., COATES V. & BIELY J. (1966) The effects of estrogen and androgen on the osmotic fragility and fatty acid composition of erythrocytes in the chicken. *Can. J. Physiol. Pharmac.* **44**, 379–87.

MARCILESE N.A., FIGUEIRAS H.D., KREMENCHUZKY S., VALSECCHI R.M., CAMBEROS H.R. & VARELA J.E. (1966) Red cell survival time in the horse, determined with D1-150 propyl-phosphoro-fluoridate P32. *Am. J. Physiol,* **211**, 281–2.

MARGOLIS J. (1957) Initiation of blood coagulation by glass and related surfaces. *J. Physiol.* **137**, 95.

MARGOLIS J. (1958) Activation of plasma by contact with glass: evidence for a common reaction which releases plasma kinin and initiates coagulation. *J. Physiol.* **144**, 1.

MARKS J., BAILEY N.T.J. & GUNZ F.W. (1950) A mechanical aid in making blood films. *J. clin. Path.* **3**, 168–74.

MARKSON L.M. (1975) Bovine leukosis. Personal communication.

MARMIENÉ I. (1972) Kai kurie Europinių stirnu (*Capreolus capreolus* L.) kraujo biocheminiai morfologiniai rodikliai įvairiame amžiuje. *Liet. vet. Akad. Darbai* **10**, 87–92.

MARMIENÉ I. & MARMA B. (1972) Tauriųjų elnių (*Cervus elaphus* L.) kraujo ir hemoglobino kiekiai bei kraujo serumo baltymų spektras. *Liet. vet. Akad. Darbai* **10**, 93–9.

MARQUARDT W.W. (1972) Radial immunodiffusion: a simple and rapid method for detection of Marek's disease antigen. *Appl. Microbiol.* **23**, 942–5.

MARQUARDT W.W. & NEWMAN J.A. (1972) A modified direct complement-fixation test for detection of Marek's disease antibodies in chicken serum. *Avian Dis.* **16**, 986–96.

MARSH G.W. & LEWIS S.M. (1969) Cardiac hemolytic anemia *Semin. Hematol.* **6**, 133–49.

MARSHAK R. & ABT D.A. (1967) The epidemiology of bovine leukosis. *Proc. 3rd int. Symp. comp. Leukemia Res.*, pp. 166–182. Paris 1967. Bibl. haemat., No. 31. Karger, Basel/New York (1968).

MARSTON H.R. (1952) Cobalt, copper and molybdenum in the nutrition of animals and plants. *Physiol. Rev.* **32**, 66–121.

MARTIN J.E., SKILLEN R.G. & DEUBLER J. (1954) The action of adrenocortico-tropic hormone on circulating eosinophils in dogs. *Am. J. vet. Res.* **15**, 489–94.

MARTINOVICH D. & WOODHOUSE D.A (1971) Post parturient haemoglobinuria in cattle. A Heinz body haemolytic anaemia. *N.Z. vet. J.* **19**, 259–63.

MASON R.G. & READ M.S. (1967) Platelet response to six agglutinating agents: species similarities and differences. *Exp. mol. Pathol.* **6**, 370.

MASON R.G. & READ M.S. (1971) Some species differences in fibrinolysis and blood coagulation. *J. Biomed. Mater. Res.* **5**, 121.

MASTRANGELO P. (1971) Study of blood cell haemoglobin concentration in domestic animals. Note 5. Buffaloes. *Acta med. vet.*, Napoli **17**, 115–21.

MATHEWS P.J. (1968) *Blood physiology of white-tailed deer on varying planes of nutrition.* M.Sc. Thesis, Louisiana State University.

MATTHEEUWS D., DE RICK A., THOONEN H. & VAN DER STOCK J. (1974) Intestinal lymphangiectasia in a dog. *J. small Anim. Pract.* **15**, 757.

MAUGHAN E. & WILLIAMS J.R.B. (1967) Haemoglobin types in deer. *Nature (London)* **215**, 404–5.

MAUK A.G., WHELAN H.T., PUTZ G.R. & TAKETA F. (1974) Anaemia in domestic cats: effect on haemoglobin components and whole blood oxygenation. *Science* **185**, 447–9.

MAXFIELD M.E., STOPPS G.J., BARNES J.R., SNEE D. & AZAR A. (1972) Effect of lead on blood regeneration following acute haemorrhage in dogs. *Amer. ind. Hyg. Ass. J.* **33**, 326.

MAXWELL M.H. (1973) Comparison of heterophil and basophil ultrastructure in six species of domestic birds. *J. Anat.* **115**, 187–202.

MAXWELL M.H. (1974) An ultrastructural comparison of the mononuclear leuco-cytes and thrombocytes in six species of domestic bird. *J. Anat.* **117**, 69–80.

MAXWELL M.H. & SILLER W.G. (1972) The ultrastructural characteristics of the eosinophil granules in six species of domestic bird. *J. Anat.* **112**, 289–303.

MAXWELL M.H. & TREJO F. (1970) The ultrastructure of white blood cells and thrombocytes of the domestic fowl. *Br. vet. J.* **126**, 583–92.

MAZURENKO N.P., MEREKALOVA Z.I., YAKOVLEVA L.S., STEPINA V.N., VINOGRADOV V.M., CHERNYAKHOVSKAYA I. YU., GUNENKOVA N.K. & PAVLOVSKAYA A.L. (1972) Study of Marek's lymphoma. 1. Virus isolation and some immuno-logical and pathomorphological studies. *Vest. Akad. med. Nauk. SSSR* **27**, 11–20.

MEADS E.B., TAYLOR P.A. & PALLISTER W.A. (1964) An unusual outbreak of sweet clover poisoning in cattle. *Can. vet. J.* **5**, 65–71.

MEARS D.C., SHEIL A.G.R. & BARNETT A.L. (1969) Preparation of canine anti-A serum. *Aust. vet. J.* **45**, 13–4.

MEDEIROS L.O., FERRI S., REINER U.R. & ARATANGY L.R. (1973) Changes in leucocyte distribution associated with age in Thoroughbred horses. *Zentbl. VetMed.* **2**, 166–71.

MEDWAY W. (1969) The pancreas and its disease. In: Medway W., Prier J.E. & Wilkinson J.S. (Eds) *A textbook of veterinary clinical pathology*, p. 86. Williams & Wilkins, Baltimore, USA.

MEDWAY W. & KARE M.R. (1959) Blood and plasma volume, hematocrit, blood specific gravity and serum protein electrophoresis of the chicken. *Poult. Sci.* **38**, 624–31.

MEDWAY W. & RAPP J.P. (1962) A case of granulocytic leukemia with thrombo-cytopenic purpura in a dog. *Cornell Vet.* **52**, 247–60.

MEDWAY W., SCHRYVER H.F. & BELL B. (1966) Clinical jaundice in a dolphin. *J. Am. vet. med. Soc.* **149**, 891–95.

MEHNER A. (1938) Beziehungen zwischen Zellgrösse und Körpergrösse. *Z. Zücht. Reihe B. Tierzüchtung und Züchtungsbiologie* **40**, 1–48. Quoted by Lucas & Jamroz (1961).

MEIER H. (1957) Neoplastic diseases of the hematopoietic system (so-called leukosis-complex) in the dog. *Zentbl. VetMed.* **4**, 633.

MEIER H. & GOURLEY G. (1957) Basophilic (Myelocyte) or Mast Cell Leukemia in a Cat. *J. Am. vet. med. Ass.* **130**, 33–40.

MELANDER Y., HANSEN-MELANDER E., HOLM L. & SOMLEV B. (1971) Seven swine intersexes with XX chromosome constitution. *Hereditas* **69**, 51–7.

MELVEGER B.E., EARL F.L. & VAN LOON E.J. (1969) Sternal bone marrow biopsy in the dog. *Lab. Anim. Care* **19**, 866.

MELVILLE G.S., WHITCOMB W.H. & MARTINEZ R.S. (1967) Haematology of the *Macaca mulatta* monkey. *Lab. Anim. Care* **17**, 189.

MERKENS J. (1938) Haemophilie bij honden. *Ned. Ind. Bladen v. Diergeneesk en Dierent* **50**, 149.

MERTZ E.T. (1942) The anomaly of a normal Duke's and a very prolonged saline bleeding time in swine suffering from an inherited bleeding disease. *Am. J. Physiol.* **136**, 360–2.

METTAM A.E. (1915) A case of lymphosarcoma in the horse: arteriosclerotic changes in heart and lungs. *J. comp. Path.* **28**, 36–43.

MEYER W. (1962) Innenkörperanämie beim Hund. *Mh. VetMed.* **17**, 181.

MEYER L.M. & BLOOM F. (1943) The bone marrow of normal dogs. *Am. J. med. Sci.* **206**, 637.

MEYER J.N. & VERHORST D. (1973) The evidence of erythrocyte acid phosphatase by starch gel electrophoresis in the pig. *Anim. Blood Grps biochem. Genet.* **4**, 129–32.

MICHAELSON S.M., SCHEER K. & GILT S. (1966) The blood of the normal beagle. *J. Am. vet. med. Ass.* **148**, 532–4.

MICHELS N.A. (1938) The mast cells. In: Downey H. (Ed.) *Handbook of hematology*, Vol. 1, pp. 231–372. Haffner Publishing Co., New York. (Reprinted in facsimile 1965.)

MICHNA S.W. & CAMPBELL R.S.F. (1969) Leptospirosis in Pigs: Epidermiology, Microbiology and Pathology. *Vet. Rec.* **84**, 135–8.

MICLAUS I., ESPERSEN G. & HJORTH P. (1973) Plasma protein composition of cattle affected with acute peritonitis. *Nord. VetMed.* **25**, 570–4.

MIGAKI G. (1969) Hematopoietic neoplasms of slaughter animals. In National Cancer Institute Monograph 32 *Comparative morphology of hematopoietic neoplasms*, pp. 121–51. National Cancer Institute, Bethesda, Maryland.

MILICEVIC M., ADDLEMAN A.D., MAYER D.T. & LASLEY J.F. (1960) Breed differences in the number and kinds of leucocytes in blood of swine. *Missouri Bull. agric. exp. Res. Sta.* **731**

MILLER E.R., ULLREY D.E., ACKERMANN I., SCHMIDT D.A., LUECKE R.W. & HOEFER J.A. (1961) Swine hematology from birth to maturity. II. Erythrocyte population, size and hemoglobin concentration. *J. Anim. Sci.* **20**, 890–7.

MILLER J.F.A.P. (1966) Immunity in the foetus and new-born foal. *Br. med. Bull.* **5**, 41–50.

MILLER JANICE M., MILLER L.D., OLSON C. & GILLETTE K.G. (1969) Virus-like particles in phytohemagglutinin-stimulated lymphocyte cultures with reference to bovine lymphosarcoma. *J. natn. Cancer Inst.* **43**, 1297–305.

MILLER R.M. & KIND R.E. (1962) Phenylbutazone toxicity in a dog. *Mod. vet. Pract.* **43** (Aug) 69.

MILLER W.J., HAUGEN A.O. & ROSLIEN D.J. (1965) Natural variation in the blood proteins of white-tailed deer. *J. Wildl. Mgmt* **29**, 717–23.

MILLS D.C.B. (1970) Platelet aggregation and platelet nucleotide concentration in different species. *Symp. zool. Soc. Lond.* No. 27, 99.

MILLS D.C.B. & THOMAS D. (1969) Blood platelet nucleotides in man and other species. *Nature (London)* **222**, 991.

MILLS J.A. & COOPERAND S.R. (1971) Lymphocyte physiology. *A. Rev. Med.* **22,** 185–220.

MILLSON G.C., WEST L.C. & DEW S.M. (1960) Biochemical and hematological observations on the blood and cerebrospinal fluid of clinically healthy and scrapie-affected goats. *J. comp. Path. Ther.* **70,** 194–8.

MIRAND E.A., MURPHY G.P., BENNETT T.P. & GRACE J.T., JR. (1968) Erythroprotein response to repeated hemorrhage in renal allotransplanted, nephrectomized or intact dogs. *Life Sci.,* **7,** pt. I, 689.

MIURA S. & OHSHIMA K. (1967) Monocytic leukaemia in cattle. I. Cytological observations of two cases. *Jap. J. vet. Sci.* **29,** 141–50.

MIYAKE Y.-I. (1973) Cytogenetical studies on swine intersexes. *Jap. J. vet. Res.* **21,** 41–9.

MOBERG R. (1955) The white blood picture in sexually mature female cattle with special reference to sexual conditions. Thesis. Stockholm, Sweden.

MOBERG R. (1965) The blood picture in connection with persistency of follicles in cattle. *Nord. VetMed.* **17,** 232.

MÖLLERBERG L. (1975) A haematologic and blood chemical study of Swedish purchased calves. *Acta vet. scand.* **16,** 170–7.

MÖLLERBERG L. & JACOBSSON S.-O. (1970) Några allmänna synpunkter på järnbristanemi hos kalv. *Svensk. VetTidskr.* **22,** 851–4.

MÖLLERBERG L., EILERS T., JACOBSSON S.O., JOHNSSON S. & OLSSON I. (1975) The effect of parenteral Fe on haematology, health, growth and meat classification in veal calves. *Acta vet. scand.* **16,** 197–204.

MOLLIN D.L. & WATERS A.H. (1971) Vitamin B_{12} and folic acid absorption and metabolism. In: Vetter H. & Belcher E.H. (Eds) *Radioisotopes in medical diagnosis,* pp. 412–36. Butterworth, London.

MOLONEY W.C., MCPHERSON K. & FLIEGELMAN LILA (1960) Esterase activity in leukocytes demonstrated by the use of naphthol AS-D chloracetate substrate. *J. Histochem. Cytochem.* **8,** 200–7.

MONCOL D.J. & BATTE E.G. (1967) Peripheral blood eosinophilia in porcine ascariasis. *Cornell Vet.* **57,** 96–107.

MONKE J.V. & YUILE C.L. (1940) The renal clearance of hemoglobin in the dog. *J. exp. Med.* **72,** 149.

MONTEMAGNO F., AGRESTI A., PERSECHINO A., MASTRANGELO P. & D'AMBROSIO G. (1972) Osservaziono sulle Metodiche di Diagnosi Ematologica nella Linfoleucosi Bovina. *Acta med. vet.* **18,** 227–33.

MOORE J.E. & JAMES G.W. (1953) A simple direct method for absolute basophil leucocyte count. *Proc. Soc. exp. Biol. Med.* **82,** 601–3.

MOOREHEAD P.S., NOWELL P.C., MELLMAN W.J., BATTIPS D.M. & HUNGERFORD D.A. (1960) Chromosome preparations of leucocytes cultured from human peripheral blood. *Expl. Cell Res.* **20,** 613–6.

MORGAN H.C. (1966) The value of erythrocyte sedimentation rate in veterinary medicine. *Vet. Med/Small Anim. Clin.* **61,** 463.

MORGAN H.C. (1967) The effect of helminth parasitism on the hemogram of the dog. *Vet. Med/Small Anim. Clin.* **62,** 218.

MORGAN R.M., GOERTEL J. & SCHIPPER I.A. (1966) Comparative hemograms of Hampshire and Duroc piglets. *SWest. Vet.* **20,** 35–41.

MORLEY A. & BLAKE J. (1975) Observer error in histological assessment of marrow hypocellularity. *J. clin. Path.* **28,** 104.

MORLEY A. & STOHLMAN F. (1969) Erythropoiesis in the dog. The periodic nature of the steady state. *Science* **165,** 1025–8.

MORRIS D. (1965) *The mammals. A guide to the living species.* Hodder and Stoughton.

MORRIS H., RISTIC M. & LYKINS J. (1971) Characterisation of opsonins eluted from erythrocytes of cattle infected with *Anaplasma marginale. Am. J. vet. Res.* **32,** 1221–8.

MORRIS M.L. JR. (1968) Nutrition. In: Catcott E.J. (Ed.) *Canine medicine.* First Catcott Edition, p. 89. American Veterinary Publications Inc., Wheaton, Illinois, USA.

MOULTON J.E. (1961) *Tumours in domestic animals*, pp. 96–7. Univ. of California Press, USA.

MOUWEN J.M.V.M., SCHOTMAN A.T.H., WENSING T. & KIJKUIT C.J. (1972) Some biochemical aspects of white scours in piglets. *Tijdschr Diergeneesk.* **97**, 65–90.

MOYE R.J., WASHBURN K.W. & HUSTON T.M. (1969) Effects of environmental temperature on erythrocyte numbers and size. *Poult. Sci.* **48**, 1683–6.

MROSS G.A. & DOOLITTLE R.F. (1967) Amino acid sequence studies on artiodactyl fibrinopeptides. II. Vicuna, elk, muntjak, pronghorn antelope, and water buffalo. *Archs Biochem. Biophys.* **122**, 674–84.

MUHRER M.E., HOGAN A.G. & BOGART R. (1942) A defect in the coagulation mechanism of swine blood. *Am. J. Physiol.* **136**, 355–9.

MUJOVIC V.M. & FISHER J.W. (1974) The effects of indomethacin on erythropoietin production in dogs following renal artery constriction. 1. The possible role of prostaglandins in the generation of erythropoietin by the kidney. *J. Pharmac. exp. Ther.* **191**, 575.

MUKHERJEE D.P. & BHATTACHARYA P. (1952) Seasonal variations in haemoglobin and cell-volume contents in rams and goats. *Indian J. vet. Sci.* **22**, 191–7.

MÜLLERTZ S. (1953) A plasminogen activator in spontaneously active human blood. *Proc. Soc. exp. Biol. Med.* **82**, 291.

MULLIGAN R.M. (1941) Quantitative studies on the bone marrow of the dog. *Anat. Rec.* **79**, 101.

MULLINS J.C. & RAMSAY W.R. (1959) Haemoglobinuria and anaemia associated with aphosphorosis. *Aust. vet. J.* **35**, 140–7.

MULNIX J.A. & SMITH K.W. (1975) Hyperadrenocorticism in a dog. A case report. *J. small Anim. Pract.* **16**, 193.

MURAYAMA M. (1966) Molecular mechanism of red cell "sickling". *Science, N.Y.* **153**, 145–9.

MURPHY R.C. & SEEGERS W.H. (1948) Concentration of prothrombin and Ac-globulin in various species. *Am. J. Physiol.* **154**, 134.

MUSTARD J.F., ROWSELL H.C., ROBINSON G.A., HOEKSEMA T.D. & DOWNIE H.G. (1960) Canine Haemophilia B (Christmas Disease). *Br. J. Haemat.* **6**, 259–66.

MUSTARD J.F., SECORD D., HOEKSEMA T.D., DOWNIE H.G. & ROWSELL H.C. (1962) Canine factor VII deficiency. *Br. J. Haemat.* **8**, 43–7.

MUTO M., OKI Y. & YAMAMOTO T. (1974) Difference in DNA polymerase activity in lymphoid tumour between avian lymphoid leukosis and Marek's disease. *Natn. Inst. Anim. Hlth Q., Tokyo* **14**, 97–102.

MUTSUMI M. (1974) Influence of adrenocorticotrophic hormone upon the circulating leukocyte count of peripheral blood in pigs. *Natn. Inst. Anim. Hlth Q., Tokyo* **14**, 104.

MYERS L.J., PIERCE K.R., GOWING G.M. & LEONPACKER R.J. (1972) Hemorrhagic diathesis resembling pseudohaemophilia in a dog. *J. Am. vet. med. Ass.* **161**, 1028.

MYLREA P.J. & BYRNE D.T. (1974) An outbreak of acute copper poisoning in calves. *Aust. vet. J.* **50**, 169–72.

NAETS J.P. & HEUSE A. (1964) Effect of anemic hypoxia on erythropoiesis of normal and uremic dogs with or without kidneys. *J. nucl. Med.* **4**, 471.

NAETS J.P. & WITTEK M. (1968) The mechanism of action of androgens on erythropoiesis. *Ann. N.Y. Acad. Sci.*, **149**, 366–76.

NAFSTAD H.J. & NAFSTAD I. (1968) An electron microscopic study of normal blood and bone marrow in pigs. *Path. Vet.* **5**, 451–70.

NAGASAWA S., TAKAHASHI H., KOIDA M., SUZUKI T. & SCHOEMAKERS J.G.G. (1958) Partial purification of bovine plasma kallikreinogen and its activation by the Hageman factor. *Biochem. biophys. Res. Commun.* **32**, 644.

NAIK S.N., BHATIA H.M., BAXI A.J. & NAIK P.V. (1964) Hematological study of Indian spotted deer (axis deer). *J. exp. Zool.* **155**, 231–5.

NAKAHARA M. (1974) Activation of dog

plasma kininogenase with glass. *Biochem. Pharmac.* **23**, 3009.

NAKHMANSON V.M. (1973) Genetic transmission of susceptibility to bovine leucosis. *Veterinariya Moscow* No. 1, 52–4.

NANDAN R., FISHER J.D., TOWERY E.P., BROWN D.R., GANOTE C.E. & JENNINGS R.B. (1975) Effects of dextrothyroxine on hyperlipidemia and experimental athersclerosis in beagle dogs. *Atherosclerosis* **22**, 299.

NATHAN D.G. & BAEHNER R.L. (1971) Disorders of phagocytic cell function. *Prog. Hemat.* **7**, 235–54.

NATT M.P. & HERRICK C.A. (1952) A new blood diluent for counting the erythrocytes and leucocytes of the chicken. *Poult. Sci.* **31**, 735–8.

NAYLOR D.C. (1971) The haematology and histopathology of *Trypanosoma congolense* infection in cattle. *Trop. Anim. Hlth & Prod.* **3**, 95–100, 159–68, 203–7.

NAZERIAN K. (1973) Oncogenesis of Marek's disease. *Cancer Res.* **33**, 1427–30.

NELSON G.S. (1966) The pathology of filarial infections. *Helminth. Abstr.* **35**, 311–36.

NESER C.P. (1923) The blood of equines. *9th & 10th Rep. Vet. Res. Onderstepoort S. Africa.* 479.

NEWELL G.W. & SHAFFNER C.S. (1950) Blood volume determination in chickens. *Poult. Sci.* **29**, 78–87.

NICHOLS B.A. & BAINTON D.F. (1975) Ultrastructure of mononuclear phagocytes. In: van Furth R. (Ed.) *Mononuclear phagocytes in immunity, infection and pathology*, pp. 17–55. Blackwell Scientific Publications, Oxford.

NICHOLS B.A., BAINTON D.F. & FARQUHAR M.G. (1971) Differentiation of monocytes. Origin, nature and fate of their azurophil granules. *J. cell Biol.* **50**, 498–515.

NIEPAGE H. (1974) Über die Brauchbarkeit des mittleren Volumens (MCV), des mittleren Hämoglobingehaltes (MCH) und der mittleren Hämoglobinkonzentration (MCHC) der roten Blutkörperchen zur Kennzeichnung von Erythrocytenpopulationen beim Hund. *Zentbl. Vet-Med. A.* **21**, 173.

NIEPAGE H. (1975) Untersuchungen über die Erythrocytengrösse beim Hund. *Zentbl. VetMed. A.* **22**, 847.

NIEWIAROWSKI S. & PROU-WARTELLE O. (1959) Rôle du facteur contact (facteur Hageman) dans la fibrinolyse. *Thromb. Diath. haemorrh.* **3**, 593.

EK, NILS (1965) Experimental salt poisoning in swine. *Nord. VetMed.* **17**, 604–13.

NIMMS R.M., FERGUSON J.A., WALKER J.L., HILDEBRANDT P.K., HUXSOLL D.L., REARDON M.J., VARLEY J.E., KOLAJA G.J., WATSON W.T., SHROYER E.L., ELWELL P.A. & VACURA G.W. (1971) Epizootiology of tropical canine pancytopenia in south-east Asia. *J. Am. vet. med. Ass.* **158**, 53–63.

NIRMALAN G., NAIR S.G. & SIMON K.J. (1967) Haematology of the Indian elephant (*Elephas maximus*). *Can. J. Physiol. Pharmac.* **45**, 986.

NIRMALAN G.P. & ROBINSON G.A. (1971) Haematology of the Japanese quail (*Coturnix coturnix japonica*). *Br. Poult. Sci.* **12**, 475–81.

NIRMALAN G.P. & ROBINSON G.A. (1973) The survival time of erythrocytes ($DF^{32}P$ label) in the Japanese quail. *Poult. Sci.* **52**, 355–9.

NIZET A. & ROBSCHEIT-ROBBINS F.S. (1950) Reticulocyte ripening in experimental anemia and hypoproteinemia. Effect of amino acids *in vitro*. *Blood* **5**, 648–59.

NORDSTOGA K. (1965) Thrombocytopenic purpura in baby pigs caused by maternal isoimmunisation. *Pathol. vet.* **2**, 601–10.

NORMAN P.S. (1958) Studies on the plasmin system. II. Inhibition of plasmin by serum or plasma. *J. exp. Med.* **108**, 53.

NOSSEL H.L., ARCHER R.K. & McFARLANE R.G. (1962) Equine haemophilia: Report of a case and its response to multiple infusions of heterospecific AHG. *Br. J. Haemat.* **8**, 335–42.

NOSSEL H. (1964) *The contact phase of blood coagulation*. Blackwell Scientific Publications, Oxford.

NOSSEL H. (1972) In: Biggs R. (Ed.) *Human blood coagulation, haemostasis and thrombosis*. Blackwell Scientific Publications, Oxford.

NOSSEL H., LANZKOWSKY P., LEVY S.,

MIBASHAN R.S. & HANSEN J. (1966) A study of coagulation factor levels in women during labour and in their newborn infants. *Thromb. Diath. haemorrh.* **16**, 185.

NOYES W.D., KITCHEN H. & TAYLOR W.J. (1966) Red cell life span of white-tailed deer *Odocoileus virginianus*. *Comp. Biochem. Physiol.* **19**, 471–3.

NURDEN A.T. (1974) Observations on platelet macroglycopeptide. *Nature (London)* **251**, 151–3.

NURDEN A.T. (1976) Personal communication.

OBARA J. & NAKAJIMA H. (1961) Iron metabolism in equine infectious anemia. *Bull. natn. Inst. Anim. Hlth, Tokyo* **41**, 45–55.

O'BRIEN J.R. (1968) Effects of salicilates on human platelets. *Lancet* **i**, 779.

O'BRIEN J.R. (1972) (Ed.) Platelet disorders. *Clin. Haematol.* **1**, 231–444.

OCHIAI T. & ENOKI Y. (1975) Oxygen transport and phosphorylated glycolytic intermediates of the ruminant blood. I. Sika deer (*Cervus nippon nippon*). *Comp. Biochem. Physiol.* **51A**, 21–6.

OGSTON D., OGSTON C.M., RATNOFF O.D. & FORBES C. (1969) Studies of a complex mechanism for the activation of plasminogen by kaolin and by chloroform: the participation of Hageman factor and additional cofactors. *J. clin. Invest.* **48**, 1786.

OKADA K. & FUJIMOTO Y. (1971) Pathological studies of Marek's disease. II. Electron microscopic observations of the cellular lesions in the peripheral nerves. *Jap. J. vet. Res.* **19**, 64–72.

O'KELLY J.C. (1974) Leucocyte values in 1-6-day-old calves of *Bos indicus* crossbred and *Bos taurus* in a tropical environment. *Aust. J. Biol. Sci.* **27**, 133–6.

OLSEN R.E. (1966) Determination of erythrocyte sedimentation rate of cattle. *J. Am. vet. med. Ass.* **148**, 801–3.

OLSON C. (1937) Variations in the cells and hemoglobin content in the blood of the normal domestic chicken. *Cornell Vet.* **27**, 235–63.

OLSON C. (1959) Avian hematology. In: Biester H.E. & Schwarte L.H. (Eds) *Diseases of poultry*, 4th Edn, pp. 53–69. The Iowa State University Press, Ames, Iowa.

OLSON C., COOK R.H. & BLORE I.C. (1950) The reaction of blood cells in experimental Listeriosis of sheep. *Am. J. vet. Res.* **11**, 29–40.

OLSON C., HOSS H.E., MILLER J.M. & BAUMGARTENER L.E. (1973) Evidence of bovine C-type (leukaemia) virus in dairy cattle. *J. Am. vet. med. Ass.* **163**, 355–7.

OLSON C., MILLER L.D., MILLER J.M. & HOSS H.E. (1972) Transmission of lymphosarcoma from cattle to sheep. *J. natn. Cancer Inst.* **45**, 1463–7.

ONIONS D.E. (1975) B- and T-cells in canine lymphosarcoma. *Vet. Rec.* **97**, 108.

ORSTADIUS K., WRETLIND B., LINDBERG P., NORDSTRÖM G. & LANNEK N. (1959) Plasma-transminase and transferase activities in pigs affected with muscular and liver dystrophy. *Zentbl. VetMed.* **6**, 971–80.

OSBALDISTON G.W. (1971) Erythrocyte sedimentation rate. Studies in sheep, dog and horse. *Cornell Vet.* **61**, 386–99.

OSBALDISTON G.W., COFFMAN J.R. & STOWE E.C. (1969) Equine isoerythrolysis—clinical pathological observations and transfusion of dam's red blood cells to her foal. *Can. J. comp. Med.* **33**, 310–5.

OSBALDISTON G.W., COFFMAN J.R. & KRUCKENBERG J.M. (1970) Biochemical differentiation of equine anemias. *J. Am. vet. med. Ass.* **157**, 322–5.

OSBALDISTON G.W. & HOFFMAN M.W. (1971) Blood coagulation values in normal sheep and in two mutant strains with hyperbilirubinemia. *Can. J. comp. Med.* **35**, 150–4.

OSBALDISTON G.W. & JOHNSON J.H. (1972) Effect of ACTH and selected glucocorticoids on circulating blood cells in horses. *J. Am. vet. med. Ass.* **161**, 53–6.

OSBALDISTON G.W., STOWE E.C. & GRIFFITH P.R. (1970) Blood coagulation. Comparative studies in dogs, cats, horses and cattle. *Br. vet. J.* **126**, 512–21.

OSBORNE C.A., PERMAN V., SAULTER J.H., STEVENS J.B. & HANLON G.F. (1968)

Multiple myeloma in the dog. *J. Am. vet. med. Ass.* **153**, 1300–19.

OSBURN B.I. & GLENN B.L. (1968) Acquired Pelger-Huët anomaly in cattle. *J. Am. vet. med. Ass.* **152**, 11–16.

OSCULATI F. (1970) Fine structural localization of acid phosphatase and arylsulfatase in the chick heterophil leucocytes. *Z. Zellforsch. mikrosk. Anat.* **109**, 398–406.

OSEBOLD J.W., CHRISTENSEN J.F., LONGHURST W.M. & ROSENS M.N. (1959) Latent *Anaplasma marginale* infection in wild deer demonstrated by calf innoculation. *Cornell Vet.* **49**, 97–115.

OSHIRO L., TAYLOR D.O.N., RIGGS J.L. & LENNETTE E.H. (1972) Replication of feline C-type virus at the plasma membrane of erythrocytes. *J. natn. Cancer Inst.* **48**, 1419–24.

OSWEILER G.D. (1968) Perirenal oedema (Amaranthus retroflexus poisoning). In: Dunne H.W. (Ed.) *Diseases of swine*, pp. 799–804. Iowa State University Press, Ames, Iowa, USA.

OSWEILER G.D., PRANKRATZ D.C., PRASSE K.W., STAHR H.M. & BUCK W.B. (1970) Porcine hemorrhagic disease. *Mod. vet. Pract.* **51**, 35–7.

OTTESEN J. (1948) Life span of red and white blood corpuscles of the hen. *Nature* **162**, 730–1.

OU D., MAHAFFEY E. & SMITH J.E. (1975) Effect of storage on oxygen dissociation of canine blood. *J. Am. vet. med. Ass.* **167**, 56.

OUDIN J. (1960) Allotyping of rabbit serum proteins. 1. Immunochemical analysis leading to the individualization of seven main allotypes. *J. exp. Med.* **112**, 107–42.

ØVERAS J. (1969) Studies on Eperythrozoon ovis infection in sheep. *Acta vet. scand. (Suppl.)* **28**.

OWEN C.A. JR., COOPER H.A. & BOWIE E.J.W. (1971) Increased fibrinolytic split products in normal dog serum. *Proc. Soc. exp. Biol. med.* **138**, 1073.

OWEN C.A. JR., BOWIE E.J.W. & COOPER H.A. (1973) Turnover of fibrinogen and platelets in dogs undergoing induced intravascular coagulation. *Thromb. Res.* **2**, 251.

OWEN C.A. JR., BOWIE E.J.W., ZOLLMAN

P.E., FASS D.D. & GORDON H. (1974) Carrier of procine von Willebrand's disease. *Am. J. vet. Res.* **35**, 245–8.

OWEN L.N. (1973) Transplantation of canine lymphocytic leukaemia. *Bibl. Haemat.* **39**, 139.

OWEN L.N., BOSTOCK D.E., BETTON G.R., ONIONS D.E., HOLMES J., YOXALL A. & GORMAN N. (1975) The role of spontaneous canine tumours in the evaluation of the aetiology and therapy of human cancer. *J. small Anim. Pract.* **16**, 155.

OWEN N.C., NEETHLING L.P. & TERBLANCHE H.M. (1971) Gyanocobalamin (Vitamin B12) absorption in normal and Haemonchus contortus infested sheep. *Jl S. Afr. vet. med. Ass.* **42**, 15–17.

OWEN R. AP.R. & HOLMES P.H. (1972) An assessment of the viability of canine blood stored under normal veterinary hospital conditions. *Vet. Rec.* **90**, 231.

OWREN P.A. (1947) The coagulation of blood. Investigations on a new clotting factor. *Acta med. scand.* Suppl. 194.

OWREN P.A. (1959b) Thrombotest: a new method for controlling anticoagulant therapy. *Lancet* **ii**, 754.

OWREN P.A. (1959a) The diagnostic and prognostic significance of plasma prothrombin and factor V levels in parenchymatous hepatitis and obstructive jaundice. *J. Lab. clin. Invest.* **1**, 131.

OXNARD C.E., SMITH W.T. & TORRES L.N. (1968) Peripheral neuropathy and hypovitaminosis B_{12} in captive monkeys. *Proc. 2nd Int. Congr. Primatol.* Atlanta Ga. **3**, 162. Karger, New York (1969).

PAAPE M.J., CARROL D.W., KRAL A.J., MILLER R.H. & DESJARDINS CLAUDE (1974) Corticosteroid, circulating leukocytes and erythrocytes in cattle. Diurnal changes and effects of bacteriologic status, stage of lactation and milk yield on response to adrenocorticotropin. *Am. J. vet. Res.* **35**, 355–62.

PAAPE M.J., SCHULTZE W.D., MILLER R.H. & SMITH J.W. (1973) Thermal stress and circulating erythrocytes, leucocytes and milk somatic cells. *J. Dairy Sci.* **56**, 84–91.

PACKER R.A. & SMITH D.A. (1968)

Spirochetal Diseases. In: Catcott E.J. (Ed.) *Canine medicine*. First Catcott edition, p. 158. American Veterinary Publications Inc., Wheaton, Illinois, USA.

PACKHAM M.A., WARRIOR E.S., GLYNN M.F., SENYI A.S. & MUSTARD J.F. (1967) Alteration of the response of platelets to surface stimuli by pyrazole compounds. *J. exp. Med.* **126**, 171–88.

PADGETT G.A. (1968) The Chediak–Higashi syndrome. *Adv. vet. Sci.* **12**, 239–84.

PADGETT G.A., LEADER R.W., GORHAM J.R. & O'MARY C.C. (1964) The familial occurrence of Chediak–Higashi syndrome in mink and cattle. *Genetics* **49**, 505–12.

PALMER C.C. (1917) Effects of muscular exercise and heat on the blood and body temperatures of normal pigs. *J. agric. Res.* **9**, 167–82.

PALMER L.S. (1916) The physiological relation of plant carotenoids to the carotenoid of the cow, horse, sheep, pig, goat and hen. *J. biol. Chem.* **27**, 27.

PALUMBO N.E., PERRI S. & READ G. (1975) Experimental induction and treatment of toad poisoning in the dog. *J. Am. vet. med. Ass.* **167**, 1000.

PAPP E. & SIKES D. (1964) Electrophoretic distribution of protein in the serum of swine with rheumatoid-like arthritis. *Am. J. vet. Res.* **25**, 1112–19.

PARKER B.N.J. & BLOWEY R.W. (1974) A comparison of blood from the jugular vein and the coccygeal artery and vein of cows. *Vet. Rec.* **95**, 14–18.

PARKER J.T. & BOONE M.A. (1971) Thermal stress effects on certain blood characteristics of adult male turkeys. *Poult. Sci.* **50**, 1287–95.

PARKER W.H. & McCREA C.T. (1965) Bracken (Pteris aquilina) poisoning of sheep in the North York Moors. *Vet. Rec.* **77**, 861–6.

PARKES B.J., BRINHOUS K.M., HARRIS P.F. & PENICK G.D. (1964) Laboratory detection of female carriers of canine hemophilia. *Thromb. Diath. haemorrh.* **12**, 368.

PARSHALL JR. C.J., VAINISI S.J., GOLDBERG M.F. & WOLF E.D. (1975) In vivo erythrocyte sickling in the Japanese sika deer (*Cervus nippon*): Methodology. *Am. J. vet. Res.* **36**, 749–52.

PASCOE R.R. (1970) Sudden death in a mare with malignant lymphoma. *Aust. vet. J.* **46**, 559–603.

PASQUIER M.-A. (1947) Teneur en calcium du sérum et du sang total de quelques mammifères. *Bull. Mus. natn. Hist. nat., Paris* 2nd ser., **19**, 249–51.

PAYNE J.M., DEW S.M., MANSTON R. & FAULKS M. (1970) The use of the metabolic profile test in dairy herds. *Vet. Rec.* **87**, 150–8.

PAYNE J.M., ROWLANDS G.J., MANSTON R. & DEW SALLY M. (1973) A statistical appraisal of the results of metabolic profile tests on 75 dairy herds. *Br. vet. J.* **129**, 370–81.

PAYNE L.N. (1971) The lymphoid system. In: Bell D.J. & Freeman B.M. (Eds) *Physiology and biochemistry of the domestic fowl*, pp. 985–1037. Academic Press, London.

PAYNE L.N. & ROSZKOWSKI J. (1972) The presence of immunologically uncommitted bursa and thymus dependent lymphoid cells in the lymphomas of Marek's disease. *Avian Path.* **1**, 27–34.

PAYNE L.N. & RENNIE M. (1973) Pathogenesis of Marek's disease in chicks with and without maternal antibody. *J. natn. Cancer Inst.* **51**, 1559–73.

PEARSE A.G.E. (1972) *Histochemistry, theoretical and applied*, 3rd Edn. Churchill London.

PECHET L. (1964) One-stage specific determination of factor II (prothrombin). In: Tocantins L.M. & Kazal L.A. (Eds) *Blood coagulation, haemorrhage and thrombosis*. Grune and Stratton, New York.

PECHET L. & ALEXANDER B. (1961) Increased clotting factors in pregnancy. *New Engl. J. Med.* **61**, 316.

PENICK G.D., DEJANOVA I., ROBERTS H.R. & WEBSTER W. (1966) Elevation of factor VIII in hypercoagulable states. *Thromb. Diath. haemorrh.* Suppl. 20, 39–48.

PENNY R.H.C. (1956) Post parturient haemoglobinuria (haemoglobinaemia) in cattle. *Vet. Rec.* **68**, 238–41.

PENNY R.H.C. (1967) The blood picture as an aid to diagnosis. *Vet. Rec.* **81**, 181–90.

PENNY R.H.C. (1974) The bone marrow of the dog and cat. *J. small Anim. Pract.* **15**, 553.

PENNY R.H.C. (1975) Intestinal haemorrhage in the pig. In: Grunsell C.S.G. & Hill F.W.G. (Eds) *The veterinary annual—fifteenth issue*, pp. 115–27. J. Wright & Sons, Bristol.

PENNY R.H.C., CARLISLE C.H., PRESCOTT C.W. & DAVIDSON H.A. (1967) Effects of chloramphenicol on the haemopoietic system of the cat. *Br. vet. J.* **123**, 145–53.

PENNY R.H.C., CARLISLE C.H. & DAVIDSON H.A. (1970) The blood and marrow picture of the cat. *Br. vet. J.* **126**, 459–64.

PENNY R.H.C. & CARLISLE C.H. (1970) The bone marrow of the dog: a comparative study of biopsy material obtained from the iliac crest, rib and sternum. *J. small Anim. Pract.* **11**, 727.

PENNY R.H.C., DAVID J.S.E. & WRIGHT A.I. (1961) Heinz-Ehrlich bodies associated with kale feeding. *Vet. Rec.* **73**, 747–8.

PENNY R.H.C., DAVID J.S.E. & WRIGHT A.I. (1964) Observations on the blood picture of cattle, sheep and rabbits fed on kale. *Vet. Rec.* **76**, 1053–9.

PENNY R.H.C., SCOFIELD A.M. & CEMBROWICZ H. (1966) Haematological values for the clinically normal bull. *Br. vet. J.* **122**, 239–47.

PENNY R.H.C., WATSON A.D.J. & MOYLE G.G. (1973) Observations of the effects of chloramphenicol and starvation on the hemopoietic system of the dog. *Clin. Toxicol.* **6**, 229.

PERK K. (1963) The camel's erythrocyte. *Nature (London)* **200**, 272.

PERK K., FREI Y.F. & HERZ A. (1964) The osmotic resistance and hemoglobin pattern of erythrocytes obtained from growing lambs. *Am. J. vet. Res.* **25**, 68–74.

PERK K., FREI Y.F. & HERZ A. (1964) Osmotic fragility of red blood cells of young and mature domestic and laboratory animals. *Am. J. vet. Res.* **25**, 1241–8.

PERK K. & LOBL K. (1960) Chemical and paper electrophoretic analysis of normal sheep serum proteins and lipoproteins. *Br. vet. J.* **116**, 167.

PERMAN V., DIRKS V.A., FANGMAN G., SNYDER MARGARET M., SORENSEN D.K., ANDERSON R.K., GOLTZ D.J., LARSON V.L. & STEVENS J.B. (1970) Statistical evaluation of lymphocyte values on Minnesota dairy cattle. *Am. J. vet. Res.* **31**, 1217–22.

PERRYMAN L.E., HOOVER E.A. & YOHN D.S. (1972) Immunological reactivity of the cat: immunosuppression in experimental feline leukemia. *J. natn. Cancer Inst.* **49**, 1357–65.

PERSSON S.G.B. (1967) On blood volume and working capacity in horses. *Acta vet. scand.* Suppl. 19.

PERSSON S.G.B., EKMAN L., LYDIN G. & TUFVESSON G. (1973a) Circulatory effects of splenectomy in the horse. 1. Effect on red-cell distribution and variability in the horse. *Zentbl. VetMed. A.* **20**, 441–55.

PERSSON S.G.B., EKMAN L., LYDIN G. & TUFVESSON G. (1973b) Circulatory effects of splenectomy in the horse. 2. Effect on plasma volume and total, and circulating red-cell volume. *Zentbl. VetMed. A.* **20**, 456–68.

PERUTZ M.F., ROSSMAN M.G., CULLIS A.F., MUIRHEAD H., WILL G. & NORTH A.C.T. (1960) Structure of haemoglobin. *Nature* **185**, 416–22.

PETERS J.L., HESS T.O., LEACH C.S., IMLAY T., GARDNER R.O., DONOVAN F.M. & KAMPEN K.R. VAN (1973) Hemic and spirometric profiles in calves used for cardiovascular research. *Am. J. vet. Res.* **34**, 1595–7.

PETERS W.P., KUFE D., SCHLOM J., FRANKEL J.W., PRICKETT C.O., GROUPE V. & SPIEGELMAN S. (1973) Biological and biochemical evidence for an interaction between Marek's disease herpesvirus and avian leukosis virus in vivo. *Proc. natn. Acad. Sci. USA* **70**, 3175–8.

PETTIT A. (1913) Procédé simple pour prelever du sang chez les petits rongeurs. *C.R. Soc. Biol. (Paris)* **74**, 11–12.

PHILLIPS G.D. (1970) The assessment of blood acid-base parameters in ruminants. *Br. vet. J.* **126**, 325–32.

PICK J.R. & EUBANKS J.W. (1965) A clinicopathological study of heterogeneous and homogeneous dog populations in North Carolina. *Lab. Anim. Care* **15**, 1, 11.

PIENING C. (1936) Chronische Myelose beim Rinde. *Berl. tierärztl. Wschr.* **52**, 504.

PIERCE K.R., JOYCE J.R., ENGLAND R.B. & JONES L.P. (1972) Acute hemolytic anemia caused by wild onion poisoning in horses. *J. Am. vet. med. Ass.* **160**, 323–7.

PILLAI R. & NAIR S.G. (1974) A critical evaluation of the methods for assessing ESR in domestic animals. *Kerala J. vet. Sci.* **5**, 56.

PIPKIN F.B. & KIRKPATRICK M.L. (1973) The blood volumes of fetal and newborn sheep. *Q. Jl exp. Physiol.* **58**, 181–8.

PISCIOTTA A.V. (1973) Immune and toxic mechanisms in drug-induced agranulocytosis. *Semin. Hematol.* **10**, 279–310.

PLAGER J.E. (1972) Intravenous, long-term infusion in the unrestrained mouse-method. *J. Lab. clin. Med.* **79**, 669–72.

PODLIACHOUK L. (1957) Les antigenes de groupes sanguins des equides et Leur transmission hereditaire. Thesis, Paris.

POLLER L. & THOMSON J. (1969) The Manchester comparative reagent. A national reference standard for anticoagulant therapy. In: Hemker H.C., Loeliger E.A. & Veltkamp J.J. (Eds) *Human blood coagulation. biochemistry, clinical investigation and therapy*, p. 290. Leiden Univ. Press, Leiden.

POLLER L., THOMSON J.M., SEAR C.H.J. & THOMAS W. (1971) Identification of a congenital defect of factor VII in a colony of beagle dogs: the clinical use of the plasma. *J. clin. Path.* **24**, 626.

POND W.G., BANIS R.J., VAN VLECK L.D., WALKER E.F. JR. & CHAPMAN P. (1968) Age changes in body weight and in several blood components of conventional versus miniature pigs. *Proc. Soc. exp. Biol. Med.* **127**, 895–900.

PONDER E., YEAGER J.F. & CHARIPPER H.A. (1928) Haematology of the Camelidae. *Zool. Sci. (N.Y. Zool. Soc.)* **11**, 1.

POOL J.G., DESAI R. & KROPATKIN M. (1962) Severe congenital hypoprothrombinaeuria in a negro boy. *Thromb. Diath. haemorrh.* **8**, 235–40.

PORTER J.A. JR. & CANADAY W.R. JR. (1971) Hematologic values in mongrel and greyhound dogs being screened for research use. *J. Am. vet. med. Ass.* **159**, 1603–6.

PORTER K.A. (1957) A sex difference in morphology of neutrophils in the dog. *Nature* **179**, 784.

PORTMAN O.W., McCONNEL K.P. & RIGDON R.H. (1952) Blood volumes of ducks using human serum albumin labelled with radio-iodine. *Proc. Soc. exp. Biol. Med.* **81**, 599–601.

POTKAY S. & ZINN R.D. (1969) Effects of collection interval, body weight, and season on the hemograms of canine blood donors. *Lab. Anim. Care* **19**, 192.

POULSEN J.S.D. (1974) Variations in the metabolic acid-base balance and some other clinical chemical parameters in dairy herds during the year. *Nord. VetMed.* **26**, 1–12.

POYNTER D., SPURLING N.W., CAFFYN Z.E.Y. & HASTINGS J.S. (1965) Haemolytic anaemia in laboratory animals caused by 2-methyl cinchoninamide. *Proc. Eur. Soc. Study Drug Toxicity* **6**, 39.

PRANKERD T.A.J. & BELLINGHAM A.J. (1975) (Eds) Haemolytic anaemias. *Clin. Haematol.* **4**, 1–260.

PRASSE K.W., CROUSER D., BEUTLER E., WALKER M. & SCHALL W.D. (1975) Pyruvate kinase deficiency anemia with terminal myelofibrosis and osteosclerosis in a Beagle. *J. Am. vet. med. Ass.* **166**, 1170–5.

PRASSE K.W., HOSKINS J.D., GLOCK R.D. & KELSO G.A. (1972) Factor V deficiency and thrombocytopenia in a dog with adenocarcinoma. *J. Am. vet. med. Ass.* **160**, 204–7.

PRESTON J.M., DARGIE J.D. & MacLEAN J.M. (1973a) Patho-physiology of ovine schistosomiasis. I. A clinico-pathological study of experimental Schistosoma mattheei infections. *J. comp. Path. Ther.* **83**, 401–15.

PRESTON J.M., DARGIE J.D. & MacLEAN J.M. (1973b) Patho-physiology of ovine schistosomiasis. II. Some observations on the sequential changes in blood volume and water and electrolyte metabolism following a single experimental infection of Schistosoma mattheei. *J. comp. Path. Ther.* **83**, 417–28.

PRESTON J.M. & DARGIE J.D. (1974) Patho-physiology of ovine schistosomiasis. V. Onset and development of anaemia in sheep experimentally infected with Schistosoma mattheei—studies with ^{51}Cr-labelled erythrocytes. *J. comp. Path. Ther.* **84**, 78–81.

PRICKETT M.E., REEVES J.T. & ZENT W.W. (1973) Tetralogy of fallot in a thoroughbred foal. *J. Am. vet. med. Ass.* **162**, 552–5.

PRIESTER W.A. & HAYES H.M. (1973) Feline leukemia after feline infectious anemia. *J. natn. Cancer Inst.* **51**, 289–91.

PRINEAS J.W. & WRIGHT R.G. (1972) The fine structure of peripheral nerve lesions in a virus-induced demyelinating disease in fowl (Marek's disease). *Lab. Invest.* **26**, 548–57.

PRITCHARD W.R., REHFELD C.E. & SAUTTER J.H. (1952) Aplastic anemia of cattle associated with ingestion of Trichloroethylene-extracted soybean oil meal (Stockman disease, Duren disease, Brabant disease). 1. Clinical and laboratory investigation of field cases. *J. Am. vet. med. Ass.* **121**, 1–8.

PRITCHARD W.R., REHFELD C.E., MIZUNO N.S., SAUTTER J.H. & SCHULTZE M.O. (1956a) Studies on Trichloroethylene-extracted feeds. I. Experimental production of acute aplastic anemia in young heifers. *Am. J. vet. Res.* **17**, 425–9.

PRITCHARD W.R., REHFELD C.E., MATTSON W.E., SAUTTER J.H. & SCHULTZE M.O. (1956b) Studies on Trichloroethylene-extracted feeds. II. The effect of feeding different levels of Trichloroethylene-extracted soybean oil meal to young heifers—experimental production of chronic aplastic anemia. *Am. J. vet. Res.* **17**, 430–7.

PRITCHARD W.R., HAMMER R., SAUTTER J.H. & SCHULTZE M.O. (1956c) Studies on trichloroethylene-extracted feeds. IV. Susceptibility of the horse to the toxic factor in trichloroethylene-extracted soybean oil meal. *Am. J. vet. Res.* **17**, 441–5.

PRITCHARD W.R., MALEWITZ T.D. & KITCHEN H. (1963) Studies on the mechanism of sickling of deer erythrocytes. *Exp. & Mol. Pathol.* **2**, 173–82.

PROUTY D.L. (1975) Hepatoencephalopathy due to portocarval shunt in a dog. *J. Am. vet. med. Ass.* **167**, 756.

PRYOR D.S. (1967) The mechanism of anaemia in tropical splenomegaly. *Q. Jl. Med.* **36**, 337–56.

PRYOR W.H. JR. & BRADBURY R.P. (1975) *Haemobartonella canis* infection in research dogs. *Lab. Anim. Sci.* **25**, 566.

PURCHASE H.G. (1972) Recent advances in the knowledge of Marek's disease. *Adv. vet. Sci. comp. Med.* **16**, 223–58.

PURCHASE H.G. & SHARMA J.M. (1974) *The differential diagnosis of lymphoid leukosis and Marek's disease.* College Station, Texas, USA American Association of Avian Pathologists.

QUAGLINO D. & FLEMANS R. (1958) Peroxidase staining in leucocytes. *Lancet,* **ii**, 1020.

QUAY W.B. (1954) The blood cells of Cetacea with particular reference to the Beluga, *Delphinapterus leucas* Pallas. *Säugetierkundliche Mitteilungen* **2**, 49.

QUICK A.J. (1935) The prothrombin in haemophilia and in obstructive jaundice. *J. biol. Chem.* **109**, 73.

QUICK A.J. (1938) The nature of bleeding in jaundice. *J. Am. med. Ass.* **110**, 1658–62.

QUICK A.J. (1941) The prothrombin concentration in the blood of various species. *Am. J. Physiol.* **132**, 239.

QUICK A.J. (1946) Experimentally induced changes in the prothrombin level of the blood. III. Prothrombin concentration of newborn pups of a mother given dicoumarol before parturition. *J. biol. Chem.* **164**, 371.

QUICK A.J., COLLENTINE G.E. JR & HUSSEY C.V. (1962) Vitamin K requirement of the growing pup. *J. Nutr.* **77**, 28.

QUICK A.J., HUSSEY C.V. & COLLENTINE G.E. JR (1954) Vitamin K requirements of adult dogs and the influence of bile on its absorption from the intestine. *Am. J. Physiol.* **176**, 239.

QUICK A.J. & STEFANINI M. (1948) The concentration of the labile factor of the prothrombin complex in human, dog and rabbit blood: its significance in the determination of prothrombin activity. *J. Lab. clin. Med.* **33**, 819.

RAAB S.O., ATHENS J.W., HAAB O.P., BOGGS D.R., ASHENBRUCKER H., CARTWRIGHT G.E. & WINTROBE M.M. (1964) Granulokinetics in normal dogs. *Am. J. Physiol.* **206**, 83.

RABINER S.F. & FRIEDMAN L.H. (1968) The role of intravascular haemolysis and the reticuloendothelial system in the production of a hypercoagulable state. *Br. J. Haemat.* **14**, 105–18.

RADEMACHER R., SODOMKOVA D. & KRAUS J. (1974) Use of bone marrow smear in the diagnosis of leucosis in Czechoslovakian Red Pied cattle. *Vet. Med., Praha* **19**, 61–70.

RAHN B. & VON KAULLA K. (1964) Pharmacological induction of fibrinolytic activity in the dog. *Proc. Soc. exp. Biol. med.* **115**, 359–61.

RAMAKRISHNAN R., SUNDARARAJ A., DAMODARAN S. & CHANDRASEKARAN K.P. (1972) Haemogram and serum proteinogram in some canine disease. *Cheiron* **1**, 11.

RAMSAY W.N.M. (1946) Plasma bilirubin in the horse. *Br. vet. J.* **102**, 206–11.

RANATUNGA P. & WANDURAGALA L. (1972) Reactions and haematology in imported Jersey cattle preimunised in Ceylon. *Br. vet. J.* **128**, 9–18.

RANDOLPH T.G. & STANTON C. (1945) A comparison of differential counts from the stained film counting chamber, using propylene aqueous stain. *Am. J. clin. Path.* **15**, 17–22.

RANNEY H.M. (1974) (Ed.) Hemoglobinopathies. *Semin. Hematol.* **11**, 383–601.

RAPACZ J., GRUMMER R.H., HASLER JUDITH & SHACKELFORD R.M. (1970) Allotype polymorphism of low density β-lipoproteins in pig serum (LDL pp. 1, LDL pp. 2). *Nature* **225**, 941–2.

RAPACZ J. & HASLER J. (1968) Allotypes (serum antigens) in farm animals. *XIth European conference on animal blood groups and biochemical polymorphism.* Warsaw, pp. 101–5. PWN—Polish Scientific Publishers.

RAPACZ J. & HASLER-RAPACZ J. (1974) Linkage between genes for different heavy-chain immunoglobulin allotypes in swine and cattle. *Anim. Blood Grps biochem. Genet.* **5**, Supplement 1, 33–4.

RASMUSEN B.A. (1964) Gene interaction and the A-O Blood Group system in pigs. *Genetics*, **50**, 191–8.

RASMUSEN B.A. (1965) Isoantigens of gamma globulin in pigs. *Science* **148**, 1742–3.

RASMUSEN B.A. (1969) Blood groups and incompatibility testing. In: Medway W., Prier J.E. & Wilkinson J.S. (Eds) *A textbook of veterinary clinical pathology*, p. 282. Williams & Wilkins, Baltimore, USA.

RASMUSEN B.A. (1972) Gene interaction and the A-O and H blood group systems in pigs. *Anim. Blood Grps biochem. Genet.* **3**, 169–72.

RASMUSEN B.A. & CHRISTIAN L.L. (1976) H blood types in pigs as predictors of stress susceptibility. *Science* **191**, 947–8.

RATNOFF O.D. (1966) The biology and pathology of the initial stages of blood coagulation. In: *Progress in haematology* **5**, 204. Grune and Stratton, New York.

RATNOFF O.D. (1974) Some recent advances in the study of hemostasis. *Circulation Res.* **35**, 1.

RATNOFF O.D. & CONLEY C.L. (1951) Studies on afibrinogenemia. II. The defibrinating effect on dog blood of intravenous injection of thromboplastic material. *Bull. Johns Hopkins Hosp.* **88**, 414.

RATNOFF O.D. & MENZIE C. (1951) A new method for the determination of fibrin in small samples of plasma. *J. Lab. clin. Med.* **37**, 316–20.

RATNOFF O.D. & MILES A.A. (1964) Activation of a vascular permeability—increasing factor in human plasma activated by Hageman factor. *Exp. Path.* **45**, 328.

RATZ F., SZEKY A. & VANYI A. (1972) Studies of the histopathologic changes of acute Marek's disease. *Acta vet. hung.* **22**, 349–64.

RAYNAUD J.P. (1961) Une epidémie d'hepatite-cirrhose du porc sévrissant à Madagascar. I. Etude des tests hépatiques chez le porc et utilisation de la vitesse de sedimentation pour un diagnostic précoce. *Revue Élev. Méd. vét. Pays trop.* **14**, 429–37.

REDA H. & HATHOUT A.F. (1957) The haematological examination of the blood of normal sheep. *Brit. vet. J.* **113**, 251–4.

REDDY P.R.K., VAN KREY H.P., GROSS W.B. & SIEGEL P.B. (1975) Erythrocyte life span in dwarf and normal pullets from growth selected lines of chickens. *Poult. Sci.* **54**, 1301–3.

REECE W.O. & SNODGRASS R.R. (1972) Effect of splenectomy on post feeding changes in packed cell volume of dogs. *Am. J. vet. Res.* **33**, 635–7.

REECE W.O. & WAHLSTROM J.D. (1970) Effect of feeding and excitement on the PCV of dogs. *Lab. Anim. Care* **20**, 1114.

REED W.O. (1949) Lymphosarcoma of the stomach of a horse. *J. Am. vet. med. Ass.* **114**, 412–13.

REEVES J.T., GROVER E.B. & GROVER R.T. (1963) Circulatory responses to high altitude in the cat and rabbit. *J. appl. Physiol.* **18**, 575–9.

REICHEL K. (1962) Klinisch-hamatologische Untersuchungen bei der leukose des Schweines. *Dt. tierärztl. Wschr.* **69**, 297–303, 331–3.

REICHEL K. (1963) Die Leukozytenzahlen beim Schwein. *Dt. tierärztl. Wschr.* **70**, 440–4.

REIHART O.F. & REIHART H.W. (1968) The hematopoietic system. In: Catcott E.J. (Ed.) *Canine medicine*, First Catcott edition, p. 339. American Veterinary Publications Inc, Wheaton, Illinois, USA.

REINHARDT W.O., ARON H. & LI C.H. (1944) Effect of adrenocorticotrophic hormone on leucocyte picture of normal rats and dogs. *Proc. Soc. exp. Biol. Med.* **57**, 19.

REKERS P.E. & COULTER M. (1948) A hematological and histological study of the bone marrow and peripheral blood of the adult dog. *Am. J. med. Sci.* **216**, 643.

RENSHAW H.W., CHATBURN C., BRYAN G.M., BARTSCH R.C. & DAVIS W.C. (1975) Canine granulocytopathy syndrome: neutrophil dysfunction in a dog with recurrent infections. *J. Am. vet. med. Ass.* **166**, 443–7.

RICH L.J. (1974) *The morphology of canine and feline blood cells*. Ralston Purina Company, St Louis, Missouri, USA.

RICHTER W. (1966) Relative aggregation tendency of erythrocytes from man and various animal species. *Acta chir. scand.* **132**, 601–12.

RICHARD C.G., POST J.E., NARONHA F. & BARR L.M. (1969) A transmissible virus induced lymphocytic leukemia of the cat. *J. natn. Cancer Inst.* **42**, 987–1014.

RICKETTS S.W. & ROSSDALE P.D. (1975) The veterinary practice laboratory. *Vet. Rec.* **97**, 320–4.

RICO A.-G., GODFRAIN J.-C., BRAUN J.-P., BENARD P. & BURGAT-SACAZE V. (1973) Dosages enzymatiques seriques en clinique canine. *Rev. Méd. vét.* **124**, 1299.

RIDGWAY S.H. (1972) *Mammals of the sea. Biology and medicine.* Thomas, Springfield, USA.

RIDGWAY S.H., SIMPSON J.D., PATTON G.S. & GILMARTIN W.G. (1970) Haematologic findings in certain small cetaceans. *J. Am. vet. med. Ass.* **157**, 566–70.

RIEGEL K., BARTELS H. & KLEIHAUER E. (1966) Comparative studies of the respiratory functions of mammalian blood. I. Gorilla, Chimpanzee and Orangutan. *Resp. physiol.* **1**, 138.

RIEK R.F. (1968) In: Weinman D. & Ristic M. (Eds) *Infectious blood diseases of man and animals*, Vol. 2, p. 259. Academic Press, New York and London.

RINGEN L.M. & DICKSON D.M. (1974) Distribution of a beta-globulin in tissues of normal and virus-infected chickens. *Am. J. vet. Res.* **35**, 689–91.

RISTIC M. (1972) Protozoal diseases. In:

Catcott E.J. & Smithcors J.F. (Eds) *Equine medicine and surgery*, 2nd Edn, pp. 137–55. American Veterinary Publications, Illinois.

RITTER H. (1965) Studien über übertragungswege bei der enzootischen Rinderleukose. *Dt. tieräztl. Wschr.* **72**, 56–60.

RIVERS J.P.W. & D'SOUZA F. (1976) Hypervitaminosis A in the tree shrew. (In preparation).

RØ J.S. & FLATMARK A. (1972) Studies on thrombin infusion in dogs. *Scand. J. Haemat.* **9**, 293–304.

ROBERTS C.J. & GRAY A.R. (1973) Studies of trypanosome resistant cattle. II. Effect on N'dama, Muturu and Zebu cattle. *Trop. Anim. Hlth & Prod.* **5**, 220–33.

ROBERTS E.J. & ARCHER R.K. (1966) Current methods for the diagnosis and treatment of haemolytic disease. *Vet. Rec.* **79**, 61–7.

ROBINSON A.J., KROPATKIN M. & AGGELER P.A. (1969) Hageman factor (factor XII) deficiency in marine mammals. *Science* **166**, 1420.

ROBINSON F.R. & ZIEGLER R.F. (1968) Clinical laboratory values of beagle dogs. *Lab. Anim. Care* **18**, 39.

ROBSCHEIT-ROBBINS F.S. & WHIPPLE G.H. (1936) Infection and intoxication. Their influence upon hemoglobin production in experimental anemia. *J. exp. Med.* **63**, 767.

RODNAN G.P., EBAUGH F.G. & FOX M.R.S. (1957) The life span of the red blood cell and the red blood cell volume in the chicken, pigeon and duck as estimated by the use of $Na_2Cr^{51}O_4$ with observations on red cell turnover rate in the mammal, bird and reptile. *Blood* **12**, 355–66.

ROGERSON P.E., JARRETT W.F.H. & MACKEY L.J. (1975) Epidemiological studies on feline leukaemia virus infection. I. A serological survey in urban cats. *Int. J. Cancer.* **15**, 781–5.

ROHOVSKY M.W. & FOWLER E.H. (1971) Lesions of experimental feline panleukopenia *J. Am. vet. med. Ass.* **158**, 872–5.

ROONEY J.R., BRYANS J.T., PRICKETT M.E. & ZENT W.W. (1966) Exhaustion shock in the horse. *Cornell Vet.* **56**, 220–35.

ROSEN M.N. & BISCHOFF A.I. (1952) The relation of hematology to condition in California deer. *Trans. N. Am. Wildl. Conf.* **17**, 482–95.

ROSENBERG S.A. (1974) (Ed.) Hodgkin's disease and other lymphomas. *Clin. Haematol.* **3**, 1–213.

ROSENFELD G., REICHMANN C.E. & ANDRADE S.O. (1971) Anemia hemolitica em bovinos alimentados com *Brachiaria* spp. (Tanner grass). IV. *Arq. Inst. biol., S. Paulo* **38**, 267–73.

ROSENTHAL R.L., DRESKIN O. & ROSENTHAL N. (1953) New haemophilia-like disease caused by deficiency of a third plasma thromboplastin factor. *Proc. Soc. exp. Biol. Med.* **82**, 171.

ROSSDALE P.D. (1966) Fellowship thesis, Royal College of Veterinary Surgeons.

ROSSDALE P.D., HUNT M.D.N., PEACE C.K., HOPES R. & RICKETTS S.W. (1975) A case of equine infectious anaemia in Newmarket. *Vet. Rec.* **97**, 207–8.

ROSSE W.F. & WALDMANN T.A. (1966) Factors controlling erythropoiesis in birds. *Blood,* **27**, 654–61.

ROSSI G. (1953) Sul tasso ematico di granulociti eosinofili in suini sani di razza Large White. (Cited *Vet. Bull.* (1955) **25**, 37.) *Annali Fac. Med. vet. Univ. Pisa* **6**, 110–19.

ROSTORFER H.H. & RIGDON R.H. (1947) The relation of blood oxygen transport to resistance to anoxia in chicks and ducklings. *Biol. Bull.* **92**, 23.

ROSZEL J., PRIER J.E. & KOPROWSKA I. (1965) The occurrence of megakaryocytes in the peripheral blood of dogs. *J. Am. vet. med. Ass.* **147**, 133–7.

ROTTMANN D. (1969) Tages rhythmische Schwankungen haematologischer Werte beim Schwein. Inaug. Diss., Hannover.

ROUND M.C. (1968) The diagnosis of helminthiasis in horses. *Vet. Rec.* **82**, 39–43.

ROUND M.C. (1971) Some aspects of naturally acquired helminthiasis of horses. *Equine vet. J.* **3**, 31–7.

ROUSE B.T., OSBORNE A.D., GRUNSELL C.S. & HOOPER R.B. (1967) Acute granulocytic leukaemia in a bitch. *Vet. Rec.* **80**, 408–9.

ROUSE B.T., WELLS R.J.H. & WARNER N.L. (1973) Proportion of T and B lymphocytes in lesions of Marek's disease: theoretical implications for pathogenesis. *J. Immun.* **110**, 534–9.

ROWLANDS G.J., LITTLE W., MANSTON R. & DEW SALLY M. (1974) The effect of season on the composition of the blood of lactating and non-lactating cows as revealed from repeated metabolic profile tests on 24 dairy herds. *J. agric. Sci. Camb.* **83**, 27–35.

ROWNTREE G. (1968) Anaemia and navel bleeding in piglets. *Vet. Rec.* **82**, 583.

ROWSELL H.C. (1963) Hemorrhagic disorders in dogs: Their recognition, treatment and importance. In: *The newer knowledge about dogs*, p. 9. Twelfth Gaines Veterinary Symposium.

ROWSELL H.C. (1968) The hemostatic mechanism of mammals and birds in health and disease. *Adv. vet. Sci.* **12**, 337.

ROWSELL H.C. (1969) Blood coagulation and haemorrhagic disorders. In: Medway W., Prier J.E. & Wilkinson J.S. (Eds) *A Textbook of Veterinary Clinical Pathology*, p. 247. Williams & Wilkins, Baltimore, USA.

ROWSELL H.C., DOWNIE H.G., MUSTARD J.F., LEESON J.E. & ARCHIBALD J.A. (1960) A disorder resembling hemophilia B (Christmas Disease) in dogs. *J. Am. vet. med. Ass.* **137**, 247–50.

ROWSELL H.C., GLYNN M.F., MUSTARD J.F. & MURPHY E.A. (1967) Effect of heparin on platelet economy in dogs. *Am. J. Physiol.* **213**, 915.

ROWSELL H.C. & MUSTARD J.F. (1963) Blood coagulation in some common laboratory animals. *Lab. Anim. Care* **13**, 752.

ROWSELL H.C. & MUSTARD J.F. (1966) Hemostasis in domestic animals. *Can. J. med. Technol.* **28**, 2.

ROYAL SOCIETY OF MEDICINE (1972) *Units, symbols and abbreviations. A guide for biological and medical editors and authors.* Ed. Ellis G., RSM, London.

ROYER M., NOIR B.A., SFARCICH D. & NANET H. (1974) Extrahepatic bilirubin formation and conjugation in the dog. *Digestion* **10**, 423.

RUDOLPH R. & HÜBNER C. (1972) Megakaryozytenleukose beim Hund. *Kleintier-Prax.* **17**, 9.

RUDOLPH VON R. & PAULSEN J. (1972) Ultrastruktur lymphatischer Zellen bei Leukose des Schafes. *Berl. Münch. tierärztl. Wschr.* **85**, 85–7.

RUDOLPH W., CRIPE W., HIRD D., RUSCH K., SOFFIA A. & VILLOUTA G. (1972) Bovine leukosis. A comparative study of three haematological diagnostic keys in Chilean cattle. *Br. vet. J.* **128**, 506–11.

RUNNELLS R.A. & BENBROOK E.A. (1944) Malignant lymphoid tumours of horses and mules. *J. Am. vet. med. Ass.* **104**, 148–50.

RUSSELL E.S., NEUFELD E.F. & HIGGINS G.T. (1951) Comparison of normal blood pictures of young adults from 18 inbred strains of mice. *Proc. Soc. exp. Biol. Med.* **78**, 761.

RYAGIN S.T. & APTEKAR I.N. (1973) Indirect immunofluorescent test for bovine leucosis. *Veterinariya Moscow*, No. 1, 46–7.

RYAN G.M. (1971a) Blood values in cows. Erythrocytes. *Res. vet. Sci.* **12**, 572–5.

RYAN G.M. (1971b) Blood values in cows. Leucocytes. *Res. vet. Sci.* **12**, 576–8.

SAAR C. (1973a) Die Knochenmarkpunktion beim Hund (1). *Tierärztl Prax* **1**, 187.

SAAR C. (1973b) Die Knochenmarkpunktion beim Hund (2). *Tierärztl Prax* **1**, 333.

SAAR C. (1974) Die Knochenmarkpunktion beim Hund (3). *Tierärztl Prax* **2**, 75.

SAAR C. (1975) Die knochenmarkpunktion beim Hund (4). *Tierärztl Prax* **3**, 335.

SABOURIN S., STANLEY P. & CHARTRAND C. (1975) Normogramme hématologique et biochimique et variations quotidiennes des paramètres de base chez le chien normal. *Can. J. comp. Med.* **39**, 397.

SAFAROVA P., KARADJOLE I., HYLDGAARD-JENSEN J., BRAUNER-NIELSEN P. & LYCIK G. (1972) Phosphoglucomutase polymorphism in porcine red cells. *Acta vet. scand.* **13**, 134–6.

SAISON R. (1968) Serum and red cell enzyme systems in pigs. *XIth European conference on animal blood groups and biochemical polymorphism* Warsaw, pp. 321–8. PWN—Polish Scientific Publishers

SAISON R. & O'REILLY M. (1971) Phosphohexose isomerase variants in pigs. *Vox. Sang.* **20**, 274–6.

SAISON R. (1973) Red cell peptidase polymorphism in pigs, cattle, dogs and mink. *Vox. Sang.* **25**, 173–81.

SAITO H., GOLDSMITH G. & RATNOFF O.D. (1974) Fletcher factor activity in plasma of various species. *Proc. Soc. exp. Biol. Med.* **147**, 519.

SAITO H. & RATNOFF O.D. (1974) Inhibition of normal clotting and Fletcher factor activity by rabbit anti-kallikrein antiserum. *Nature* **248**, 597.

SALZMAN E.W. (1963) Measurement of platelet adhesiveness. *J. Lab. clin. Med.* **62**, 724–35.

SAMPSON J., HESTER H.R. & GRAHAM R. (1942) Studies on baby pig mortality. II. Further observations of acute hypoglycaemia in newly born pigs (so-called baby pig disease). *J. Am. vet. med. Ass.* **100**, 33–7.

SANCHEZ-MEDAL L. (1971) The hemopoietic action of androstanes. *Prog. Hemat.* **7**, 111–36.

SANGER V.L., MAIRS R.E. & TRAPP A.L. (1964) Hemophilia in a foal. *J. Am. vet. med. Ass.* **144**, 259–64.

SAROR D. & COLES E.H. (1973) The blood picture of White Fulani (Zebu) and White Fulani/Friesian (crossbred) dairy cows. *Bull. epizoot. Dis. Afr.* **21**, 485–7.

SATO A. & SEKIYA N. (1926) A simple method for differentiation of myeloid and lymphatic leucocytes in human blood. *Tohoku J. exp. Med.* **7**, 111–15.

SAUER R.M. & FEGLEY H.C. (1960) The role of infectious and non-infectious diseases in monkey health. *An. N.Y. Acad. Sci.* **85**, 866.

SAUNDERS C.N., KINCH D.A. & IMLAH P. (1966) Thrombocytopenic purpura in pigs. *Vet. Rec.* **79**, 549–50.

SAUNDERS C.N. & KINCH D.A. (1968) Thrombocytopenic purpura of pigs. *J. comp. Path.* **78**, 513–23.

VON SCHAEWEN H. (1974) Die korrelation Fibrinogenzeit / Fibrinogenkonzentration bei Hund, Pferd und Huhn und die Korrelation Fibrinogengehalt/Gerinnselfestigkeit beim Hund. *Berl. Münch. tierzärztl. Wschr.* **86**, 91.

SCHALM O.W. (1965) *Veterinary hematology.* 2nd Edn. Baillière Tindall & Cassell, London.

SCHALM O.W. (1967) *Veterinary haematology.* Lea & Febiger, Philadelphia.

SCHALM O.W. (1969) Leukopenia and resurgence of granulopoiesis in the cat. *Calif. Vet.* **23**, 16–20.

SCHALM O.W. (1972) *Refresher course for veterinarians on blood disorders.* Proc. No. 17—Postgraduate Committee on Veterinary Science, University of Sydney.

SCHALM O.W. (1972) Interpretations in feline bone marrow cytology. *J. Am. vet. med. Ass.* **161**, 1418–25.

SCHALM O.W. (1974) Multiple myeloma in a dog. *Calif. Vet.* **28**, 4, 30.

SCHALM O.W. (1975) Granulopoiesis. 1. Leukemoid reaction in blood. *Canine Pract.* **2**, May–June, 18.

SCHALM O.W. & GRIBBLE D.H. (1974) Viral inclusions in blood cells and hemograms in canine distemper. *Calif. Vet.* **28**, 12, 23.

SCHALM O.W. & HOLLIDAY T.A. (1975) Hematology of lead poisoning in the dog. *Calif. Vet.* **29**, 2, 22.

SCHALM O.W., HUGHES J. & HARDY D. (1967) Dynamics of the neutrophil leukocyte and a unique response in acute indigestion in the cow. *Calif. Vet.* **21**, 20–3.

SCHALM O.W., JAIN N.C. & CARROLL E.J. (1975) *Veterinary haematology*, 3rd Edn. Lea & Febiger, Philadelphia.

SCHALM O.W. & LING G.W. (1971) The blood platelets (thrombocytes). III. The hemorrhagic syndrome in thrombocytopenia. *Calif. Vet.* **25**, 8, 10.

SCHALM O.W. & SMITH R. (1963) Some unique aspects of feline hematology in disease. *Small anim. Clin.* **3**, 311–22.

SCHALM O.W. & STROMBECK D.R. (1974) Pancytopenia in a dog due to *Ehrlichia canis. Canine Pract.* **1**, Nov–Dec, 13.

SCHECTER R.D., SCHALM O.W. & KANEKO J.J. (1973) Heinz body hemolytic anemia associated with the use of urinary antiseptics containing methylene blue in the cat. *J. Am. vet. med. Ass.* **162**, 37–44.

SCHEIDEGGER H.R. (1973a) Veränderungen des Roten Blutbildes und der Serumeisen-Konzentration bei Simmentaler Kälbern. *Schweizer. Arch. Tierheilk.* **115**, 483–97.

SCHEIDEGGER H.R. (1973b) Verhalten des fötalen Hamoglobins bei Simmentaler Kälbern. *Schweizer. Arch. Tierheilk.* **115**, 499–506.

SCHEIDEGGER H.R., GERBER H. & MARTIG J. (1974) Das Weisse Blutbild von Aufzucht und Milchmastkälbern. *Schweizer. Arch. Tierheilk.* **116**, 87–94.

SCHERMER S. (1958) *Die Blutmorphologie der Laboratoriumstiere.* Barth, Leipzig.

SCHERMER S. (1967) *The blood morphology of laboratory animals.* F.A. Davis Co, Philadelphia.

SCHIFFMAN S. & LEE P. (1974) Preparation, characterization and activation of highly purified factor XI: evidence that a hitherto unrecognised plasma activity participates in the interaction of factors XI and XII. *Br. J. Haemat.* **27**, 101–14.

SCHILLER I., BERGHIND N., TERRY J.R., REICHLIN R., TRUEHART R. & COX G. (1964) Hypercholesterolaemia in pet dogs. *Archs. Path.* **77**, 389.

SCHMID D.O. & OTTO F. (1971a) Zur Serologie der Lymphozytenantigene beim Schwein. *Zentbl. VetMed.* **B18**, 147–52.

SCHMID D.O. & OTTO F. (1971b) Zur Serologie der Granulozytenantigene beim Schwein. *Zentbl. VetMed.* **B18**, 205–10.

SCHMID D.O. & CWIK S. (1972) On leucocyte serology in pig and cattle. *Anim. Blood Grps biochem. Genet.* **3**. Suppl. 1, 11–12.

SCHNAPPAUF H., STEIN H.B., SIPE C.R. & CRONKITE E.P. (1967) Erythropoietic response in calves following blood loss. *Am. J. vet. Res.* **28**, 275–8.

SCHROEDER W.F. & RISTIC M. (1968) Blood serum factors associated with erythrophagocytosis in calves with anaplasmosis. *Am. J. vet. Res.* **29**, 1991–5.

SCHRÖFFEL J. (1965) Genetic determination of the serum 'thread proteins' and the slow α_2-globulin polymorphism in pigs. In: Matousek J. (Ed.) *Blood groups of animals*, pp. 321–9. Publishing house of the Czechoslovak Academy of Sciences, Prague.

SCHRÖFFEL J. (1966) New genetic variants of transferrins and haptoglobins in pigs. *Nature*, **210**, 1274–5.

SCHULZ H. (1968) *Thrombocyten und Thrombose im elektronenmikroskopischen Bild.* [Electron Microscopy of Blood Platelets and Thrombosis], p. 46. Springer, Berlin.

SCHULTZ R.D. (1974) Immunologic disorders in the dog and cat. *Vet. Clin. N. Am.* **4**, 153–74.

SCHULZE W. & SCHÜTZLER H. (1958) Knochenmarkuntersuchungen beim Schaf mit besonderer Berücksichtigung der Technik der Brustbeinpunktion. *Dt. tierärztl. Wschr.* **65**, 150–6.

SCHUMACHER A. (1965) Zur submikroskopischen Struktur der Thrombozyten, Lymphozyten und Monozyten des Haushuhnes (*Gallus domesticus*). *Z. Zellforsch. mikrosk. Anat.* **66**, 219–32.

SCORZA J.V. (1971) Some haematological observations on Tropidurus Torduatus (Sauria, Inguanidae) from Venezuela. *J. Zool. Lond.* **165**, 557–61.

SCOTT A.M. (1975) Blood typing in horses. *Vet. A.* **15**, 181–4.

SCOTT A.M. (1973) Red cell groups of horses. *Proc. 3rd. Int. Conf. Equine Infectious Diseases.* Paris, pp. 384–93. Karger, Basel.

SCOTT M.I.R. (1941) Methylene blue as an antidote for nitrite poisoning in sheep. *Aust. vet. J.* **17**, 71–2.

SCOTT D.W., SCHULTZ R.D., POST J.E., BOLTON G.R. & BALDWIN C.A. (1973) Autoimmune haemolytic anemia in the cat. *J. Am. anim. Hosp. Ass.* **9**, 530–9.

SEAL U.S. (1969) Carnivora systematics: a study of haemoglobins. *Comp. Biochem. Physiol.* **31**, 799.

SEAL U.S., SWAIN W.R. & ERICKSON A.W. (1967) Haematology of the Ursidae. *Comp. Biochem. Physiol.* **22**, 451.

SEAL U.S. & ERICKSON A.W. (1969) Hematology, blood chemistry and protein polymorphism in the white-tailed deer (*Odocoileus virginianus*). *Comp. Biochem. Physiol.* **30**, 695–713.

SEAL U.S., OZOGA J.J., ERICKSON A.W. &

VERME L.J. (1972a) Effects of immobilization on blood analyses of white-tailed deer. *J. Wildl. Mgmt* **36**, 1034–40.

SEAL U.S., VERME L.J., OZOGA J.J. & ERICKSON A.W. (1972b) Nutritional effects on thyroid activity and blood of white-tailed deer. *J. Wildl. Mgmt* **36**, 1041–52.

SEAMER J. (1956) Piglet anaemia. A review of the literature. *Vet. Revs. Annot.* **2**, 79–93.

SEAMER J. & SNAPE T. (1970) Tropical canine pancytopaenia and *Ehrlichia canis* infection. *Vet. Rec.* **86**, 375.

SEARCY G.P., MILLER D.R. & TASKER J.B. (1971) Congenital hemolytic anemia in the Basenji dog due to erythrocyte pyruvate kinase deficiency. *Can. J. comp. Med.* **35**, 67.

SECKINGTON I.M. (1969) The practical application of haematology—2. *Equine vet. J.* **1**, 198–201.

SECKINGTON I.M., HUNTSMAN R.G. & JENKINS G.C. (1967) The serum folic acid levels of grass-fed and stabled horses. *Vet. Rec.* **80**, 158–61.

SEEGERS W.H., COLE E.R., HARMISON C.R. & MARCINIAK E. (1963) Purification and some properties of autoprothrombin C. *Can. J. Biochem. Physiol.* **41**, 1047.

SEELEMANN M., HEESCHEN W. & KRÜGER K.E. (1963) Die leukose des rindes—ein tierzuchterisches problem. *Berl. Münch. tierärztl. Wschr.* **76**, 489–508.

SEFFNER W. (1972) Osteomalacia skeletal change in dairy cows with post parturient haemoglobinuria. *Mh. VetMed.* **27**, 729–30.

SELYE H. (1965) *The mast cells.* Butterworths, Washington.

SEYMOUR JONES E., McCALL K.B., ELVELIJEM C.A. & CLARK P.F. (1947) The effect of diet on the haemoglobin, erythrocyte and leucocyte content of the rhesus monkey (*Macaca mulatta*). *Blood* **2**, 154–63.

SHADDUCK J. & WEIKERT J. (1963) Acute disseminated histoplasmosis accompanied by anemia. *Speculum* **16**, 5.

SHANKS P.L. (1968) Anaemia and navel bleeding in piglets. *Vet. Rec.* **82**, 526–7.

SHARMA J.M. (1974) Resistance to Marek's disease in immunologically deficient chickens. *Nature (London)* **247**, 117–18.

SHARMA D.P., MALIK P.D. & SAPRA K.L. (1973) Age-wise and species-wise haematological studies in farm animals. *Indian J. anim. Sci.* **43**, 289–95.

SHARMA R.N., MOHANTY G.C. & RAJYA B.S. (1972) Skin manifestations of Marek's disease. *Curr. Sci.* **41**, 708–10.

SHARMA J.M. & STONE H.A. (1972) Genetic resistance to Marek's disease. Delineation of the response of genetically resistant chickens to Marek's disease virus infection. *Avian Dis.* **16**, 894–906.

SHARMA J.M., WITTIER R.L. & BURMESTER B.R. (1973) Pathogenesis of Marek's disease in old chickens: lesion regression as the basis for age-related resistance. *Infect. Immun.* **8**, 715–24.

SHARP A.A. & DIKE G.W.R. (1964) Haemophilia in the dog. Treatment with heterologous anti-haemophilic globulin. *Thromb. Diath. haemorrh.* **10**, 494.

SHEMIN D. (1948) The biosynthesis of porphyrins. *Cold Spring Harb. Symp. quant. Biol.* **13**, 185–91.

SHEPHERD V.J., DODDS-LAFFIN W.J. & LAFFIN R.J. (1972) Gamma A myeloma in a dog with defective hemostasis. *J. Am. vet. med. Ass.* **160**, 1121–7.

SHERWOOD L., SCHMIDT D.A., BRETT I.J. & HOWARD D.L. (1966) Canine hemophilia due to antihemophilic factor deficiency: a case report. *Mich. St Univ. Vet.* **26**, 52.

SHIFRINE M., MUNN S.L., ROSENBLATT L.S., BULGIN M.S. & WILSON F.D. (1973) Hematologic changes to 60 days of age in clinically normal beagles. *Lab. Anim. Sci.* **23**, 894.

SHIFRINE M. & STORMONT C. (1973) Hemoglobins, haptoglobins and transferrins in Beagles. *Lab. Anim. Sci.* **23**, 704.

SHIVELY J.N., FELDT C. & DAVIS D. (1969) Fine structure of formed elements in canine blood. *Am. J. vet. Res.* **30**, 893.

SHOPE R.E. (1964) Swine Influenza. In: Dunne H.W. (Ed.) *Diseases of swine*, 2nd Edn, pp. 109–26. State Univ. Press, Ames, Iowa.

SHOPE R.E., MACNAMARA L.G. & MAN-

GOLD R. (1955) Report on the deer mortality, epizootic hemorrhagic disease of deer. *New Jers. Outdoors* **6**, 16–21.

SIDDONS R.C. (1974a) Experimental nutritional folate deficiency in the baboon (*Papio cynocephalus*). *Br. J. Nutr.* **32**, 579.

SIDDONS R.C. (1974b) The experimental production of vitamin B_{12} deficiency in the baboon (*Papio cynocephalus*). A 2-year study. *Br. J. Nutr.* **32**, 219.

SIDDONS R.C. (1974c) Vitamin B_{12} antagonism by monocarboxylic acids and analides of cyanocobalamin. *Nature (London)*, **247**, 308–9.

SIEGAL A.M., CASEY H.W., BOWMAN R.W. & TRAYNOR J.E. (1968) Leukaemia in a rhesus monkey (*Macaca mulatta*) following exposure to whole body proton irradiation. *Blood* **32**, 989–96.

SIKES D., HAYES F.A. & PRESTWOOD A.K. (1969) Electrophoretic distribution of serum proteins of normal and arthritic white-tailed deer (*Odocoileus virginianus*). *Am. J. vet. Res.* **30**, 143–8.

SIKES D., KISTNER T.P., EVE J.H. & HAYES F.A. (1972) Electrophoretic distribution and serologic changes of blood serum of arthritic (rheumatoid) white-tailed deer (*Odocoileus virginianus*) infected with *Erysipelothrix insidiosa*. *Am. J. vet. Res.* **33**, 2545–9.

SIMMS B.T. (1940) Erythrocyte sedimentation studies in dogs. *J. Am. vet. med. Ass.* **96**, 77.

SIMON M. & HRUBAN V. (1971) Lymphocyte typing in pigs: evidence for antigen Ll. *Anim. Blood Grps biochem. Genet.* **2**, 95–100.

SIMONYAN G.A. (1974) Reticulosarcomatosis in cattle. *Veterinariya Moscow*, No. ii, 57–60.

SIMPSON C.F. (1968) Ultrastructural features of the turkey thrombocyte and lymphocyte. *Poult. Sci.* **47**, 848–50.

SIMPSON C.F. (1974) Relationship of *Ehrlichia canis*-infected mononuclear cells to blood vessels of lungs. *Infect. Immun.* **10**, 590.

SIMPSON C.F. & TAYLOR W.J. (1974) Ultrastructure of sickled deer erythrocytes. I. The typical crescent and holly leaf forms. *Blood* **43**, 899–906.

SINAKOS Z. & CAEN J.P. (1967) Platelet aggregation in mammalians (human, rat, rabbit, guinea pig, horse, dog); a comparative study. *Thromb. Diath. haemorrh.* **17**, 99.

SINCLAIR K.B. (1964) Studies on the anaemia of ovine fascioliasis. *Br. vet. J.* **120**, 212–22.

SINGH B. (1970) Studies on the pathology of bovine lymphosarcoma/leukaemia in Indian buffaloes. Ph.D. thesis, Punjab Agric. Univ., Ludhiana.

SINGH H., KHANNA N.D. & PRABHU S.S. (1970) Variation in the frequency of occurrence of blood group factors in Hariana and Jersey–Sindhi crossbred cattle. *J. Genet.* **60**, 146–51.

SIPPEL W.L. (1952) White blood cell count in hog cholera. *Vet. Med.* **47**, 497–501.

SIRCHIA G. & LEWIS S.M. (1975) Paroxysmal nocturnal haemoglobinuria. *Clin. Haematol.* **4**, 199–229.

SIRS J.A. (1966) Oxygen dissociation of sheep haemoglobins A and B in solution. *Nature (London)* **211**, 533–4.

SIRS J.A. (1975) Erythrocyte flexibility, blood fibrinogen and surgery. In: Nicolaides A.N. (Ed.) *Thromboembolism*, pp. 59–78. Medical & Technical Publishing Co Ltd., Lancaster.

SJØLIN K.E. (1965) Lack of Christmas factor in horse plasma. *Nature (London)* **178**, 153.

SLADE C.L., TAYLOR L.M. JR., WECHSLER A.S. & MCKEE P.A. (1973) Postsurgical hemorrhage in dogs anticoagulated with Ancrod (Arvin). *Ann. Surg.* **178**, 721.

SLAPPENDEL R.J., VAN ARKEL C., MIEOG W.H.W. & BOUMA B.N. (1972) Response to heparin of spontaneous disseminated intravascular coagulation in the dog. *Zentbl. VetMed. A*, **19**, 502.

SLAPPENDEL R.J. & VAN DIJK J.E. (1973) Diffuse intravasale stolling (DIS) II Spontane DIS bij de hond. *Tijdschr. Diergeneesk.* **98**, 615.

SLAPPENDEL R.J., VAN ERP C.L.G.M., GOUDSWAARD J. & BETHLEHEM M. (1975) Cold hemagglutinin disease in a toy Pinscher dog. *Tijdschr. Diergeneesk.* **100**, 445.

SLAPPENDEL R.J., DE MAAT C.E.M., RIJNBERK A. & VAN ARKEL C. (1970) Spontaneous consumption coagulopathy in a dog with thyroid cancer. *Thromb. Diath. haemorrh.* **24**, 129–35.

ŠLESINGR L. (1967) Hämatologische Ergebnisse bei gesunden Schweinen die in Bilanzkäfigen gehalten wurden. *Berl. Münch. tierärztl. Wschr.* **80**, 291–3.

SLOAN H.J. & WILGUS H.S. (1930) Heart probe—a method for obtaining blood samples from chickens. *Poult. Sci.* **10**, 10–16.

SMALL E. & RISTIC M. (1967) Morphologic features of haemobartonella felis. *Am. J. vet. Res.* **28**, 845–51.

SMITH B.L. & BEATSON N.S. (1970) Bovine enzootic haematuria in New Zealand. *N.Z. vet. J.* **18**, 115–20.

SMITH B., WOODHOUSE D.A. & FRASER A.J. (1975) The effects of copper supplementation on stock health and production. *N.Z. vet. J.* **23**, 109–12.

SMITH H.A., JONES T.C. & HUNT R.D. (1972) *Veterinary pathology.* 4th Edn, p. 213. Lea and Febiger, Philadelphia, USA.

SMITH I.M. (1959) The blood picture of Ankole Longhorn cows. *Br. vet. J.* **115**, 27–30.

SMITH J.E. & KIEFER S. (1973) Comparative erythrocyte metabolism: breed differences using canine cells. *Enzyme* **14**, 76.

SMITH J.E. & AGAR N.S. (1975) The effect of phlebotomy on canine erythrocyte metabolism. *Res. vet. Sci.* **18**, 231–6.

SMITH J.E. & AGAR N.S. (1976) Studies on erythrocyte metabolism following acute blood loss in the horse. *Equine vet. J.* **8**, 34–7.

SMITH N. & ENGELBERT V.E. (1969) Erythropoiesis in chicken peripheral blood. *Can. J. Zool.* **47**, 1269–73.

SMITH R.D., RISTIC M., HUXSOLL D.L. & BAYLOR R.A. (1975) Platelet kinetics in canine ehrlichiosis: evidence for increased platelet destruction as the cause of thrombocytopenia. *Infect. Immun.* **11**, 1216.

SMITH R.H., EARL C.R. & MATHESON N.A. (1974) The probable role of S-methylcysteine sulphoxide in kale poisoning in ruminants. *Biochem. Soc. Trans.* **2**, 101–4.

SMITHIES O. (1955) Zone electrophoresis in starch gels; group variations in the serum proteins of normal human adults. *Biochem. J.* **61**, 629–41.

SOAVE O.A. & BOYLE C.C. (1965) A comparison of the hemograms of conditioned and non-conditioned laboratory dogs. *Lab. Anim. Care* **15**, 359.

SOLIMAN M.K. & EL-AMROUSI S. (1966) Erythrocyte fragility of healthy fowl, dog, sheep, cattle, buffalo, horse and camel blood. *Vet. Rec.* **78**, 429.

SOLIMAN M.K., EL AMROUSI S. & AHMED A.A.S. (1966) Cytological and biochemical studies on the blood of normal and spirochaete-infected ducks. *Zentbl. VetMed.* Reihe B **13**, 82–6.

SOLIMAN M.K., AHMED A.A.S., EL AMROUSI S. & MOUSTAFA I.H. (1966) Cytological and biochemical studies on the blood constituents of normal and spirochete-infected chickens. *Avian Dis.* **10**, 394–400.

SOLIMAN M.K., EL-AMROUSI S. & KHAMIS M.Y. (1965) The influence of tranquillisers and barbiturate anaesthesia on the blood picture and electrolytes of dogs. *Vet. Rec.* **77**, 1256.

SOLOMON G.E., HILGARTNER M.W. & KUTTE H. (1974) Phenobarbital-induced coagulation defects in cats. *Neurology* **24**, 920–4.

SORENSEN D.K. (1972) Hemorrhagic diseases. In: Catcott E.J. & Smithcors J.F. (Eds) *Equine medicine and surgery*, 2nd Edn, pp. 358–62. American Veterinary Publications, Illinois.

SORENSON D.K., MARTINSONS E., HIGBEE J.M., HOYT H.H., NELSON G.H., BERGELAND M.E., MOON H.W., BALL R.A. & NELSON N.D. (1961) Demonstration of clinical and diagnostic aspects—hog cholera and salmonellosis. In: Mainwaring G.T. & Sorenson D.K. (Eds) *Symposium on hog cholera*, p. 29. University of Minnesota, St. Paul, Minnesota.

SORVETTULA O. & ANDERSSON P. (1968) The influence of mastitis, local peritonitis and distomatosis on the lymphocyte picture of bovine blood. *Acta vet. scand.* **9**, 302–7.

SPAULDING G.L., WILKINS R.J., TILLEY L.P., JOHNSON G.F., KAY W.J. & INDRIERI R.J. (1975) Defibrination syndrome following therapy for heartworm disease. *J. Am. Anim. Hosp. Ass.* **11**, 310.

SPLITTER E.J. (1950) *Eperythrozoon suis*, the etiologic agent of ictero-anemia of an anaplasmosis-like disease of swine. *Am. J. vet. Res.* **11**, 324–30.

SPLITTER E.J., ANTHONY H.D. & TWIEHAUS M.J. (1956) Anaplasma ovis in the United States. Experimental studies with sheep and goats. *Am. J. vet. Res.* **17**, 487–91.

SPOONER R.L. (1966) The cattle blood typing service. *A.B.R.O. Report*, January 1966.

SPOONER R.L. (1967) Blood groups in animals and their practical application. *Vet. Rec.* **81**, 699–708.

SPOONER R.L. (1977) Personal communication.

SPRANGER J P.C. & HIME J.M. (1961) Bone marrow biopsy from the femur of the dog. *Vet. Rec.* **73**, 1080–1.

SPURLING N.W. (1971) Studies on a defect of the blood coagulation system in a breeding colony of Beagles. Canine factor-VII deficiency. Thesis Institute of Biology, London.

SPURLING N.W. (1973) Canine factor-VII deficiency. *Proceedings of IVth international congress on thrombosis and haemostasis,* Vienna. Abstract volume p. 439.

SPURLING N.W., BURTON L.K., PEACOCK R. & PILLING T. (1972) Hereditary factor-VII deficiency in the Beagle. *Br. J. Haemat.* **23**, 59–67.

SPURLING N.W., BURTON L.K. & PILLING T. (1974a) Canine factor-VII deficiency: experience with a modified thrombotest method in distinguishing between the genotypes. *Res. vet. Sci.* **16**, 228–39.

SPURLING N.W., PEACOCK R. & PILLING T. (1974b) The clinical aspects of canine factor-VII deficiency including some case histories. *J. small Anim. Pract.* **15**, 229.

SQUIBB R.L., GURMAN M., AGUIRRE F. &

SCRIMSHAW N.F. (1953) Ten constituents of the blood stream of well-fed white rats, chickens, swine, sheep and horses in Guatemala. *Am. J. vet. Res.* **14**, 484–6.

SQUIRE R.A. (1969) Spontaneous hematopoietic tumors of dogs. In: Lingeman C.H. & Garner F.M. (Eds) *Symposium on comparative morphology of hematopoietic neoplasms. Natn. Cancer Inst. Monogr.* No. 32, p. 97.

SQUIRE R.A., BUSH M., MELBY E.C., NEELEY L.M. & YARBROUGH B. (1973) Clinical and pathologic study of canine lymphoma: clinical staging, cell classification, and therapy. *J. natn. Cancer Inst.* **51**, 565.

STAMATOVIĆ S., BRATANOVIĆ U. & SOFRENOVIĆ DJ. (1965) Das klinische Bild der durch Verfütterung von Adlercarn (*Pteris aquilina*) experimentell hervorgerufenen Haematuria vesicalis der Rinder. *Wien. tierärztl. Mschr.* **52**, 589–96.

STANDERFER R.J., RITTENBERG M.B., CHERN C.J., TEMPLETON J.W. & BLACK J.A. (1975) Canine erythrocyte pyruvate kinase. II. Properties of the abnormal enzyme associated with hemolytic anemia in the Basenji dog. *Biochem. Genet.* **13**, 341–51.

STANDERFER R.J., TEMPLETON J.W. & BLACK J.A. (1974) Anomalous pyruvate kinase deficiency in the Basenji dog. *Am. J. vet. Res.* **35**, 1541–3.

STASNEY J. & HIGGINS G.M. (1937) A quantitative cytologic study of the bone marrow of the adult dog. *Am. J. med. Sci.* **193**, 462.

STEENSGAARD J. (1968) On the normal activities of glucose-6-phosphate dehydrogenase and 6-phospho-gluconate dehydrogenase in bovine erythrocytes. *Acta vet. scand.* **9**, 223–41.

STEFANO H.S. DI, MARUCCI A.A. & DOUGHERTY R.M. (1973) Immunohistochemical demonstration of avian leukosis virus antigens in paraffin embedded tissue. *Proc. Soc. exp. Biol. Med.* **142**, 1111–13.

STEFANINI M. (1951) Activity of plasma labile factor in disease. *Lancet* **i**, 606.

STEGEMANN D. (1962) Tagesrhythmus der Eosinophilenwerte im Blut beim Schwein. Inaug. Diss., Hannover.

STEIN C.D. & MOTT L.O. (1942) Studies on congenital transmission of equine infectious anaemia. *Vet. Med.* **37**, 370.

STEINBERG D. (1963) Fatty acid mobilization—mechanisms of regulation and metabolic consequences. In: Grant J.K. (Ed.) *The control of lipid metabolism*, p. 111. Academic Press, London.

STEINER K. (1973) Mechanism of methaemoglobin formation in chronic copper poisoning of ruminants. Inaugural dissertation, 88 pages. *Tierärztliche Fakultät, München.*

STEPHENSON E.H., CLOTHIER E.R. & RISTIC M. (1975) *Ehrlichia canis* infection in a dog in Virginia *J. Am. vet. med. Ass.* **167**, 71.

STERZ I. & WEISS E. (1973) Elektronenmikroskopische Untersuchungen zur Phagozytose und Vermehrung des Virus der Klassischen Geflügelpest (KP) in Thrombozyten infizierter Hühner. *Zentbl. VetMed.* B, **20**, 613–21.

STEVENS J.B., ANDERSON J.F., PERMAN V. & SCHLOTTHAUER J. (1974) Metabolic and cellular profile testing. A modern approach to health management. *Minn. Vet.* **14**, 20–7, 30.

STEVENS R.W.C. & RIDGEWAY G.J. (1966) A technique for bleeding chicken from the jugular vein. *Poult. Sci.* **45**, 204–5.

STEWART G.A. & CLARKSON G.T. (1968–69) Serum iron and total iron binding capacity in the horse. *Vict. vet. Pract.* **27**, 25–6.

STEWART G.A., CLARKSON G.T. & STEEL J.D. (1970) Hematology of the racehorse and factors affecting interpretation of the blood count. *Proc.* 16*th A. Conv. Am. Ass. equine Pract.* 17–35.

STEWART G.A. & STEEL J.D. (1974) Haematology of the fit racehorse. *Jl S. Afr. vet. Ass.* **45**, 287–91.

STEWART J. & HOLMAN H.H. (1940) The blood picture of the horse. *Vet. Rec.* **52**, 157.

STEWART W.B., STEWART J.M., IZZO M.J. & YOUNG L.E. (1950) Age as affecting the osmotic and mechanical fragility of dog erythrocytes tagged with radioactive iron. *J. exp. Med.* **91**, 147–59.

STEWART W.B., VASSAR P.S. & STONE R.S.

(1953) Iron absorption in dogs during anemia due to acetylphenylhydrazine. *J. clin. Invest.* **32**, 1225.

STITES D.P. & LEIKOLA J. (1971) Infectious mononucleosis *Semin. Hematol.* **8**, 243–60.

STOCK J.v.D. & DE SCHEPPER J. (1968) The urinary excretion of bilirubin after increased plasma haemoglobin concentration in dogs. *Experientia* **25**, 814.

STOCKWELL A., PERUTZ M.F., MUIRHEAD H. & GLAUSEN S.C. (1961) A comparison of adult and fetal horse hemoglobins. *J. molec. Biol.* **3**, 112–16.

STOHLMAN F. JR. (1970) (Ed.) *Hemopoietic cellular proliferation.* Grune and Stratton, New York.

STOLPE J. (1970) Untorsuchungen zur thrombozytenzahl der trabrennpferde. *Mh. VetMed.* **25**, 510.

STORMONT C. (1951) An example of a recessive blood group in sheep. *Genetics* **36**, 577–8 (Abstr.).

STORMONT C. (1958) On the applications of blood groups in animal breeding. *Xth Int. Congr. Genetics*, Vol. **1**, 206–24. McGill University, Montreal.

STORMORKEN H. (1975a) Species differences of clotting factors in ox, dog, horse and man. Proaccelerin and accelerin. *Acta physiol. scand.* **39**, 121.

STORMORKEN H. (1957b) Species differences of clotting factors in ox, dog, horse and man. Prothrombin. *Acta physiol. scand.* **41**, 101.

STORMORKEN H. (1957c) Species differences of clotting factors in ox, dog, horse and man. Thromboplastin and proconvertin. *Acta physiol. scand.* **41**, 301.

STORMORKEN H., EGEBERG O. & AUSTAD R. (1965) Haemophilia A in Samoyed dog. *Scand. J. Haemat.* 2· 174–8.

STORMORKEN H., SVENKURUD R., SLAGSVOLD P., LIE H. & LUNDEVALL J. (1963) Thrombocytopenic bleedings in young pigs due to maternal isoimmunisation. *Nature, Lond.* **198**, 1116–17.

STRAFUSS A.C. & ZIMMERMANN W.J. (1967) Hematologic changes and clinical signs of trichinosis in pigs. *Am. J. vet. Res.* **28**, 833–8.

STRAUB OTTO C., SCHALM OSCAR W.,

HUGHES J.P. & THEILEN GORDON H. (1959) Bovine hematology. II. Effect of parturition and retention of fetal membranes on blood morphology. *J. Am. vet. med. Ass.* **135,** 618–22.

STRAUB O.C., WEILAND F. & FRENZEL B. (1974) Ergebnisse von hämatologischen und serologischen Untersuchungen bei natürlichen und experimentellen Rinderleukose-Übertragungsversuchen. *Dt. tierärztl. Wschr.* **81,** 581–3.

STREET A.E. (1970) Biochemical tests in toxicology. In Paget G.E. (Ed.) *Methods in toxicology,* p. 313. Blackwell Scientific Publications, Oxford.

STRIKE T.A. (1970) Haemogram and bone marrow differential of the chinchilla. *Lab. Anim. Care* **20,** 33.

STUART M.J. (1975) Inherited defects of platelet function. *Semin. Hematol.* **12,** 233–53.

STUBBS E.L. & BOYER C.I. (1954) Studies of sheep blood. *Vet. Ext. Q. Univ. Pa.* **136,** 20–3.

STURKIE P.D. (1965) *Avian physiology,* 2nd Edn. Baillière, Tindall & Cassell, London.

STURKIE P.D. & NEWMAN H.J. (1951) Effects of estrogen and thyroxine upon plasma proteins and blood volume in the fowl. *Endocrinology* **49,** 565–70.

STURKIE P.D. & TEXTOR K. (1958) Sedimentation rate of erythrocytes in chickens as influenced by method and sex. *Poult. Sci.* **37,** 60–3.

STURKIE P.D. & TEXTOR K. (1960) Further studies on sedimentation rate of erythrocytes in chickens. *Poult. Sci.* **39,** 444–7.

SUN N.C.J., BOWIE E.J.W., TITUS J.L. & OWEN C.A. JR. (1974) Effect of induced chronic intravascular coagulation on plasminogen activator in dogs. *Thromb. Diath. haemorrh.* **32,** 189–202.

SURGENOR D. MACN. (1974) (Ed.) *The red blood cell,* Vol. 1. Academic Press, New York and London.

SUTTON R.H. (1970) Eperythrozoon ovis— a blood parasite of sheep. *N.Z. vet. J.* **18,** 156–64.

SUTTON R.H. & HOBMAN B. (1975) The value of plasma fibrinogen estimations in cattle. A comparison of leucocyte and neutrophil counts. *N.Z. vet. J.* **23,** 21–7.

SUZUKI Y., STORMONT C., MORRIS B.G., SHIFRINE M. & DOBRUCKI R. (1975) New antibodies in dog blood groups. *Transplant Proc.* **7,** 365.

SWEENY P.R. & CARLSON H.C. (1968) Electron microscopy and histochemical demonstration of lysosomal structures in chicken thrombocytes. *Avian Dis.* **12,** 636–44.

SWENSON M.J. (1951) Effect of a vitamin B_{12} concentrate and liver meal on the histopathology of chicks fed on all-plant protein ration. *Am. J. vet. Res.* **12,** 224–9.

SWIATEK K.R., KIPNIS D.M., MASON G., CHAO K.L. & CORNBLATH M. (1968) Starvation hypoglycaemia in newborn pigs. *Am. J. Physiol* **214,** 400–5.

SWISHER S.N. (Ed) (1976) Immune hemolytic anaemias. *Semin. Haematol.* **13,** 251–358.

SWISHER S.N., BULL R. & BOWDLER J. (1973) Canine erythrocyte antigens. *Tissue Antigens* **3,** 164.

SWISHER S.N. & YOUNG L.E. (1961) The blood grouping system of dogs. *Physiol. Rev.* **41,** 495.

SWISHER S.N., YOUNG L.E. & TRABOLD N. (1962) *In vitro* and *in vivo* studies of the behaviour of canine erythrocyte–isoantibody systems. *Ann. N.Y. Acad. Sci.* **97,** 15.

SYKES P.E. (1966) Hematology as an aid in equine track practice. *Proc. 12th A. Conv. Am. Ass. equine Pract.* 159–167.

SZABO ST, SZENT-IVANYI TH. & SZEKY A. (1956) Haemolytic disease of newborn pigs. *Acta vet. Hung.* **6,** 313–31.

TABER R.D., WHITE K.L. & SMITH N.S. (1959) The annual cycle of condition in the Rattlesnake, Montana, mule deer. *Proc. Mont. Acad. Sci.* **19,** 72–9.

TAKETA F. (1974) Organic phosphates and haemoglobin structure–function relationship in the feline. *Ann. N.Y. Acad. Sci.* **241,** 524–37.

TALIAFERRO W.H. & KLÜVER C. (1940) The haematology of malaria (*Plasmodium brasilianum*) in Panamanian monkeys. I. Numerical changes in leucocytes. *J. infect. Dis.* **67,** 162.

TALIAFERRO W.H. & TALIAFERRO L.G. (1955) Reactions of the connective tissue in chickens to *Plasmodium gallinaceum* and *Plasmodium lophurae*. I. Histopathology during initial infections and superinfections. *J. infect. Dis.* **97**, 99–136.

TAMMEMAGI L. (1966) Iron dextran in the treatment of anaemia associated with bovine babesiosis. *Aust. vet. J.* **42**, 260–1.

TANAKA T. & ROSENBERG M.M. (1954) Relationship between hemoglobin levels in chickens and certain characters of economic importance. *Poult. Sci.* **33**, 821–7.

TANIS R.J., TASHIAN R.E. & YU Y-S.L. (1970) Properties of carbonic anhydrase isoenzymes isolated from porcine erythrocytes. *J. biol. Chem.* **245**, 6003–9.

TARTOUR G., ADAM S.E.I., OBEID H.M. & IDRISS O.F. (1974) Development of anaemia in goats fed with *Ipomoea carnea*. *Br. vet. J.* **130**, 271–9.

TARTOUR G., OBEID H.M., ADAM S.E.I. & IDRIS O.F. (1973) Haematological changes in sheep and calves following prolonged oral administration of *Ipomoea carnea*. *Trop. Anim. Hlth & Prod.* **5**, 284–92.

TASKER J.B., SEVERIN G.A., YOUNG S. & GILLETTE E.L. (1969) Familial anemia in the Basenji dog. *J. Am. vet. med. Ass.* **154**, 158–65.

TASKIN J. (1935) Un cas grave d'hémophilie chez une chienne. *Bull. Acad. vét. Fr.* **8**, 595.

TAYLOR L.A. & CRAWFORD L.M. (1968) Aspirin-induced gastrointestinal lesions in dogs. *J. Am. vet. med. Ass.* **152**, 617.

TAYLOR W.J., EASLEY C.W. & KITCHEN H. (1972) Structural evidence for heterogeneity of two hemoglobin chain gene loci in white-tailed deer. *J. biol. Chem.* **247**, 7320–4.

TAYLOR W.J. & SIMPSON C.F. (1974) Ultrastructure of sickled deer erythrocytes. II. The matchstick cell. *Blood* **43**, 907–14.

TEGER-NILSSON A.C. & BLOMBÄCK B. (1974) Rate of thrombin-fibrinogen reaction in some mammalian species. *Thromb. Res.* **5**, 223.

TEGERIS A.S., EARL F.L. & CURTIS J.M. (1966) Normal hematological and bio-chemical parameters of young miniature swine. In: Bustad L.K., McClellan R.O. & Burns M.P. (Eds) *Swine in biomedical research*, pp. 576–96. Battelle-Northwest, Richland, Washington.

TELFER T.P., DENSON K.W. & WRIGHT D.R. (1956) A new coagulation defect. *Brit. J. Haemat.* **2**, 308–16.

TENNANT B.C., ASBURY A.C., LABEN R.C., RICHARDS W.P.C., KANEKO J.J. & CUPPS P.T. (1967) Familial polycythemia in cattle. *J. Am. vet. med. Ass.* **150**, 1493–1509.

TENNANT B.C., HARROLD D., REINA-GUERRA M. & LABEN R.C. (1969) Arterial pH, PO_2 and PCO_2 of calves with familial bovine polycythemia. *Cornell Vet.* **59**, 594–604.

TENNANT B.C., HARROLD D. & REINA-GUERRA M. (1972) Physiologic and metabolic factors in the pathogenesis of neonatal enteric infections in calves. *J. Am. vet. med. Ass.* **161**, 993–1007.

TENNANT B.C., HARROLD D., REINA-GUERRA M., KENDRICK J.W. & LABEN R.C. (1974) Hematology of the neonatal calf. Erythrocyte and leukocyte values of normal calves. *Cornell Vet.* **64**, 516–32.

THEILEN G.H., DUNGWORTH D.L., LENGYEL J. & ROSENBLATT L.S. (1964) Bovine lymphosarcoma in California. 1. Epizootiologic and hematologic aspects. *Health Lab. Sci.* **1**, 96–106.

THEILEN G.H., DUNGWORTH D.L., HARROLD J.B. & STRAUB O.C. (1967) Bovine lymphosarcoma transmission studies. *Am. J. vet. Res.* **28**, 373–86.

THEILEN G.H., DUNGWORTH D.L., JAMAJAMI T.G., MUNN R.J., WARD J.M. & HARROLD J.B. (1970) Experimental induction of lymphosarcoma in the cat with C-type virus. *Cancer Res.* **30**, 401–8.

THEILEN G.H. & FOWLER M.E. (1962) Lymphosarcoma (lymphocytic leukemia) in the horse. *J. Am. vet. med. Ass.* **140**, 923–30.

THEILEN G.H., SCHALM O.W., STRAUB O.C. & HUGHES J.P. (1959) Bovine hematology. I. Leukocyte response to acute bovine mastitis. *J. Am. vet. med. Ass.* **135**, 481–5.

THOMAS D.B. (1973) Antibodies specific

for human T lymphocytes in cold agglutinin and lymphocytotoxic sera. *Eur. J. Immunol.* **3**, 824.

THOMAS R.E. & KITTRELL J.E. (1966) Effect of altitude and season on the canine hemogram. *J. Am. vet. med. Ass.* **148**, 1163.

THOMAS E.D., PLAIN G.L. & THOMAS D. (1965) Leukocyte kinetics in the dog studied by cross circulation. *J. lab. clin. Med.* **66**, 64–74.

THORNTON I., KERSHAW G.F. & DAVIES M.G. (1972) An investigation into subclinical copper deficiency in cattle. *Vet.* **90**, 11–12.

THORNTON J.R., BUTLER D.G. & WILLOUGHBY R.A. (1973) Blood urea nitrogen concentrations and packed cell volumes of normal calves and calves with diarrhoea. *Aust. vet. J.* **49**, 20–2.

THORP F. & HARSHFIELD G.S. (1939) Onion poisoning in horses. *J. Am. vet. med. Ass.* **94**, 52–3.

TIETZ W.J. JR., BENJAMIN M.M. & ANGLETON G.M. (1967) Anemia and cholesterolemia during estrus and pregnancy in the beagle. *Am. J. Physiol.* **212**, 693.

TILLETT W.S. & GARNER R.L. (1933) The fibrinolytic activity of haemolytic streptococci. *J. exp. Med.* **58**, 485.

TISDALL MARGARET & CROWLEY J.P. (1971) The pattern of disappearance of foetal haemoglobin in young calves. *Res. vet. Sci.* **12**, 583–4.

TOBIAS G. (1964) Congenital porphyria in a cat. *J. Am. vet. med. Ass.* **145**, 462–3.

TOCANTINS L.M. (1938) The mammalian blood platelet in health and disease. *Medicine* **17**, 155.

TODD A.C., MCGEE W.R., WYANT Z.N. & HOLLINGSWORTH K.P. (1951) Studies on the hematology of the Thoroughbred horse. V. Sucklings. *Am. J. vet. Res.* **12**, 364–7.

TODD A.S. (1964) Localization of fibrinolytic activity in tissues. *Brit. med. Bull.* **20**, 210.

TODD J.R., MILNE A.A. & HOW P.F. (1967) Hypocuprosis without clinical symptoms in single-suckled calves. *Vet. Rec.* **81**, 653–6.

TODD J.R. & THOMPSON R.H. (1963) Studies on chronic copper poisoning. II. Biochemical studies on the blood of sheep during the haemolytic crisis. *Br. vet. J.* **119**, 161–73.

TOLLE A. (1965) Zue Beurteilung quantitativer hämatologischer Befunde im Rahmen der Leukose-Diagnostik beim Rind. *Zentbl. VetMed*, **B12**, 280–90.

TOPP R.C. & CARLSON H.C. (1972a) Studies on avian heterophils. III. Histochemistry. *Avian Dis.* **16**, 369–73.

TOPP R.C. & CARLSON H.C. (1972b) Studies on avian heterophils. III. Phagocytic properties. *Avian Dis.* **16**, 374–80.

TORTEN M. & SCHALM O.W. (1964) Influence of the equine spleen on rapid changes in the concentration of erythrocytes in peripheral blood. *Am. J. vet. Res.* **25**, 500–4.

TRAININ Z., MAIROM R., KLOPFER U. & MEIDAN G. (1973) Levels of IgM and IgG in the sera of normal and leukaemic calves. *J. comp. Path.* **83**, 87–90.

TRAUTWEIN G. & STOBBER M. (1965) Leukämische Mastzellenretikulose beim Rind. *Zentbl. VetMed.* **A12**, 211–31.

DE TRAY D.E. & SCOTT G.R. (1957) Blood changes in swine with African swine fever. *Am. J. vet. Res.* **18**, 484–90.

TRUM B.F. (1952) Normal variances in horse blood due to breed, age, lactation, pregnancy and altitude. *Am. J. vet. Res.* **13**, 514–19.

TSAPOGAS M.J. & FLUTE P.J. (1964) Experimental thrombolysis with streptokinase and urokinase. *Br. med. Bull.* **20**, 223.

TSCHOPP TH.B. (1970) Aggregation of cat platelets *in vitro*. *Thromb. Diath. haemorrh.* **23**, 601–20.

TSCHUDI P., ARCHER R.K. & GERBER H. (1975) The cells of equine blood and their development. *Equine vet. J.* **7**, 141–7.

TUCKER E.M. (1963) Red cell life span in young and adult sheep. *Res. vet. Sci.* **4**, 11–23.

TUCKER E.M. (1966) The life span and other physiological properties of sheep red cells containing type A, B, or C (N) haemoglobin. *Res. vet. Sci.* **7**, 368–78.

TUCKER E.M. (1974) A shortened life

span of sheep red cells with a glutathione deficiency. *Res. vet. Sci.* **16**, 19–22.

TUMBLESON M.E. & KALISH P.R. (1971) Serum biochemical and hematological parameters in crossbred swine from birth through eight weeks of age. *Can. J. comp. Med.* **36**, 202–9.

TUMBLESON M.E., BURKS M. & WINGFIELD W.E. (1973) Serum protein concentrations, as a function of age, in female dairy cattle. *Cornell Vet.* **63**, 65–71.

TUMBLESON M.E., CUNEIO J.D. & MURPHY D.A. (1970) Serum biochemical and hematological parameters of captive white-tailed fawns. *Can. J. comp. Med.* **34**, 66–71.

TUMBLESON M.E., TICER J.W., DOMMERT A.R., MURPHY D.A. & KORSCHGEN L.J. (1968b) Serum proteins in white-tailed deer in Missouri. *Am. J. vet. clin. Path.* **2**, 127–31.

TUMBLESON M.E., WOOD M.G., DOMMERT A.R., MURPHY D.A. & KORSCHGEN L.J. (1968a) Biochemic studies on serum from white-tailed deer in Missouri. *Am. J. vet. clin. Path.* **2**, 121–5.

TURNER A.W. & HODGETTS V.E. (1959) The dynamic red cell storage function of the spleen in sheep. I. Relationship to fluctuations of jugular haematocrit. *Aust. J. exp. Biol. med. Sci.* **37**, 399–419.

TURNER J.H. (1959) Experimental strongyloidiasis in sheep and goats. I. Single Infections. *Am. J. vet. Res.* **20**, 102–10.

TURPIE A.G.G., McNICOL G.P. & DOUGLAS A.S. (1971) Platelets: haemostasis and thrombosis. In: Goldberg, A. & Bram, M.C. *Recent advances in haematology*, pp. 249–301. Churchill Livingstone, Edinburgh and London.

TYSLOWITZ R. & DINGEMANSE E. (1941) Effect of large doses of estrogens on the blood picture of dogs. *Endocrinology* **29**, 817.

UGLIALORO A. & ALDER H.L. (1957) The correlation between packed cell volume and erythrocyte number in canine blood. *Am. J. vet. Res.* **18**, 909–11.

ULLREY D.E., MILLER E.R., LONG C.H., & VINCENT B.H. (1965) Sheep hematology from birth to maturity. I. Erythrocyte population, size and hemoglobin concentration. *J. Anim. Sci.* **24**, 135–40.

ULLREY D.E., YOUATT W.G., JOHNSON H.E., KU P.K. & FAY L.D. (1964) Digestibility of cedar and aspen browse for the white-tailed deer. *J. Wildl. Mgmt* **28**, 791–7

ULLREY D.E., YOUATT W.G., JOHNSON H.E., FAY L.D. & BRADLEY B.L. (1967) Protein requirements of white-tailed deer fawns. *J. Wildl. Mgmt* **31**, 679–85.

ULLREY D.E., YOUATT W.G., JOHNSON H.E., FAY L.D., SCHOEPKE B.L., MAGEE W.T. & KEAHEY K.K. (1973) Calcium requirements of weaned white-tailed deer fawns. *J. Wildl. Mgmt* **37**, 187–94.

UNDRITZ E. (1946) Über das Vorkommen von Sichelzell—Erythrozyten und anderer Blutzellen—Varaintem unter normalen Verhältnissen und als Anomalie bei Mensch und Tier. *Arch. Julius Klaus-Stift. Vererb-Forsch.* **21**, 288–95.

UNDRITZ E. (1952, 1973) *Sandoz Atlas of Haematology*, Basle, Switzerland.

UNDRITZ E., BELKE K. & LEHMANN H. (1960) Sickling phenomenon in deer. *Nature (London)* **187**, 333–4.

UPCOTT D.H. & HERBERT N. (1965) Some haematological data for red deer (*Cervus elaphus*) in England. *Vet. Rec.* **77**, 1348–9.

UPCOTT D.H., HERBERT C.N. & ROBINS M. (1971) Erythrocyte and leucocyte parameters in newborn lambs. *Res. vet. Sci.* **12**, 474–7.

UPCOTT D.H., HERBERT C.N. & ROBINS M. (1973) Erythrocyte and leukocyte parameters in fetal and neonatal piglets. *Res. vet. Sci.* **15**, 8–12.

UR A. (1974) The blood coagulation curve of some mammals. *Res. vet. Sci.* **16**, 204–7.

URBAIN A., CAHEN R., PASQUIER M.-A. & NOUVEL J. (1936) Sur le nombre d'hématies de quelques ongulés. *C.r. Séanc. Soc. Biol.* **122**, 1208–10.

URBAIN A., CAHEN R. & PASQUIER M.-A. (1938a) Teneur en cholestérol du sérum de quelques mammifères. *C.r. Séanc. Soc. Biol.* **127**, 475–7.

URBAIN A., CAHEN R., PASQUIER M.-A. & Servier J. (1938b) Teneur en chlore du sérum de quelques mannifères sauvages et domestiques. *C.r. Séanc. Soc. Biol.* **128**, 144–6.

URBAIN A. & PASQUIER M.-A. (1941a) Teneur en sucres réducteurs du sang total de quelques mammifères sauvages. *C.r. hebd. Séanc. Acad. Sci., Paris* **212**, 510–11.

URBAIN A. & PASQUIER M.-A. (1941b) Teneur en potassium du sang total, des globules et du sérum de quelques mammifères sauvages. *C.r. hebd. Séanc. Acad. Sci., Paris* **213**, 83–5.

URBAIN A. & PASQUIER M.-A. (1948) Teneur en magnésium du sérum et du plasma de quelques mammifères. *Bull. Mus. natn. Hist. nat., Paris* 2nd ser., **20**, 232–4.

USACHEVA, I.N. (1957) Peripheral blood and bone marrow indices in healthy dogs. *Bull. exp. Biol. Med.* **44**, 1133.

VACCA C., MONTEMAGNO F., PERSECHINO A. & PIZZUTI G.P. (1972) Nuovi orientamenti sulla eritrosedimentazione. *Atti Soc. ital. Sci. vet.* **26**, 219–21.

VACCA C., MONTEMAGNO F., PERSECHINO A. & PIZZUTI G.P. (1974) Erythrocyte sedimentation in cattle and buffaloes. *Folia vet. Latina* **4**, 24–39.

VAGHER J.P., PEARSON B., BLATT S. & KAYE M. (1973) Biochemical and hematologic values in male Holstein-Friesian calves. *Am. J. vet. Res.* **34**, 273–7.

VAHERI A. & RUOSLAHTI E. (1973) Expression of the major group-specific antigen (gs-a) of avian type-C viruses in normal chicken cells and tissue. *Int. J. Cancer* **12**, 361–7.

VAIDYA M.B., VAGHARI P.M. & PATEL B.M. (1970) Haematological constituents of blood of goats. *Indian vet. J.* **47**, 642–7.

VAIMAN M., RENARD CHRISTINE, LA PAGE P., AMETEAU J. & NIZZA P. (1970) Evidence for a histocompatibility system in swine (SL-A). *Transplantation* **10**, 155–64.

VALENTINČIĆ S. (1971) Beitrag zur Kenntnis des normalen Blutbildes beim Reh und seiner Änderung durch Wurmbefall. *Tag. -Ber. dt. Akad. Landwirtsch. -Wiss. Berlin* No. 113, 245–55.

VALENTINE W.N. (1971) (Ed.) Hereditary enzymatic deficiencies of erythrocytes. *Semin. Hematol.* **8**, 307–440.

VALENTINE W.N. (1972) Red cell enzyme deficiencies as a cause of hemolytic disorders. *A. Rev. Med.* **23**, 93–100.

VALIKHOV A.F., NADTOCHEI G.A., VAGANOVA N.B., BURBA L.G., SIMONYAN G.A. & SURIN B.I. (1974) C-type virus in cultures of lymphocytes from leucotic cows. *Veterinariya Moscow* No. 4, 43–5.

VALLEJO-FREIRE A. (1951) A simple technique for repeated collection of blood samples from guinea pigs. *Science* **114**, 524–5.

VALLI V.E.O., McSHERRY B.J., ROBINSON G.A. & WILLOUGHBY R.A. (1969) Leukophoresis in calves and dogs by extracorporeal circulation of blood through siliconised glass wool. *Res. vet. Sci.* **10**, 267–78.

VALLI V.E.O., HULLAND T.J., McSHERRY B.J., ROBINSON G.A. & GILMAN J.P.W. (1971a) The kinetics of haematopoiesis in the calf. I. An autoradiographical study of myelopoiesis in normal, anaemic and endotoxin treated calves. *Res. vet. Sci.* **12**, 535–50.

VALLI V.E.O., McSHERRY B.J., HULLAND T.J., ROBINSON G.A. & GILMAN J.P.W. (1971b) The kinetics of haematopoiesis in the calf. II. An autoradiographical study of erythropoiesis in normal, anaemic and endotoxin treated calves. *Res. vet. Sci.* **12**, 551–64.

VAN CREVALD S. (1958) Haemorrhagic diathesis in congenital heart disease—influence of operation under hypothermia and of whole blood transfusions. *Annls. paediat.* **190**, 342.

VANDER J.B., HARRIS C.A. & ELLIS S.R. (1963) Reticulocyte counts by means of fluorescence microscopy. *J. Lab. clin. Med.* **62**, 132–40.

VAN DYKE D.C., SHKURKIN C., PRICE D., YANO Y. & ANGER H.O. (1967) Differences in distribution of erythropoietin and reticuloendothelial marrow in hematologic disease. *Blood* **30**, 364–74.

VAN KAMPEN K.R., JAMES L.F. & JOHNSON A.E. (1970) Hemolytic anemia in sheep fed wild onion (Allium validum) *J. Am. vet. med. Ass.* **156**, 328–32.

VAN LOON E.J. & CLARK B.B. (1943) Hematology of the peripheral blood and bone marrow of the dog. *J. Lab. clin. Med.* **28**, 1575.

VAN PELT R.W. (1970) Synovial effusion changes in idiopathic septic arthritis in calves. *J. Am. vet. med. Ass.* **156**, 84–92.

VAN DER WALT K. & OSTERHOFF D.R. (1969a) Blood transfusion in cattle with special reference to the influence of blood groups. I. Single transfusions into young animals and pregnant cows. *Jl S. Afr. vet. med. Ass.* **40**, 107–20.

VAN DER WALT K. & OSTERHOFF D.R. (1969b) Blood transfusion in cattle with special reference to the influence of blood groups. II. Repeated blood transfusions. *Jl S. Afr. vet. med. Ass.* **40**, 265–75.

VAUGHAN J.M. (1969) A case of equine lymphosarcoma. *Vet. Rec.* **84**, 474–5.

VAUGHN H.W., KNIGHT R.R. & FRANK F.W. (1973) A study of reproduction, disease and physiological blood and serum values in Idaho elk. *J. Wildl. Dis.* **9**, 296–301.

VENKATARATNAM A. & CLARKSON M.J. (1962) The blood cells of the turkey. *Res. vet. Sci.* **3**, 455–9.

VENZLAFF W. Quoted by Sturkie (1965).

VERHORST D. (1973) Polymorphism in glucose-6-phosphate dehydrogenase in the German Large White. *Anim. Blood Grps biochem. Genet.* **4**, 65–8.

VERMA S.K. & TYAGI R.P.S. (1974) The effect of Caesarian section and normal parturition upon the concentration of blood electrolytes, glucose and total protein in goats. *Res. vet. Sci.* **16**, 162–6.

VERMEERSCH G. & VANSCHOUBROEK F. (1974) Haematology of the veal calf. *Vlaams diergeneesk. Tijdschr.* **43**, 14–29.

VIDEBAEK A. (1975) (Ed.) Polycythaemia and myelofibrosis. *Clin. Haematol.* **4**, 261–481.

VOGEL J. (1961) Quoted by Sturkie (1965).

VOGT W. (1966) Demonstration of the presence of two separate kinin-forming systems in human and other plasma. In: Erdös E.G., Back N., Sicuteri F. & Wilde A.F. (Eds) *Hypotensive Peptides*, p. 185. Springer-Verlag, Berlin.

VOHRADSKY F. (1974) Observations on some blood constituents in British Friesian cattle imported to Ghana. *Acta vet. Brno* **43**, 221–4.

VOLLER A. & HAWKEY C.M. (1976) Unpublished observations.

VOLLER A., RICHARDS W.H.G., HAWKEY C.M. & RIDLEY D.S. (1969) Human malaria (*Plasmodium falciparum*) in owl monkeys (*Aotus trivirgatus*). *J. trop. Med. Hyg.* **72**, 153.

VRIESENDORP H.M., DUYZER-DEN HARTOG B., SMID-MERCK B.M.J. & WESTBROEK D.L. (1974) Immunogenetic markers in canine paternity cases. *J. small Anim. Pract.* **15**, 693.

WADDILL D.G., ULLREY D.E., MILLER E.R., SPRAGUE J.I., ALEXANDER E.A. & HOEFER J.A. (1962) Blood cell populations and serum protein concentrations in the fetal pig. *J. Anim. Sci.* **21**, 583–7.

WALDMAN R., REBUCK J.W., SAITO H., ABRAHAM J.P., CALDWELL J. & RATNOFF O.D. (1975) Fitzgerald factor; a hitherto unrecognised coagulation factor. *Lancet* **i**, 949–51.

WALKER J. & DZIEMIAN A.J. (1950) Biochemical and physiological data on the normal goat. *Chem. Corps. Med. Div. Res. Rep.* No. 31. Army Chem. Cent. Maryland.

WALTER H., BRAKE J.M. & SELBY F.W. (1965) Aspects of the aging of the avian (nucleated) red blood cell *in vivo*. *Expl. Cell Res.* **37**, 420–8.

WASHBURN A.H. & MEYERS A.J. (1957) The sedimentation of erythrocytes at an angle of 45 degrees. *J. Lab. clin. Med.* **49**, 318.

WASHBURN K.W., EIDSON C.S. & LOWE R.H. (1971) Association of hemoglobin type with resistance to Marek's disease. *Poult. Sci.* **50**, 90–3.

WASHBURN K.W. & GUILL R.A. (1972) Comparison of hematology between Leghorn-type and heavy-type egg production strains. *Poult. Sci.* **51**, 946–50.

WASHBURN K.W. & HUSTON T.M. (1968) Effect of environmental temperature on iron deficiency anemia in Athens-Canadian randombred chicks. *Poult. Sci.* **47**, 1532–5.

WASS W.M. & HOYT H.H. (1965a) Bovine congenital porphyria. I. Studies on heredity. *Am. J. vet. Res.* **26**, 654–8.

WASS W.M. & HOYT H.H. (1965b) Bovine congenital porphyria. II. Hematologic studies, including porphyrin analyses. *Am. J. vet. Res.* **26**, 659–67.

WATSON A.D.J., DUFF B.C. & ALLAN G.S. (1975) Erythrocyte aplasia in a dog. *Aust. vet. J.* **51**, 94–6.

WATSON A.D.J. & WRIGHT R.G. (1974a) The ultrastructure of inclusions in blood cells of dogs with distemper. *J. comp. Path.* **84**, 417–27.

WATSON A.D.J. & WRIGHT R.G. (1974b) Ultrastructure of cytoplasmic inclusions in circulating lymphocytes in canine distemper. *Res. vet. Sci.* **17**, 188–92.

WATSON P.F. & HAWKEY C.M. (1976) The effect of age and anaesthetics on the blood picture of the cuis, *Galea musteloides*. *Lab. Anim.* **10**, 279–84.

WATT J.G. (1967) Fluid therapy for dehydration in calves. *J. Am. vet. med. Ass.* **150**, 742–50.

WEATHERALL D.J. (1969) The control of human hemoglobin synthesis and function in health and disease. *Prog. Hemat.* **6**, 261–304.

WEATHERALL D.J. & CLEGG J.B. (1972) *The thalassaemia syndromes*, 2nd Edn. Blackwell Scientific Publications, Oxford.

WEBER A., ANDREWS J., DICKINSON B., LARSON V., HAMMER R., DIRKS V., SORENSEN D. & FROMMES S. (1969) Occurrence of nuclear pockets in lymphocytes of normal, persistent lymphocytic and leukaemic adult cattle. *J. natn. Cancer Inst.* **43**, 1307–15.

WEBER A., BENDIXEN H. JR., HAMMER R., JESSEN C. & POMEROY K. (1974) Correlative studies of the frequency of blood lymphocytic nuclear pockets and persistent lymphocytosis in cattle. *Am. J. vet. Res.* **35**, 537–41.

WEBER Y.B. & BLISS M.L. (1972) Blood chemistry of Roosevelt elk (*Cervus canadensis roosevelti*). *Comp. Biochem. Physiol.* **43A**, 649–53.

WEBER Y.B. & GIACOMETTI L. (1972) Sickling phenomenon in the erythrocytes of wapiti (*Cervus canadensis*). *J. Mammal.* **53**, 917–19.

WEBSTER M.E. & RATNOFF O.D. (1961) Role of Hageman factor in the activation of vasodilator activity in human plasma. *Nature* (*London*) **192**, 180.

WEBSTER W.P., DODDS W.J., MANDEL S.R. & PENICK G.D. (1975) Biosynthesis of factors VIII and IX: organ transplantation and perfusion studies. In: Brinkhous K.M. & Hemker H.C. (Eds) *Handbook of hemophilia*, p. 149. Excerpta Medica, Amsterdam.

WEED R.I., CRUMP S.L. & SWISHER S.N. (1965) Evaluation of a technique for counting dog and human platelets. *Blood* **25**, 261.

WEIDEN P., STORB R., KOLB H.J., GRAHAM T., ANDERSON J. & GIBLETT E. (1974) Genetic variation of red blood cell enzymes in the dog: use of soluble glutamic oxaloacetic transaminase as proof of chimerism. *Transplantation* **17**, 115.

WEIKEL J.H. JR., NELSON L.W. & RENO F.E. (1975) A four year evaluation of the chronic toxicity of megestrol acetate in dogs. *Toxic. appl. Pharmac.* **33**, 414.

WEILAND F. & STRAUB O.C. (1975) Frequency of surface immunoglobulin bearing blood lymphocytes in cattle affected with bovine leukosis. *Res. vet. Sci.* **19**, 100–2.

WEILER O., DELAIN E. & LACOUR F. (1971) Studies on a viral nephroblastic nephroblastoma of the chicken; an electron microscope comparison of the sequence of development of the virions in different organs. *Eur. J. Cancer* **7**, 491–4.

WEINER D.J. & BRADLEY R.E. (1972) The hemogram and certain serum protein fractions in normal Beagle dogs. *Vet. Med. Small Anim. Clin.* **67**, 393.

WEISBERGER A.S. (1964) The sickling phenomenon and heterogeneity of deer hemoglobin. *Proc. Soc. exp. Biol. Med.* **117**, 276–80.

WEISS L. & TAVASSOLI M. (1970) Anatomical hazards to the passage of erythrocytes through the spleen. *Semin. Hematol.* **7**, 372–80.

WEISS R.A., FRIIS R.R., KATZ E. & VOGT

P.K. (1971) Induction of avian tumor viruses in normal cells by physical and chemical carcinogens. *Virology* **46**, 920–38.

WEISSE I., KNAPPEN F., SCHRANK H. & KLUPP H. (1971) Das blutbild der englischen Beagle-Hunde in Abhängigkeit von Alter and Geschlecht. *Arzneimittel-Forsch.* **21**, 1703.

WELCH D.C. & DELLARS R.W. (1973) Suspected adenoviral infection in adult dairy cattle. *J. Am. vet. med. Ass.* **163**, 741.

WELLDE B.T., JOHNSON A.J., WILLIAMS J.S., LANGBEHN H.R. & SADUN E.H. (1971) Haematologic, biochemical and parasitologic parameters in the night monkey, *Aotus trivirgatus. Lab. Anim. Sci.* **21**, 575.

WELS A., SCHNAPPAUF H. & HORN V. (1967) Blutvolumenbestimmung bei Hühnern mit Cr^{51} und T-1824. *Zentbl. Vet-Med.* **14**, Reihe A, 741–6.

WESTEN H. (1974) Bone marrow examination in experimental animals. *Proc. Eur. Soc. Study Drug Toxicity* **14**, 313.

WHEPPER K.D. (1972) In: Lepow I.H. & Ward P.A. (Eds) *Inflammation: mechanism and control.* Academic Press, London.

WHITAKER H.K. (1974) The viral etiology of feline and canine lymphosarcoma. *Diss. Abstr. Internat.* **34B**, No. 9, 4543.

WHITE D.J.G., BRADLEY B., CALNE R.Y. & BINNS R.M. (1973) The relationship of the histocompatibility locus in the pig to allograft survival. *Transplant. Proc.* **5** (1) 317–20.

WHITE J.M. & DACIE J.W. (1971) The unstable hemoglobins—molecular and clinical features. *Prog. Hemat.* **7**, 69–109.

WHITE M. & COOK R.S. (1974) Blood characteristics of free-ranging white-tailed deer in southern Texas. *J. Wildl. Dis.* **10**, 18–24.

WHITE V.M. (1970) Sweet clover poisoning in cattle (a review). *Vet. Med.* **65**, 804–7.

WHITEHAIR C.K. (1970) Nutritional deficiencies. In: Dunne H.W. (Ed.) *Diseases of swine*, 3rd Edn, pp. 1015–44. State Univ. Press, Ames, Iowa.

WHITLOCK R.H., LITTLE W. & ROWLANDS G.J. (1974) The incidence of anaemia in dairy cows in relation to season, milk yield and age. *Res. vet. Sci.* **16**, 122–4.

WHITNEY J.C. (1957) Atrophic myositis in a dog: the differentiation of this disease from eosinophilic myositis. *Vet. Rec.* **69**, 130.

WHITTEN C.F. (1967) Innocuous nature of the sickling (pseudo-sickling) phenomenon in deer. *Br. J. Haemat.* **13**, 650–5.

WICKRAMASINGHE S. (1975) *Human bone marrow.* Blackwell Scientific Publications, Oxford.

WIDAR J., ANSAY M. & HANSET R. (1974) Polymorphism of adenosine deaminase in the pig: allelic variation in erythrocytes. *Anim. Blood Grps biochem. Genet.* **5**, 115–24.

WIDAR J. & ANSAY M. (1975) Adenosine deaminase in the pig: tissue specific patterns and expression of the silent ADA° allele in nucleated cells. *Anim. Blood Grps biochem. Genet.* **6**, 109–16.

WIDAR J., ANSAY M. & HANSET R. (1975) Allozymic variation as an estimate of heterozygosity in Belgian pig breeds. *Anim. Blood Grps biochem. Genet.* **6**, 221–34.

WIDDOWSON E.M. & McCANCE R.A. (1956) The effect of development on the composition of the serum and extracellular fluids. *Clin. Sci.* **15**, 361–5.

WIDDOWSON R.W. & NEWTON T.A. (1965) A new approach to boar progeny testing. In: Matousek J. (Ed.) *Blood Groups of animals*, pp. 137–48. Publishing House of the Czechoslovak Academy of Sciences, Prague.

WIESNER E., REX J.O. & WIESNER B. (1968) Blood coagulation in cattle fed sweet clover. II. Feeding experiments. *Mh. VetMed.* **23**, 788–90.

WIGHT P.A.L. (1970) The mast cells of *Gallus domesticus.* I. Distribution and ultrastructure. *Acta anat.* **75**, 100–13.

WIGHT P.A.L. & MACKENZIE G.M. (1970) The mast cells of *Gallus domesticus.* II. Histochemistry. *Acta anat.* **75**, 263–75.

WIGNALL W.N., BANKS A.W., HACKETT E. & IRVING ELIZABETH A. (1961) Dicoumarol poisoning of cattle and sheep in South Australia. *Aust. vet. J.* **37**, 456–9.

WILBER C.G. & ROBINSON P.F. (1958) Aspects of blood chemistry in the white-tailed deer. *J. Mammal.* **39**, 309–11.

WILDE J.K.H. (1961) A technique of bone marrow biopsy in cattle. *Res. vet. Sci.* **2**, 315–19.

WILDE J.K.H. (1964) The cellular elements of the bovine bone marrow. *Res. vet. Sci.* **5**, 213–27.

WILDE J.K.H. (1966) Changes in bovine bone marrow during the course of East Coast Fever. *Res. vet. Sci.* **7**, 213–24.

WILKINS J.H. (1962) A review of the radiation syndrome in domestic animals. Part I—Lethal studies. *Jl R. Army vet. Cps* **33**, 74–82.

WILKINS J.H. (1963a) A review of the radiation syndrome in domestic animals. Part II—Clinical signs and symptoms. *Jl R. Army vet. Cps* **34**, 11–20.

WILKINS J.H. (1963b) A review of the radiation syndrome in domestic animals. Part III—Pathological aspects. *Jl R. Army vet. Cps* **34**, 64–73.

WILKINS J.H. & HODGES R.E.D.H. (1962) Observations on normal goat blood. *Jl R. Army vet. Cps* **33**, 7–10.

WILKINS R.J., HURVITZ A.I. & DODDS-LAFFIN W.J. (1973) Immunologically mediated thrombocytopenia in the dog. *J. Am. vet. med. Ass.* **163**, 277–82.

WILLEMART J.P. & SCHRICKE E. (1972a) Marek's disease. Occurrence in France of the cutaneous form of the disease in broilers. *Recl Méd. vét. Éc. Alfort* **148**, 1351–61.

WILLEMART J.P. & SCHRICKE E. (1972b) Appearance in France of cutaneous leucosis in broiler fowl. *Bull. Acad. vét. Fr.* **45**, 367–9.

WILLIAMS D.M., LYNCH R.E. & CART-WRIGHT G.E. (1973) Drug-induced aplastic anemia. *Semin. Hematol.* **10**, 195–223.

WILLIAMS E.I. (1966) Brucellosis eradication: collection of blood samples. *Vet. Rec.* **79**, 815.

WILLIAMS E.I. & JONES E.W. (1968) Blood transfusion during patent bovine anaplasmosis. *Am. J. vet. Res.* **29**, 703–10.

WILLIAMS J.R.B. (1951) The fibrinolytic activity of urine. *Brit. J. exp. Path.* **32**, 530–37.

WILLIAMS W.J., BEUTLER E., ERSLEV A.J. & WAYNE RUNDLES R. (1972) *Hematology*. McGraw-Hill Book Co, New York.

WILLIAMSON H.M. (1974) Normal and abnormal electrolyte levels in the racing horse and their effect on performance. *Jl S. Afr. vet. Ass.* **45**, 335–40.

WILLSON J.E. & BROWN D.E. (1965) Leukemoid reaction resembling myelogenous leukemia in a dog. Failure of the leukocyte alkaline phosphatase test to aid in the differential diagnosis. *Cornell Vet.* **55**, 55–63.

WILSON G.D.A., HARVEY D.G. & SNOOK C.R. (1972) A biochemical and pathological study of kidney diseases in slaughtered pigs. *Br. vet. J.* **128**, 512–22.

WINGFIELD W.E. & TUMBLESON M.E. (1973) Hematologic parameters, as a function of age, in female dairy cattle. *Cornell Vet.* **63**, 72–80.

WINQUIST G. (1954) Morphology of the blood and the haemopoietic organs in cattle under normal and some experimental conditions. *Acta anat. Suppl.* 21–1 ad., vol. **22**, 1–159.

WINTER A.J. (1962) Studies on nitrate metabolism in cattle. *Am. J. vet. Res.* **23**, 500–5.

WINTER A.R. (1935) Influence of egg production on haemoglobin content of chicken blood. *Poult. Sci.* **14**, 316.

WINTER H. (1964a) Lipid reaction of leucocyte granules in sheep and man. *J. comp. Path. Ther.* **74**, 205–9.

WINTER H. (1964b) The myelogram of normal sheep. *J. comp. Path. Ther.* **74**, 457–69.

WINTER H. (1965a) Automatic red cell counting in sheep. *J. comp. Path. Ther.* **75**, 205–14.

WINTER H. (1965b) Comparison of haematological stains in sheep and man. *Aust. vet. J.* **41**, 14–16.

WINTER H. (1965c) The bone marrow cells of sheep. *Pap. Univ. Qd.* **I**, No. 3.

WINTER H. (1966a) Volume distribution curves of erythrocytes obtained by automatic counting. *J. Path. Bact.* **91**, 273–6.

700 *References*

WINTER H. (1966b) Changes of the red blood cell hemogram in posthemorrhagic anemia in sheep. *Am. J. vet. Res.* **27**, 891–7.

WINTER H. (1967) Diagnosis of babesiosis by fluorescence microscopy. *Res. vet. Sci.* **8**, 170–4.

WINTERS W.D. & SNOW H.D. (1974) Precipitating antibodies to canine lymphosarcoma associated antigens. *Am. J. vet. Res.* **35**, 1333–5.

WINTROBE M.M. (1933) Variations in the size and hemoglobin content of erythrocytes in the blood of various vertebrates. *Folia haemat.* **51**, 32–49.

WINTROBE M.M., LEE G.R., BOGGS D.R., BITHELL T.C., ATHENS J.W. & FOERSTER J. (1974) *Clinical hematology.* 7th Edn. Lea and Febiger, Philadelphia.

WIRTH D. (1950) *Grundlagen einer Klinischen Hämatologie der Haustiere.* Vienna, Urban & Schwarzenburg.

WISECUP W.G., HODSON H.H., LOVETT R.L., PRINE J.R. & HANLY W.C. (1968) Anaemia in chimpanzees (*Pan troglodytes*) resulting from serial collection of blood. *Am. J. vet. Res.* **29**, 1823–30.

WITTER R.L., SHARMA J.M., SOLOMON J.J., CHAMPION L.R. & ALFORT E.C. (1973) An age-related resistance to chickens to Marek's disease: some preliminary observations. *Avian Path.* **2**, 43–54.

WITTMAN W. (1968) Untersuchungen zür Ätiologie der Rinderleukose. *Arch. exp. VetMed.* **22**, 509–19.

WITTWER F. & BÖHMWALD H. (1974) Leucocyte count in normal female Friesian cattle of various ages in the Valdivia area, Chile. *Archiv. de Medicina Vet.* **6**, 32–6.

WOLF P. (1953) A modification of Stefanini's method of estimating factor V using human oxalated plasma. *J. clin. Path.* **6**, 34.

WOLSTENHOLME G.E.W. & O'CONNOR M. (1973) (Eds) *Haemopoietic stem cells.* Ciba Foundation Symposium 13 (New Series). Elsevier Associated Scientific Publishers, Amsterdam.

WOLTERINK L.F., DAVIDSON J.A. & REINCKE E.P. (1947) Hemoglobin levels in the blood of Beltsville Small White poults. *Poult. Sci.* **26**, 559. As reported by Sturkie (1965).

WOMACK J.E. (1972) Red cell survival in the gerbil (*Meriones unguiculatus*). *Comp. Biochem. Physiol.* **43A**, 801.

WORLLEDGE S.M. (1973) Immune drug-induced hemolytic anemias. *Semin. Hematol.* **10**, 327–44.

WOROWSKI K. (1968) The hypercoagulability in mercury chloride intoxicated dogs. *Thromb. Diath. haemorrh.* **19**, 236–41.

WRETLIND B., ORSTADIUS K. & LINDBERG P. (1959) Transaminase and transferase activities in blood plasma and in tissues of normal pigs. *Zentbl. VetMed.* **6**, 936–70.

WRIGHT I.G. (1973) Observations on the haematology of experimentally induced *Babesia argentina* and *B. bigemina* infections in splenectomised calves. *Res. vet. Sci.* **14**, 29–34.

WRIGHT J.N. (1962) Blood incompatibilities in the dog. *Cornell Vet.* **52**, 523–33.

WRIGHT M.A. (1961) Haemoglobinuria from excessive water drinking. *Vet. Rec.* **73**, 129–30.

WUEPPER K.D. (1972) In Lepow I.H. & Ward P.A. (Eds.) *Inflammation, mechanism and control.* Academic Press. London.

WURZEL H.A. & LAWRENCE W.C. (1961) Canine hemophilia. *Thromb. Diath. haemorrh.* **6**, 98.

YAKELEY W.L. & STREETER R.J. (1972) Transient thrombasthenia in a dog (a case report). *Vet. Med/Small Anim. Clin.* **67**, 1193.

YAMADA Y. & SONODA M. (1970a) Neutrophils of ovine peripheral blood in electron microscopy. *Jap. J. vet. Res.* **18**, 83–9.

YAMADA Y. & SONODA M. (1970b) Eosinophils of ovine peripheral blood in electron microscopy. *Jap. J. vet. Res.* **18**, 117–23.

YAMADA Y. & SONODA M. (1972a) Electron microscopy of agranulocytes in the peripheral blood of normal sheep. *Jap. J. vet. Sci.* **34**, 235–41.

YAMADA Y. & SONODA M. (1972b) Basophils

of ovine peripheral blood in electron microscopy. *Jap. J. vet. Sci.* **34**, 29–32.

YAMAMOTO H., YOSHINO T., HIHARA H. & ISHITANI R. (1972) Histopathologic comparison of Marek's disease with avian lymphoid leukosis. *Natn. Inst. Anim. Hlth Q. Tokyo* **12**, 29–42.

YAZAN Y. & KNORRE Y. (1964) Domesticating elk in a Russian national park. *Oryx* **7**, 301–4.

YIN E.T. & DUCKERT F. (1961) The formation of intermediate product I in a purified system. The role of factor XI or of its precursors and of a Hageman factor —PTA fraction. *Thromb. Diath. haemorrh.* **6**, 224–34.

YOUATT W.G. & ERICKSON A.W. (1958) Notes on the haematology of Michigan black bears. *J. Mammal.* **39**, 588.

YOUATT W.G., VERME L.J. & ULLREY D.E. (1965) Composition of milk and blood in nursing white-tailed does and blood composition of their fawns. *J. Wildl. Mgmt* **29**, 79–84.

YOUNG L.E., CHRISTIAN R.M., ERVIN D.M., DAVIS R.W., O'BRIEN W.A., SWISHER S.N. & YUILE C.L. (1951) Hemolytic disease in newborn dogs. *Blood* **6**, 291–313.

YOUNG L.E., ERVIN D.M. & YUILE C.L. (1949) Hemolytic reactions produced in dogs by transfusion of incompatible dog blood and plasma. 1. Serologic and hematologic aspects. *Blood* **4**, 1218.

YUNIS J.J. (1969) (Ed.) *Biochemical methods in red cell genetics.* Academic Press, New York and London.

ZALUSKY R., GHIDONI J.J., McKINLEY J., LEFFINGWELL T.P. & MELVILLE G.S. (1965) Leukaemia in the rhesus monkey (*Macaca mulatta*) exposed to whole body neutron irradiation. *Radiat. Res.* **25**, 401.

ZANDER A.R., BOOPALAM N. & EPSTEIN R.B. (1975) Surface markers on canine lymphocytes. *Transplant. Proc.* **7**, 369.

ZANJANI E.D., COOPER G.W., GORDON A.B., WONG K.K. & SCRIBNER V.A. (1967) The renal erythropoietic factor (REF) IV. Distribution in mammalian kidneys. *Proc. Soc. exp. Biol. Med.* **126**, 540–2.

ZANJANI E.D., GORDON A.S., WONG K.K. & McLAURIN W.D. (1969) The renal erythropoietic factor (REF). X. The question of species and class specificity. *Proc. Soc. exp. Biol. Med.* **131**, 1095–8.

ZAWIDSKA A.A., JANZEN E. & GRICE H.C. (1964) Erythremic myelosis in a cat: A case resembling Di Guglielmo's syndrome in man. *Path. Vet.* **1**, 530–41.

ZINKL J. & KANEKO J.J. (1973) Erythrocyte 2,3-diphosphoglycerate in normal and porphyric fetal, neonatal and adult cattle. *Comp. Biochem. Physiol.* **45A**, 699–704.

ZOOK B.C., McCONNELL G. & GILMORE C.E. (1970) Basophilic stippling of erythrocytes in dogs with special reference to lead poisoning. *J. Am. vet. med. Ass.* **157**, 2092–9.

INDEX

In addition to using this index, reference should be made to the detailed contents list at the beginning of each chapter.

720   *Index*

Iron (*cont.*)
    sheep schistosomiasis and   329
    turnover rate   39
    Prussian blue reaction   591–2
    serum concentration, in disease   31
Irradiation
    equine aplastic anaemia and   208
    piglet white cell changes and   282
Isoerythrolysis   186, 188, 198
Isozymes, serum, porcine   299–300
Itikawa and Ogura Schiff reagent preparation method   588
ITP *see* Purpura, thrombocytopenic, idiopathic

Jaundice, neonatal, G-6-PD deficiency and   65
Jersey cattle
    blood values   226, 227
        enzymes   227
    enzootic leucosis, familial aspects   256
Johne's disease, bovine, white cell response   253

Kale poisoning
    bovine anaemia and   242–3
    sheep   324–5
Karyotype, porcine   284–5
Kasten fluorescent Feulgen reaction   589
Kidney
    disorders, polycythaemia and   91
    Wilms tumours, myeloblastosis virus-induced   527, 528
Kids
    anisocytosis   337, 339
    lymphocytes   341–2
    red cells   339
        fragility   338
    reticulocytes   339
    white cells, total count   341
Kittens
    aplastic anaemia, leukaemia and   461
    red cells, normal values   444, 445
    salmonellosis   470
    white cells, normal values   445
Koch's blue bodies   332
Koilonychia   35
Kurloff bodies   130
Kwashiorkor   42
    protein malnutrition and   49

Lactation, bovine metabolic profile effects   267–8

Lactobacillus leichmannii, serum vitamin B_{12} levels and   47
Lagomorpha
    antithrombin levels   141
    factor V levels   142
    factor VIII levels   146
    factor IX levels   147
    factor X levels   148
    factor XII levels   150
    fibrinogen levels   140
    partial thromboplastin test   154
    plasminogen activator levels   156
    prothrombin levels   142
Lambs
    blood groups   310
    eosinophils   316
    iron deficiency   322
    neutrophils   316
    plasma proteins   319
    red cells
        life span   308
        potassium levels   311
    trichostrongylosis   326
    white cells   315
Landsteiner ABO blood group system   11
Lantana camara, toxicity, bovidae   241
Lead poisoning   37
    bovidae   238
    canine   398
    equine   204
Lee and White whole blood clotting time   597–8
Leishman stain   562, 563
    reticulocytes   586, 587
    white cells   579–81
Leishmaniasis, canine   412
Leptospira pomona   244
    sheep anaemia and   332
Leptospirosis
    bovine anaemia and   244
    canine   396, 401, 428
        anaemia and   391
    equine   204
    porcine   288
Leucocytes *see* White cells
Leucocytosis   10, 78–9
    canine   400–1
    equine   210–12
        causes   211
    feline   466–70
    neutrophil   78
Leucopenia   9, 77
    canine   401–4
    equine   209–10
        causes   211

Poultry
  basophils 510–12
  blood
    differences from mammalian 484
    normal values 484–8
  blood coagulation 500–2
  blood samples
    collection techniques 553–4
    practicable volumes 539
  embryos, blood sample collection 554
  eosinophils 507, 509–10
  erythroblastosis 524–6
  ESR 486–7
    technique for 574
  granulocytopoiesis 512
  H virus-induced tumours 519–20, 531–5
  haemoglobins 492–5
  heterophils 506–7, 508
  L-S virus-induced tumours 519–30
  lymphocytes 502–4, 513
  lymphoid tumours 523–4
  lymphosarcoma 522–3
  monocytes 504–6, 513–14
  myelocytoma 528–9
  red cells 488–97
    counts 571–2
  reticulocytes 496–7
  thrombocytes 497–502
  white cells 502–17
  see also Ducks; Geese; Guinea fowl; Quail
Pre-albumins, porcine 299
Pre-eclampsia 69
Pregnancy
  bovidae
    blood value effects 227–8
    metabolic profile effects 268
  daily iron requirements 33
  folate deficiency and 44
  porcine red cell changes and 273, 274
  'pseudo-anaemia' and 50
  serum iron levels 31
Prekallikrein, Fletcher factor deficiency and 152
Primates
  carnivora and, factor VII species specificity lack 144
  non-human
    antithrombin levels 141
    factor V levels 142
    factor VII levels 145
    factor VIII levels 146
    factor IX levels 147
    factor X levels 148

    factor XI levels 149
    factor XII levels 150
      plasminogen and 151
    fibrinogen levels 140
    fibrinolysis inhibitors 156, 157
    Fletcher factor levels 152
    haemoglobin polymorphism 111
    haemoglobin A 111
    haemoglobin S 111
    leucocytosis and neutrophilia 121
    leukaemia 125
    lymphoproliferative disorders 125
    neutrophil hyperlobulation 121
    partial thromboplastin test 154
    plasminogen activator levels 156
    plasminogen levels 155
    platelets
      aggregation 132
      characteristics 131
    prothrombin levels 142
    red cells 111–13
    white cells 122–5
      histochemical reactions 123–4
  red cells, normal 106
  see also various sub-orders, families and species
Proaccelerin 100, 142, 143
Proboscidea
  factor V levels 142
  factor VIII levels 146
  factor IX levels 147
  factor X levels 148
  fibrinogen levels 140
  partial thromboplastin test 154
  plasminogen activator deficiency 156
  platelet characteristics 131
  prothrombin levels 142
  red cells, normal 106, 108, 109
  white cells 120, 129
Proconvertin *see* Factor VII
Procyonidae
  Hb, PCV and MCHC 108
  neutrophil/lymphocyte ratio 126
  normal 106, 109
  WBC, neutrophils and lymphocytes 120
Proerythroblasts
  equine 173
  feline 447
  poultry 496
Profile testing 20
Progestogens, canine erythropoiesis and 397
Pronormoblasts, equine 173
Prosimii
  haemorrhagic anaemia 112
  Hb, PCV and MCHC 108